AFRICAN AMERICAN MEN'S HEALTH

Professor Valiere Alcena M.D., M.A.C.P

∞ INFINITY
PUBLISHING

ISBN 978-1-4958-2094-6
eISBN 978-1-4958-2095-3
Copyright © 2017 by Professor Valiere Alcena M.D., M.A.C.P

Published December 2017

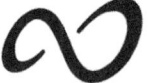

INFINITY PUBLISHING
1094 New DeHaven Street, Suite 100
West Conshohocken, PA 19428-2713
Toll-free (877) BUY BOOK
Local Phone (610) 941-9999
Fax (610) 941-9959
Info@buybooksontheweb.com
www.buybooksontheweb.com

CONTENTS

—◄◄▌∫▐►►—

PREFACE

African American Men are discriminated against in all aspects of the health care system in the United States of America. They receive questionable to very poor medical care when they present to ememergy rooms. Their pain symptoms are very often neglected. They are frequently made to wait for long period of time before being seen by physicians. Even when they have good insurance it is quite frequently very difficult for them to get appoitments to see competent physicians. Ofentimes they are not offered cardiac catherizations when they are admitted to the hospital with chest pain. To give a few examples. Of course there are exceptions, but in general African American men tend to receive inferior medical care as compared to American Caucasians men.

INTRODUCTION

This book is being written to bring to light the plight and strugles African American Men face on a daily basis with regards to health care disparity and dicrimination.

African American men are discrimanated against constantly when they present either to Emergency rooms, clinics, and physicians offices all the time.

This noble profession of medicine has not yet found a way to end racial discrimination in medicine against blacks and another minorities in this country. Some caucasian physicians bring their racial biases to work with them every day to the ERs, Clinics, Hospitals, and their offices, which more often than not results in the poor delivery of medical care to thier black and other minority patients.

There are many dedicated Caucasian physicians who don't discriminate against blacks and other minorities and who provide excellent medical care to all people, and these physicians are good examples of what physicians are supposed to be, and they are a credit to the nobleness of the great profession of medicine.

In Adition, I write this book to advocate for better medical care for all Minorities in the United States of America and to ask those who choose to discriminate against minorities in the delivery of medical care to STOP IT.

CHAPTER 1

HYPERTENSION IN AFRICAN AMERICAN MEN

—◄◄◄‖∫‖►►►—

Hypertension is one of the most common diseases in the world and a disease that is associated with other diseases such as obesity, diabetes mellitus, and high lipid in the blood. When left untreated or poorly treated, it causes conditions like stroke, coronary artery disease, heart attack, congestive heart failure, kidney failure, blindness, and dementia.

Seventy-six millions of adults in the U.S. have hypertension, 1 in 3 white adults have hypertension and 1in 2 blacks in the U.S. has hypertension. 1.5 billion People in the world have high blood pressure.

In 2015, 42.1% Blacks, 28% whites, 26% Hispanics and 24.7% Asians had hypertension in the U.S.

Hypertension is more common in Negroes/Blacks and other minorities as compared to whites and other racial groups in the world, and the disease begins at an earlier age in these subgroups and is much more aggressive. 1 out of every 2 Negroes/Black Americans has hypertension. Worldwide, 7.5 million people die of high blood pressure every year. "Every year, hypertension contributes to one out of every seven deaths in the United States and nearly half of all cardiovascular disease related deaths, including stroke." If all hypertensive patients were treated sufficiently to reach the goal specified in current clinical guidelines, 46,000 deaths might be averted each year in the U.S."

"Thirty percent of patients with hypertension in the U.S. are not being treated pharmacologically, and only 52% of individuals with hypertension have their blood pressure under control." The direct and indirect cost of hypertension is $93.5 billion per year. Sources: CDC, MMWR. 2011; 60:103-108, National Health and Nutrition Examination Survey (NHANES).

More blacks and other minorities have hypertension than do whites. The incidence of the disease is 41% among black Americans and 27% among white Americans.

Forty-eight percent of black males and 41.4 percent of black more in the U.S. have high blood pressure. The incidence of high blood pressure in blacks in the U.S. is higher than in any other ethnic group in the world. Blacks represent 14.5 % or forty-two million one hundred and sixty thousand (42,160,000) of the U.S. population and 15.6 million blacks in the U.S. have high blood pressure.

High blood pressure develops at an earlier age in blacks and other minorities and the complications it causes are more severe and aggressive compared to whites. Fifty percent of blacks with hypertension die of stroke and eighty percent die of heart disease.

Among the U.S. population with high blood pressure, 78.7 percent are aware that they have the disease, 69% are being treated for the disease, 52 % have the blood pressure under control, and 48% do not have the blood pressure under control. Roughly 63% of whites, 58% of Hispanics, and only 40% of blacks have normal blood pressure readings when taking medications for high blood pressure. Source: U.S. Department of Health and Human Services.

Since 2005, the death rates for high blood pressure rose from 25.2% in 1995 to 56.4% in 2005. In 2005, the death rates per 100,000 from high blood pressure were 15.6 for white males, 52.1 for black males, 15.1 for white females, and 40.3 for black females.
Source: American Heart Association –Heart Disease and stroke Statistics Update 2009.

What is hypertension?

The kidney is the organ responsible for the development of hypertension. Hypertension occurs when the systolic part of the blood pressure is higher than normal and the diastolic part of the blood pressure is higher than normal.

What is the systolic blood pressure?

The systolic blood pressure is the upper number in the blood pressure reading machine.

What is the diastolic blood pressure?

The diastolic blood pressure is the lower number in the blood pressure reading machine

What is a normal systolic blood pressure?

A normal systolic blood pressure ranges from 100 to an upper limit of 130

What is normal diastolic blood pressure?

A normal diastolic blood pressure ranges from 60 to an upper limit of 80

CLASSIFICATION OF BLOOD PRESSURE IN ADULTS AGE 18 YEARS AND OLDER

New blood pressure Classifications

Classification	Systolic		Diastolic
Normal	<120	and	<80
Pre-hypertension	120-139	or	80-89
Stage 1	140-159	or	90-99
Stage 2	160+		100+

Source JAMA Volume 289, No 19 May 21, 2003 the JNC-7 Report

What instruments are needed to take the blood pressure?

The instruments that are needed to take the blood pressure are:

1. A blood pressure cuff, which is attached to a manometer on which is listed different numbers from 20 mm/Hg to 300 mm/Hg.
2. A stethoscope, which is placed on a pulsating artery, most often at the bend and on the inside part of the arm.

What are some of the pitfalls in taking the blood pressure?

If the cuff is too small the blood pressure can be falsely high, as much as 10 to 20 mm/Hg systolic or diastolic. If the cuff is too large, the reverse can happen, namely the blood pressure can be too low by as much as 10 to 20 mm, /Hg. The person taking the measurement should make sure the blood pressure cuff is neither too large nor too small. That person should also make sure that the blood pressure cuff is functioning properly before using it. In particular, the blood pressure cuff should not be leaking, because if it is leaking air, then it is sure to give a false reading.

Both errors can have a serious negative impact in the care of a person being treated for hypertension, in that either she can receive too much or too little medication, which in either case can be harmful.

A small cuff should be used for a person with a small arm, a medium-size cuff for a person with a medium-sized arm and a large cuff for a person with a large arm. There are also very large cuffs made to suit the needs of very obese individuals, and as just stated above, using an undersized cuff to take the blood pressure of a person with a very large arm can cause a false reading in the blood pressure of that person.

An example of such an error in a blood pressure reading is a person with a large arm with a blood pressure reading of 140/90 measured with an undersized cuff, when in fact the blood pressure is 130/80 when a large blood pressure cuff is used.

This type of error must be avoided because the man's psyche can be quite seriously affected when she has been told that her blood pressure is high when in fact the pressure is perfectly normal when it is taken with the proper cuff. When the person in this situation applies for life insurance, this particular error can adversely affect her ability to be insured. If insurance is obtained, higher premiums are likely to be charged because of the falsely taken blood pressure.

One should make sure that the stethoscope being used to take the blood pressure is in good working order, because if it is not, this can also cause improper blood pressure readings. One should be certain that there are no holes in the diaphragm of the stethoscope - the bottom part - and be certain to check the rubber tubing for holes and cracks. If these problems are found in the stethoscope or the blood pressure machine, it should not be used because air will escape while the doctor is trying to listen to the blood pressure, resulting in false blood pressure readings.

Automatic blood pressure machines are suitable if one knows how to use them. The blood pressure should always be taken in three positions:

1. When the person is lying down.
2. When the person is sitting down.
3. When the person is standing up for at least 3 to 5 minutes.

Why is it important to take blood pressure in this manner?

It is important to take the blood pressure in this manner because most active individuals are either sitting up or standing up most of the time during the day and lie down only to sleep at night or to take a nap during the day. Several antihypertensive medications work best when the person is standing up. It is, therefore, important to know what these individuals' blood pressure readings are when they are standing up, sitting down or lying down. If an individual is bleeding or dehydrated, his or her blood pressure will drop when he or she is sitting up or standing up compared to when he or she is lying down.

The pulse rate of the person who is sitting up or standing up who has lost a lot of blood or fluid is likely to go up. This is the cause of orthostatic hypotension. That is, the pulse goes up and the blood pressure goes down. The pulse rate going up is a much more sensitive sign of orthostatic hypotension than the blood pressure dropping by itself. Of course, this maneuver depends on the age of the person because the older the individual, the weaker will be the tone within the wall of their vessels.

When one stands up, this can itself cause one's blood pressure to drop. Such individuals tend to have what is called a wide pulse pressure and all this has to be taken into consideration when one is talking about volume loss that is either blood or fluid from the body.

It takes a minimum of 1200 to 1800 cc of either fluid or blood loss for orthostatic hypotension to occur.

Again, it depends on the age and the size of the man, because an older individual who has lost between 800 and 1000 cc of either blood or fluid may have his blood pressure drop significantly. This is because a person's intravascular volume becomes contracted as the person ages.

Therefore, a diagnosis of orthostatic hypotension has to be made taking into account the person's size and age. A younger individual is more likely to tolerate the loss of 1800 cc of either blood or fluid with only slight evidence of orthostasis, compared to an older individual who might in fact develop cardiovascular collapse due solely to 1800 cc of either blood or fluid loss.

Other conditions that can cause an acute drop in blood pressure include:

1. Too much anti-hypertension medications
2. Acute heart attack;
3. Certain abnormal rhythms of the heart - either too fast or too slow a heart rate;
4. Severe infection in the blood, such as sepsis;
5. Oversensitivity of the carotid bodies, which are located in both sides of the neck, can frequently cause orthostatic hypotension to occur.

Vasovagal reaction can also cause a person's blood pressure to drop. In fact, it can also cause the person to collapse based on certain emotional factors, foe example when someone receives bad news such as the loss of a loved one or some other major crisis. Such events can cause a person to collapse because of vasovagal reaction. In addition, a vasovagal reaction in an older person with underlying cardiac disease can actually cause her blood pressure to drop when having a bowel movement, due to the straining that activates the vasovagal reaction mechanism.

In addition, acute and severe vomiting with retching can also cause an older individual to collapse because of the activation of the vasovagal reaction mechanism of the human body.

The system just described is closely associated with the control of posture in the human body, referring specifically to the carotid body is located in the neck- sensitivity. Many other factors or conditions exist that can cause a person's blood pressure to drop which can result in collapse.

It is mandatory and necessary to take blood pressure in the elderly in both arms, and when feasible, lying down, sitting down and standing up as described above. The reason for this is that as a person gets older, he or she loses muscle elasticity within the blood vessels, resulting in what is called wide pulse pressure (the term for a large difference between the systolic and diastolic blood pressure).

A drop in blood pressure can occur in the standing position as a natural physical phenomenon in elderly individuals.

This phenomenon is partly responsible for the higher systolic blood pressure seen frequently in the elderly. Although it is important to treat hypertension in the elderly, it is prudent to make all efforts not to be too aggressive with antihypertensive medications in the elderly so as not to cause too great a drop in the systolic blood pressure. The elderly need the systolic blood pressure to remain in the range of 130 to 140 for proper perfusion to take place in the brain.

As the blood vessels of the veins get stiffened and narrowed due to plaques that occur due to aging, a higher systolic pressure head is needed to push blood to the brain circulation to deliver the necessary oxygen for proper brain functions.

Dropping the systolic blood pressure too low in the elderly can lead to a stroke and this is something that must be avoided. On the other hand, if the systolic blood pressure is allowed to remain too high in the 170 to 180 range, for example for too long a period, the result can be a stroke, a heart attack, or congestive heart failure, and even death can result.

The root causes of essential hypertension in people are many, but chief among them are the followings:

1. Genetic predisposition
2. Salt sensitivity
3. Salt-rich diet
4. Obesity
5. Stress
6. Genetic component of the salt sensitivity being transferred from the forebears of men in Africa to those who are now living in the New World and also those who are still living in Africa.

Among these factors, salt sensitivity and fluid retention are the most important as the genesis of hypertension. Salt sensitivity and fluid retention is a genetic phenomenon. The gene responsible for causing salt retention and sensitivity originated in Africa. Salt retention in the body of blacks living under the severest conditions that existed in Africa millions of years ago, and to some degree still existing today, was and is necessary for survival.

Working in the hot sun in the fields of Africa was associated with massive salt loss due to sweating through the skin that existed then and that exists today for those who still have to toil the land under the hot sun in Africa and tropical courtiers of the world. This massive salt loss leads to water loss resulting in dehydration.

To prevent death, which would have been the result of this severe water loss, the body developed a gene located in the kidneys to retain salt in the body, thereby retaining water and preserving life.

Incidentally, on October 1, 2009, scientists at the University of California - Berkeley published information about the discovery of Ardi 4 feet tall that lived 4.4 million years ago in Ethiopia. Once more, this discovery confirms that the human race began in Africa and that all human beings are to one degree or another Africans, no matter the skin color or other physical characteristics.

This lifesaving gene located in the kidneys, was a necessity in the Old World in Africa, but is a detriment to health in the New World and results in the disease of essential hypertension. The salt-sensitive gene is extremely strong and highly penetrating. The diet contributes significantly to the development of many of the most common diseases. The interplay of hypertension, diabetes mellitus, obesity and high cholesterol, referred to as metabolic hypertension, or Syndrome X, is quite common in people Worldwide. All four components of hypertension are genetically transmitted.

When babies start out in life with this abnormal genetic package, by the time they grow up and are forced to live through all the psychosocial and other stresses of living in this fast paced world they are certain to suffer from the adverse effects of metabolic hypertension.

The history of salt sensitivity and secondary fluid retention resulting in elevation of blood pressure did not start millions of years ago as a disease, but rather as a God-given measure to maintain life and prevent deaths, as described above.

Living conditions in ancient Africa millions of years ago, and to a significant extent in present-day Africa, are quite harsh with people working in extremely high temperatures. Under these conditions, the human body loses a lot of salt through the skin and in so doing loses water along with salt through the skin as sweat.

Wherever salt goes in the human body, water goes with it. When a person loses salt and too much water with it, the body can become dehydrated quickly. Once the intravascular system is depleted of fluid the body risks being collapsed.

It takes between 1800 cc to 2500 cc of fluid lost ordinarily to cause the blood pressure to fall in a 70 kg man.

Once the kidneys sense that the blood pressure is falling, their normal tendency is to prevent salt from going out of the body in the urine, thereby attempting to maintain the blood pressure in the normal range. Through this mechanism, salt remains in the body and keeps water with it to maintain blood pressure and to prevent the body from collapsing.

The kidneys are able to do this because there are special genes that are located in the kidneys that enable them to hold on to salt.

This gene, called G protein-coupled receptor kinase 4, (GRK4γ,) was discovered in 2002 at the University of Virginia and Georgetown University after eighteen years of research using specimens taken from kidneys of some Caucasian American, Ghanaian, and Japanese individuals. The same quantity of GRK4 was found in all three racial groups.

This study documents that GRK4 is responsible for the salt retention that occurs in essential hypertension and therefore is the basis of this disease. Source: Proceedings of National Academy of Sciences (2002; 99:3872-3877).

As far as the kidney is concerned, people are still living in the same conditions that the forbearers of the human race lived in Africa six millions years ago and need to hold onto salt constantly to preserve the human body from dehydration.

Essential hypertension has the same genesis in people of all racial stripes, without regard to skin color. All human beings are salt sensitive to one degree or another.

Blacks, Hispanics and Asians are more salt sensitive than other racial groups. Blacks and Hispanics are salt sensitive because they are born with low renin.

Asians are salt sensitive because they eat a salt rich diet that suppresses their rennin level.

These three racial groups when there are hypertensives have what is called high volume high blood pressure.

The kidney is the center of the cause of essential hypertension and the center where some of the most important medications are used to treat high blood pressure work. Two examples of these medications are thiazide diuretic and angiotensin receptor blocker.

Hypertension causes significant problems for people because it affects such important organs as the heart, brain, kidneys, and eyes - the four organs commonly referred to as the end organs. The damage done to people's heart by hypertension causes arteriosclerotic plaques to be deposited within their coronary arteries resulting frequently in heart attacks and death, congestive heart failure and hypertensive heart disease.

Hypertension can also cause the heart to become enlarged because the heart has to pump against a high load, the high load being the high blood pressure. Over time, the muscles around the heart become hypertrophied, resulting in enlarged ventricles. Once hypertrophy sets in, because the heart muscle only has a finite length to which it can be stretched, it can no longer stretch, and the heart then begins to pump ineffectively. The infectivity of the heart muscle reflects in what is referred to as cardiomyopathy with secondary congestive heart failure. Many people develop congestive heart failure due only to high blood pressure.

At this point, the heart is unable to push the blood away from the ventricles (heart chambers), the blood/ water backs up into the lungs and accumulates as fluid, and then congestive heart failure causing shortness of breath, tiredness and other symptoms of congestive heart failure.

If not treated quickly it can result in what is referred to as pulmonary edema (acute congestive heart failure), the result of which, when it is not treated quickly and acutely, is immediate death.

In the less dramatic way, the enlarged heart sets in and the person suffering from it begins to develop lassitude, inability to walk down the block without stopping several times, inability to sleep at night on one pillow and constant coughing at night.

This condition is referred to as nocturnal coughing. All these are signs that the heart is failing. If the person gets to a physician quickly, the condition can be discovered and treatment can be started with appropriate medication to prevent the aforementioned acute condition from occurring.

Another organ that suffers immensely from the effect of hypertension is the kidney. Hypertension damages the kidney resulting in kidney failure.

The way this happens is that the pressure rises within the vessels that run through the substance of the kidneys. All the different tissues of the kidney need blood vessels of different sizes to carry blood and oxygen to them.

As the pressure rises within the kidneys, there are structures within the kidneys referred to as glomeruli, which are small capillary blood vessels, which need to be fed blood and oxygen. As the blood pressure rises, these very delicate capillary blood vessels begin to rupture. They are rupturing without the person realizing that this is occurring.

After a while, these vessels rupture and die out and the tissues to which they are responsible to bring blood and oxygen will no longer be there and, as a result, these areas of the kidneys die. Eventually, the person loses so many glomureli that the kidneys cannot function properly affecting the renal tubules, (the filtering system inside the kidneys) resulting in renal insufficiency/kidney failure.

Once all the glomeruli die, the kidneys can fail suddenly. Once the kidneys fail, waste materials accumulate within the body, resulting in swelling of the legs with smelly breath and salty skin, and a condition referred to as chronic renal failure with uremia develops. At this point either peritoneal dialysis or hemodialysis on a chronic basis must be used to clean the blood free of toxic materials to maintain life.

If a person is fortunate enough that he or she can get a kidney transplant, and the transplant succeeds, then he or she can go back to normal kidney function and a normal life. High blood pressure that goes untreated can damage the kidney to the point of kidney failure. Typically, the kidneys fail slowly, losing function gradually.

Another organ that is very sensitive to the effects of hypertension is the eye. When the blood pressure rises in the body, the pressure also rises within the vessels in the eyes. The vessels inside the eyes are quite fragile and as a result they can get damaged easily. The damage that occurs to the vessels inside the eyes of untreated or poorly treated hypertension causes different degrees of leakage to occur. If left untreated, blindness is usually the result. Hypertension is also associated with an increased incidence of glaucoma, a common disease of the eye seen hundred of millions people throughout the world.

The brain is yet another organ that suffers the effects of hypertension to varying degrees. Over time, the effects of elevated blood pressure cause plaques to develop within small vessels and large vessels of the brain. The damage that occurs within the small vessels in the brain results in multiple small vessel infarctions. This condition inevitably leads to the condition referred to as multi-infarct syndrome. Multi-infarct syndrome is the most common cause of senility in people in the world (organic brain syndrome).

Hypertension affects 1.5 billion people in the world. The incidence of hypertension is highest among people of immediate African ancestry as compared to Whites. 1 in 2 black Americans are hypertensive.

Blacks and other minorities across the world are more prone to the development of early senility due to untreated hypertension or poorly treated hypertension. Elevated blood pressure can cause three different types of major strokes to occur (cerebrovascular accident). The first type is called ischemic stroke; the second type is called hemorrhagic stroke; and the third type is known as embolic stroke.

Ischemic stroke occurs because of the chronic narrowing of the affected vessel with plaques and/or the rupture of plaques within the affected vessels, resulting in bleeding, with clot formation acutely closing off the vessel, cutting off blood flow, resulting in a stroke.

Elevated blood pressure can cause hemorrhagic stroke to occur due to chronic damage that takes place affecting the vessels, resulting in acute rupture of those vessels, causing hemorrhage to occur inside the brain. Hypertension-associated embolic stroke can occur because of hypertensive heart disease with enlargement of the heart. This can cause atrial fibrillation to develop, and if the atrial fibrillation is not treated with anticoagulants such as Heparin, Coumadin, Prodaxa, or Xarelto to prevent clot formation, then the clot can get dislodged from the atrium to the brain, causing an embolic stroke.

Frequently, hypertension is intertwined with obesity, diabetes mellitus, and elevated lipids in the same individuals. These conditions interplay in a significant percentage of people.

About of 69% of black American men are overweight/ obese. Overall, 73% of black men and women are overweight/obese in the U.S. Two third of the adults in the U.S. are obese/overweight and one third of children in the U.S. are obese/overweight, and 3.3 billion people in the world are obese/overweight.

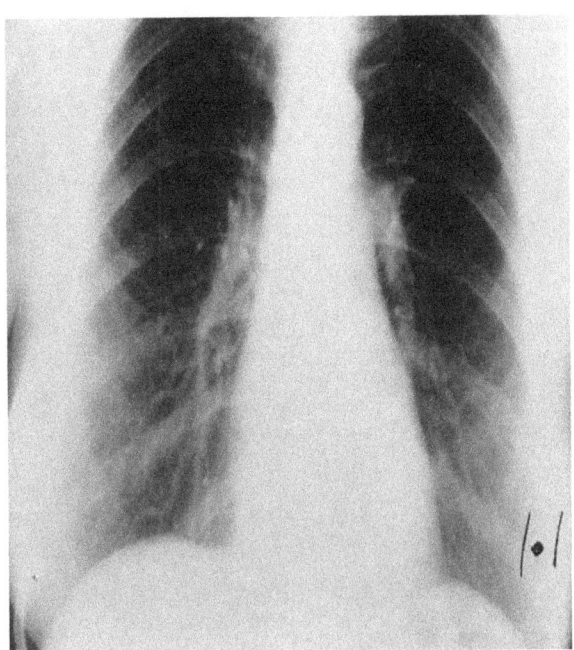

Figure 1:1– *normal chest x-ray in a patient*

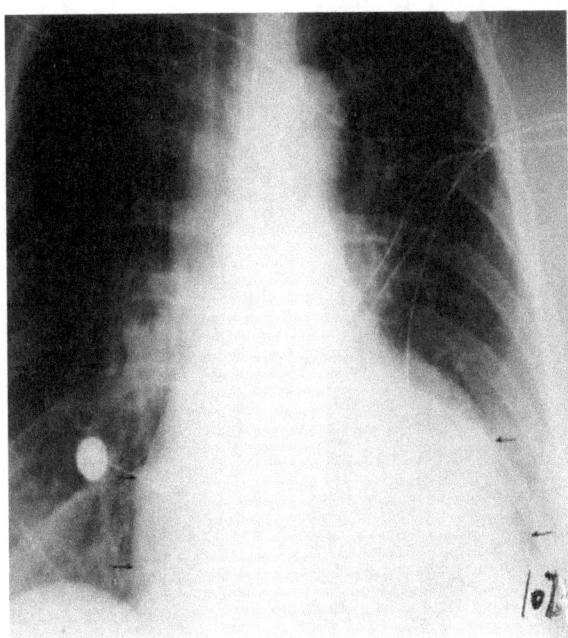

Figure 1:2–An abnormal chest x-ray in a patient with hypertensive cardiovascular disease, showing heart failure as a result of chronic hypertension with secondary coronary artery disease, leading to an enlarged heart and heart failure, with arrow showing enlarged border of the right heart and arrows showing enlarged border of the left heart with pleural effusion (fluid in lower left lung).

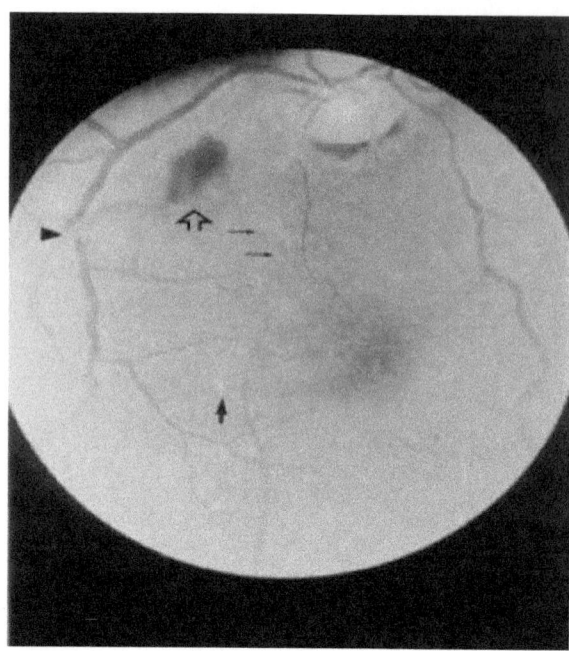

Figure **1:3**–*Showing different degrees of abnormalities in the eye of a hypertensive patient (hypertensive retinopathy). Small arrow showing silver wiring; big arrow showing hard yellow exudates; open arrowhead showing hemorrhage; arrowhead showing A-V nicking.*

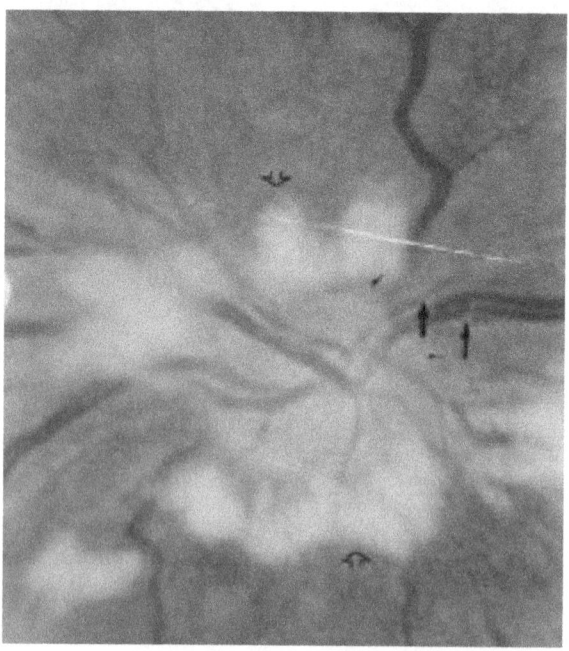

Figure **1:4**–*Showing different types of abnormalities in the eye of a hypertensive patient (hypertensive retinopathy). Small arrows showing early papilledema, one big arrow pointing to engorgement of (larger vessel). The other big arrow pointing to arterial attenuation (smaller vessel): open arrowheads showing cotton wool exudates.*

If the blood pressure in a person is 138/88, and he or she is overweight, and he or she has a family history of hypertension (that is, either her mother or father has hypertension), then the approach to this upper normal limit of blood pressure is to repeat the blood pressure during an office visit in about one month.

If in the second visit, the blood pressure is again 138/88, and then the treatment is 4 g sodium, 90 g protein, 160 g carbohydrate, 31 g fat diet per day along with exercise to try to lose the weight and thereby prevent the blood pressure from creeping up even higher.

The usual daily American diet contains an average of 7 g of sodium. The diet of African Americans is likely to contain on the average 10 g of sodium. This is so because of the so-called soul food or other types of salt-rich foods that many blacks like to eat. The salt adds taste to these foods. Whites also eat a lot of salt because they consume many fast foods and the diet of Asians is very rich in salt.

These foods typically are rich in salt, and if one is accustomed to eating food that is salty, no matter what type of food one eats one tends to add more salt in order to satisfy one's taste for salt. The vast majority of African Americans live under substandard economic conditions in which they consume fast foods, because that is the type of foods most can afford. Fast foods, in general, are of poorer quality. To enhance taste, a lot of fat and salt are added to these types of foods.

Fast foods, therefore, end up containing much more salt than would normally be the case. The greater the level of poverty, the more likely is a diet of poor quality. Since the diet is of poor quality, a lot of spices and salt are added in order to enhance the taste and make the foods more palatable. This is not a negative comment. This is a comment based on known facts. In fact, this is the genesis of the so-called "soul-food", which is really a legacy left over from slavery days.

During the time of slavery, slaves were forced to eat foods that were of poor quality and so they devised all sorts of ingenious ways of preparing meats and other foods to make them more palatable. To prevent the meats and other foods from getting spoiled, they cured these foods with juices from sours (a bitter orange), lime juice, plenty of salt and other spices, crushed hot peppers etc.

Slaves would then put the meat on a rope in the sun to dry to prevent it from getting spoiled. They would then eat it gradually. No doubt these foods tasted very good, but unfortunately they were very bad for their bodies particularly because of the salt content. These foods are still bad for the human body today especially when eaten on a regular basis. So, when the statement is made that the poorer the individual, the poorer the quality of food is likely to be, that is a statement of fact, because the foods that are of higher quality cost much more money which is unaffordable for poor people. One can only eat what one can afford, balanced with the numerous other financial demands with financially limited resources.

The DASH Diet ("Dietary Approaches to Stop Hypertension") recommends eating nuts, legumes, seeds, fruits and vegetables four to five times per week, along with a low fat dairy intake. The results show lowering of both systolic and diastolic blood pressures (Source: *Internal Medicine News*, June 1, 2003). The present recommended daily salt intake is 1.5 grams or a maximum of 2.3 grams per of sodium. Therefore, adherence to a good diet is very important as both prevention and management of hypertension.

Treatment of high blood pressure should be started early. Once the blood pressure reaches 140/90 in a salt-sensitive person, treatment with medication ought to be started, particularly if the person is obese. The best and most effective medication for hypertension is a water pill (diuretic). It does not matter what the racial make-up of the person is, so long as his or her kidneys are functioning. Water pills work to control high blood pressure by preventing salt from being reabsorbed by the kidneys back into the blood stream, taking water with it, which results in raising the blood pressure. Some of the common diuretics that are available in the United States are:

Hydrocholorothiazide
Clorthalidone
Dyazide
Moduretic
Aldactone
Lozol
Maxzide
Lasix
Bumex
Torsemide etc.

All these medications are effective in removing salt and water from the body. The cost of Hydrochlorothiazide at 25 mg per day is low (30 generic tablets cost $10.00). However, if one were to buy a more expensive medication, the blood pressure would be treated much less effectively (using it as mono-therapy meaning by itself) and yet the person would spend four times more money for that medication. A good example is Procardia XL 30 mg, 30 tablets Brand costs $75.00. Another example is Zestril 10 mg 30 tablets Brand cost $52.00. Because it is an angiotensin-1-converting enzyme (ACE) inhibitor (meaning that it needs the presence of an elevated level of renin to be effective in bringing down the blood pressure), it does not work in blacks to treat hypertension.

The reason Zestril and other ACE don't work to treat blood pressure is blacks, Asians, Hispanics and other minorities is because these people genetically have low renin in their blood. Zestril and other ACE inhibitors such as Accupril, Capoten, Vasotec, Monopril, Altace, Mavik, etc. are great medications to treat hypertension when used in some whites. These medications are also extremely effective in the treatment of congestive heart failure and certain cardiac arrhythmias.

Overall, the basic reason for essential hypertension is salt retention and the water retention that goes with it and this phenomenon applies to all individuals who suffer from essential hypertension, which accounts for about 98% of people with hypertension without regards to ethnicity. The gene responsible for essential hypertension has been discovered and it is located in the kidneys and it is the same in all individuals without regard to race.

Therefore, all individuals who suffer from hypertension and have functioning kidneys need water pills to treat their hypertension.

Water pills work to control high blood pressure by preventing salt from being reabsorbed by the kidneys back into the blood stream. A water pill / diuretic forces salt out in the urine taking water with it. This decreases the amount of water in the intravascular compartment resulting in lowering of the blood pressure.

The first medication that must be used in the treatment of high blood pressure in a person with functioning kidneys is a thiazide diuretic.

There is a substance made by the human kidney called renin. Renin, once made by the kidneys, enters into a biochemical reaction leading ultimately to another substance called aldosterone, which causes salt retention leading to water retention, which in turn causes expansion of water within the intravascular compartment, leading to elevation of blood pressure.

This system is called the renin angiotensin aldosterone system.

However, blacks, Hispanics, Asians, and other people of color have low renin in their bloods as a genetic fact. So prescribing medications that work to attack the renin angiotensin system to decrease blood pressure in these individuals is useless and makes no clinical sense. Furthermore, these medications have a lot of side effects and are very expensive.

Examples of these medications are beta-blockers, such as Inderal, Lopressor, Tenormin, Toprol XL to name a few, and ACE inhibitors such as Capoten, Zistril, Vasotec, etc. Beta-blockers are excellent medications for treating angina, migraine headaches, cardiac arrhythmias, congestive heart failure, etc., in people of all ethnic make-ups and work very well in these circumstances.

The only situation in which a beta-blocker might have some effect in a salt-sensitive person in controlling hypertension is when the person is under stress and is secreting a lot of adrenalin. The beta-blocker might transiently shut off the sympathetic system in this setting to decrease the blood pressure.

However, when a salt-sensitive low-renin-secreting person's kidneys fail and the person develops chronic renal failure, the renin level goes up by necessity, and then a beta-blocker becomes a necessity in the treatment of hypertension because the renin level is always elevated in chronic renal failure.

Another circumstance in which the beta-blocker might work to decrease blood pressure although the individual may be classified as salt-sensitive is in reno-vascular hypertension.

When plaques or fibrous substances within the vessels obstruct the circulation of the kidneys, then the renin level at that point is elevated. In this circumstance, beta-blockers would work via the renin angiotensin system and the beta-receptors within the kidneys to decrease the blood pressure.

Beta-Blockers also work to decrease high pressure in pheochromocytoma.

Pheochromocytoma is a benign tumor of the adrenal gland that secretes catecholamine resulting in elevated blood pressure.

Still another important use for a beta-blocker occurs when a person's blood pressure is critically high - for example, in the 200/120 range. In this situation, Labetalol IV can be used to acutely bring the blood pressure down.

The reason that Labetalol works to acutely decrease blood pressure when given intra-venously is that via the rennin-angiotensin system, angiotensin-2 is released causing stimulation of the adrenal medulla resulting in the release of catecholamines, which raises the blood pressure. Labetalol blocks the release of catecholamine and decreases the blood pressure.

However, this is a minor effect of the rennin-angiotensin system on the overall causation of high blood pressure. This is the reason that beta blockers given by mouth do not work to decrease blood pressure. There are specific circumstances when beta-blockers are used to treat specific medical conditions that cause blood pressure to go up. Source: "Beta-blockers for hypertension going out of style", Cleveland Clinic Journal of Medicine, Volume 76, Number 9, September 2009.

The ASCORT-BPLA (Anglo-Scandinavian Cardiac Outcomes Trial –Blood Pressure Lowering Arm) shows that beta-blockers, as monotherapy, do not work to treat high pressure.

Some of the beta-blockers in use in the U.S. are:

Inderal
Tenormin
Corgard
Timolol
Labetalol
Visken
Tenormin
Toprol XL
Coreg
Bystolic

As has been just stated, ACE inhibitors are very good medications in the treatment of the blood pressure in Caucasians and in the treatment of cardiomyopathy with associated congestive heart failure, myocardial infarction in diabetics with associated high blood pressure, diabetics with microalbuminuria and in all individuals, regardless of their ethnic background, who suffer from these conditions.

ACE inhibitors can be used with caution in blacks with chronic renal failure to treat high blood pressure because in this setting, the renin level is high. The reason for the caution is because ACE inhibitors can cause an increase in the BUN and serum potassium, and the elevated serum potassium is a major problem unless the patient is on chronic dialysis, in which case the potassium can be removed during dialysis.

It is best to treat Blacks, Hispanics, Asians and other racial minorities with high blood pressure with an angiotensin -2-receptor blocker (ARB) because ARB blocks the entire rennin angiotensin Aldosterone system to prevent the production of Aldosterone which, when elevated, causes salt and water retention resulting in elevation of blood pressure. ARB works effectively in all ethnic groups. Everything that an ACE can do, ARB does it better for high blood pressure, microalbuminuria in diabetics, post myocardial infarction, congestive heart failure etc.

The following are some of the ARBs in use in the U.S.:

Cozzar
Avapro
Diovan
Aceon
Atacand
Benicar
Micardis

As already mentioned, the second most common form of hypertension is reno- vascular hypertension, which represents about 2% of all types of hypertensions. As individuals age, plaques may develop within the blood vessels carrying blood to the kidneys, resulting in elevation of renin, causing a state referred to as hyperenemia and high blood pressure.

Frequently, in renovascular hypertension, a sound referred to as a "bruit" can be heard over the flanks of the patient's abdomen using the stethoscope, either on the right side or the left side of the abdomen. However, in a certain percentage of patients with renovascular hypertension, a bruit is not heard. In this situation, either the so-called Capoten test or renal angiography has to be done to determine whether renovascular obstruction exists or not.

The other family of medications in use in the U.S. to treat high blood pressure is calcium channel blockers. These medications work by relaxing the smooth muscles in the human body. Relaxing the muscles causes the blood pressure to drop. Constriction of blood vessels causes blood pressure to rise. In order for any muscle to contract, calcium is needed for the contraction to occur and the absence of calcium inside the blood vessels results in relaxation of muscle.

The following are some of the calcium channel medications in use in the U.S.:

Verapamil
Cardizem CD
Vasotec
Procardia
Adalat
Caduet

These medications are expensive, but they are very effective to treat hypertension not only in all ethnic groups.

Still another family of anti-hypertension medications in use in the U.S. is Alpha-blockers such as:

Hytrin
Cardura
Clonidine
Aldomet
Hydralazine

Aliskiren is a newly approved family of medications. Angiotensin -2 is a vasoconstrictor, which causes the release of catecholamine from the adrenal medulla and prejunctional nerve endings and causes the secretion of aldosterone to occur resulting in reabsorption of salt raising the blood pressure. This reaction occurs under the influence of rennin, which is made by the kidney. Aliskiren works to decrease blood pressure by blocking renin directly.

None of the anti-hypertensive medications listed above works as monotherapy to treat high blood pressure. For any of these medications to work to treat high blood pressure, a water pill (Thiazide diuretic) must be added to the regimen. As explained above, the reason it is necessary to use a diuretic in the treatment of high blood pressure is that the basis of essential hypertension is salt retention and water retention resulting in high volume hypertension with expansion of the intra-vascular compartment with elevation of the blood pressure.

Modiuretic, Dyazide, Maxzide, etc contain triamterene, which prevents potassium loss in the urine. In addition, potassium chloride can be prescribed by mouth along with the water pills, if on testing the blood, the potassium is found to be low. It is the standard practice to prescribe potassium supplement for any elderly patient on water pills to prevent low serum potassium. Elderly individuals frequently have a diet that contains less than 80 mg of potassium per day.

In addition, elderly individuals have a higher propensity of losing potassium in their urine when taking water pills. For these, and all the other aforementioned reasons, when an elderly person is on water pills and particularly if that elderly person is on Digitalis, close attention must be paid to the serum potassium.

Potassium replacement ought to be provided to prevent potassium loss which alone can cause severe cardiac dys-arrhythmias.

The argument that water pills cause blood sugar to rise is, in fact, a false argument because replacing potassium restores insulin receptor sensitivity, which then keeps the blood sugar at a normal level. The benefit of having well-controlled blood pressure far outweighs the questionable slight increase in cholesterol that might be seen in some rare instances in individuals taking water pills.

All that needs to be done is to advise the individual to stay on a low-fat diet and monitor the serum cholesterol as often as possible.

The incidence of high blood pressure is on the decrease in whites, but is on the increase in blacks and is continuing to increase steadily in this group.

There is a rare tumor of the adrenal gland called pheochromocytoma that secretes substances called catecholamines. Catecholamine causes a characteristic elevation in blood pressure. Because 95% of the time when a person has high blood pressure, it is due to the so-called essential hypertension, it is more cost effective to do a few simple tests following a complete physical examination and start treatment for the blood pressure. It is inappropriate to do extensive and expensive tests before trying treatment with antihypertensive medications in a man with hypertension.

The basic tests that are necessary in the initial evaluation of hypertension in blacks include:

1. Complete blood count
2. Blood chemistries, such as blood sugar, blood urea nitrogen, serum electrolytes, serum creatinine, lipid profiles such as cholesterol, triglycerides, high-density lipoprotein, low-density lipoprotein
3. Urinalysis
4. EKG
5. Chest x-ray.

The tests for pheochromocytoma are expensive and very tedious to do. It requires serum catecholamines; 24 hours urine catecholamines, and a specific diet that must be adhered to for several days before these tests can be done. It is simpler to do an abdominal CT scan to evaluate the adrenal glands looking for abnormality, rather than doing these very extensive blood tests looking for pheochromocytoma, which is quite rare. Most of the time, people with pheochromocytoma have sustained elevated blood pressure rather than the blood pressure that goes up and down as is being taught in medical schools and residency training.

To determine the extent of damage that the hypertensive state has done to the different end organs of hypertensive women, a series of basic tests ought to be done. The end organs are the brain, heart, eyes, and kidneys.

These basic tests are not only inexpensive, but also clinically rationale. The Complete Blood Count (CBC) can tell whether a person is anemic or not, and in renal failure associated with long-time hypertension, the red blood cell count is low because the kidneys are damaged and not able to make erythropoietin. Erythropoietin is a hormone made by the kidneys to stimulate the production of red cells by the bone marrow - the organ within which red blood cells are made in adults.

The urinalysis is abnormal in kidney disease associated with hypertension. When high blood pressure damages the kidneys, the urine specific gravity is low. The urine is likely to have protein in it and the urine sediment, when examined with the microscope, is likely to have substances called casts, indicating intrinsic kidney damage.

In the blood chemistry tests, the BUN, the creatinine, the serum potassium and the bicarbonate may all be abnormal in high blood pressure-associated kidney disease. If the blood sugar is elevated, this means the patient, in addition to having hypertension, may have diabetes mellitus. The serum lipids such as cholesterol, triglycerides, LDL, are elevated and if the man is hypertensive, the blood sugar is elevated, and if the man happens to be obese, this is also very important; this is called syndrome X or metabolic hypertension.

Metabolic hypertension or syndrome X is a very serious condition in which there is interplay between obesity, hypertension, hyperlipidemia, and diabetes in the same individual. This very deadly combination needs to be handled extremely expertly and carefully. The chest x-ray is important to determine whether the heart is enlarged or not, or whether the lungs have fluid in them, a condition known as congestive heart failure. If the heart is enlarged, it gives the physician a very good idea as to how long the person has been hypertensive. The electrocardiogram (EKG) is very important, in that it allows the physician to have an idea as to the different types of damage that the high blood pressure may have caused to the heart muscle over a long period.

These basic tests having been done, then the physician has sufficient information at hand to organize a sensible, rational, safe, and cost-effective treatment plan for the hypertensive patient. Examining the eyes using the ophthalmoscope allows the physician to see the fundi of hypertensive women, which shows small blood vessels in the eyes, and if found to be damaged, reveals that these women have been hypertensive for a long time and most probably without effective treatment.

In order for people to keep their blood pressures normal, in addition to appropriate medications such as diuretics, they must follow a diet that is low in salt, fat, and simple carbohydrates and high in fiber, protein, vitamins, iron, and minerals. They also must control their weight and exercise regularly.

The rate of glomerular filtration inside the kidneys and the so-called renal plasma flow are both increased by anywhere from 30% to 50%.

People must endeavor to exercise regularly, stop smoking, and abstain from abusing alcohol, if they are to decrease their incidence of high blood pressure. These measures can lead to decreasing some of the adverse consequences of high blood pressure such as stroke, heart attack, and kidney failure.

All these factors contribute to decrease the median survival age in black women of 77 years compared to the white women's median survival age of 81 years as well as black men's median survival age of 70 years compared to that of white men's median survival age of 76 years.

There is a need for a change of lifestyle of individuals to help decrease the incidence of hypertension. This change in lifestyle is not always realistic because of the poor economic circumstances of most poor people in the U.S. and in the world.

The stress brought on by a multitude of problems associated with poverty plays a major role in the elevation of blood pressure. If the stress that is common in poor people is not significantly diminished, it makes it that much more difficult to control the elevation of their blood pressures.

Hypertension is among the leading causes of morbidities and mortalities in people in the U.S. and in the world. However, education and an understanding of this most serious disease can delay its onset by many years, and therefore, can decrease its incidence in all racial groups.

It is important to understand that essential hypertension has the same genesis in all racial groups and therefore must be treated the same in all these groups.

Doing otherwise guarantees the development of major difficulty in controlling blood pressure in all ethnic groups. Treating high blood pressure in all individuals with a proper regimen of medications is essential to decrease hypertension-associated deaths.

Hypertension is an easily treatable disease if the right medication or medications are provided to hypertensives. Treatment with the right medications would mean that this highly treatable disease would be dealt with much more effectively; the result is the prevention or at least the significant decrease of the devastation it causes on the health of people in the U.S. and in the world.

CHAPTER 2

STROKES IN AFRICAN AMERICAN MEN

Stroke is one of the leading diseases that kills and disables people in the United States and around the world. Each year, 795,000 people suffer a new or recurrent stroke in the United States; 600,000 of these strokes are first strokes and 185,000 are recurrent strokes. Worldwide, 12.7 million people suffer a stroke yearly because of high blood pressure. Source: WHO.

Every 53 seconds someone suffers a stroke in the U.S. and every 3.3 minutes someone dies of a stroke. Altogether, 7 million Americans have had a stroke. Each year, 60,000 more women than men have a stroke. Every year, 143,579 people die from stroke in the U.S. Stroke is the fourth leading cause of death in the U.S. Worldwide, 15 million people have a stroke each year, 5 million people die from a stroke, and 5 million people are permanently disabled from a stroke. Stroke is the second leading cause of deaths in the world.

The rates of stroke are higher in blacks and other minorities than in whites, and stroke develops in blacks and other minorities at a younger age than it does in whites. Eighty-seven percent (87%) of strokes are of the ischemic type, 10% are of the intracerebral hemorrhage type, and 3 % are of the subarachnoid hemorrhage type.

Blacks and other minorities have twice the incidence of a first stroke compared to whites. The rates of stroke in ages 45-84 are 6.6 per 1,000 in black males and 3.6 in white males.

For black females in the same age range, it is 4.9 per 1,000 and 2.2 in white females. Source: National Heart, Lung, and Blood Institute, 2006, Bethesda, M.D.

According to report presented on 2/7/13 at the American Stroke association's conference in Honolulu, people who eat deep fried foods and who drink a lot sugary drinks have a high incidence of stroke. In addition, people who eat traditional southern diet have a 41% increase of stroke and African Americans who eat this diet have a 63% higher risk of stroke.

"The so-called Stroke Belt" of the U.S. consists of Alabama, Arkansas, Georgia, Indiana, Kentucky, Louisiana, Mississippi, North Carolina, South Carolina, Tennessee and Virginia, according the National Heart, and Lung, and Blood Institute," 10 of which are Southern states.

Stroke is responsible one of every 16 deaths in the U.S. Stroke is the third leading cause of deaths in the U.S. after heart disease and cancer.

Every year, 140,000 people die of a stroke in the U.S. and 5 million people die of stroke in the world. About 7.6% of the individuals who suffer ischemic strokes and 37.5% of those who suffer a hemorrhagic stroke die within 30 days.

In 2004, the overall death rate from stroke was 50.0 percent: 74.9 percent for black males, 48.1 percent for white males, 65.5 percent for black females, and 47.2 percent for white females. Source: NCHS, CDC.

There are 4,600,000 survivors of strokes in the U.S. Negroes/Blacks and other minorities have the highest prevalence of large vessels/small vessel strokes than whites. The incidence of intracranial strokes is 19% in black women and 6% in white women. The incidence of lacuna strokes is 10% in black women and 2.7% in white women. Black males have 19% prevalence of small vessel stroke compared to 6% for white males and black males have 10% of lacuna strokes compared to 2.7% for white males.

Small vessel strokes (TIA) and large vessel strokes are associated with a high incidence of dementia. Therefore, the incidence of stroke related dementia is highest for blacks than any other racial group.

Because blacks and other minorities have a higher incidence of high blood pressure than any other racial groups and poorer treatments or no treatments at all for this disease, they suffer more strokes and other serious complications of high blood pressure.

Risk factors for stroke include:

1. Being men or women
2. Hypertension
3. Diabetes mellitus
4. Hyperlipidemia/High cholesterol
5. Obesity
6. Metabolic syndrome
7. Hypercoagulable state
8. Primary polycythemia
9. Essential thrombocythemia
10. Kidney failure
11. Sickle cell disease
12. Atrial fibrillation
13. Cancer
14. Cigarette /Tobacco smoking
15. Trousseau syndrome
16. Elevated Lipoprotein-a
17. Elevated homocysteine
18. Vitamin B12 deficiency
19. Folic Acid deficiency
20. Low protein C level in the blood
21. Low protein S level in the blood

22. Nephrotic syndrome
23. Secondary polycythemia
24. Decreased anti-thrombin lll level in the blood
25. Obstructive sleep apnea
26. Taking birth control pill
27. Taking Estrogenic hormone
28. Elevated anti- phospholipin anti body
29. Elevated circulating lupus anticoagulant
30. AIDS
31. Factor V liden mutation
32. Prothrombin G20210A mutations
33. Hyperviscosity in patients with multiple myeloma
34. Hematocrit level 40% or greater in patients with chronic renal failure can cause stroke to occur
35. Hematocrit level 40% or greater in patients with sickle cell anemia can cause stroke to occur
36. Racial discrimination
37. Poverty
38. Stress
39. Pregnancy
40. Alcoholism
41. Elevated factor VIII level
42. Elevated fibrinogen level
43. Vasculitis of the brain
44. Low anti-thrombin III
45. Systemic Lupus Erythematosus etc.

What is a stroke?

A stroke occurs when an obstruction of blood flow occurs within the blood vessel, preventing blood flow to an area of the brain, which then becomes damaged.

This damage results in what is called a stroke. Another terminology frequently used to describe a stroke is a "cerebrovascular accident".

This obstruction of blood flow can be either caused by plaques within a vessel or by a clot from the heart brought through the vessel by the bloodstream to the brain. Another type of stroke occurs when a vessel inside the brain ruptures and leaks blood inside the brain. The rupture of a vessel in the brain is either due to a vessel filled with atherosclerotic plaques or the elevation of blood pressure within the vessel, which causes the membrane of this vessel to rupture and leak blood into the brain, leading to a stroke.

This type of stroke is called a "hemorrhagic stroke". Brain aneurysms, which are a meshwork of vessel malformations due to genetic defects, can rupture and leak blood into the brain when the blood pressure is too high.

Aneurysms of the brain can rupture and cause a hemorrhagic stroke within the brain whether the blood pressure of the individual is elevated or not.

Another frequent cause of bleeding into the brain is hemangiomas, or arteriovenous malformations. These are a group of small arteries and veins in a mesh, which form an abnormal network of vessels, which can bleed easily in the brain, leading to hemorrhagic stroke.

There is a form of stroke called a transient ischemic attack (TIA). In TIA, there is a transient occlusion of a small vessel by a clot or a clump of platelets, which are trapped within the vessel, preventing free flow of the blood to pass to deliver oxygen to that part of the brain. This temporary lack of oxygen to the brain causes a clinical condition, which can temporarily lead to loss of consciousness, seizures, weakness, lassitude, and a feeling of being sick, which sometimes can last for several hours or several days.

Frequently these people have what is called "pre-syncope" or a full-blown "syncopal episode" because of the TIA. This condition usually occurs in the setting of what is referred to as multi-infarct syndrome, which is the result of many years of either poorly treated or untreated hypertension. In multi-infarct syndrome, different parts of the brain deep within it are affected with this condition.

The most common types of stroke or cerebrovascular accident include:

1. Arteriosclerotic or ischemic stroke 61% of all strokes.
2. Lacunae stroke 20%
3. Embolic stroke, which represents 24% of all strokes.
4. Hemorrhagic stroke associated with high blood pressure 10% of all strokes.
5. Ruptured aneurysms.
6. Bleeding arteriovenous malformations.
7. Transient ischemic attacks.
8. Subarachnoid hemorrhage 7% of all strokes.
9. Occlusion of carotid arteries by plaque, causing stroke to occur because of lack of blood flow to the brain.

Arteriosclerotic-type strokes and hypertension-associated strokes are the two most common types seen. Stroke is one of the leading diseases that cause deaths among people of all ethnic backgrounds. The combination of salt sensitivity, salt retention and water retention and the elevated high blood pressure are responsible for such a high incidence of strokes.

As far as the risk of having a stroke is concerned, even people who are rich and have the best of everything face the same fate if they fail to take good care of themselves. That is to say, obesity, diabetes mellitus, hypertension, stress, and domestic turmoil also affect individuals of good financial means, high education, and esteemed professions as well.

The human brain is in total control of all activities associated with being a human being. The ability of the brain to think is what differentiates the human animal from all other animals.

The following outlines, in part, some of the facilities that the human brain controls:

1. The ability to think
2. The ability to gather information and process such information logically, rationally to formulate judgments rightly or wrongly.
3. The ability to breathe
4. The ability to see
5. The ability to hear
6. The ability to smell
7. The ability to feel
8. The ability to taste
9. The heartbeat and other crucial functions of the heart
10. Lung functions
11. Hunger
12. Lack of desire for food
13. Thirst
14. Lack of desire to drink
15. Sleep
16. Insomnia
17. Happiness
18. Unhappiness
19. Moods
20. Good moods
21. Bad moods
22. Elation
23. Motivation
24. Lack of motivation
25. Hardworking habits
26. Laziness
27. Neatness
28. Sloppiness
29. Anger
30. Aggressive behavior
31. Antisocial behavior
32. Pleasant and friendly behavior
33. Lying as a habitual behavior
34. Honesty
35. Dishonesty
36. Criminal behavior and other antisocial behaviors
37. Sexual orientations/preferences
38. Sexual desires
39. Erectile functions for both men and women
40. Ejaculatory functions and satisfactions for both men and women
41. Bowel functions
42. Urinary functions

43. Chewing
44. Swallowing
45. Sneezing
46. Coughing
47. Yawning
48. Lying down
49. Sitting
50. Bending
51. Standing
52. Walking
53. Running
54. All other motor body functions
55. Writing
56. Reading
57. Speaking etc.

Different parts of the human brain are in control of these different functions, so when the brain is damaged by a stroke, or accidents of one type or another, infections or other abnormalities that interfere with its normal functions, one, or several of these vital functions become impaired in one way or another.

Hypertension causes a stroke to occur through two basic mechanisms:

1. Increased blood pressure in the vessels within the brain which causes the inside part of these vessels to become damaged, and over time, the damaged areas of these vessels trap platelets and other material as they pass through the blood. A nidus of these different materials develops within these vessels and the result is plaque formation.

The formation of plaques within these vessels leads to narrowing of these vessels, impeding blood flow. Superimposed on the plaque frequently is a clot which can acutely close off a vessel, resulting in a cerebrovascular accident stroke. A plaque within a vessel can cause a stroke through different mechanisms:

The plaque can cause the vessel to become narrowed, impeding blood flow and oxygen delivery to a particular part of the brain. (b) The plaque that sits inside that vessel can break off, causing either an embolus or a clot to start forming, resulting in a stroke as has just been outlined.

2. Another mechanism through which hypertension causes stroke is acute intracerebral bleeding secondary to very elevated blood pressure causing rupture of a blood vessel, resulting in bleeding within the brain. Bleeding inside the brain can result in a coma because of edema (swelling) within the brain, and if the coma lasts too long, then the result can be death of the affected person. Another type of stroke syndrome that can occur, is people who have been hypertensive for a long time, and in particular if the blood pressure has not been treated or not treated properly as mentioned before, is multiple small vessel infarctions (microvascular disease) of the brain.

The following are radiological examples of strokes.

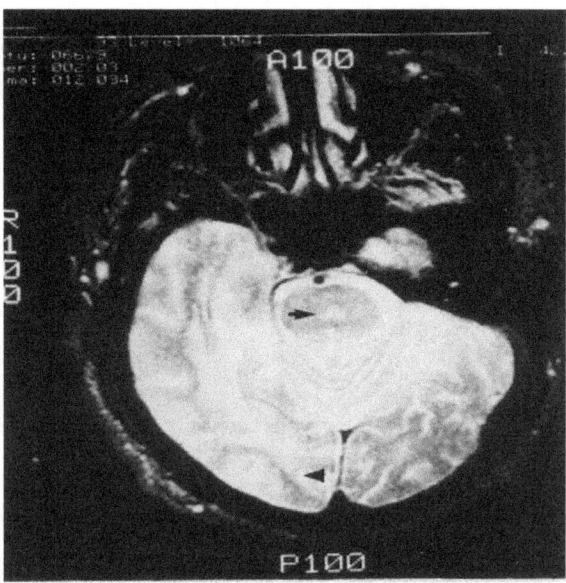

Figure 2:1–MRI *of the brain in a person patient with hypertension: small infarct in the pond (arrow) and right occipital white matter (arrowhead).*

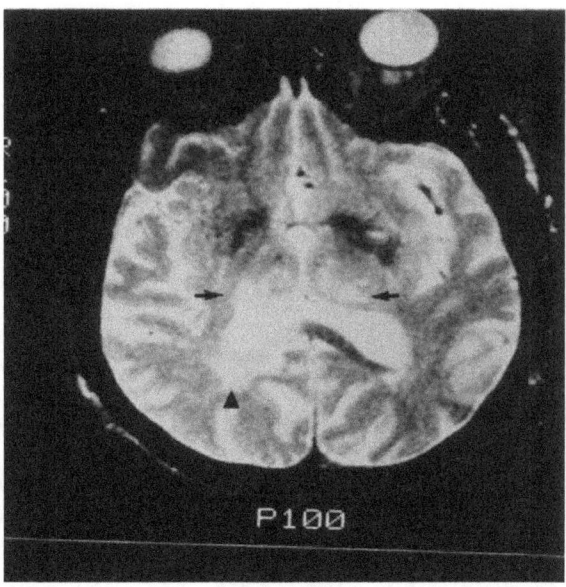

Figure 2:2–MRI *of the brain in a person with hypertension: infarction of thalamus (arrows) and right parietal white matter (arrowhead).*

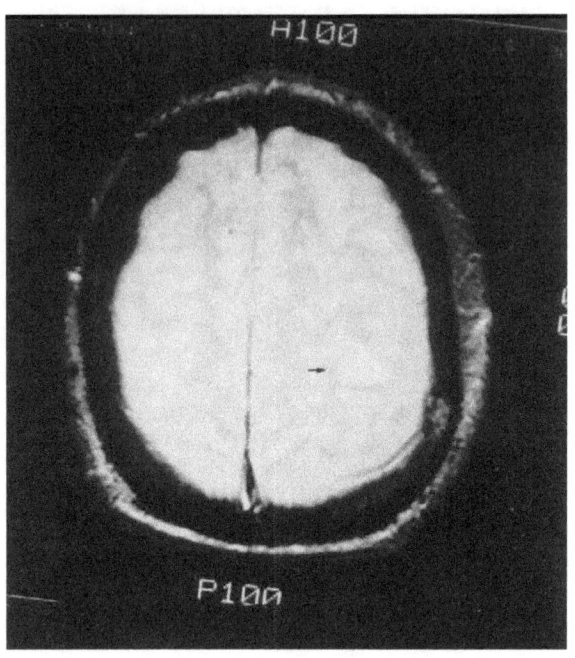

Figure 2:3–MRI *of the brain in a person with hypertension: left parietal small infarction (arrow).*

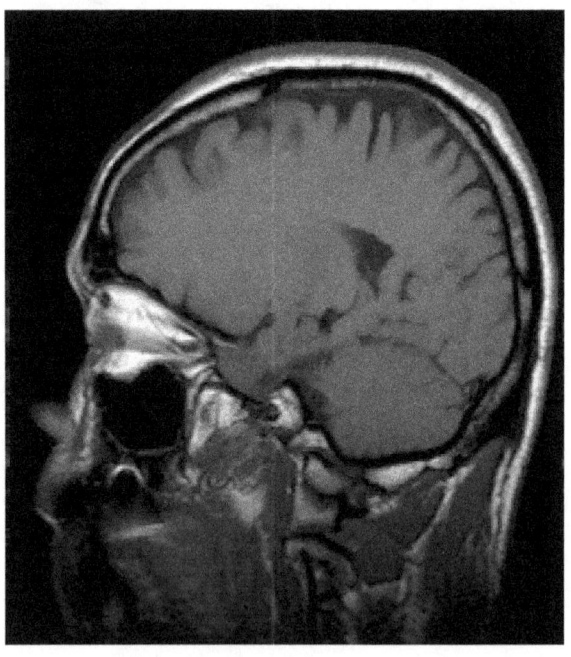

Figure 2:4 -Brain MRA of a person a stroke

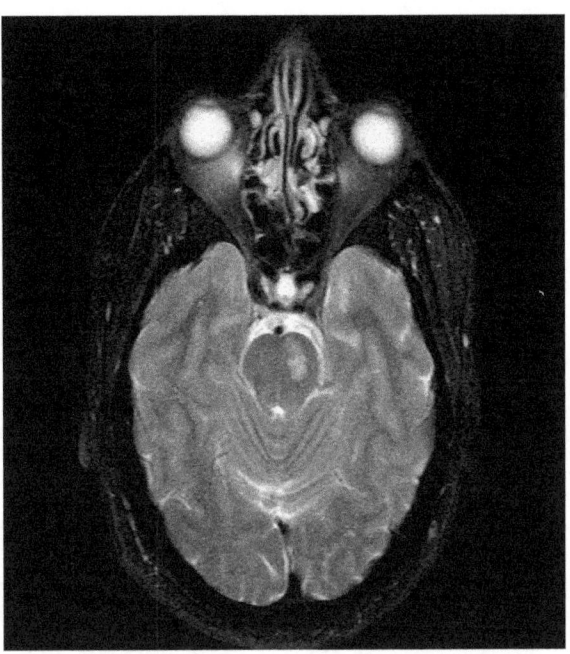

Figure 2:5 -Brain MRA of a person with a stroke

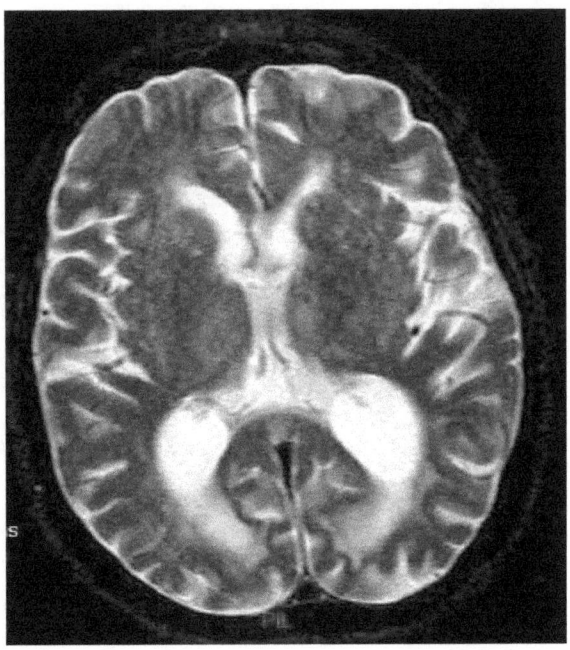

Figure 2:6 -Brain MRA in a person with ischemic and hemorrhagic stroke

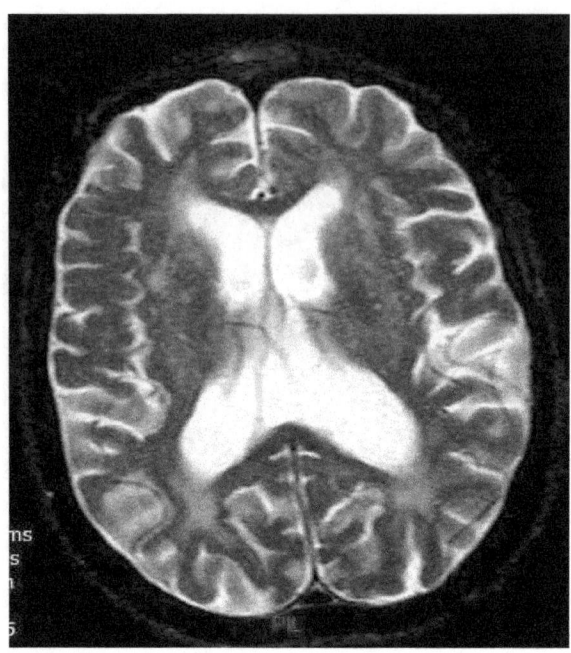

Figure 2:7 -Brain MRA in person with ischemic/hemorrhagic stroke

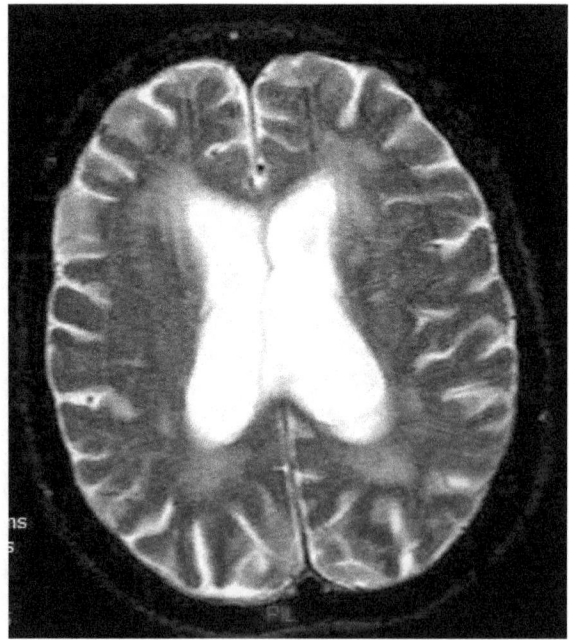

Figure 2:8 -Brains in MRA & MRI in a person with hemorrhagic stroke

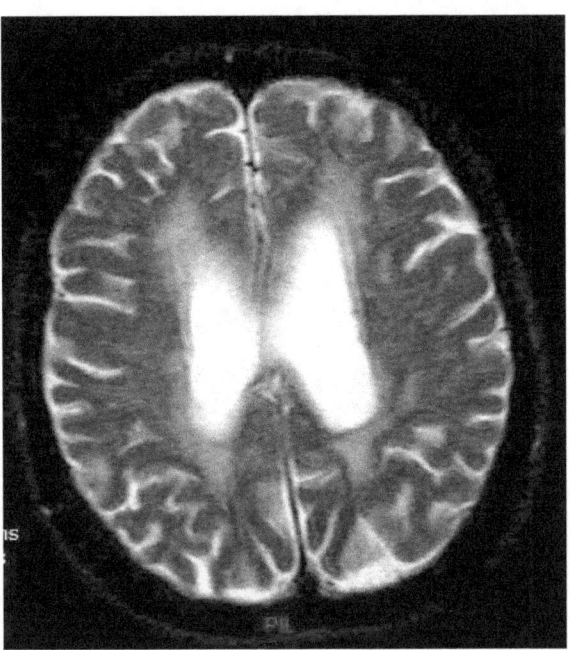

Figure 2:9 -Brains MRI & MRA in a person with hemorrhagic stroke

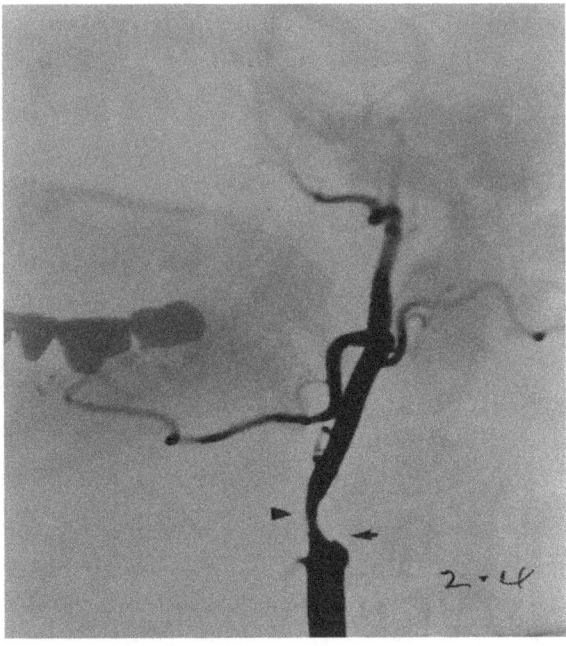

Figure 2:10–Arteriosclerotic disease of carotid artery in a peson with hypertension causing transient ischemic attacks (pre-stroke syndrome). Carotid angiogram: occlusion of internal carotid artery at its origin (arrow); narrowing of proximal internal carotid artery (arrowhead).

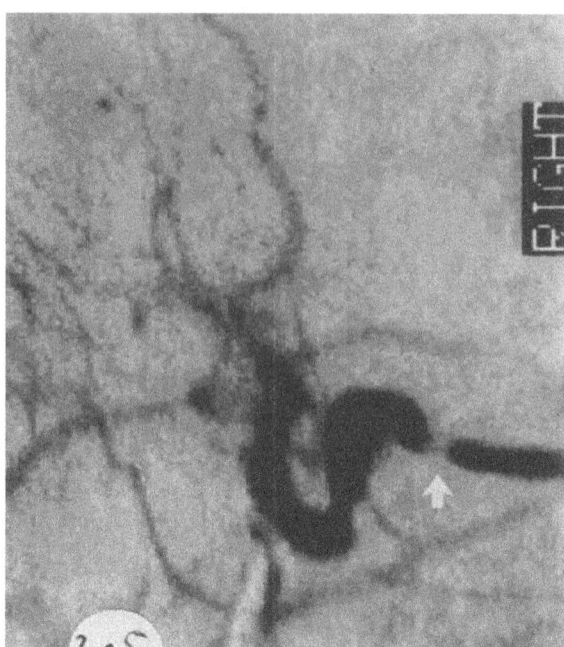

Figure 2:11–*Cerebral angiogram 95% occlusion of internal carotid artery in a person with hypertension (arrow).*

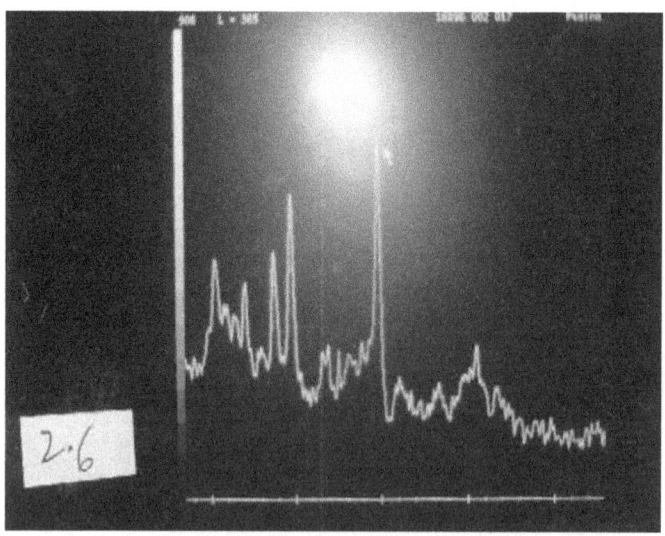

Figure 2:12 — SPECT MRI *of the brain of a person with Alzheimer's disease showing hypo perfusion of the frontal lobe of the brain.*

These small vessels are located deep inside the brain and supply blood to very vital structures within the brain. This condition is associated with early memory loss resulting in organic brain syndrome. Multiple small vessel infarctions are second only to Alzheimer's disease as a cause of senility. In fact, it is probably more common than Alzheimer's in terms of causing senility because there are so many more hypertensive patients than people who have Alzheimer's. It is common to see 40-year-old black men who have been hypertensive since their 30s or 20s who are having difficulty remembering very simple things because of multiple small vessel infarctions of the brain, as seen on brain MRI (magnetic resonance imaging). (CT of the brain does not show this syndrome very well.)

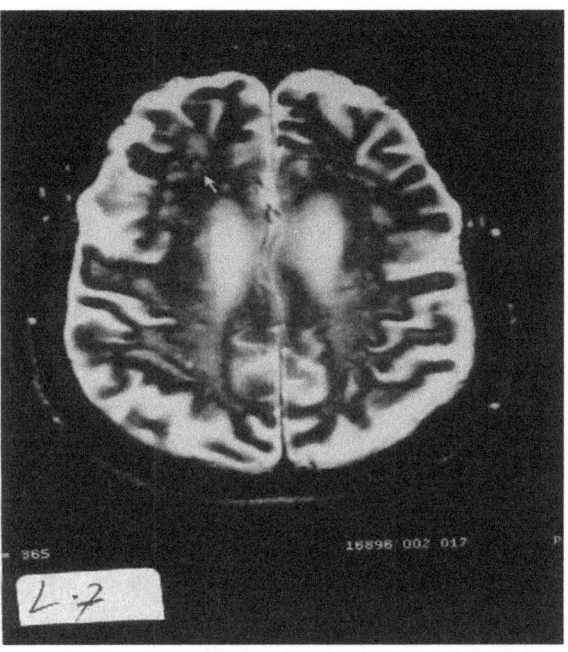

Figure 2:13–MRI *of the brain of a person with Alzheimer's disease and longstanding hypertension showing multiple small vessel infarctions of the brain.*

In evaluating memory loss in a 40- to 60-year-old hypertensive person, the following tests need to be done:

1. A complete history and physical examination by a competent internist, primary care physician or neurologist
2. CBC with differential
3. SMA20
4. Urinalysis
5. Thyroid tests such as T4, TSH, and T3
6. B12/ Folate levels
7. Complete lipid profile
8. Lipoprotein-a level
9. Homocysteine level
10. Protein S level
11. Protein C level
12. Anti-thrombin III level
13. Factor V Liden evaluation
14. Anti-phospholipin antibody evaluation

15. Prothrombin mutation evaluation
16. ANA
17. VDRL
18. HIV test
19. Chest x-ray
20. EKG
21. Brain CT
22. MRI/MRA of the brain
23. Carotid Ultrasound etc.

If the tests mentioned above are normal and the neurological examination is normal, then a SPECT scan of the brain must be done to look for hypo perfusion in the frontal lobe of the brain. (Hypo perfusion in the frontal lobe of the brain is seen in Alzheimer's disease on SPECT MRI of the brain.). Enlargement of the temporal horns of the lateral ventricles when present on MRI of the brain is diagnostic of AD

Each one of these tests is done for a particular reason. The history gives the physician a profile as to what sorts of exposures or conditions the patient may have had.

The physical examination allows the physician the opportunity to find abnormalities that may shed light on the poor memory. The complete blood count tells the physician if the white blood cell count is either too low or too high. Both too low and too high white blood cell counts may be associated with conditions that might explain the memory loss. It is important to realize that there is a difference in the level of white blood cell (WBC) counts in Caucasians compared to Blacks and Hispanics.

The normal white blood cell count in whites is 4,500 to 10,000. In Blacks and Hispanics, the normal white blood cell count is from 3,500 to 10,000. In Blacks from the Caribbean, and Ashkenazi Jews, the normal WBC may be as low as 2.500. If the WBC is found to be 3,500 or even lower in a Black person, and the differential count is normal, then there may not be a need to do anything further other than ANA, ESR and rheumatoid factor to rule out collagen vascular disease or connective tissue diseases.

However, low WBC/leukopenia is a very important finding and may have serious medical implications. It is up to each individual physician to decide what to do when the WBC is in a particular clinical setting.

The red blood cell count tells the physician whether the poor memory is due to low red cell count (anemia) or too high red blood cell count (polycythemia). When the red blood cell count is too low, oxygen cannot be delivered easily to the body's vital organs, including the brain. Poor oxygen delivery to the brain is one of the causes of poor memory (organic brain syndrome).

When the red blood cell count is too high such as in polycythemia the high viscosity of the blood results in stagnation of blood flow within blood vessels making it difficult for oxygen to get to the brain for proper perfusion.

The thicker the blood, the more difficult it is for oxygen to get to the memory center in the brain for good memory to occur. The platelet count, which is part of the CBC, is also very important.

If the platelets drop to less than 10,000 (normal platelet count is 130,000 to 400,000), spontaneous bleeding can occur anywhere in the body, including the brain. Bleeding in the brain can result in serious brain malfunctions including stroke and poor memory.

If the platelet count is too high - 750,000 to 1,000,000 or greater - both stroke and bleeding can occur within the brain, resulting in poor brain functioning including poor memory. **(This occurs only if the high platelet count is associated with a myeloproliferative disorder.)**

Abnormalities in the differential blood count may indicate many different abnormalities, including leukemia or lymphoma, both of which frequently affect the brain, resulting in poor brain functioning.

The blood chemistry and its component parts are very important in determining whether a person's poor memory is due to abnormality or abnormalities of the body's chemistry.

Abnormalities in the electrolytes can cause poor brain function. The electrolytes are sodium, potassium, chloride, and bicarbonate. Severe acidosis (too low bicarbonate) or severe alkalosis (too high bicarbonate) can lead to abnormalities that can cause brain abnormalities and brain malfunction. Too high blood sodium (a condition called hypernatremia), the normal sodium being 135 to 140, can cause brain malfunction, including confusion, to occur. Too low blood sodium 110–120 can cause low blood pressure, confusion, poor memory, and, at times, seizures to occur.

One of the frequent abnormalities in the blood chemistries that can cause brain malfunction is too low blood sugar, known as hypoglycemia. The normal blood sugar is between 60 and 112. When the blood sugar falls to less than 60 or lower, this situation can lead to confusion, poor memory, or seizure. Starvation is a common cause of low blood sugar. Medications such as blood sugar-lowering pills and insulin are the most common medications that frequently cause too low blood sugar to occur.

When the blood sugar is too high 400 or greater it can lead to a condition called diabetic ketoacidosis, which can cause severe brain malfunction and, if not treated quickly and properly, can cause the person to go into a coma and die. What happens in diabetic ketoacidosis is that the person is unable to use sugar as fuel, due to lack of insulin; therefore, fat is being used as fuel, resulting in breakdown products of fat, which are ketone bodies. These ketone bodies are toxic to the body, leading to severe brain malfunctioning, including confusion and sometimes seizures.

There is another condition involving high blood sugar called non-ketotic hyperglycemia, which frequently can lead to coma if left untreated for very long. In this condition, there is no high level of ketones, but the blood sugar rises very high, and sometimes greater than 2,000, and frequently in people who never before had trouble with elevated blood sugar.

High blood sugar acts as diuretic and affected individuals pass a large quantity of urine daily and experience extreme thirst. After a while, the volume of urine that he or she passes is far in excess of the fluid he or she takes in, resulting in severe dehydration, including dehydration of the brain, causing coma to develop, and death if left untreated.

When the kidneys are malfunctioning, many abnormalities can be detected in the blood and in the urine, but some of the earliest and most important abnormalities that can be seen when the kidneys start to fail are:

1. High BUN
2. High creatinine
3. High potassium
4. High phosphate
5. Low bicarbonate
6. Anemia
7. Too much protein in the urine
8. Low 24-hour urine creatinine clearance
9. Low GFR
10. High micro albumin level in the urine

When the kidneys fail, waste products, which are very toxic cannot be removed from the blood, resulting in malfunctioning of the brain including confusion and seizures.

Another important series of blood chemistry tests that are used by physicians to detect diseases in the human body are the liver function tests. In particular, liver function tests such as serum calcium, serum phosphate, serum LDH, serum SGOT, serum SGPT, GGTP, serum uric acid, serum bilirubin, and alkaline phosphatase and prothrombin time and uric acid.

Abnormalities seen in these different tests may indicate association with different diseases such as hepatitis, cancer involving the liver, etc. Complete liver failure causes mental confusion and, at times, seizures. If the urinalysis is abnormal, it may indicate infection in the bladder or kidneys. If sugar is found in the urine, it may indicate diabetes mellitus.

If a substance called acetone is found in the urine, this may indicate dehydration or the presence in the body of the condition called diabetic ketoacidosis as mentioned above, seen in people who are diabetic, when the diabetes is out of control.

If protein is found in the urine, it may indicate different degrees of kidney failure. When sediment of the urine is examined under the microscope, different crystals may be seen in association with kidney stones. Materials called casts of different types may be seen in these sediments representing association with different diseases of the kidneys. Prominent among these diseases include hematuria, (blood in the urine both gross and microscopic), urinary tract infection, kidney stone, sickle cell disease, cancer of the bladder, cancer of the kidney.

When the kidneys fail, urine output ceases and different degrees of mental confusion can be seen and if dialysis is not carried out to cleanse the blood of toxic substances, coma may ensue, which may result in death. Blood tests to evaluate the functions of the thyroid glands are very important. Both hypothyroidism (low function of the thyroid gland) and hyperthyroidism (high function of the thyroid gland) can cause mental aberration, resulting at times in memory loss, confusion, and many times, coma.

Evaluating serum magnesium, serum phosphorus, parathyroid hormone and vitamin D3 levels are extremely important to rule out secondary hyperparathyroidism and Rickett's disease/osteomalasia.

Low Vitamin B12 can cause a multitude of problems, such as numbness, pain and needle symptoms over the legs and the fingers. Memory loss and neurological damage can occur because of low B12. If the B12 level remains low for five years or more, permanent brain and neurological damage are certain to occur.

The conditions that can cause low Vitamin 12 include:

Diet deficient in vitamin B12
Atrophic gastritis
Malabsorption
Tropical sprue
Non-tropical sprue
Crohn's disease
Ulcerative colitis
Blind loop syndrome
Fish tape worm infestation
Gastrectomy
Pernicious anemia
Xerostomia
Inhalation of Nitrous oxide
Chronic pancriatitis with secondary malabsorption

More recently, a condition has been discovered the low B12 syndrome occurring in the elderly population. It is, therefore, very important to do a B12 level when evaluating a person for memory loss. It is also important if one has evidence physically that a person is suffering from B12 deficiency and the B12 level comes back normal, to do a urine or blood test for methylmalonic acid. It is a very sensitive test because if someone has B12 deficiency the methylmalonic acid will be elevated.

A test for syphilis, using the RPR or VDRL, is very important because syphilis, when involving the brain, can cause severe brain damage resulting in memory loss, etc. The VDRL test is used to detect syphilis in the human body; if it is positive, it is very important to do the confirmatory blood test, FTA-ABS (Fluorescent Treponoma Antibody-Absorption Test). In true syphilitic infection, this test stays positive for life.

When neurosyphilis is suspected, then a CT scan ought to be done, and if the CT scan appears normal, then a lumbar puncture ought to be conducted to examine the cerebrospinal fluid for the presence of syphilis.

In the evaluation of poor memory (organic brain syndrome) the HIV Type I or Type II test is very important and ought to be done. Frequently, in AIDS, loss of memory is a presenting symptom. This is due either to HIV infection of the brain tissue itself or infections of the brain such as toxoplasmosis, Cryptococcus of the brain or herpes infection of the brain etc;

In evaluating poor memory or organic brain syndrome, the chest x-ray is very important because the chest x-ray may show evidence of cancer in the lungs, which if allowed to spread to the brain, can result in memory loss, confusion and, at times, coma.

There are many infectious processes that can be seen in the lungs on chest x-rays which may affect the function of the brain, resulting in poor memory, confusion and sometimes coma.

Doing an electrocardiogram in evaluating a patient with poor brain function is important because the EKG may show evidence of recent myocardial infarction during which the patient may have become hypotensive and that situation may have affected brain function transiently. The EKG may show cardiac arrhythmias or other rhythm abnormalities that may interfere with proper pumping of the heart, preventing adequate oxygen delivery to the brain, causing transient ischemic attack, and its associated brain malfunctions.

When a person presents to the emergency room or to the doctor's office with symptoms of brain malfunction manifesting as acute confusion or acute memory loss, this could at times be due to a syncopal episode. A syncopal episode can be caused by a number of different things, among them malfunctioning of the heart, which can oftentimes be seen on an EKG or 24-hour holter monitor.

When a person presents with symptoms that are consistent with stroke, several things need to be done. A thorough history ought to be taken from the patient if she is able to speak, and if she cannot speak, the history should be taken from a family member. The next thing to do is to carry out a complete physical examination. It is crucial that the patient's airway be quickly evaluated to be certain she is breathing properly and that she has control over her saliva to prevent aspiration.

It is also crucial that all precautions are taken to watch out for seizures that can occur because of the damage to the brain. Oxygen ought to be administered, IV access ought to be established, and a Foley catheter ought to be inserted. Blood must be drawn for blood tests such as CBC, SMA20, PT, PTT, ANA, ESR, B12, serum folate, lipid profile, serum liprotein -a level, serum homocysteine level, serum immunoglobulin levels and serum protein electrophoresis.

Other tests that need to be done are a chest x-ray, EKG, urinalysis and a brain CT. In acute stroke, the CT scan of the brain is used right away to see whether there is blood within the substance of the brain or whether the brain is swollen, the ventricles of the brain are pushed to one side or another, or whether there is a brain tumor.

Any one of these findings can cause symptoms consistent with a stroke. Sometimes evidence of old strokes can be seen on the same brain CT scan. When contrast material is injected into the patient's blood stream, through an arm vein, more can be seen within the brain, such as metastatic brain tumor or fungal infection such as toxoplasmosis, as seen in patients with AIDS.

Frequently, nothing is seen on a non-contrast brain CT in someone who has an acute stroke. That is not to say that the person does not have a stroke. It simply means it takes one to two weeks to see evidence of a non-bleeding stroke on a brain CT, but doing it eliminates the presence of both acute bleeding and brain tumor.

Elimination of these findings in the brain when someone presents with an acute stroke is not only important in diagnosing the cause of the acute stroke, but it also allows the treating physician the possibility to proceed with a test such as a lumbar puncture to rule out sub-acute bleeding.

It also allows the treating physician to use medications such as TPA (tissue plasminogen activator), heparin and aspirin, if he or she thinks that this is an evolving stroke. Heparin or TPA can help to prevent an acute stroke in this setting. The CT scan of the brain does all these things, in addition to being a diagnostic instrument. MRI of the brain can be used to evaluate the brain immediately after a stroke and it will show either the stroke or whatever else may be causing the patient's symptoms of a stroke.

Once the initial evaluations of the patient are completed, blood must be drawn for CBC, PT, PTT SMA20 (blood chemistry profile), lipid profile and urinalysis.

Depending on the severity of the stroke, a Foley catheter may be inserted into the bladder to insure that the patient can pass her urine and monitor her urine output.

If the blood pressure is very high, heparin ought not to be used to avoid bleeding into the brain. In this case, the blood pressure must be brought down very carefully to avoid worsening the stroke or to prevent the precipitation of a new stroke by dropping the blood pressure too fast.

If bleeding in the brain has been ruled out, then the patient ought to be given 325 mg of aspirin to chew and swallow. If she is not able to do these things, she then can be given the aspirin in suppository form rectally.

The decision that must be made is whether the patient should be given heparin intravenously or whether she should be given tPA IV in an attempt to dissolve the clot that is causing the stroke.

These are very difficult decisions and can only be made by the treating physicians who are at the bedside.

Then, one might ask why not do an MRI right way on everybody who has a stroke, bypassing the need for a brain CT Scan for one thing, the brain MRI is very expensive; it costs about $1,500 with contrast and $950.00 without contrast.

Brain CT with no contrast costs about $520. Another reason is that not every community hospital has MRI available and not everybody is suitable for an MRI study. Some people are claustrophobic; they just do not want to go into the MRI machine, and some people are too obese to fit into an MRI machine. The maximum weight that can fit in the MRI machine is about 300 lbs. Sometime in the future they might be able to make a machine that can fit these individuals.

Some facilities now have open MRI available which makes it easier for individuals who are claustrophobic to be able to undergo the MRI test. In addition, there are certain individuals who have metals implanted in them due to a previous accident or other surgical procedure, making them unsuitable for the MRI machine.

The list of metals found in the body that can prevent an MRI from being done is quite long, but the most important ones include:

1. Aneurysm and hemostatic clips
2. Biopsy needles
3. Carotid artery vascular clamps
4. Dental implant devices and materials
5. Halo vests
6. Heart valve prosthesis
7. Intravascular coils, filters, and stents
8. Ocular implants
9. Orthopedic implants, materials, and devices
10. Otologic implants
11. Pellets and bullets
12. Penile implants
13. Vascular access ports etc. as published in the literature

Some of these devices may, in fact, be dislodged or moved by the magnetic field of the MRI machine, with possible disastrous consequences. All of the above tests and procedures may be necessary, at any one time, in any patient who presents with a stroke.

Blacks and other minorities are at higher risk of having strokes compared to whites because of their higher incidence of hypertension, obesity, and diabetes mellitus. Blacks and other minorities are five times more likely to have a stroke and dying from that stroke compared to whites.

Some of the predisposing factors for developing a stroke:

1. Blacks and other minorities are many times more likely to be hypertensives than whites are and hypertensive blacks and other minorities are less likely to seek medical care for their hypertension. When treatment is given, it is less likely to be appropriate and, therefore, less effective.
2. The incidence of obesity is quite high among blacks. Approximately 81% of black women in the United States are obese/overweight and 68% of black men are obese/overweight, two third of the adults in the U.S. are obese/overweight and obesity plays a major role in the elevation of blood pressure.
3. The high salt content diet that many people eat plays a major role in the elevation of the blood pressure and its devastating propensity in causing stroke.
4. Another factor that plays a role in an increased incidence of stroke in is stress. Most blacks and other minorities are under stress because of racial discrimination, their poorer educational status, poorer economic status, poorer social status, and their overall poorer living conditions, which cause a constant state of stress, resulting in elevation of adrenalins such as epinephrine and norepinephrine. These can cause a rise in blood pressure with subsequent development of stroke.

Until these conditions are vastly improved in blacks and minorities, the incidence of stroke in blacks and other minorities in the world and in the United States, can be expected to continue unabated.

People can decrease their incidence of dying from stroke simply by decreasing the amount of salt, fat, and simple carbohydrates in their foods and by exercising regularly.

Stress is something over which blacks and other minorities in the world have no control over. Presently, blacks other minorities and poor people in the world eat the types of foods they can afford to eat. In the U.S. 50 million people go hungry every day, and 17 million children in the U.S. go hungry daily. Worldwide, 1 billion people go hungry every day. Twenty five thousands people die every day in the world because of hunger and fifteen million children die every year in the world because of hunger and in total, thirty five million people die every year in the world because of hunger.

It is a known fact that the poorer the individual, the less likely it is that he or she is able to afford the proper nutritional types of foods that are necessary to maintain good health. Sometimes it is not so much the quantity or quality of the food itself, but a combination of poor quality, high quantity, and poor preparation. The way one prepares one's food goes a long way in keeping one healthy.

Many blacks and other minorities in the world do not have access to foods of good quality. However, there are many simple things that can be done to prepare the foods in a healthier way.

They should be careful to avoid some of the negative consequences of eating foods that are too salty, greasy, or too studded with simple carbohydrates. They ought to try to eat a lot of vegetables and fruits and whole grains if at all possible. Obviously this not always possible and to satisfy hunger, people eat what they have access to.

Treatments of strokes include aspirin, heparin, tPA, control of hypertension and physical therapy with rehabilitation therapy. These are used in different stages of the stroke syndrome.

One of the important things to do for the stroke patient is to provide him or her with prophylactic anticoagulant treatment with either Coumadin or heparin to prevent DVT (deep vein thrombophlebitis).

Patients who suffer hemorrhagic strokes ought not to be given anticoagulation to prevent DVT or pulmonary embolism because this type of treatment would cause more bleeding into the brain. In these cases, a sequential compression device ought to be used in their legs to prevent DVT and a Greenfield filter ought to be placed in their inferior vena cava to prevent the migration of clot into the lung, which can cause pulmonary embolism.

Every year in the USA, 2.5 million people have DVT (clot in the leg) and 600,000 people develop pulmonary embolism (Source: *Internal Medicine World Report*, Vol. 18 No. 6, and June 2003). The direct and indirect cost of stroke in 2010 was $73.5 billion.

In summary, it is clear that diet and weight management, exercise, and appropriate anti-hypertensive are important factors in the prevention of high blood pressure and stroke and in the prolongation of the life of people.

CHAPTER 3

HIGH CHOLESTEROL IN AFRICAN AMERICAN MEN

World wide the incidence of high cholesterol is the highest in Europe (54% for both sexes), Americas (48% for both sexes), Africa 22.6%, and Asia 29.0 %. Source: WHO

Approximately 106,700 million individuals in the U.S. have high cholesterol: 50,800,000 males and 55,900,000 females have high cholesterol; 47.9% white males and 49.7% white females have high cholesterol; 44.8 negro/black males and 42.1 negro/black females have high cholesterol. Seven million children/adolescents in the U.S. have high cholesterol.

High cholesterol is one of the leading risk factors for coronary artery heart disease. The different types of abnormal lipids that can be found in the blood of people are:

Hyperlipidemia
High cholesterol
High triglycerides/high cholesterol
High low-density cholesterol (LDL)
Low high-density cholesterol (HDL)
High cholesterol/LDL ratio
High VLDL cholesterol

All these abnormal lipids are genetically transmitted from parents to their children to one degree or another.

According to a recent report that appeared in the *New England Journal of Medicine*, Vol. 342 No. 12 (March 23, 2000), four new markers of inflammation were found to be predictors of future development of coronary heart disease. These are hs-CRP, serum amyloid A., interleukin-6, and sICAM-1. According to the authors, the hs-CRP was the most sensitive predictor when found to be elevated.

Hyperlipidemia (too much fat in the blood) is, generally speaking, a genetically transmitted disease. If a person's mother or father has too much fat in his or her blood, this trait is likely to be transmitted to his or her children, resulting in hyperlipidemia, which can lead to the development of coronary heart disease resulting in heart attack and possible early death. Hyperlipidemia is categorized as:

High blood cholesterol
High blood triglycerides
High low-density lipoprotein
Low high-density lipoprotein
Cholesterol/HDL ratio, which is LDL/HDL, greater than 7.13

In a man, if the LDL/HDL ratio is greater than 7.13, that is a high risk factor.

Each one of these different components of hyperlipidemia represents an independent risk factor when abnormal, resulting in coronary heart disease.

Normal blood cholesterol is from 130 to 200 mg/dl. A normal blood triglyceride level is 60–150 mg/dl. Normal HDL is 35–80 mg/dl. Normal LDL is less than 130 mg/dl. Normal cholesterol/HDL is less than 3.4. Normal LDL/HDL is less than 2.8 these ratios are for men. In women, normal cholesterol /HDL ratio is less than 3.27 and the LDL/HDL less than 2.34.

Most people believe that blood cholesterol level is the only thing that matters when addressing abnormal fat levels in the blood. This is wrong because a person may have perfectly normal total blood cholesterol and yet have significant hyperlipidemia, predisposing that person to coronary artery disease. One must be aware that the quick cholesterol test may be misleading if normal. Normal blood cholesterol by itself is not enough to tell if a person has abnormal genetically transmitted lipid. There are five basic cholesterols in the blood:

1. Total cholesterol
2. High-density lipoprotein (HDL)
3. LDL cholesterol
4. Triglycerides
5. VLDL (Very low-density lipoprotein)

HDL is the cholesterol that takes the regular cholesterol from the blood, carries it into the bowel and the colon, mixes it with stool, and carries it out of the body. If the HDL is low - less than 45 mg/dl - then there is not enough of it in the blood to complex with bad cholesterol to remove it from the body. This is a genetic abnormality transmitted from parents to children. More appropriately, these lipid abnormalities are called hyperlipoproteinemias. When both the fasting total cholesterol and the LDL are elevated, this is type 2a hypercholesterolemia.

When the fasting total cholesterol, the LDL cholesterol, and the triglycerides are elevated, this is type 2b hypercholesterolemia. When the total cholesterol is high and when the level of triglycerides is very high, that is type 3 -hyperlipidemia. When the triglycerides are very high and the VLDL is high, that is type 4 -hyperlipidemia.

High chylomicrons, high VLDL, high triglycerides, and cholesterol manifest type 5 hyperlipidemia.

Type 1 hyperlipoproteinenemia is manifested by high chylomicrons.

Secondary hyperlipoproteinemia is seen in association with several medical conditions, such as diabetes mellitus, hypothyroidism, uremia, and nephrotic syndrome, alcoholism with acute or chronic pancreatitis, ingestion of oral contraceptive, etc.

First, high triglycerides and VLDL may be evident on the skin and under the eyes as deposits (xantomas). Second, VLDL, triglycerides, and high cholesterol may be high in diabetic women who develop ketoacidosis. Third, high triglycerides, high cholesterol, diabetes mellitus, and hypertension may be present persistently in obese people (Syndrome X).

The use of birth control pills or ingestion of any estrogen-containing pills can raise the level of VLDL and triglycerides. One of the dangers of taking estrogen-containing pills is the possibility of high level of lipids.

Alcohol abuse is also associated with elevated lipids in the blood, such as triglycerides and, in particular, a high level of very-low-density lipoprotein and chylomicrons. In addition, Type 5 hyperlipidemia and sometimes Type 4 hyperlipidemia may be associated with increased alcohol abuse. Type 5- hyperlipidemia may cause acute pancreatitis, which is a very serious medical condition and if left untreated can be fatal.

Hyperlipidemia causes coronary artery disease because in a high lipid state, lipid is deposited within the lumen of coronary arteries, causing gradual narrowing of these vessels and resulting in coronary occlusive heart disease. When the vessels around the heart become narrowed, the condition called angina pectoris frequently develops. Angina pectoris is manifested by chest pain because of lack of oxygen delivery to the heart muscle.

Elevated LDL-C cholesterol is associated with aortic valve calcium deposit and aortic stenosis. Source: JAMA November 5, 2014 Volume 312, Number 17

As just stated, the pain occurs when tissue is deprived of oxygen, causing a series of substances, called kinins, to be secreted in and around that tissue, which causes the burning pain to occur. A good example of what kinins are is what one develops in a blister in one's finger or toe. If one bursts the blister right away, the liquid that forms within it causes a burning sensation to occur in the finger or toe because this liquid contains kinins.

High lipoprotein A is also associated with coronary heart disease. A high level of homocysteine level is also associated with coronary heart disease. Both these conditions are genetically transmitted and can cause thrombosis to occur anywhere in the body.

When one is having a heart attack, what happens frequently is that the clot forms acutely because of the plaque within the vessels that cracks or a fissure within the vessel that develops, resulting in the crack.

The result is that bleeding occurs acutely within that vessel, causing a clot to develop. The clot closes the vessel, acutely cutting off blood flow to the part of the heart muscle for which this vessel is responsible for delivering oxygen, and the result is an acute heart attack. The muscle that is damaged may die acutely due to lack of flow of blood to that muscle.

Cardiac dysrhythmias can develop, resulting in all sorts of rhythm disturbances such as atrial arrhythmias, ventricular tachycardia and ventricular fibrillation, etc., which can lead to the death of the individual who just had the heart attack. If a person presents to the emergency room with acute chest pain and a physician administers tPA acutely to dissolve the clot based on the symptoms and the EKG findings, the death of the involved muscle can be prevented.

This can frequently result in the survival of the patient by preventing the heart attack from occurring. It is safe to say that from the time that the patient presents with the symptoms up to several hours later, in certain circumstances, the tPA can still be of value if administered.

In 2011, coronary artery disease claimed the lives of 7.5 million people in the world and 425,425 people in the United States. There is a high rate of cardiovascular-associated deaths in people due to the following factors: Sources: WHO and CDC

1. High blood pressure
2. Obesity
3. High lipids in the blood
4. Smoking
5. Diabetes mellitus
6. Poor diet with too much fat, carbohydrates, and salt. Two-third of people is obese/ overweight in the United States and obesity is a major risk factor for coronary artery disease.
7. Genetic predisposition, gender, stress, poverty, poor education, poor economic status, marital problems, raising children and caring for a family, etc.

All these factors together play a major role in the causation of an increased rate of coronary artery disease.

The following is a list of some factors that can decrease the incidence of coronary occlusive disease secondary to high lipids:

1. Maintenance of an ideal weight.
2. Regular exercise.
3. Non-abuse of alcohol.
4. A diet of plenty fruits and vegetables.
5. Preparation of foods only with vegetable oils.
6. Avoidance of butter.
7. Use of skim milk.
8. Removal of the skin from the chicken to remove as much fat as possible.
9. Use of margarine that is low in fat.
10. Avoidance of red meat as much as possible.
11. Decreased ingestion of pork, bacon, cheese, sausages, egg yolk, all foods that are too rich in fat.

12. Avoidance of too much simple carbohydrate-containing foods because simple carbohydrates are converted into fat in the liver, which ultimately results in fat deposition in the tissues in the human body resulting in obesity.
13. Decreased consumption of foods with high sugar content such as cakes and pies.
14. Avoidance of fast foods as much as possible because they contain too many fat and simple carbohydrates.
15. Minimization of the ingestion of high cholesterol foods such as lobster, crabs, shrimps, and oysters by individuals who already have high cholesterol.
16. Avoidance of cooking foods with coconut oil because coconut is too rich in cholesterol.
17. Eating foods with high fiber, such as collard greens when prepared without ham, hocks, hock tails, and bacon. Vegetable oil, a little bit of hot sauce, and a little bit of wine make the greens taste just as good.
18. Eating foods with complex carbohydrates, such as yams, plantain, sweet potato, green bananas, and pasta. These foods are very high in cellulose, which turns into fiber, which is good for the body. These foods also contain good vitamins and satisfy hunger. Yet, they will not result in gain weight because the human body is not capable of breaking down complex carbohydrates. People in the underdeveloped world eat these types of food and they, by and large, do not suffer from the same degree of obesity as people in the United States. The incidence of high lipids is quite low in the underdeveloped world because a lot of vegetables and fruits are consumed instead of fast foods frequently consumed in the so-called "developed world". Fat-containing foods that are a great part of the diet in the United States and other developed countries predispose their inhabitants to all sorts of diseases such as cancer, coronary artery disease, and diabetes.
19. Using vegetable oils and olive oil that contain polyunsaturated fat in cooking.
20. Sparing use of mayonnaise, which is very rich in cholesterol.

Treatments of hypercholerolemia:

The rate -limiting enzyme that controls the synthesis of cholesterol in the liver is 3-Hydroxy-Methyl-glutaric- Co -enzyme A (HMG-CoA). Once this enzyme is blocked, LDL receptors increase, preventing the re-absorption of cholesterol from the blood.

The medications in use to treat high cholesterol are called Statins and they include:

1. Zocor
2. Lipitor
3. Lescol
4. Mevacor
5. Crestor
6. Niacin
7. Pravastatin
8. Livalo
9. Repatha has just been approved by the FDA to be used IM to lower cholesterol

Some of the most important parts of the treatment of high cholesterol, high triglycerides and hyperlipidemia in general are diet, exercise and weight loss. However, once the cholesterol reaches a level at which the diet is not sufficient, then the clinical thing to do is to provide the patient with medication.

Medications in use to treat high triglycerides are:

1. Lopid (gemfibrozil)
2. Tricor (fenofibrate)
3. Cholestyramine
4. Colestipol (bile acid rasins)
5. Trilipix
6. Lipofen

The usual dose of Cholestyramine is 8–12 grams 2 or 3 times per day by mouth. The usual dose of Colestipol is 10–15 grams 2 or 3 times per day by mouth. Lopid (gemfibrozil) decreases triglycerides and VLDL (very low-density lipoprotein) and increases HDL. The usual dose of Lopid is 600 mg by mouth 2 times per day. The usual dose of Tricor is 145 mg or 43 mg daily by mouth.

The usual dose of Trilipix is 135 mg by mouth nightly and the usual dose of Lipofen is150 mg by mouth nightly.

It is important that these fat-lowering medications and, in particular, the Statin be taken one half hour after dinner every night and the reason is that fat is circadian, which means there is more fat in the blood at night. The more fat there is in the blood at the time the Statin is being taken, the better the chance of removing the most fat from the bloodstream.

It is important to realize that these medications work best when given in the evening because cholesterol works via the circadian system. That is to say, that cholesterol level is highest in the evening in the body. The usual doses of these medications are 10–20 mg a half hour after dinner nightly for Lovastatin, 10– 40 mg for Provestatin, and 5–20 mg for Simvastatin. The maximum dose of Lovastatin can go as high as 80 mg daily, Provestatin as much as 40 mg and the Simvastatin as high as 40 mg.

These medications are quite expensive, but they are very effective in bringing down the total cholesterol, LDL, and triglycerides and raising the HDL, thereby decreasing incidence of coronary disease and arterial occlusive disease all over the body.

All these medications, and in particular the HMG CoA reductase inhibitors, can cause mild liver function test abnormality and for that reason it is important to monitor the liver function tests every six weeks to two months. It is very important to emphasize that these medications must be used in conjunction with a low-fat, low simple-carbohydrate diet along with a good exercise program.

Another known side effect of these medications is muscle and joint pain. This occurs because of muscle breakdown and secondary inflammation. In some cases, this can lead to rhabdomyolysis, which, if not recognized quickly and treated, can lead to kidney failure. If these symptoms are persistent and severe, the medication ought to be stopped and the patient's doctor contacted.

The test to do to confirm this problem is serum CPK. When muscles are swollen, the CPK level in the blood goes up. Niacin is also a very good medication to treat high cholesterol. The usual starting dose is 500 mg at bedtime. The maximum dose of Niacin is 2000 mg at bedtime. Niacin has many side effects and prominent among them are flushing and diarrhea etc.

Along the same line, it has been shown that drinking one or two glasses of wine at night, either red or white, with dinner, increases the level of the HDL (the good cholesterol). It is not advisable that people drink or abuse alcohol, but these studies clearly show that moderate ingestion of alcohol, in particular red wine, seems to have a significant advantage in increasing the level of the HDL cholesterol.

Diet plays a major role in the prevention of obesity and the prevention and control of hypertension. Diet also plays a major role in both preventing and controlling the levels of cholesterol and triglycerides in the blood. The so-called soul food that blacks like to eat so much is a legacy of slavery that began 500 hundred years ago in the United States.

However, soul foods have too much fat, simple carbohydrates, and salt, and are too spicy. These foods taste good, but they are unhealthy. Therefore, it is fine to eat them every now and then, but when a person eats them on a daily basis, it increases his or her chances of becoming obese and raising his or her blood pressure and cholesterol.

A combination of obesity, high blood pressure, and high level of fat in the blood is responsible in part for the high incidence of coronary artery disease and deaths of people in the United States. To prevent this high occurrence of coronary artery disease and deaths, the diet of most people must clearly be modified. Diet is very ethnic in its origin. People of different ethnic backgrounds have different tastes for different foods, and that is fine, except that one has to understand that everything has to be done in moderation.

If a person eats fat and simple carbohydrate and salt-laden foods too often, that person is likely to pay the consequences with an increased incidence of coronary artery disease, hypertension, diabetes, and stroke. Poor people in large measure suffer from these conditions because of poor education, poor living conditions, poor diet, and overall poor economic conditions.

An understanding of these issues and doing the things that are necessary either to modify or change them will go a long way to prevent the high incidence of high cholesterol, coronary heart disease, diabetes mellitus, micro vascular systemic arterial occlusive disease, macrovascular systemic arterial occlusive disease, and stroke seen in people in the world.

CHAPTER 4

OBESITY IN AFRICAN AMERICAN MEN

Obesity is a serious medical problem and has reached epidemic proportion in the world. In 2015, a total of 107.7 million children and 603.7 adults were obese and high BMI accounted for 4.0 million deaths globally. Source:N Engl J MED 377.1 NEJM.ORG July 6,2017

"In the United States, approximately 70% adults and 33% children and adolescents are overweight and obese." Source: JAMA November 27, 2013 Volume 310. Number 20"

There are 79 million adults and 13 million children who are obese in the U.S.

"Approximately 38 percent of American adults were obese in 2013 and 2014, up from 35 percent in 2011 and 2012."

"Study Shows Obesity Rate Exceeds 10 Percent Worldwide
"The New York Times 6/12, 2017 reports more than 10 percent of people in the world are obese, according to a study published in the New England Journal of Medicine. Researchers found that obesity rates at least doubled in 73 countries between 1980 and 2015, and "continuously increased in most other countries." The researchers analyzed "some 1,800 data sets from around the world," and "found that excess weight played a role in four million deaths in 2015, from heart disease, diabetes, kidney disease and other factors."

"USA Today 6/12, 2017 reports the researchers concluded that about 30 percent of the world's populations is obese or overweight, having a BMI of at least 25."

"CNBC 6/12, 2017 reports on its website that the US has the highest rate of obesity among children and young adults at almost 13 percent, while Egypt has the highest adult obesity rate at 35 percent, according to the same study."

"CNN 6/12, 2017 reports on its website that the researchers also found that "obesity levels were higher among women than men across all age groups, which correlates with previous findings on obesity." The US had the greatest number of obese adults, 79.4 million, while China had the second greatest number, 57.3 million. Bangladesh and Vietnam have the lowest obesity rates of 1 percent."

According to a recent report by the CDC, September 2015, "the rates of obesity in the remains study around the country. The analysis revealed that Arkansas, West Virginia and Mississippi were the states with the highest adult obesity. Hawaii, the District of Columbia and Colorado had the lowest rates.

According to the CDC, over a third of U.S. adults are obese and around 17% of children are obese. The study indicates the obesity rate is nearly 48 percent for African-American adults, 43 percent Latino adults 33 percent for white adults.

The report also indicates that 23 of the 25 states with highest rates of obesity are in the South and Midwest."

Blacks and other minorities are affected disproportionately by obesity compare to whites and other racial groups in the world. Thirty seven percent of Black men are obese in the U.S.

Two-thirds of the U.S. population is overweight / obese. In 2007-2008, 32.2 % of adult men and 35.5 % of women in the U.S. were obese. Source: JAMA January 20, 20010, Vol 303, No 3.

"Research has increasingly shown that being obese or overweight increases the risk of cancer recurrence and reduces survival in cancer patients, with an estimated 84,000 cancer diagnoses each year that can be attributed to obesity."

"With nearly three in four Americans obese or overweight, obesity has become a tremendous public health challenge that also impacts cancer care and prevention today."
Source: Oncology Times November 10, 2014

According to a recent report from Columbia University that came out 8/15/2013 "Obesity Kills More Americans Than Previously Thought. One in five Americans, Black and white, dies from obesity".

Worldwide, there are an estimated 1 billion total obese people, and three million people die annually in the world because overweight/obesity. 440,000 deaths occur annually because of obesity in the U.S. Obesity if the fifth leading cause of deaths in the world annually.

According to the WHO, by 2020 there will be 2.3 billion overweight people in the world and 700 million individuals will be obese. Annually, obesity is responsible for 440,000 deaths in the U.S. and costs $270 billion dollars per year.

In attempt to help curb the obesity epidemic in the U.S. the FAD approved to new medications to treat obesity. Qsymia (Phentermine plus topiramate extended – release) and Belviq (Lorcaserin) were approved in 2012.

Obesity, when it is not associated with malfunction of the endocrine system, is always the result of eating too much. Eating too much is a major psychological disorder.

The most effective diet is a diet that is low in carbohydrates, fats, and high in protein. Source: THE THIRD WORLD TROPICAL DIET HEALTH MAITENANCE AND MEDICAL MAGEMENT PROGRAM WRITTEN BY VALIERE ALCENA M.D. F.A.C.P PUBLISHED BY ALCENA MEDICAL COMMUNICATION INC, Copyright© 1994, ISBN 0-9633365-0-9

A diet that is low in fat and high in protein is good and will lower both weight and cholesterol. The same is true of a diet that is low in simple carbohydrates and high in protein. This raises the question: can these two types of diets help people maintain the weight they have lost on a longterm basis?

When a person eats foods that have too much fat and carbohydrates, and the body is unable to break them all down, the remaining fat and carbohydrates are stored in the liver where they are distributed to different tissues of the abdomen, hips, thighs, and other parts of the body. The fat and carbohydrates that are broken down are used as fuel to provide needed energy for proper functions of the body.

In order for this process to work properly, one needs a well-functioning basal metabolism. The basal metabolism is a process through which the body burns calories that are ingested in the body. If the basal metabolism is high, one burns calories too fast and stays thin.

If the basal metabolism is too low, one burns calories too slow and stays fat. Slow basal metabolism, when not associated with medical problems such as hypothyroidism, is always the result of a genetically transmitted abnormality, which is passed on from parents to offspring.

There are several medical conditions that are associated with obesity, among them are:

1. Hypothyroidism
2. Syndrome X
3. Cushing's disease (when the adrenal gland secretes too much adrenal hormone)
4. Gigantism a condition where a person becomes overgrown, too big and too large, due to hyper functioning of the pituitary gland.

When a person is obese and the aforementioned endocrine conditions have been ruled out as a cause, he or she is not taking steroids or estrogen replacement medication, then he or she is obese because of a combination of low basal metabolism associated with ingestion of too much foods containing fat and simple carbohydrates.

Prevalence of obesity in the United States

72.7 percent of blacks are overweight/obese
63.2 percent whites are overweight/obese
37.0 percent of black males are obese/overweight

Obesity is defined as being 20% over one's ideal weight and a BMI >30.

"IDEAL WEIGTHS FOR MEN"

HEIGHT FEET	INCHES	SMALL FRAME	MEDIUM FRAME	LARGE FRAME
5	2	128-134	131-141	138-150
5	3	130-136	133-143	140-153
5	4	132-138	135-145	142-156
5	5	134-140	137-148	144-160
5	6	136-142	139-151	146-164
5	7	138-145	142-154	149-168
5	8	140-148	154-157	152-172
5	9	142-151	148-160	155-176
5	10	144-154	151-163	158-180
5	11	146-157	154-166	161-184
6	0	149-160	157-170	164-188
6	1	152-164	160-174	168-192
6	2	155-168	164-178	172-197
6	3	158-172	167-182	176-202
6	4	162-176	171-187	181-207

"Weight in pounds, based on ages 25-59 with the lowest mortality rate
(indoor clothing weighing 5 pounds and shoes with 1" heels)

"Table II—Modified classification of overweightness on obesity by BMI "

	Obesity Class	BMI kg/m2
Underweight		<18.5
Normal		18.5 – 24.9
Overweight		25.0 – 29.9
Obese	I	30.0 – 34.9
	II	35.0 – 39.9
"Extremely Obese	III	>40

In the United States of America, many factors interplay in causing this high degree of obesity. For instance, the diet industry spends somewhere from 40 to 50 billion dollars a year selling different products and types of dietary programs. The medical profession devotes very little time and resources in the prevention and treatment of obesity. The food industry spends somewhere around 36 billion dollars a year advertising the different food products and agricultural materials they produce and encouraging people to eat more.

The main reason that the medical profession in the United States spends very little time in the prevention and management of obesity is because insurance companies could not care less about obesity and will not pay the medical profession the monies that are necessary to prevent and treat obesity.

The federal and state governments are not doing very much either, because those two governments spend somewhere around 50 thousand dollars a year on nutritional and other educational programs addressing obesity, which is a pitiful type of gesture considering that 68.8 billion dollars were spent in 1990 to treat the different complications associated with obesity.

These complications include breast cancer, colon cancer, cancer of the uterus, heart disease, adult-onset diabetes, Gall Stones, Cholecystitis, Pancreatitis secondary to Gall Stones hypertension, strokes, high cholesterol, deep vein thrombophlebitis, pulmonary embolism secondary to deep vein thrombophlebitis, etc.

Many factors interplay in the excessive degree of obesity. The main factor is low basal metabolism. Low basal metabolism is inherited from parents to offspring. Genetic traits are adaptable, penetrating, and "transmittable". Obese women the world over inherited the obesity gene from their African ancestry. This gene is disseminated among people and their children. The human race and all its original DNA genetic traits began in Africa around 4.4 million years ago. Source: Ardipithecus (Ardi) Fossils, reported by a group from the University of Minnesota.

Another factor that plays a significant role in the development of obesity in people is diet. People who live in the third world who, by necessity, are forced to eat a meager diet are less obese than people who live in the developed countries, such as the United States. In the under-developed world, people eat plenty of fresh fruits, green vegetables, grains, yams, plantains, bananas, and less red meat, and plenty of fish.

People in the so-called "third world" exercise more because they often have to walk long distances to the farm or marketplace and walk to the river to fetch water etc. Some of them spend long hours working under the hot sun in the farms and some work long hours in sweatshops. Still others work at home doing all sorts of chores around their houses. All these activities cause them to lose calories, which is quite important in maintaining their weights.

A combination of these factors leads to less obesity/overweight in people who live in the under-developed world. Nevertheless, they still carry the gene and are able to pass it on, even though they themselves manage to work off the extra fat that was to be deposited into their tissues as predetermined by their hereditary trait.

In addition, it must be understood that fat people are likely to give birth to fat babies. Babies born to fat parents are destined to become fat children, fat adolescents, and fat adults. The low basal metabolism gene, which is responsible for obesity is always passing on to the offspring of obese people.

Typically, diet in the under-developed world is a diet that is high in protein, low in fat, high in vitamins and fibers, and low in simple carbohydrates. This combination of foods contains high complex carbohydrates. Examples of high complex carbohydrates foods include brown rice, pretzels, pasta, yams, sweet plantains, potatoes, dumpling, corn, cereals, breads, grains, tortillas, waffle grits, millet, oats, wheat germs, granola, cornmeal, shredded wheat flour etc.

High complex carbohydrates when eaten, is broken down very slowly in the body and provides a lower, but longer level of energy. That is what makes them ideal food products, in that a person can eat high complex carbohydrates to satisfy hunger and also to provide vitamins and fiber for regular gastrointestinal functioning, particularly for proper bowel movements. Therefore, they do not lead to an increased level of calories, which can cause a person to become obese.

On the other hand, simple carbohydrates, such as sugar-containing foods, when eaten can be broken down in the liver and some of them distributed into the tissues and muscles, resulting in obesity in individuals who consume them in large quantities.

Examples of foods and liquid that contain simple carbohydrates include:

Refined sugar
Sodas
All sugar containing drinks
Cake
Donuts
Bagels
White bread
White rice
Pan Cake
Waffle
Biscuits
Ice cream
Chocolates
Mayonnaise
Butter
Candies
Syrup
Wine
Wiskeys
Rum
Bourbon
Brandy
Beers
All alcoholic drinks
All sandwiches that have cheese, butter, meat, eggs and mayonnaise

Tacoes
Pizza
All fast foods /junk foods
All cereals that have sugar etc;

Example of foods containing high complex carbohydrates includes:

Brown rice
Bagels
Pretzels
Pasta
Yam
Breadfruit
Akee
Sweet potatoes
Cassava
Plantain
Bananas
Dumpling
Corn
Sugar free cereals
Brown bread
Whole wheat bread
Whole grains of all types
Grit
Millet
Oats
Wheat germ
Granola
Corn meal
Shredded wheat
Honey
Flour etc.

Fat containing foods are not healthy and contribute to the development of obesity.

Examples of fat containing foods include:

Red meats
Pork
Lamb
Lobsters
Shrimps
Crabs
Oysters

Goat meat
Ham
Sausages
Hamburger
Cheeseburger
Pizza
Hot dogs
Bacon
Eggs
Butter
Mayonnaise
Cheese
Coconuts oil
Coconut milk
Lard
Non vegetable oil
Pig feet
Hog tails
Chitlins etc.

Foods and liquid that are good to eat and drink include:

Chicken
Turkey
Duck
Fish
Veal
Vegetables
Fruits
Milk
Water
Seltzer water
Coconut water
Tea (herbal tea is better for menstruating females, because it does not have tannic acid which can block iron absorption making iron deficiency anemia worst)
Coffee
Sugar substitutes
Nuts
Tuna fish
Sardines

The afore-outlined foods, when prepared in vegetable oil, either boiled or broiled and not fried, satisfy hunger, provide needed vitamins such as Vitamin A, Vitamin K, the B Vitamins, including B6, B12, etc. All of them are important nutrients for the body.

Breast cancer, uterine cancer, colon cancer, cancer of the stomach, and cancer of the pancreas, cancer of the kidney, cancer of the rectum and cancer of the esophagus are all associated with eating too much fatty, spicy, and smoked foods.

The following diseases are associated with obesity.

1. Diabetes mellitus type 2
2. Atherosclerotic heart disease
3. Hypertension
4. Stroke
5. Arthritis
6. Depression
7. High cholesterol
8. Breast cancer
9. Uterine cancer
10. Colon cancer
11. Cancer of the pancreas
12. Stomach cancer
13. Rectal cancer
14. Prostate cancer
15. Sleep apnea
16. Cardiac arrhythmia
17. Gall bladder disease etc.

The first disease on the list, adult-onset diabetes mellitus, is closely associated with obesity.

What is the relationship between the onset diabetes mellitus and obesity?

When a person is obese, his or her fat cells are resistant to the effect of insulin, creating an insulin-resistant state in his or her body. In this setting, the insulin cannot penetrate these fat cells to bring about the metabolism of sugar. Consequently, blood sugar rises. The rising blood sugar creates all sorts of symptoms, which are very disturbing to the affected person. Since the insulin has difficulty entering into the fat cells, it remains elevated in her bloodstream.

The high insulin level, in turn, forces the obese person to crave for sweets-containing foods to satisfy him or her, resulting in a vicious cycle. The more obese a person is, the higher the level of insulin in his or her bloodstream. The higher the level of insulin in his or her bloodstream, the more he or she craves sweets-containing foods, which are high in simple carbohydrates.

The afore-outlined foods, when prepared in vegetable oil, either boiled or broiled and not fried, satisfy hunger, provide needed vitamins such as Vitamin A, Vitamin K, the B Vitamins, including B6, B12, etc. All of them are important nutrients for the body.

Breast cancer, uterine cancer, colon cancer, cancer of the stomach, and cancer of the pancreas, cancer of the kidney, cancer of the rectum and cancer of the esophagus are all associated with eating too much fatty, spicy, and smoked foods.

The following diseases are associated with obesity.

1. Diabetes mellitus type 2
2. Atherosclerotic heart disease
3. Hypertension
4. Stroke
5. Arthritis
6. Depression
7. High cholesterol
8. Breast cancer
9. Uterine cancer
10. Colon cancer
11. Cancer of the pancreas
12. Stomach cancer
13. Rectal cancer
14. Prostate cancer
15. Sleep apnea
16. Cardiac arrhythmia
17. Gall bladder disease etc.

Evaluations of obesity include:

History and physical examination
Weight measurement
Height
BMI measurement
CBC
Complete blood chemistry profile
Hgb A1C
T4 and TSH
EKG
Brain MRI
Lipid profile
Growth hormone level

The first disease on the list, adult-onset diabetes mellitus, is closely associated with obesity.

What is the relationship between the onset diabetes mellitus and obesity?

When a person is obese, his or her fat cells are resistant to the effect of insulin, creating an insulin-resistant state in his or her body. In this setting, the insulin cannot penetrate these fat cells to bring about the metabolism of sugar. Consequently, blood sugar rises. The rising blood sugar creates all sorts of symptoms, which are very disturbing to the affected person. Since the insulin has difficulty entering into the fat cells, it remains elevated in her bloodstream.

The high insulin level, in turn, forces the obese person to crave for sweets-containing foods to satisfy him or her, resulting in a vicious cycle. The more obese a person is, the higher the level of insulin in his or her bloodstream. The higher the level of insulin in his or her bloodstream, the more he or she craves sweets-containing foods, which are high in simple carbohydrates and rich in calories. The more he or she eats these calorie-rich foods, the fatter he or she becomes, raising his or her blood sugar even higher.

What is the relationship between atherosclerotic heart disease and obesity?

Obesity is associated with atherosclerotic heart disease, in that the persistent high level of insulin that is present in the bloodstream of the obese person causes plaques to develop within vessels throughout his or her body, including the coronary arteries around the heart. When these arteries are occluded, blood flow is impeded, preventing proper oxygen delivery to the muscles of the heart, causing pain in the chest to occur. Because there are plaques in the coronary arteries, sudden closure of one or several of these coronary arteries can result in a heart attack and, frequently, death.

Obesity as just outlined is quite common in people in the U.S. Obesity is very highly associated with hypertension, which is also quite common. When a person is obese, the obesity is frequently associated with diabetes mellitus, hyperlipidemia, and hypertension.

This combination of diseases is frequently referred to as syndrome X, or more recently renamed as metabolic hypertension. (Syndrome W is used as well to refer to this condition.) Blacks retain more salt in their bodies than other people do, and as a result, blacks retain more fluid, and the fluid retention causes elevation in their blood pressures. When a person who is obese loses weight, frequently, his or her blood pressure decreases, and the need for medication decreases proportionately.

Obesity is also commonly associated with stroke. Many of the conditions that are frequently seen in people who are obese, such as diabetes mellitus, hypertension and hyperlipidemia, are also seen in people who suffer from stroke, and frequently the underlying reason for the stroke seen in these people is the obesity. The reason why obesity, diabetes, hyperlipidemia, and hypertension are associated with stroke is because all these conditions can cause atherosclerosis to occur.

Once vessels in the brain develop plaques, these vessels become narrowed, thereby preventing the proper flow of blood and oxygen to the brain tissues. When one of these vessels becomes acutely closed, a stroke is usually the result.

Obesity is frequently associated with breast cancer in women. In particular, there is a frequent association of breast cancer in obese in women ages 38 to 49. The type of breast cancer seen in this group of women is extremely aggressive and very resistant to treatments, resulting in a high percentage of deaths.

Obesity is also associated with uterine cancer in a high percentage of women and prostate cancer in men.

Osteoarthritis of the shoulders, lower back, knees, and ankles is frequently seen in obese women. The obesity causes a great deal of mechanical stress on these areas of the body, resulting in wear and tear, causing severe pain, and suffering.

Obese people also feel the pressure of society, which seems to favor thinner people. This negative attitude causes some obese people to become depressed a great deal of the time. Depression is more common in obese people. Obese people have difficulty in finding boyfriends and girlfriends and experience more difficulties in finding suitable employment, frequently facing discriminations of all sorts in a society obsessed with thinness and beauty. Obesity is a serious medical problem with significant impact on the overall health of people who are afflicted with the condition.

Because of obesity, these people suffer from psychosocial deprivation, economic deprivation and the interplay of these problems results in unnecessary early death from heart disease, cancer, hypertension, diabetes mellitus, stroke, kidney failure, and suicide.

Treatments of obesity include:

Low simple carbohydrates foods
Low simple carbohydrates drinks
High complex carbohydrates foods
High protein diet
Low fat diet
Low salt diet
Vegetable rich foods
Fruits rich foods
Regular exercise
Medications: Xenical, Oristat, Phentermine, Belviq, Qsymia
The FDA has just approved Contrave to treat obesity.

The FDA has just approved Saxenda to treat people who are obesity/overweight who have hypertension.

Gastric bypass surgery
The ReShape Integrated Dual Balloon System is newly approved non-surgical device that takes 30 minutes to be placed into the stomach. It can remain in the stomach up to 6 months. "It is indicated for adults who have a body mass index of 30 to 40 and 1 or more obesity related conditions such as hypertension, elevated cholesterol levels, or diabetes".

People are pre-disposed to obesity either from genetics or behavior, must fight against the disease by having a diet that is low in fat, salt, and simple carbohydrates, high in protein, green vegetables, fruits, non-shellfish, chicken, veal, and low in red meats, sausages, bacon, pork, ham, egg yolks, white breads, and cakes.

The poorer economic situation of poor people in the U.S. and the world makes it almost impossible to carry out these recommendations to eat healthier foods.

The unemployment rate in the U.S. for Negroes / Blacks was 9.2% compared to 4.4% for whites as of September 2015.

In general, fast foods are not healthy because they contain too much fat, salt, and simple carbohydrate, all of which can contribute to obesity when eaten in excess.

It is important for people to exercise at least three times per week. It is not necessary to spend money going to expensive gymnasiums to exercise. These exercise centers charge a lot of money, which are largely unaffordable for most poor people. For those who can afford the cost, they are likely to benefit from going regularly.

However, walking one hour daily also helps to burn off significant calories. Aerobic exercise, push-ups, bicycling, gardening, walking the dog, and other forms of exercise can all result in weight loss without incurring the cost of an expensive gymnasium. Bariatric surgery is an effective treatment modality in many instances.

Paying to join the so-called diet programs is frequently useless and dangerous. These programs are expensive and, according to the U.S. Government, have questionable motives in saying that they are trying to help people to lose weight.

In addition, these programs may be medically dangerous if entered into without proper medical supervision.

Learning a new way to prepare foods and a change in eating habits by eating smaller portions of foods is important. Decreasing the consumption of fat and sugar laden foods and eating less fast food, will go a long way in decreasing the rate of obesity among people in the U.S. and in the world.

People ought to pay attention to the basics and adhere closely to a healthy lifestyle of frequent exercise, good diet, low alcohol consumption, and frequent visits to the physician's office for proper health screening. In addition, people must change their mind set and develop a better understanding of their circumstances by doing the things that are necessary to get a good education.

Education is the only guaranteed **FORMULA** to achieving financial success and a better life in American Society. Education not only allows a person to feel better about himself or herself, but it increases an individual's self esteem and allows him or her to understand better the pitfalls that exist in society, thus being better able to avoid them. As part of the package of education, is the attainment of professional skills that are necessary to facilitate people to get jobs that pay good wages.

Understanding these facts, following them and taking the necessary precautions are the best ways to go about solving the problems associated with obesity and its devastating consequences on people. Consider that the annual cost of obesity in the U.S. may exceed $215 billion. Source: The Brooking Institute, May 3, 2011 and, $270 billion according to some reports in 2012.

CHAPTER 5

DIABETES MELLITUS IN AFRICAN AMERICAN MEN

World wide in 2015, about 400 millions people or 8.3% of the world population had diabetes mellitus, and of that number, 22 million have type 1 diabetes. About 10% of pregnant women worldwide develop gestational diabetes. Source: WHO

"Diabetes kills one person every six seconds and affects about 400 millions people worldwide". According to the International Diabetes Federation 11/14/2015

By 2035 the number of people with diabetes is expected to reach 590 million worldwide.

Twenty nine million people or 9.3 % of the U.S. population have diabetes mellitus; 1.7 million of them have type 1 diabetes and the rest have type 2 diabetes and 30.8% of them use insulin. 86 millions people in the U.S. have pre-diabetes. Gestational diabetes mellitus is the third form of diabetes. Each year 130,000 women develop Gestational diabetes in the U.S.

"HealthDay 7/18, 2017 reports that the CDC "report [pdf] found that nearly one in four adults with diabetes didn't even know they had the disease, and less than 12 percent with prediabetes knew they had that condition." CDC Director stated, "More than a third of US adults have prediabetes, and the majority don't know it." In a news release, the Director added, "Now, more than ever, we must step up our efforts to reduce the burden of this serious disease." "

Type 1 diabetes accounts for 5% of all cases of diabetes mellitus. Type 1 diabetes is an autoimmune disease in which the body develops antibodies against the beta cells that produce insulin in the pancreas. There are 2 types of type 1 diabetes. Juvenile diabetes occurs mainly in children mainly and Latent Autoimmune Diabetes occurs mainly in Adults.

Both forms of type 1 diabetes can be seen in children as well as in adults. I addition, because of the epidemic of obesity many adolescent have developed type diabetes as well. "In 2013, diabetes was associated with US $548 billion in health care expenditures globally."

The tests that are available to diagnose type 1 diabetes are

"C peptide
Diabetes mellitus auto -antibodies panel
Islet cell antibodies tests
Glutamic acid Decarboxylase antibodies tests
Insulin antibodies tests"

There are 86 millions people with pre-diabetes (1 in 3 people in U.S. are pre-diabetics): 13% or 2.8 million Blacks in the U.S. have diabetes mellitus. Diabetes mellitus is tow to three times more common in blacks compared to whites. According to the CDC, there are 7 million undiagnosed diabetics in the U.S.

As a consequence of obesity, 3,700 young people under the age of 20 are diagnosed every year with adult onset type diabetes. Source: CDC.

Diabetes mellitus has increased 600% in the United States since 1958 and it is estimated that the incidence of diabetes mellitus will rise by 35% in the next ten years. The genetics of diabetes mellitus Type II works out this way.

Roughly, one-half of the first-degree relatives of diabetics are said according to recent reports to have or will develop abnormal glucose tolerance, and about one-fourth will become diabetic. Another way of stating the genetics is that about 4/10 of siblings of diabetics and 1/3 of the offspring of diabetics have the propensity to become diabetic.

Type I diabetes is a different disease altogether from Type II diabetes and it is said to be caused by either an autoimmune disease or some sort of a viral disease, but no one is quite sure. Type I diabetes usually starts in childhood, but, it can also be seen in young adults. According to the latest figures in 2012, the cost of diabetes in the U.S. was 245 billion dollars. Source: American Diabetics Association. Worldwide, $465 billion were spent for the treatments of diabetes mellitus in 2011. $65.2 billion were spent for treatment of diabetes in Latin America and the Caribbean in 2011.

The risk of death is roughly two times higher in black diabetics than in non-diabetic other racial groups. Diabetes is the sixth leading cause of death in the U.S. Every year, 3.2 million people die in the world because of diabetes.

What is diabetes mellitus?

Diabetes mellitus is a condition in which the body is incapable of using sugar as a fuel due to lack of insulin. Three basic abnormalities cause diabetes mellitus.

1. Lack of insulin secretion from the pancreas,
2. Abnormal insulin secretion from the pancreas, and
3. Insulin resistance.

In the first instance, the beta cells of the Islets of Langerhans of the pancreas have been destroyed either by an autoimmune process or by a viral organism resulting in a total lack of insulin in the body, sometimes since early infancy or childhood, resulting in juvenile diabetes. In the second instance, the pancreas still has the ability to produce insulin, but needs to be forced to secrete it. In the third instance, the pancreas simply cannot make any more insulin, period. That is Type II diabetes. In the third instance, insulin has to be given either subcutaneously or intravenously. This is called insulin-requiring diabetes mellitus type II.

The normal blood glucose is from 65 to about 109 mg/dL. Diabetes mellitus is a condition in which the blood glucose is higher than normal, when the blood glucose is drawn following a period of fasting for about 8 to 12 hours. As just mentioned, the normal blood glucose is between 65 to 109 mg/dL.

If the fasting blood sugar is 110 to 124, this is pre-diabetes. If the fasting blood sugar is 125 or higher, this is frank diabetes.

If the screening hemoglobin A1C is 5-6, diabetes is not present. If the hemoglobin A1C is 6.2-6.5, pre-diabetes is present. If the hemoglobin is A1C is 6.6 or greater, frank diabetes is present. In diabetes mellitus, when the blood sugar is well controlled from 5-6 weeks, the A1C is normal.

However, if the blood sugar remains poorly controlled for up to 90 days, the A1C is abnormally high. A1C is hemoglobin A with glucose attached to a terminal amino acid of the beta chains of the molecule.

Another way to test the blood of an individual to see if she or he is diabetic is for the physician to order what is called a two-hour post-prandial glucose test (Post-prandial means after eating). Two hours after eating a meal containing sugar, a tube of blood is drawn from the individual and if the blood glucose is elevated, between 140 mg/dL and 190 milligrams per deciliter or (mg/dl), then that individual is said to have glucose intolerance or early diabetes mellitus. Except for evaluation of pregnant women and screening patients for episodic hypoglycemia, glucose tolerance test will no longer be carried out to diagnose diabetes mellitus.

By the time a person with type II diabetes becomes abnormally elated, he or she has been diabetic for about 10 years and he or she has already lost 80% the beta cells in his or her pancreas. In addition, if the blood sugar is not well controlled, he or she is using fat as fuel. When fat is used in the body as fuel, ketone bodies (broken down products of fat) are produced which further damages the remaining 20% of beta cells in his or her pancreas, making the situation worse.

The genetic locus for insulin-dependent diabetes mellitus is on chromosome 6. The genetic locus for non-insulin diabetes mellitus is unknown. Usually insulin-dependent diabetes (juvenile diabetes) or type I diabetes, occurs before age 40. On the other hand, non-insulin-dependent diabetes (Type II diabetes) occurs after 40, although there are exceptions.

However, most of the time insulin-dependent diabetes mellitus appears before age twenty, but it can also occur later in life. Non-insulin-dependent diabetes can also occur in the late teens and early adulthood.

It is not an absolute rule, but age 35 to 40 is usually the cut-off point for someone to present with Type I diabetes mellitus. If a person is age 35 or over, the diagnosis is most likely going to be adult-onset diabetes, or Type II diabetes. If a person is between childhood and age 35, the diagnosis is most likely going to be insulin-dependent diabetes or type I. Again, there are crossovers and there are exceptions.

Recently, a group of obese adolescents ages 10–19 has been reported to have Type II diabetes mellitus.

There are different types of Type II diabetes mellitus. The most common type is due to the inability of the pancreas to secrete sufficient insulin. Other types are due to insulin resistance because of obesity. Often, in people who have chronic pancreatitis, the pancreas may ultimately fail, resulting in Type II diabetes mellitus.

Primary hemochromatosis always leads to type II diabetes.
Cushing's disease can cause chemically induced secondary diabetes, although it can be transient.

Another common form of diabetes is gestational diabetes seen in pregnancy. It is more common in black, Hispanic, Asian American, Pacific Islander, and Native American women than in white women. It is very important to control the blood sugar very tightly in pregnant women using insulin to prevent complications in the infant. A multitude of birth defects is known to occur in infants born to diabetic mothers.

Diabetic mothers are known to give birth to large babies and sometimes, some of these babies can be born with a very large head, making vaginal delivery difficult, if not impossible. About 10% of women with gestational diabetes go on to continue to have type II diabetes after delivery. Some 20–50% of women who had gestational diabetes will become diabetic 5–10 years later.

Endocrine pancreatic failure occurs in obese individuals resulting in type II diabetes. This happens because the pancreas over secretes insulin due to insulin resistance, which the obese state causes. In obesity, the insulin is not able to penetrate the fat cells effectively; the result is that the pancreas keeps secreting insulin as though there is a need for it, and after an extended period, it uses up its store of insulin.

Steroids can cause blood sugar to rise in people who have occult or pre-diabetes. Alcoholics who suffer from chronic pancreatitis can also develop diabetes mellitus as result of pan-pancreatic failure.

People who have occult diabetes mellitus or pre-diabetes can develop overt diabetes with markedly elevated blood sugars when under stress or in the case of infection.

Stress causes an excess secretion of adrenalin, which works counter to the effect of insulin, allowing a rise in blood sugar. (Adrenalin is an anti-insulin hormone).

Individuals, who are known diabetics, when under stress, experience a constant rise in their blood sugars, necessitating an increase in the doses of their insulin or oral hypoglycemic medications.

Since blacks and other minorities live under constant racial discrimination, their blood sugars are harder to control.

This, plus many other factors causes Black, Hispanic and Native American diabetics to develop a higher rate of complications compared to whites and other racial groups.

What is happening in the body of a person that causes him or her to become diabetic?

The pancreas is an organ that is located on the left side of the abdomen.
The pancreas has several functions to perform within the body for proper health. Among these functions is the production of insulin.

What is insulin?

Insulin is a hormone that is produced by the pancreas. The beta cells of the pancreas produce insulin in the Islands of Langerhans.

How is the pancreas able to produce insulin?

The pancreas is able to produce insulin by means of a group of cells located within the area of the pancreas referred to as the Islands of Langerhans. These cells have the ability to produce the hormone called insulin. Once produced, the insulin is secreted into the bloodstream.

What is the role of the insulin in the body?

The job of the insulin is to metabolize breakdown sugar (Glucose) so that the body can use it as fuel. The insulin actually forces the glucose into cells where it is used for the multitude of functions that are necessary for the body to function properly.

Glucose plays many roles in the human body under the influence of insulin.

1. Sugar is used as a fuel for the body to function properly. The human body gets the bulk of its energy from the breakdown of sugar under the influence of insulin.
2. Sugar is needed in order for the blood to carry oxygen to the different tissues and organs of the human body, most importantly - the brain. Without sugar, human beings cannot carry the appropriate amount of oxygen to the brain, which is needed

to remain alert. Insulin is needed to push the sugar into these tissues and organs for proper body functions.

When the body is not able to use sugar because of lack of insulin, it is forced to use fat for fuel. Fat is a very bad fuel to be used for energy because it is not effective. When one uses fat it produces breakdown products called ketone bodies that are very toxic when dumped into the bloodstream. The accumulation of these ketone bodies in the body because of the inability to use sugar is a condition known as ketoacidosis, which can be life-threatening if it goes unrecognized and untreated.

There exists another common reason for diabetes mellitus Type II diabetes, which is hemochromatosis. Hemochromatosis is a condition described in the chapter on Anemia. Hemolytic anemias cause iron overload and secondary hemochromatosis. The gene for primary hemochromatosis is located on the long arm of chromosome 6 on the HLA locus.

Recently, several more genes have been discovered that cause primary hemochromatosis. In addition, deficiency of Hepcidin causes hemochromatosis/iron over load. More recently, a genetic test has been developed that identifies the gene called C282Y. This gene is known to cause hemochromatosis. Many individuals who have Type II diabetes believe that they inherited the diabetic gene that was passed on to them by their parents, when, in fact, it is the hemochromatosis gene that was passed on to them, which results in their iron overload.

The excess iron accumulates in the pancreas, damaging the area where the beta cells are produced and preventing it from being able to make enough insulin, resulting in hyperglycemia and a form of Type II diabetes.

The percentage of blacks and other minorities who have hemochromatosis is not well known. However, it used to be thought that primary hemochromatosis was a disease seen mainly in European Caucasians and Scandinavians, which turned out not to be altogether the case.

Many blacks and other minorities have genetically transmitted primary hemochromatosis, although most blacks are negative for the C282Y gene. The C282Y gene that causes hemochromatosis has been identified in a black person by the author. See Valiere Alcena, MD, FACP, "Prevalence of Iron Overload in African-Americans: A Primary Care Experience; A Clinical Observation," *Prestige Medical News, Feb. 7, 2003.*

The serum ferritin test when elevated may mean that a person has hemochromatosis, costs about $18.00 and is routinely available.

Clinically, hemochromatosis is manifested the same way in non-Caucasians as it is in Caucasians, and the severity of the clinical disease is as intense in Caucasians as it is in blacks. What used to be called African Iron Overload Syndrome is, in fact, real primary hemochromatosis in blacks due to hepcidin deficiency. There is no such thing as African Iron Over load Syndrome. This syndrome never existed Some of the early signs of diabetes mellitus include:

Recurrent fungal vaginal infection
Recurrent fungal toenails infection
Recurrent fingernail infection, (paronychia infection in the bed of the nails)
Recurrent groin fungal infection
Infection in the foreskin of the penis
Blurry vision
Thirst
Recurrent infection under the breasts (especially in women with large breasts)
Infertility
Lack of libido
Numbness and tingling in toes and fingers
Frequent spontaneous abortions
Erectile dysfunction etc

All of these symptoms may also be due to occult or overt diabetes, etc. Some of the overt signs of diabetes, in addition to those listed above are urinary frequency, excessive consumption of fluid, dryness of the mouth, weight loss and frequent urinary tract infection.

Diabetes is a very complicated and complex disease that affects all organs in the human body one way or another. However, the organs that suffer most from the devastation of diabetes are the so-called end organs. These end organs consist of:

1. The eyes
2. The heart
3. The kidneys
4. The brain
5. The peripheral vascular system
6. The peripheral nervous system
7. The general nervous system

Other organ systems that are frequently affected by diabetes mellitus, causing severe pain and suffering, are the nervous system, causing peripheral neuropathy with pain, numbness, and coldness in the toes, feet, and fingers. If severe enough, diabetic neuropathy can cause affected people to be unable to walk. The skin is one of the most frequently affected organs in patients with diabetes. Diabetes affects the colon by causing constipation. Diabetes affects the stomach by causing gastro paresis with frequent indigestion, bloating, and burning in the stomach. Diabetes affects the urinary system by causing urinary retention.

The eyes are affected by diabetes because of the damage that the elevated blood sugar causes to take place inside the eyes. This damage results in bleeding within the eyes, a condition called diabetic retinopathy (see figures 1 and 2). Diabetic retinopathy is a condition that, if left untreated, can lead to blindness. The treatment for diabetic retinopathy is laser surgery.

The heart is affected by diabetes by causing hardening of the arteries, known as atherosclerosis. Atherosclerosis causes narrowing of the coronary arteries, resulting in ischemic heart disease, which causes angina pectoris, and frequently results in myocardial infarction (heart attack).

The kidneys are affected by diabetes through damage to the kidney tubules and glomureli, resulting in diabetic nephropathy of different degrees. Diabetic nephropathy can cause protein loss, microalbuminuria and, ultimately, nephrotic syndrome. The result of this constellation of abnormalities is elevated serum BUN, creatinine, potassium, and renal insufficiency, which usually result in end-stage renal failure. End-stage renal failure is treated with dialysis.

Forty nine percent of blacks with end stage kidney failure needing dialysis are receiving dialysis because of the effects of diabetes.

The brain is affected by diabetes by way of atherosclerosis of the arteries inside the brain, causing narrowing of these vessels, and preventing easy flow of blood and oxygen which can result in strokes.

The following are some of the acute symptoms that may signify that a person is diabetic:

1. Weight loss
2. Thirst
3. Blurred vision
4. Urinary frequency
5. Frequent tiredness and a feeling of unwellness, which if very nonspecific, may be due to diabetes mellitus.

If these symptoms are not recognized, and the diagnosis is established and treatment is begun, then the patient may go on to develop diabetic ketoacidosis, which can lead to a comatose state and, ultimately, death.

There is a subgroup of diabetes called hyperosmolar nonketotic diabetes mellitus: a condition in which the individual loses so much water that the blood sugar can exceed 1,000. In addition, sometimes the blood sugars can go up to 1,500 to 2,000.nanogram/dL. because the person has lost so much water that the brain becomes dehydrated, and the patient can go into a coma without having diabetic ketoacidosis. This is a very serious condition and if it is not recognized right away and treatment given with appropriate and careful fluid replacement and insulin, then the person may develop acute kidney failure because of marked dehydration, and death can result.

Some of the late signs and symptoms of diabetes are.

1. Blindness
2. Chronic kidney failure
3. Coronary artery disease
4. Recurrent leg and feet ulcers with frequent loss of lower limbs
5. Peripheral neuropathy

6. Sexual impotence
7. Loss of libido
8. Gastroparesis.
9. Infertility
10. Constipation
11. Recurrent fungal infections of the skin, sinuses, etc.

Another frequent problem that develops is urinary tract infection because diabetes damages the smooth muscle and nerves within the bladder, causing poor contraction of the bladder, preventing complete excretion of urine.

The residual urine that stays in the bladder serves as a culture medium allowing for bacterial growth, and the result is recurrent urinary tract infection and all its many potential complications.

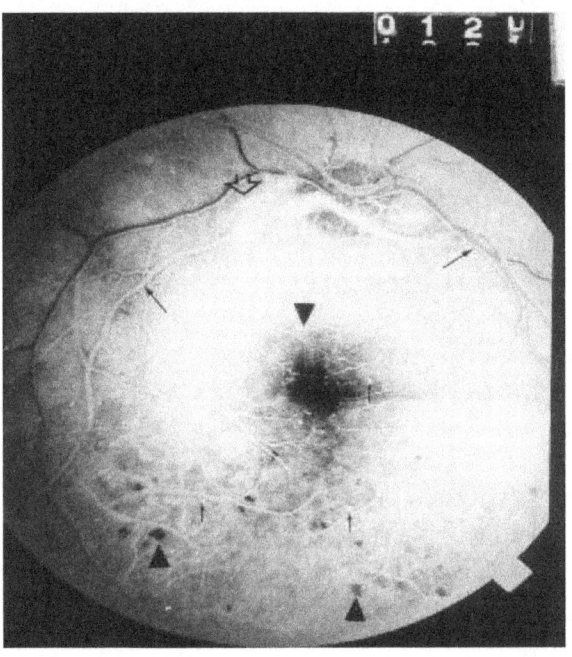

Figure 5:1–*Showing different degrees of abnormalities in the eye of a patient with diabetes mellitus (diabetic retinopathy); Fluorescein angiogram shortly after injection of dye in patient's eye. Dye in arteries (white) and just starting to enter veins (large arrow). White area off NH is neovascular tuff (open arrow). White spots are hemorrhages (arrow heads). Tiny white dots are microaneurysms (small arrow).*

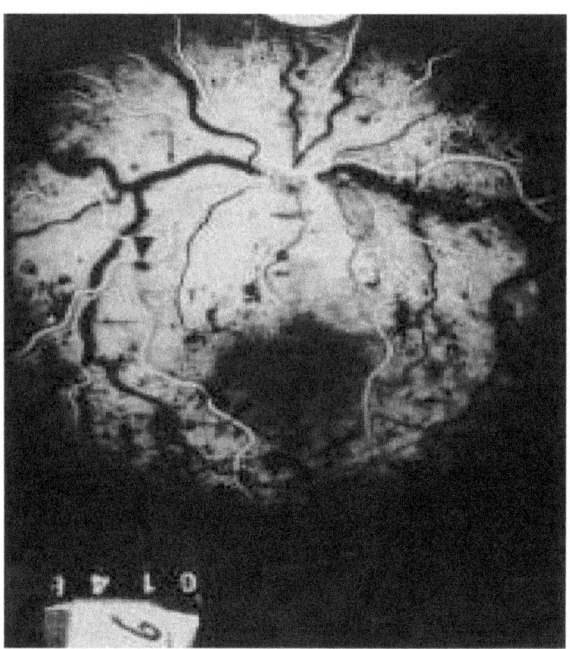

Figure 5:2–Showing different degrees of abnormalities in the eye of a patient with diabetes mellitus (diabetic retinopathy). The large arrows showing dilated veins and Arrowheads showing hemorrhages inside the eye.

Why is the incidence of diabetes mellitus so high?

The answer lies partly in the fact that obesity is more common in Blacks Hispanics, and Native Americans are more obese than Whites and Asians are, and obesity has a high association with diabetes mellitus.

Both obesity and certain forms of adult-onset diabetes mellitus are genetically transmitted diseases and it is therefore not surprising that these two diseases are so closely linked and so highly prevalent in blacks. Obesity causes a state of insulin resistance to exist, meaning that in the natural situation, the insulin that the obese person's pancreas secretes has a great deal of difficulty penetrating the fat cells to carry out proper metabolism (breaking down) of sugar. When that happens, the blood sugar stays above normal in the blood, causing a state of glucose intolerance, which is the earliest form of diabetes mellitus.

Another possible explanation for this high incidence of diabetes mellitus in Blacks Hispanics and Native Americans is stress. When added to the underlying obesity, stress associated with racial discrimination and its multitude of related problems, as well as the problems of daily living in the United States, it becomes clear why the blood sugar of many blacks is so much higher and so much more difficult to bring under control compared to their white counterparts. When an individual is under stress, that person secretes adrenalin in excess, and adrenalin is an anti-insulin hormone.

Another way of saying this is that the adrenalin prevents the insulin from doing its work, which is to break down sugar. The result is that the sugar level rises.

Any other type of stressful situation, such as an acute heart attack, an acute infection such as urinary tract infection, pneumonia, or any accident can cause the level of adrenalin to go up, resulting in an elevation of blood sugar.

The dietary habits of some Blacks, Hispanics, and Native Americans play a major role in their being overweight and play a major role in their being insulin-resistant. These blacks have a diet that is rich in fat and simple sugars. Poverty plays a major role in most blacks' inability to afford better foods. Therefore, they eat the foods they can afford. The types of foods that they can afford are frequently of poor quality. Even when the food is of very good quality, the manner in which it is prepared makes it too rich in fat and carbohydrates.

Food tends to be very ethnic in character. The foods that many blacks like to eat, the socalled "soul food", has its origin in Africa and is a the legacy from slavery. During slavery, slaves were not able to eat high-quality foods. Therefore, they compensated by preparing the foods in a way to make it more palatable by curing it with a fruit called "sour". This fruit is very juicy and is a bitter orange.

When plenty of salt, hot pepper and other spices are added, the food is more palatable and its taste improves, but not necessarily its quality. This is the legacy of the so-called "soul food", which is frequently eaten by some blacks, but is detrimental to their health. Whites and Asians eat these foods less frequently and when they do, they eat them as delicacies.

Fast foods like hamburgers, cheeseburgers, hot dogs, fried chicken, spareribs, pizza, pancakes, waffles, donuts etc.; have proliferated in U.S. society and are easy to purchase. People, young and old, eat these types of foods very often, they are getting fat and many of them are developing type II diabetes. Those foods, although popular, are definitely not very nutritious and certainly not particularly healthy.

It is perfectly fine to eat fast foods if done infrequently, but if one makes it a habit to feast on these foods on a regular basis, then the health consequences can be dire indeed.

Obesity and diabetes are intertwined, and as just outlined, they are both genetically transmitted diseases and interact together. When they interact together in the same individual, it makes it much more difficult to provide medical care for such a person who is both obese and diabetic.

Insulin is a hormone that the body needs in order to break down glucose, to provide energy, and to carry oxygen to the brain and tissues in the body. Stress causes a person to secrete a series of other hormones called counter-regulatory hormones, which includes adrenalin and nor-adrenalin, and other catecholamines. When secreted in large amounts as described above, adrenalin and nor-adrenaline can negate the effect of insulin, making it much more difficult to lower a person's blood sugar.

Most of these counter-regulatory hormones, including Cortisol, have effects that would counter the insulin's ability to do its work properly in the body.

An obese person has a good deal of difficulty using insulin because the obesity state renders his and or her insulin-resistant. Individuals who are obese and diabetic and living under stressful conditions have a constant interplay of over-secretion of adrenalin as well as an inability for insulin to penetrate the fat cells in order to lower their blood sugars. All these factors make the management of their diabetes extremely difficult.

What can people do to decrease their incidence of diabetes and what can those people who are genetically pre-determined to develop diabetes do to delay the onset of this disease?

The first thing for people to do is to learn about their family health history. They should ask questions about their parents and their grandparents who might have been diabetic. They should also find out if their siblings are diabetic. If their mothers or fathers died at an early age, they ought to inquire from their aunts and uncles whether diabetes existed in their immediate families.

If they have access to the treating physicians who cared for their parents, they ought to inquire as to the health records of their parents to ascertain whether the physicians treated their parents for diabetes. Knowing the family history may in many instances save lives. If either parent has diabetes, or more so, if both parents are diabetic, then these blacks must be ever so careful and must see their physicians for frequent evaluation of their blood sugars. Having this knowledge can go a long way in helping these blacks take the necessary precautions to delay the onset of diabetes and its devastating complications.

Some of the precautions that people need to take to decrease their chances of becoming diabetics and, if already diabetics, to better control their blood sugars include:

1. A diet rich in fruits, vegetables, protein, high in complex carbohydrates, and low in fat, simple sugar, and salt.
2. Regular exercise to burn calories, thereby decreasing weight and increasing insulin-sensitivity, which in turn decreases blood sugar.

The increase in insulin sensitivity decreases the level of insulin in the blood, which in turn decreases obese people's appetite and decreases the craving for carbohydrate-containing foods. High insulin levels in the blood of obese individuals are part of the reason why these individuals have such a craving for carbohydrates, resulting in a vicious cycle. The more obese people are, the more insulin-resistant they become, and the more insulin-resistant they are, the more they feel a need to eat simple carbohydrate-containing foods.

Insulin is an anabolic hormone, meaning that the more insulin is injected exogenously into the obese diabetics, the more the obese diabetics consume, and the more obese they become. The only way to break this vicious cycle is to treat the obese diabetics with a strict dietary program that can decrease their weight and thereby increases the insulin sensitivity.

If possible, the best way to treat obese diabetics is with oral hypoglycemic agents and diet. Insulin should be used to treat obese diabetics only when it is necessary. Using a combination of oral hypoglycemia and insulin is used frequently to treat diabetics to bring down their blood sugars.

There is a long list of oral hypoglycemic agents available on the market to treat people with type II diabetes.

The following is a partial list of these medications.

1. DiaBeta
2. Glucotrol
3. Glucotrol XL
4. Amaryl
5. Avandia
6. Actos
7. Glucophage
8. Glucophage XR
9. Glucovance
10. Diabinese
11. Januvia
12. Onglyza
13. Kombiglyze XR
14. FARXIGA
15. BYDUREON injectable
16. Trulicity (dulaglutide) was just approved by the FDA for once per week injection to treat type 2 diabetes mellitus.

Type I diabetes is treated only with insulin because the pancreas of diabetics with type I diabetes is not able to secrete any insulin at all.

The following oral hypoglycemic agents, Glucophage, Glucophage XR, Avandia and Actos and Januvia, work to lower blood sugar by increasing insulin sensitivity and uptake from the blood to cells and tissues. Glucovance, which is a combination of Glucophage and Glyburide, on the other hand, works by both stimulating the pancreas to secrete insulin while facilitating insulin uptake in the blood to cells and tissues to lower the blood sugar. Because of that, these oral hypoglycemic agents can be used in conjunction with insulin, as well as with other oral agents to control blood sugar.

Diabeta, Glucotrol, Glucotrol XL, Amaryl, and Diabinese work to lower blood sugar by stimulating the pancreas to secrete insulin into the bloodstream to control blood sugar.

In addition to controlling blood sugars, all these agents work to allow the body to use sugar properly as fuel for normal body functions.

Some Type II diabetics are insulin-requiring meaning that they need to be given insulin in order to survive. In this sub- group of diabetics, the pancreas is no longer able to produce insulin in any amount.

There is another group of diabetics who are non-insulin-requiring, meaning that they still have enough beta cells left in their pancreas that can be stimulated by oral agents to secrete insulin into the bloodstream to break down the glucose as just described. The way one finds out which group of diabetics is insulin requiring and which group is not, is by trial and error.

The different doses of oral hypoglycemic agents used to treat diabetics are as follows: The usual starting dose of Diabeta (glyburide) is 2.5 mg–5 mg each morning with breakfast; a maximum dose of 20 mg per day divided into 10 mg twice per day can be used.

The usual dose of Glucotrol (glipizide) is 5 mg each morning with breakfast, but a maximum dose of 40 mg can be given per day in divided doses. The usual dose of Glucotrol is 5 mg with breakfast each morning, but a maximum dose of 20 mg per day can be given in divided doses to control the blood sugar. The usual starting dose of Amaryl is 1–2 mg per day with breakfast. A maximum dose of 8 mg per day may be used in divided doses to control the blood sugar.

The usual starting of Avandia is 4 mg per day with breakfast. A maximum dose of 8 mg of Avandia can be used in two divided doses to control the blood sugar.
The usual dose of Actos is 15–30 mg per day.

A maximum dose of 45 mg can be used to control the blood sugar. The usual dose of Glucophage (metformin) is 500 mg three times per day, but a maximum dose of 2.550 mg per day can be used to control the blood sugar.

The usual dose of Glucophage XR (metformin) is 500 mg with supper, but up to 2000 mg with supper may be used to control the blood sugar. The usual starting dose of Glucovance is 1.25 mg Diabeta with 250 mg of Glucophage (1.25/250 mg), but 5/500 mg twice per day of Glucovance may be used to control the blood sugar. The usual dose of Diabinese is 250 mg per day, but up to 500 mg per day can be used to control the blood sugar.

The dose of these hypoglycemic agents must be decreased significantly in elderly people to prevent hypoglycemia, because elderly people are more likely to have fewer fats in their body and are less likely to have a good diet. These two factors, along with the long-acting effects of the agents, can cause severe and prolonged hypoglycemia in elderly women if the doses of these medications are not well monitored.

Another important factor to consider when treating elderly people with oral hypoglycemic agents is the status of their kidney functions. Renal insufficiency is very likely in an older individual, which dictates that less insulin is needed to maintain the normoglycemic state.

This is so because 15% of the body's sugar is metabolized (made in the kidneys), and as the kidneys become sick and insufficient, the less able they are to produce that amount of sugar, making the need for insulin less, therefore the need for oral hypoglycemic agents also much less.

There are many different insulin preparations available to treat diabetes mellitus, some of them, such as Humulin N or NPH, are long-acting, and some of them, such as Humulin R regular insulin, are short-acting. Some insulin preparations are intermediate acting. There is also a mixture of regular insulin with long-acting insulin called 70/30. The patient's physician and the patient determine the types of insulin that are appropriate for her.

The following is a list of some of the insulin preparations in use to treat Diabetes Mellitus.

Humulin N
Lantus
Humulin R
NovoLog
Novolog 70/30
Bydureon once weekly injection (is GLP-1 receptor antagonist newly approved by the FDA)

In the acute setting, in a person who presents with elevated blood sugar, dehydration, thirst and other associated acute symptoms of diabetes, she must be treated inside a hospital with fluid replacement, electrolyte replacement, and either IV regular insulin drip or subcutaneous insulin to bring the blood sugar down and correct the dehydration and the electrolyte abnormalities. If he or she presents in diabetic ketoacidosis, he or she must be treated with IV fluid, and regular insulin either intravenously or subcutaneously. If he or she is in shock, and cannot perfuse his or her skin well, the regular insulin must be given intravenously to assure its entry into the bloodstream to bring down the blood sugar and correct the ketoacidosis.

The management of diabetes mellitus and its associated problems is very complex and it takes an experienced physician to properly treat them. A diet poor in simple sugar, carbohydrates, in association with exercise and weight management are crucial and necessary parts in the treatment of diabetes mellitus.

Type I diabetes mellitus (juvenile diabetes) is treated with insulin, diet, exercise, and weight management. Oral agents that work to control the blood sugar by stimulating the pancreas are not appropriate in the treatment of juvenile diabetes because there is no insulin in the pancreas for these oral agents to secrete in the bloodstream.

In the hospital setting, blood sugar is tested several times per day and insulin dosages are adjusted according to the level of sugar in the blood.

At home, there are different types of blood sugar meters available commercially for patients who are diabetic to test their blood sugar, which allow them to adjust their insulin dosages or the dosages of their oral hypoglycemic agents on instructions from their physicians.

Diabetics ought to have their eyes examined to be certain that they do not have diabetic retinopathy. They also ought to see the podiatrist in order to have proper foot care and avoid cuts in their toes that can lead to diabetic ulcers with the potential for the loss of a limb.

The reason that diabetics do not heal very easily is due in part to poor circulation, which is secondary to the damage that diabetes causes to veins, arteries, and smaller vessels in their feet, which results in poor blood and oxygen delivery to tissues in their extremities.

Another reason why diabetics do not heal easily is that when a cut occurs, the polynuclear white blood cells of the diabetics do not migrate well towards the site of the infection. The result is that the infection is much more difficult to treat.

It is a good idea also for diabetics to get in contact with the American Diabetic Association to become familiar with all the different programs that are available to them.

In addition, wearing an arm bracelet identifying themselves as diabetics is a very good idea so that they can be easily identified as diabetics in the event they become ill in the street or on the job, either because of hypoglycemia (low blood sugar) or hyperglycemia (high blood sugar).

In such a case, the bracelet will show that the wearer is diabetic and can be quickly given a piece of candy, a glass of orange juice or soda while waiting for medical help to arrive. It is also a good idea for diabetics always to carry in their pocketbooks a candy bar. In the event they feel dizzy and weak or feel like they are going to develop a hypoglycemic episode, which consists primarily of dizziness, sweatiness, or a feeling of impending doom, they can prevent the hypoglycemic episode by eating the candy bar.

Hypoglycemia (low blood sugar) that occurs on a repeated basis is very dangerous because sugar is needed to carry oxygen into the brain. When the patient is having repeated episodes of hypoglycemia, the brain is being deprived of oxygen.

In other words, when the diabetic person feels sick, it is best for him or her to ingest sugar because it is an easy way to raise the level of the blood sugar.

In addition, during each episode of hypoglycemia high level of adrenalin is secreted resulting stimulation of the heart, which can lead to ischemia resulting in heart attacks and cardiac arrhythmia and death.

Therefore, tightly control blood sugar is no longer recommended.

On the other hand, it is much more difficult to treat the condition of low blood sugar or hypoglycemia if it is the result of medications such as oral anti-diabetic medications. In particular, hypoglycemia associated with oral agents that the diabetic might be taking must be treated in a hospital setting because it could take days to raise the level of the blood sugar. This is because the half-life of some of these hypoglycemic agents can be quite long.

Recent literature supports the approach that it makes no sense to over treat diabetics with Insulin or oral hypoglycemic medications to control blood sugar tightly. There is no proof that this over treatment reduces vascular damage in diabetics. On the other hand, clear evidence exists to show that recurrent hypoglycemic episodes damage the brain, which can lead to dementia.

Diabetes mellitus, while not a curable disease, is definitely a treatable disease. There are plans underway for pancreatic transplants and if these become successful, then the disease can, at that point, be considered curable. Insulin pumps are also already in use. These pumps add a great deal to the treatments of diabetics requiring insulin.

There is also research underway to try to determine the cause of Type I diabetes and the hope is that someday, the answer will be found. Meanwhile, it is important for diabetics to learn as much about diabetes mellitus as they can, and in the case of obese diabetics, it is important that they make every effort to get the excess weight under control to help better control their diabetes, decrease the multitudes of end organs damage, and thereby prolong their lives.

The cost diabetes and all its associated complications amounts to $322 billions Annually in the U.S.

CHAPTER 6

CORONARY HEART DISEASE IN AFRICAN AMERICAN MEN

Cardiovascular disease (CVD) is a combination of hypertension, coronary heart disease, and stroke. 34% of individuals in the U.S. have CVD. 16 million have coronary artery disease. 5.8 million have stroke, 73 million have hypertension and 5.3 million have congestive heart failure. CVD is the leading cause of deaths in the U.S. Every year, more than 900,000 individuals die of CVD in the U.S. Worldwide, 17.3 million people die from CVD every year and hypertension is the cause of 8,000,000 of these deaths. The annual cost of CVD in the U.S. is $450 billion. The total annual cost of CVD worldwide is $863 billion.

"Ischemic heart diseases and stroke are the top 2 leading causes of death worldwide in 2011, responsible for 7 million and 6.2 million deaths, respectively."
Source: WHO

Heart disease is the leading cause of death in the U.S. 12,900,000 million individuals has coronary heart disease costing 130 billion dollars per year. About 7,600,000 million of these individuals have had heart attacks. Every year, there are 1.1 million heart attacks in the U.S. and 450,000 of them are recurrent heart attacks (Source: *Morbidity and Mortality: 2002 Chart Book on Cardiovascular, Lung and Blood Diseases.* Bethesda, Maryland National Heart, Lung and Blood Institute, May 2002). Some 6,600,000 individuals in the U.S. suffer from angina pectoris (chest pain). Every day 2,600 people die of cardiovascular disease in the U.S.; this represents on an average one death every 33 seconds.

In the year 2000, there were 2,400,000 deaths in the U.S. from different causes and 1,415,000 of these deaths were due to cardiovascular disease of different types. Each year over 600,000 people die from coronary heart disease in the U.S. Cardiovascular heart disease is the number one killer in the U.S.

The incidence of cardiovascular disease is much higher in Negroes /blacks than it is in whites and other racial groups. In 2005, 44.6 percent of Negros/Black males and 37.2 of white males had CVD and 35 percent of white females and 49 per cent of Negros/black females had CVD.

Every day, 2,400 people in the U.S. die of CVD. This is an average of one death every 37 seconds. The death rates from CVD are much higher for blacks than for whites and other racial groups. Source: NCHS. Compressed mortality files underlying cause of death. Coronary heart disease is much more common in blacks than in whites and other non-blacks in the U.S.

In 2006, 81,100,000 individuals in the U.S. had CVD: 17,600,000 had Chronic Heart Disease (CHD), 8,500,000 had acute heart attack, 10,200,000 had angina pectoris, 6,400, 000 had stroke, 73,600,000 had high blood pressure, and 5,800,000 had congestive heart failure.

In 2012, 16.8 million Americans have CHD, 8.7 million men and 8.1 million women. In 2012, 1.2 million Americans had a new or recurrent heart attack. 770,000 had a new heart attack and 430,000 had a recurrent heart attack.

About 17,600,000 individuals living today have a history of heart attack or angina pectoris or both. This represents 9,200,000 males and 8,400,000 females.

The incidence of CHD and deaths from CHD are higher in blacks, Hispanics, American Indians, and Alaska Natives than in Asians and whites and other racial groups.

The black community is not homogenous: about 10% of blacks in the U.S. were born outside the U.S. and as such have different dietary habits.

Blacks, Hispanics, Asians and Whites born outside the U.S. have a healthier diet than Blacks, Hispanics, Asians and Whites born in the U.S. do. A good example of that is the French; they have less CHD than Americans do.

Every 37 seconds some one has a heart attack and every 60 seconds some dies of a heart attack in the U.S.

Every year, 295,000 cardiac arrests occurred out of the hospital in the U.S. In 2006, 425,425 deaths resulted from CHD in the U.S. making CHD the leading yearly killer in the United States.

Although Black Americans, Hispanics and other minorities are less likely to be diagnosed with CHD, they die more frequently of CHD compared to White Americans.

In 2006, the death rates from CHD per 100,000 people were 206.4 Black American Males vs. 176.3 White American males and 130.0 Black American females vs. 101.5 White American females. Source: American Heart Association.

In 2011, 450,000 people died of CHD in the U.S. Worldwide, CHD is the leading cause of deaths, responsible for 1 in 5 men and 1 in 6 women deaths, totaling 7.2 million deaths.

Worldwide 17.3 million people died of CHD in 2014. 1/3 of the deaths or 8.6 millions occurred in women and ½ of the deaths occurred in men. 15, 800,000 people in the U.S. have CHD in 1n 2014 and about 1 million people died of CHD in the U.S.

In 2006, 5,800,000 individuals had congestive heart failure in the U.S. (water in the lungs) and there are 500,000 new cases of congestive heart failure every year.

World wide 22 million people have CHF with 2 million new cases every year.

The rates of congestive heart failure are several times more common in American Blacks than in Whites and other racial groups.

In addition, congestive heart failure occurs at an earlier age in Blacks compared to Whites and other racial groups.

"African Americans between the ages of 45 and 65 have a 70% higher rate of CHF, with mortality rates of 2.5 times more than the Caucasian population" Source: CDC, 2011

Why is there such a high incidence of coronary artery heart disease (CAD) and deaths from CAD in the USA and around the world?

Now a new concept of "Nonobstructive Coronary Artery Disease and Risk of Myocardial Infarction" is being proposed. "Nonobstructive CAD, compared with no apparent CAD, was associated with a significant greater 1 year risk of MI and all-cause mortality." Source: JAM November 5, 2014 Volume 312, Number 17

Obesity contributes to CAD. Over all, 76% of African Americans are over weight/overweight; fifty three percent of African American women are obese and 77% of them are overweight; about 38% of African American men are obese. 75.7% of Hispanic women are overweight/obese. 59.5 % of white women are overweight/obese. 81.7 % of Hispanic males are overweight/obese. 69.9% of white males and 74.0% of black males are overweight/obese. See chapter on obesity above.

Hypertension also contributes to CAD in blacks: In 2010, there were 736, 000,000 people with hypertension in the USA. While forty percent of African Americans have hypertension, blacks are more likely to ignore their symptoms of hypertension. Worldwide 1 billion have hypertension. See chapter on hypertension.

The symptoms of hypertension are:

Headache
Dizziness
Shortness of breath
Chest pain
Palpitations
Tiredness
Blurry vision etc;

Blacks and other minorities are less likely to get proper medical attention when presenting to the emergency room seeking medical help because some of the health care professionals working in the ER believe that most blacks complain of vague and hysterical symptoms when they present in the ER. (Of course, more often than not, this assumption is false).

Blacks are less likely to be offered cardiac catheterization to evaluate them for the possibility of coronary artery disease. When blacks are found to have coronary occlusive disease, they are less likely to be offered coronary bypass to treat their coronary artery disease. Blacks live under conditions that oftentimes are more stressful than whites are. These multitudes of stresses predispose blacks to conditions that create a perfect formula for the development of CAD heart attacks and sudden death.

The combination of obesity, hypertension, diabetes mellitus, high cholesterol and insulin resistance, referred to as syndrome X or metabolic syndrome plays a major role in the causation of coronary artery disease in blacks in the USA.

The diet of African Americans is, for the most part, less healthy than that of whites, due partly to their deprived economic circumstances. Because, generally, blacks are poorer than whites, the result is a lifestyle that predisposes them to poorer cardiac health.

The diet of most blacks and other minorities is too rich in fats, simple carbohydrates, salt, and too poor in protein, fibers, fruits and vegetables. The poor diet of most blacks is guaranteed to give rise to many serious medical problems including heart disease.

The cholesterol level of people of color is usually higher than that of whites. The higher rates of obesity seen in blacks and other minorities compared to whites predispose them to higher rates of morbidity and mortality.

Stress as a psychological state is generally more prevalent in blacks and other minorities than in whites. The higher rate of stress seen in blacks and other minorities predisposes them to a much higher incidence of CAD.

The incidence of cigarette smoking is generally higher in blacks and other minorities than in whites. The higher rate of smoking as seen in blacks and other minorities predisposes them to higher incidence of CAD.

The incidence of alcohol abuse, percentage-wise, is higher in whites than in whites, but all the chronic medical problems associated with alcohol abuse is seen more frequently in blacks compared to their white counterparts. Chronic alcohol abuse is associated with an increased incidence of CAD.

The incidence of IV drug abuse is higher in blacks and other minorities than in whites. IV drug abuse is a major risk factor for overall poor heart health. The result is that the overall rate of heart disease morbidity/mortality is higher in blacks and other minorities than in whites.

When blacks and other minorities present to emergency rooms as previously mentioned with symptoms of heart disease, they are less likely to be taken seriously compared to white patients. Their pain is usually attributed to other factors.

They are less likely to be admitted to a coronary care unit and they are less likely to be offered cardiac catheterization, angioplasty, or coronary bypass.

The individuals who receive the quickest attention and the highest priority in the health care system in the USA are white males. This is so, in part, because more often than not, the physicians making the decisions as to who gets what type of care are white male doctors in training (interns, residents, and fellows). These young physicians work at the front line in the emergency rooms and inside the hospitals.

It is a wellknown secret of the profession, white Physicians are more attentive to white patients than they are to black and other minority patients. Racism quite frequently enters into life and death decisions made by physicians who take an OATH to provide needed health care for all.

Not too long ago, the American Medical Association apologized for one hundred twelve years of racial discrimination towards black Americans.

The availability of health insurance also plays a major role in the type of care that is offered to blacks when they present seeking health care. The number of uninsured in the U.S. in 201 is 37 million. When the number of people unemployed is factored in, the actual number of people uninsured in the U.S. is closer to 40 million.

The percentage of uninsured is higher in black and other minority Americans than in white Americans. Thirty six percent of black Americans ages 19-29 are uninsured while twenty three percent of white Americans of the same ages are uninsured.

Many people who are uninsured are working. Economic status determines insurance status. In August 2015, the unemployment number in the U.S. was 5.1%. During that same time, the unemployment rate for Blacks was 9.5%, 6.6% for Latinos, 3.4% for Asians and 4.4% for whites.

Many millions people live below the poverty line in the U.S. In fact, 24.7% black Americans live below the poverty line.

Risk factors for coronary heart disease include:

1. Hypertension
2. Obesity
3. Diabetes mellitus
4. Poor dietary habits
5. Hyperlipidemia (high cholesterol, high triglycerides, high LDL, low HDL, high cholesterol / HDL ratio)

6. High lipoprotein A in the blood
7. High lipoprotein A in conjunction with high LDL in the blood
8. High homocysteine level in the blood
9. Alcohol abuse
10. Stress
11. Type A personality
12. Tobacco smoking
13. Hereditary predisposition
14. Racial discrimination
15. Poverty
16. Lack of health insurance
17. Sickle cell disease
18. Hemochromatosis/Iron overload
19. Sleep apnea etc.

How does hypertension cause coronary heart disease?

Hypertension takes various routes in causing heart disease. First, the fact of having a high pressure within vessels while the blood passes through those vessels causes the lumen of the vessels to get damaged. The areas of the blood vessels' lumen that get damaged trap debris as the blood passes through them and platelets and lipid particles settle onto the damaged areas inside the vessels, resulting in the formation of a nidus.

Once a nidus is formed, then more of such materials are deposited on these areas, resulting in formation of plaques. The plaques grow larger and larger, causing narrowing of the vessels, particularly in the coronary arteries. The narrowed coronary arteries prevent blood and oxygen delivery to heart muscle, causing symptoms of coronary heart disease.

Another mechanism through which hypertension causes cardiovascular heart disease is sustained high blood pressure which lasts for a long time and remains untreated for a long time, resulting in a hypertrophied (enlarged) heart muscle. The enlarged heart, in time, becomes unable to pump blood properly and fails resulting in congestive heart failure. The reason that the enlarged heart fails is that muscle fibers have a finite stretching ability, and once the muscle fibers of the heart are stretched to the maximum, then the heart becomes like a big floppy bag with very poor function, resulting in the development of many serious and disabling symptoms of cardiovascular disease, including cardiac rhythm abnormalities.

Diabetes mellitus also has a high association with coronary artery heart disease.

How does diabetes mellitus cause coronary heart disease?

The high level of blood sugar in the circulating blood damages blood vessels, including the vessel around the heart, namely the coronary arteries.

Once the effects of diabetes damage the lumen of the coronary arteries, then plaques easily form, resulting in coronary disease and the symptoms of coronary heart disease.

Sorbitol is a sugar whose level becomes quite elevated in uncontrolled diabetes and Sorbitol has a very toxic effect on different vessels in the body as well as different peripheral nerves in the body, causing a multitude of vascular and nerve damage. Obesity also has a high association with the development of coronary artery heart disease.

How does obesity cause coronary heart disease?

Obesity is associated with coronary heart disease by being associated with diabetes mellitus, hyperlipidemia, and hypertension. Some prefer to call this metabolic syndrome, metabolic hypertension, syndrome W or syndrome X. A sedentary life style is highly associated with obesity, increasing the evidence of coronary heart disease. In addition, obesity is associated with coronary heart disease because obesity creates a state of insulin resistance in the human body.

The insulin resistance results in an elevated level of insulin in the circulation of the human body. This excess insulin works in a negative way to cause more plaques to develop in arterial vessels of these obese patients. In other words, too much insulin in the circulation is atrogenic. The higher the level of circulating insulin is in the blood, the higher the likelihood that affected people might develop coronary occlusive disease. The more obese a person is, the more insulin-resistant he or she is likely to be, the more insulin-resistant he or she is, and the higher the level of circulating insulin in his or her blood.

Once plaques form in these arteries, the vessels' narrowing process begins, leading to all the possible problems associated with this process.

How does a poor diet contribute to a high incidence of atherosclerotic heart disease?

A fat-rich diet leads to higher lipid levels and its propensity to cause coronary artery heart disease. The higher carbohydrate-containing diet results in obesity and its propensity to the development of heart disease.

The high salt in the diet of many people contributes to the development of hypertension and all of its associated problems. The average black eats about 7 grams of salt per day. "The average white eats 3.436 mg of salt per day. The recommended daily salt intake is 1.5 grams of salt per day. Decreasing the salt intake to 1.5 grams of salt per day can save more 100,000 lives per year in the U.S."

Moreover, according to a report by the AMA issued in April of 2010, most of the salt eaten by Americans comes from processed foods and, as a result, the health care system can save 24 billion dollars per year by decreasing the salt intake to 1.5 grams per day.

Decreasing salt intake will result in the decreased occurrence of hypertension, coronary artery disease, heart attacks, congestive heart failure, stroke, and kidney failure.

The high carbohydrate content in the diet of many people is also associated with both the development and poor control of diabetes mellitus, which ultimately contributes to the development of coronary artery heart disease.

Having high cholesterol and high triglycerides (hyperlipidemia) is a genetically transmitted condition from parent or parents to their children. However, diet plays a major role in how high the level of cholesterol, triglycerides, and low-density lipoprotein goes. The high-density lipoprotein (HDL) goes up with exercise and moderate intake of wine - 2–3 glasses of red or white wine or 1–2 drinks of hard liquor per day.

Alcohol in wine causes a decrease in coronary artery disease by raising HDL cholesterol. Substances found in the skin of the grapes that are used to make wine such as polyphenoles and flavonoids and other antioxidants decrease the incidence of coronary heart disease. These substances are also found in olives and green peas. Apparently, these substances play some role in preventing local inflammatory reaction within coronary arteries, which is an important factor in reducing the formation of coronary occlusive disease. The French, however, show that the effect of alcohol on decreasing the stickiness of the platelets is important in preventing clot formation. It is not altogether clear whether white wine has a similar effect.

How does high cholesterol cause coronary heart disease?

One hundred and two million American adults have high cholesterol: 44.8% of black men and 47.9% of black women have high cholesterol in the U.S. The number of blacks dying of CAD yearly in the U.S. is approximately 104,000 and high cholesterol plays a significant role in causing these deaths. Therefore, it is very important that blacks have their cholesterol level tested on a regular basis.

There are five parts to the clinically lipid profile:

1. Cholesterol
2. Triglycerides
3. High-density lipoprotein
4. Low-density lipoprotein
5. HDL/cholesterol ratio

Each one of these five parts of the lipid profile, when abnormal, is a risk factor for the development of coronary heart disease. The cholesterol is abnormal when it is too high, greater than 200 (there are certain situations in clinical medicine when too low cholesterol is also abnormal, in particular in malabsorption). The triglycerides are abnormal when the level is too high. The HDL is abnormal when it is too low. The low-density (LDL) is abnormal when it is too high. The ratio of HDL to cholesterol is abnormal when it is too high.

Poor and lower-middle-class individuals in the U.S. and in the world have limited income, so their food-buying power is also limited to purchasing foods that are poor in quality. Consequently, the health benefit of these foods is limited. These foods satisfy hunger, but have very little nutritional value. Foods such as bologna, bacon, sausages, pig's feet, cow's feet, cheeseburgers, pizza, hamburgers, chitterlings, and collard greens cooked with ham hogs are greasy and too rich in fats and salt to have any substantial nutritional value. As just stated, these foods do satisfy hunger, and that is a positive thing, but in the long run they can cause high cholesterol.

In addition, they can contribute to obesity, high blood pressure, all of which can lead to the development of coronary artery disease, heart attacks, congestive heart failure, stroke, kidney failure, glaucoma, and other lethal consequences.

Foods such as pork, beef, goat meat, eggs, ham, lobster, shrimp, crabs, oysters, cheeses, avocado, coconut, etc., are rich in cholesterol and when eaten in large quantities and too frequently can cause elevation in blood cholesterol.

Once the lipid level is high in the blood, regardless of how it gets there, it causes plaque to form. Once plaque is formed, coronary arteries become narrowed, resulting in coronary artery heart disease, all its associated symptoms, and other consequences.

How can a high level of lipoprotein–A in the blood causes a heart attack to occur?

Lipoprotein-A is a large lipoprotein, which is made by the liver and secreted into the blood. When the level of lipoprotein-A is elevated in the blood, if the LDL cholesterol is also elevated, the two work synergistically to bring about the development of plaques within the coronary arteries around the heart, resulting in coronary artery heart disease. In addition, the elevated lipoprotein-A by itself can cause a clot to develop in the coronary arteries without the formation of plaques, resulting in an acute myocardial infarction.

This reaction occurs because lipoprotein-A competes with plasminogen, displaces it, overwhelms it and renders it helpless in preventing clots from forming. (The main role of plasminogen is to prevent fibrin/clot from forming.) In addition, lipoprotein-A attaches itself to heparin, cells, and tissues creating a state of hypercoagulability making clot formation occur spontaneously, which can result in death.

Elevated lipoprotein-A can also cause a clot to form in the low pressure (venous system) resulting in Deep Vein Thrombophlebitis/Pulmonary Embolism.

About 20% of the U.S. population has elevated lipoprotein-A, but the percentage of lipoprotein -A is much higher in blacks than whites. The percentage of Lipoprotein-A is higher in Jamaicans and other Caribbean blacks than in black Americans and other racial groups. Overall, 20% of the U.S. population has high lipoptrotein-A.

Elevated lipoprotein A can also cause multiple stroke syndromes in the brain causing TIA, seizures and dementia.

High homocysteine level in the blood is toxic to blood vessels and can cause plaques to form inside vessels in both the high pressure and low-pressure systems in the human body.

Alcohol abuse can cause coronary artery occlusive disease to develop, because when alcoholics are drunk, they frequently become agitated. The agitated state creates a hyperdynamic situation, resulting in rapid heart rate and elevation of blood pressure. This transient, but frequent high blood pressure causes two things to happen: first, the high blood pressure damages the inside of coronary arteries, resulting in plaque formation and eventual narrowing of these vessels; and second, the frequent elevation of blood pressure causes enlargement of the heart, resulting in hypertensive heart disease, which in time causes congestive heart failure.

Another form of heart disease that frequently develops in alcoholics is alcoholic cardiomyopathy - enlargement of the muscles and different chambers of the heart. The toxic effect of alcohol itself causes damage to muscles of the heart. The result of alcohol-associated heart disease is congestive heart failure and cardiac arrhythmias of different types and severities.

Stress can cause heart disease to develop via several mechanisms: first, stress causes the level of adrenalin in the blood to rise; second, the rise in the level of adrenalin causes the blood pressure to rise; third, the rise in adrenalin can also cause both acute heart attack as well as cardiac arrhythmias to develop, with lethal consequences.

Blacks live under constant racism associated stress in America and this kind of stress increases the incidence of hypertension, coronary artery heart disease, stroke, kidney failure, high cholesterol, obesity, diabetes mellitus, alcoholism, drug addiction, tobacco smoking, depression, poverty, increased rate of suicide, etc.

Type A personality (an aggressive and restless person who is always on the go) is also associated with the development of coronary heart disease via some of the mechanisms just outlined.

Tobacco smoking can cause coronary occlusive disease because of the effects of nicotine on the coronary vessels resulting in the development of plaques inside these vessels.

Heredity is associated to a very high degree with coronary heart disease because if a man's mother or father has coronary heart disease or died of a heart attack, chances are she also is at a high risk of encountering the same fate, if appropriate medical care is not sought by her to forestall the possibility of her developing CAD.

Poverty is associated with an increased incidence of coronary artery heart disease because all the factors just outlined are seen in greater numbers in poor blacks than in people of higher financial means.

A large percentage of the 47 million or so people in the USA who have no health insurance are blacks and other minorities. Many of these individuals are employed and yet they have no health insurance because they simply do not have enough money to pay for it.

According to recent reports, there are 18 million children in this country living below the poverty line; a good percentage of these children are black children, other minority children and white children.

Tragically, roughly 14 million children in the USA go to bed hungry every night.

When people are poor, they are concerned about being able to find the bare necessities of daily living, such as where to find food to eat, and they will eat any food that is edible regardless of its nutritional value.

The quality of the food does not enter into the equation of their lives; they are more concerned about being able to afford the rent and utility bills- electric, oil and gas - to keep a roof over their heads and their homes warm in the winter. These are important and essential factors in the overall lives of poor people in the U.S. and the world.

Poverty is associated with a greater number of poor health habits, all of which can lead to the development of major medical problems such as hypertension, high cholesterol, obesity, diabetes mellitus, cancer, atherosclerotic heart disease, heart attack, congestive heart failure, stroke, osteoarthritis, etc. People of better financial means also suffer from these same medical problems, but because they are more likely to have health insurance and can see a physician with ease, these problems are dealt with more quickly and more efficiently.

Blacks and other minorities tend to go to physicians with diseases of all sorts when these diseases are already in their advanced stages. They frequently ignore their symptoms and go to physicians when the medical problems are frequently more challenging to address. Symptoms of coronary artery disease and a heart attack in women are quite different than they are in men. Most women, when they are having a heart attack, do not have chest pain, but often describe their symptoms of myocardial infarction as an aching, pressure, tightness in the chest, nausea, vomiting, and indigestion.

Other acute symptoms of heart attack are weakness, shortness of breath, fatigue, dizziness and cold sweat (Source: *Circulation,* 2003; 108: 2619–2623).

Typical symptoms of acute coronary syndrome include:

1. Chest pain often the most common symptom of arteriosclerotic heart disease.
2. Shortness of breath.
3. Pain in the left shoulder radiating down the left arm, associated with numbness and shortness of breath.

4. A combination of the three symptoms mentioned above and worsening of these symptoms on exertion. This complex of symptoms is often referred to as Angina Pectoris.

5. Irregular, rapid heartbeats and too slow heartbeats also known as Bradycardia / Tachycardia

6. Chest pain associated with dizziness, sweating, and shortness of breath which can often mean not just angina, but often that the patient is in the process of having an acute heart attack.

7. Shortness of breath along with accumulation of fluid in the lungs and ankles can be a result of cardiovascular disease and a particular condition known as Congestive Heart Failure.

How to diagnose coronary heart disease:

In order to arrive at a diagnosis of cardiovascular heart disease, the physician must:

1. Take a good medical history.
2. Carry out a good physical examination.
3. Perform an electrocardiogram (EKG).
4. Follow up with a chest x-ray.

Based on these tests, the physician may institute a treatment protocol involving beta-blocker, nitroglycerin, and aspirin, if there is no contraindication to aspirin. Then, arrangements can be made for the person to undergo a stress test, provided the person is not having active chest pain. If the cardiac stress test, along with the echocardiogram, suggests the possibility of a coronary occlusive disease, i.e., arteriosclerotic heart disease, then the patient may be referred to a cardiologist for a cardiac catheterization.

In the acute setting, when the patient presents to an emergency room, all of the steps just listed, namely the history, the physical exam, the EKG, and the chest x-ray can be done in an emergency room setting to begin the process of evaluating the patient's symptoms for an acute cardiac event.

In evaluating the patient with chest pain in the ER, a new blood test (troponin-1) can be done. Troponin-1 is a substance that is secreted by heart muscle that has just become damaged. This test becomes elevated within six hours of an acute myocardial infarction, and remains elevated for about two weeks. The troponin-1 is therefore quite sensitive to help the physician pick up an acute myocardial infarction. The normal troponin-1 is 0–0.4NG/ml.

The other blood tests available to assist the physician to ascertain whether the patient has had a myocardial infarction or is having a myocardial infarction are the creatinine phosphokinases, known as CPK, in particular the total CPK and the MB CPK.

In acute heart attack where there is heart muscle damage, the total CPK and MB CPK are elevated. In most laboratories, the normal MB is as high as 4–5%. Most hospital laboratories are set up to do electrophoresis on the CPK MB fraction.

The CPK MB electrophoresis is read as either positive or negative. If it is positive for MB, then you get the total MB level to follow. The first cardiac enzyme to rise when an acute heart attack has occurred is the troponin-1; it rises 1–6 hours after heart muscle damage. Ordinarily the CPK is tested three times during an acute hospitalization for an acute heart attack. Usually the total and MB CPK go up between 12 and 24 hours and start coming back down in about 24–48 hours.

The blood levels of lactic dehydrogenase (LDH) and the (SGOT) Serum Glutamic Pyruvic Transaminase go up after a heart attack. The first enzyme to go up following a heart attack is the troponin-1; follow by the CPK, then the SGOT and then the LDH. The first to go down after a heart attack is the CPK, followed by the SGOT, followed by the LDH and the troponin-1. It usually takes the troponin-1 about two weeks to go down to normal.

Elevated B-type Natriuretic Peptide (BNP) "Myocardial ischemia is a strong trigger of B-type natriuretic peptide (BNP) release. As ischemia precedes necrosis in acute myocardial infarction, we hypothesized that BNP might be useful in the early diagnosis and risk stratification of patients with acute chest pain." Source: The American Journal of Medicine May 2011, Volume 124, and Number 5.

There are classic abnormalities that are seen on the EKG tracing when an acute myocardial infarction is about to occur, or has just occurred, hours before the person presents either to the emergency room or to the doctor's office. What is often seen is what is referred to as coronary insufficiency. The EKG might show what is called inversion of the T-wave on different parts of the EKG along with ST depression. A more classic example is called ST elevation, an elevation of the ST segment of the EKG from the base line.

Physicians are able to map out the circulation of the heart, as it relates to coronary artery, based on the 12-lead EKG. For instance, in a myocardial infarction occurring in the inferior wall of the heart, one expects to see abnormalities in leads 2, 3 and AVF. If it is happening in the lateral wall, then one sees abnormalities in leads 1, AVL and maybe V1, V2. If it is taking place in the anterior wall of the heart, then one can see findings in lead leads V1-V6. The right coronary artery supplies blood and oxygen to the inferior wall of the heart and the left anterior descending coronary artery supplies blood and oxygen to the left part of the heart, etc., etc.

It is very important for a physician to know how to read an EKG properly in order to know if a person is just about to have a heart attack or just had it hours before. This is very important because by infusing tPA (tissue plasminogen activator) in an individual's blood, the clot that is occluding the involved coronary artery causing the myocardial infarction can be dissolved, thereby preventing the heart attack from taking place.

In fact, up to six hours after a heart attack has occurred, if the patient presents to the emergency room, tPA can still dissolve the clot that has caused the heart attack, thereby opening up the vessel and preventing further muscle damage.

Limiting the severity of the heart attack, by infusing tPA can in many instances help to save the life of a patient. Often, the history regarding when the patient started to experience chest pain, shortness of breath, sweating or just severe pressure in the chest, along with the EKG finding, is all that is needed to prevent a heart attack from occurring.

If the EKG findings and history are not consistent with a myocardial infarction, then the person is said to be having angina, unstable angina, or pre-infarction angina or acute myocardial syndrome. A physician is able to determine if a person has had or is having a myocardial infarction, angina, unstable angina, or pre-infarction angina based strictly on the experience and clinical judgment of the physician, along with the findings on the EKG and the cardiac enzyme blood tests.

Every year, a significant percentage of people are admitted to intensive coronary care units complaining of chest pain, which, in fact, were not cardiac-related chest pain or myocardial infarctions. On other hand, many people get sent home because the physicians, either in the emergency rooms or in their offices, saw these people and did not believe they had heart-related chest pain, resulting in them having heart attacks at home and sometimes dying.

The literature amply confirms that blacks and other minorities receive less attention when they present to an emergency room with chest pain compared to their white counterparts. As described above, blacks and other minorities also get referred less often for invasive cardiac tests, such as cardiac catheterization, to determine whether they have coronary occlusive disease to explain their complaints of chest pain.

To underline this issue even more strongly, the recent literature shows that the lifetime risk of heart attacks at age 40 is 1 in 2 for men and 1 in 3 for women. Even as late as age 70, the incidence of coronary artery disease and heart attacks is 1 in 3 for men and 1 in 4 for women.

These statistics are much worse in blacks and other minorities. It is also important to realize that cardiovascular disease is the number one cause of death in blacks and other poor people, and the number one cause of death in the U.S. and in the world.

Several possible scenarios exist when a black person presents to the emergency room with chest pain:

1. Blacks and other minorities may be seen in the emergency room for the complaint of chest pain, evaluated and sent home.
2. Whites may be seen in the emergency room for complaint of chest pain, evaluated and admitted for further evaluation and observation on a telemetry unit.
3. Whites may be seen in the emergency room for chest pain, evaluated and the physician may think that the patients have pre-infarction or unstable angina and are admitted for treatments in the coronary care unit. In this case, he or she will be treated with heparin, aspirin, nitroglycerine, a Beta-blocker and oxygen.
4. In addition, three sets of cardiac enzymes and troponin-1 tests are ordered. An EKG is taken also for three days to be sure that a myocardial infarction has not occurred.

In the setting of number 1 and 2 above, an echocardiogram may be done to rule out other causes of chest pain such as mitral valve prolapsed, myocarditis, pericarditis, etc.

5. A person who presents to the emergency room with chest pain and other symptoms of a heart attack and is found to be having a heart attack by EKG findings and sometimes by the first elevated CPK value or the troponin-1 value will be admitted to the coronary care unit.

6. In the coronary care unit, IV nitroglycerine or nitroglycerine paste will be given.

7. In addition, Beta blocker, angiotensin inhibitor/or angiotensin receptor blocker along with nasal oxygen, Aspirin, pain medication and tPA will be given if there is no contraindication. As mentioned above, in this particular setting, the tPA can be lifesaving in that it can dissolve the clot that is causing the heart attack, thereby allowing blood flow and oxygen to go to the muscle of the heart and preventing further damage. Depending on the clinical circumstances, cardiac catheterization may be carried out.

The clinical scenarios outlined above unfortunately are not always afforded to blacks and other minorities in the U.S. and in the world.

Across the USA in the world blacks and other minorities get worse medical care when they present to emergency rooms with complaints of heart disease than do whites.

Once a myocardial infarction has been ruled out, after three sets of enzymes and an EKG that is unremarkable, then further decision has to be made as to how to proceed in evaluating this person. One common approach is to do a nuclear Adenosine or MIBI stress test, Persantine MIBI test or a stress echocardiogram. If any one of these tests is found to be negative, then the assumption is that the patient does not have severe coronary occlusive disease. That patient is frequently sent home and taken off acute myocardial-type medications such as beta-blockers and nitrates. These tests, although they are excellent, are not 100% full-proofs.

There have been situations when a nuclear imaging test of the heart was normal, and yet the patient went on in a matter of days or weeks to have a heart attack. What can be said is that if the nuclear stress test or the stress echocardiogram is negative, the patient probably does not have major occlusive coronary heart disease.

These stress tests can miss a 30–40% occlusion of a coronary artery. For several reasons, a fissure or crack can occur in a 30–40% plaque inside a coronary artery, causing bleeding and clot formation resulting in closure of that vessel and an acute heart attack.

Human beings carry in their mouths anaerobic bacteria that produce enzymes tha can cause this fissure or crack to occur in a coronary.

It is said that certain species of mycoplasma bacteria can contribute to the development of coronary artery disease. It may be wise to test the blood for the presence of the antibody to mycoplasma. In addition, if the antibody test is positive, then erythromycin can be used to treat these patients. When a person has only a 30–40% occlusion of a coronary vessel, this vessel has not had sufficient time to develop collateral vessels, so when this person suffers an occlusive incident, there are no collateral vessels in the immediate vicinity to protect the affected myocardium and keep it alive.

So, in this setting a 30–40% coronary occlusive disease is worse than an 80% occlusion in that the 80% occlusion has had plenty of time to develop collateral vessels, which can protect the heart muscle in the event of a heart attack to keep the heart muscle alive.

The other scenario is that if the patient continues to have chest pain and yet there is no clear evidence of acute myocardial infarction, then that patient is a candidate to be taken immediately to cardiac catheterization in order to visualize the vessels around the heart, to see if indeed the patient has major coronary occlusive disease. It is not safe to do a stress test on someone who is having active chest pain.

Doing the regular treadmill stress test in evaluating someone for coronary insufficiency has some value, but because it has such a high incidence of false positivity and also such a high incidence of false negativity, it has become less and less appropriate in the setting of acute evaluation of chest pain. Especially in women, there is a very high incidence of false negative treadmill stress test. For that reason, nuclear cardiac imaging has replaced the treadmill stress test.

The regular treadmill stress test is appropriate for a younger individual in the 35-to-40-year-old bracket that is being evaluated to fly planes, or race a car, starting a jogging program or something of that sort.

As just mentioned there are several sensitive stress tests available to evaluate the heart:

1. The MIBI Myoview stress test.
2. IV Persantine or IV Adenosine.
3. IV Dobutamine
4. Resting Thallium distribution stress test.
5. Stress echocardiogram
6. Cardiac PET/CT is a new test that is extremely sensitive in detecting plaques in
7. coronary arteries.

Any one of these tests can be used to evaluate the heart. In certain circumstances, a gated blood pool, known also as MUGA, is done in evaluating the heart.

The Persantine MIBI stress test and Adenosine stress test are suitable for individuals who are able to exercise. Roughly two days prior to having these stress tests, certain medications and certain beverages have to be stopped. Among them are beta-blocker medications to name a few, Tenormin, Atenolol, Metoprolol, Propanolol, Coreg, etc. Some calcium channel blockers need to be stopped as well such as Cardizem, Nifedipine, and Verapamil, etc. Certain medications such as Aminophylline and Theophylline must be stopped. Beverages such as coffee, tea, and any caffeine or decaffeinated beverages also ought to be stopped prior to having these tests done.

The cardiac nuclear department has a long list of things that people cannot do that they distribute prior to having these tests done, so patients know precisely what not to do. This is done because it is important that the heart is able to pump forcefully without interference. The higher the heart rate during exercise, the more stress there is on the heart, and the more stress there is on the heart the better the evaluation of the heart.

Anything that suppresses the contractile effort of the heart has a negative impact on the evaluation of the result of the stress test.

Individuals who are going to have the Persantine stress test also ought to take certain precautions as mentioned above. If the patient is taking Dipyridamole, which is still being used in certain settings, this medication must be stopped before undergoing a Persantine stress test.

The MIBI nuclear stress test or the Adenosine stress test is done in such a way as to be able to tell both angina and/or previous myocardial muscle damage. The Sestamibi test or the thallium test has the same clinical properties as potassium. That being the case, potassium will only be picked up by live heart muscle as a physiological fact.

Taking advantage of this known fact, the physician injects the MIBI substance into the blood of the person being tested, and after it mixes with his or her own blood, this minute nuclear material functions as a tracer in her blood to allow the stress test to be carried out. The entire process is computerized, allowing color pictures of the heart to be taken along with a lot of other important values such as the ejection fraction of the heart.

These nuclear cardiac stress tests enable cardiologists to differentiate between normal heart muscles, scarred heart muscles and heart muscles that are not receiving sufficient blood and oxygen. During the exercise, the area of the heart that is supplied by the plaque-containing coronary artery does not receive sufficient blood and oxygen, resulting in an area of emptiness or lightness compared to the rest of the pictured heart muscles.

Because at rest the oxygen demand is less, that same area when pictured again normalizes; then this is an area of poor blood flow made worse by the stress of the work imposed on the heart, simulating the natural phenomenon referred to as angina or coronary insufficiency. Physicians can, in fact, tell exactly which coronary artery or arteries are diseased with plaques based on the result of the MIBI stress test.

On the other hand, if the abnormal area remains unchanged, both at rest and during exercise when pictured, it means that this person has had a previous myocardial infarction, either known or unknown. The reason that the area remains unchanged, showing an area of defect, is that the muscle that is showing as a defect is scarred and is dead muscle.

Dead tissue cannot pick up potassium, and Sestamibi and thallium have some of the same chemical properties as potassium, as previously mentioned.

Another nuclear stress test that is frequently employed to diagnose occlusive coronary artery disease is the Persantine MIBI stress test. This test is suitable for individuals with infirmities that prevent them from being able to exercise on a treadmill. Some of these individuals are women who suffer from arthritis of the lumbar spine or arthritis of the knees, who are markedly obese, have had a stroke or are somewhat more advanced in age and so are not able to exercise.

The difference between the regular MIBI stress test and the Persantine MIBI stress test is that Persantine is given to the person undergoing the test to dilate the coronary arteries acutely. The acute dilatation causes the heart to beat very fast, resulting in a stressful situation for the heart. The result is the same as exercising on the treadmill to raise the heart rate. Another advantage of the Persantine stress test is that Beta-blockers and calcium channel blocker medications can be continued while the patient is having the test.

The findings discussed under the heading Sesta MIBI stress test are the same as the Persantine stress test and have the same meaning. If the stress MIBI is negative, that is evidence that the man who was tested probably does not have significant occlusive coronary artery disease. This is, however, not always the case; although these stress tests are very sensitive tests, every now and then there can be a false negative test.

If the person continues to have chest pain, then the right thing to do is first to do an abdominal ultrasound to evaluate the gall bladder, because gall bladder disease, such as gallstones, can cause chest pain that is similar to chest pain seen in coronary heart disease. Interestingly, medications such as nitroglycerin, which relieves angina chest pain, can also relieve gall bladder disease pain, confusing the whole situation.

Gall bladder disease due to gallstones is quite common among women, in particular black and other minority women who are 30–40 years old, obese, and fertile.

Blacks and other minorities are more likely to develop obesity and therefore more prone to develop gallstones. In addition, blacks and other minorities are more likely to be carrying abnormal hemoglobins, which predispose them to a higher propensity to the formation of gallbladder disease. They are more likely to form bilirubin stones.

Sickle cell hemoglobin, hemoglobin C, beta thalassemia, alpha thalassemia, and different combinations of these abnormal hemoglobins cause hemolysis, resulting in the formation of bilirubin gallstones. It is the dumping of bilirubin in the bloodstream that ultimately leads to bilirubin gallstones causing gall bladder disease to be so frequently seen in this subgroup of women who suffer from hemolytic anemia of different types.

If the abdominal sonogram is negative, ruling out gallstones, then an upper G.I. series must be done to look for diseases such as hiatal hernia with or without reflux esophagitis or ulcers of different types and degrees in the stomach.

Any one of these can cause chest pain similar to the chest pain caused by coronary artery heart disease. Hiatal hernia with reflux is frequently seen as a cause of severe chest pain. This particular condition is called GERD (gastro-esophageal reflux disease).

Frequently, the physician does not have the luxury of waiting to do an evaluation of the gallbladder or the stomach in a person who is having pain in the chest with a negative stress test. In this case, she must go directly for a coronary angiogram to be certain that coronary artery disease is not the cause of the pain.

It would be rather dangerous to wait to do a prolonged G.I. work-up while the patient is having pain that could be risking the possibility of a heart attack while the patient is waiting for these tests to be done. As just stated, before undertaking this invasive procedure, however, the physician must be sure that all other possible causes of chest pain have been ruled out, including mitral valve prolapsed, which can be seen on an echocardiogram, and a costochondritis, which can be detected on physical examination.

Pulmonary embolism must also be ruled out by doing an ultrasound of the extremities, with D-dimer blood test or by doing a lung scan. Other tests to conduct are the ESR and ANA to rule out inflammatory processes such as myocarditis, pericarditis and pleuritis. A chest x-ray ought to be done to rule out pneumonia, which can also cause chest pain.

If the patient has a fever, then a series of viral blood tests ought to be done to rule out viral disease as a cause of the fever and chest pain.

Costochondritis is a condition that causes pain in the ribs and upper chest wall. When the physician touches these areas with the examining finger, they are tender. Conditions such as arthritis or bursitis of the left or right shoulder with radiating pain down the arm must also be considered.

Chest pain can also be due to cancer of the lung, and therefore a chest x-ray must be done to rule out that possibility.

Many other conditions that can cause chest pain, but the point is that the physician must keep an open mind and properly evaluate for these possibilities before proceeding to more invasive tests to explain the chest pain. It is neither too expensive nor too time consuming to conduct these evaluations.

As just stated, before offering a patient cardiac catheterization, a thorough medical evaluation must first be completed, unless she continues to have chest pain and the clinical impression is that she faces an impending myocardial infarction. In such a case, naturally the physician ought to proceed immediately to do a cardiac catheterization.

Ordinarily, cardiac catheterization for the possibility of coronary occlusive disease is undertaken when a patient has a positive stress test and he/she has failed medical management and the patient is of an age where cardiac catheterization will not be contraindicated. In addition, if the patient has major risk factors such as smoking, hypertension, hyperlipidemia, diabetes mellitus, obesity and a family history of coronary artery disease, in conjunction with the aforementioned factors, then this patient should be offered cardiac catheterization.

If a patient agrees to undergo a cardiac catheterization to determine whether there is an impending myocardial infarction and/or to determine whether the chest pain in question is due to coronary insufficiency, he or she must be given informed consent, to explain the risks and benefits of the procedure.

Cardiac catheterization is a procedure done by highly qualified cardiologists who do this procedure as a subspecialty of cardiology. The procedure is done in a special operating room, which is well equipped with all sorts of modern equipment to provide care for the heart under different circumstances.

A making a large needle-size puncture in the groin, where the femoral artery is located, does the procedure. The area is shaved and properly cleansed with Betadine, and then appropriate local anesthetic is injected in the area. Time is allowed for the anesthetic to take effect, and then a puncture is made with a needle through which a catheter is threaded that goes to the heart, where it can be moved to different parts of its chambers. A dye is then injected through the catheter, which is able to display the coronary arteries around the heart.

A multitude of very important information is obtained during the cardiac catheterization including the displaying of the coronary arteries.

The displaying of the coronary arteries may show evidence of plaques and narrowing in the coronary arteries. If the cardiac catheterization is negative for occlusive coronary disease, it means no gross coronary artery disease is present. Other conditions can cause chest pain that can be seen during cardiac catheterization. Coronary spasm can be seen or induced during cardiac catheterization.

Coronary spasm can cause chest pain and when it occurs acutely, it can cut off blood and oxygen flow to the heart muscle, sometimes resulting in acute myocardial infarction.

Recently, a new condition has been described in which people who suffer from long-time hypertension can develop this type of hypertensive cardiovascular disease with enlargement of the left ventricle and increased end diastolic pressure, suggesting that these people have what is called "small vessels myocardial disease" causing chest pain. Obese people, because of their greater propensity for having hypertension, are quite prone to having this particular condition.

During the cardiac catheterization, abnormalities of the valves of the heart can be discovered. Several other muscular abnormalities of the heart can also be discovered.

After completion of the cardiac catheterization, the results are evaluated and the determination is made as to whether the abnormalities found can explain a person's symptoms. In the case of chest pain, the key finding is coronary artery narrowing due to plaques of different degrees.

Normal and abnormal cardiac catheterization photographs

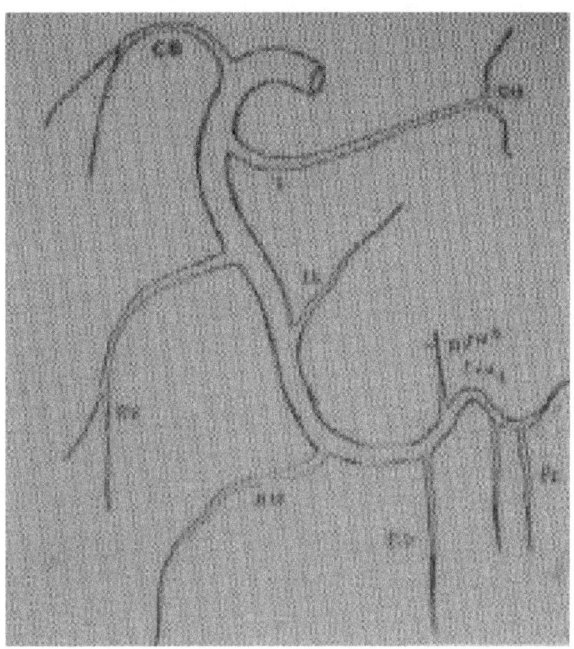

Figure 6:1-A normal coronary artery in a person

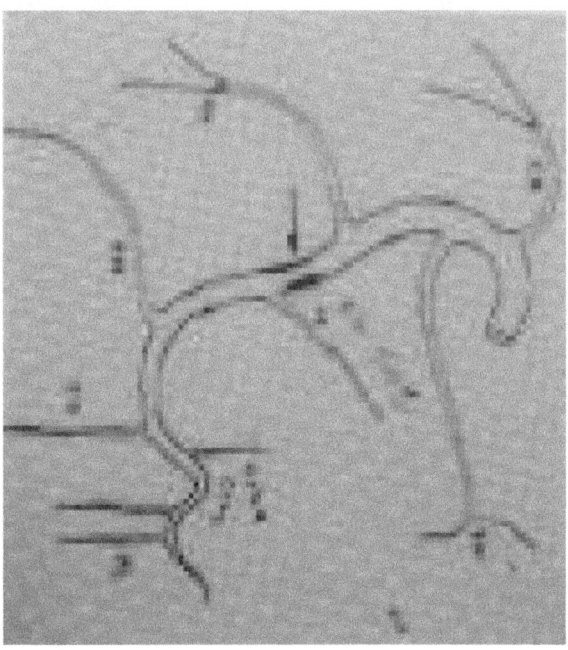

Figure 6:2–Big arrow shows 50–60% occlusion in the mid-portion of a right coronary artery of a person.

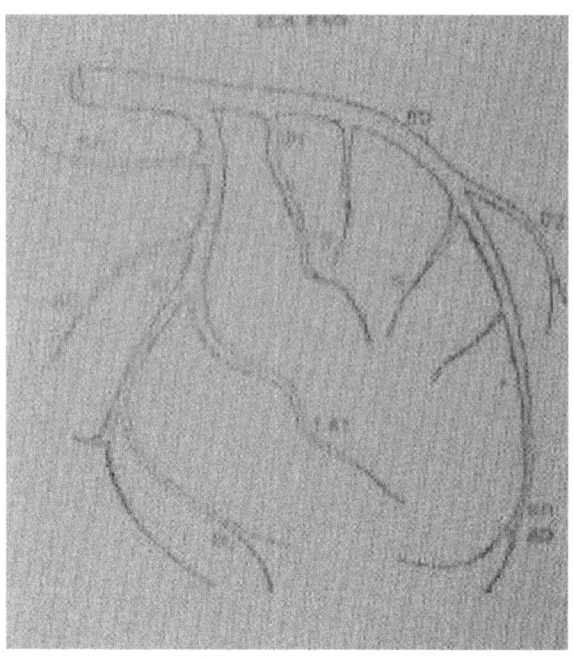

Figure 6:3–*A normal left coronary artery in a person.*

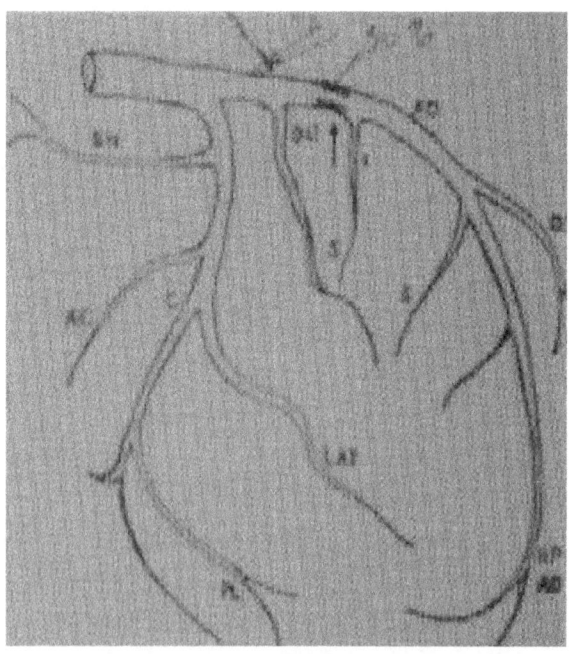

Figure 6:4 *A 50% occlusion of a left anterior descending coronary artery, in patient with both high cholesterol and hypertension.*

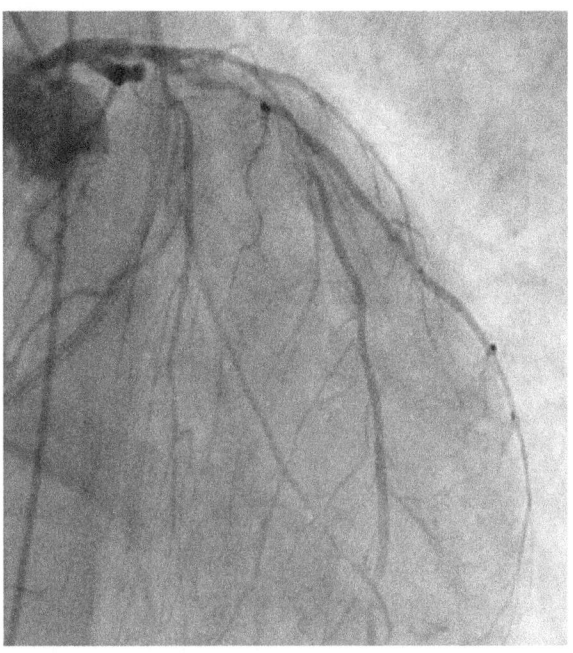

Figure 6:5 *80% Occlusion of the left coronary artery LAD*

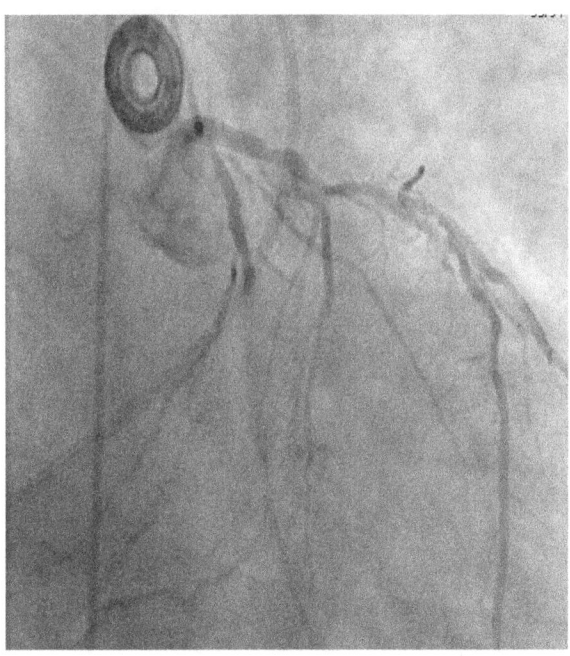

Figure 6:6 *95% Occlusion of the left coronary artery LAD*

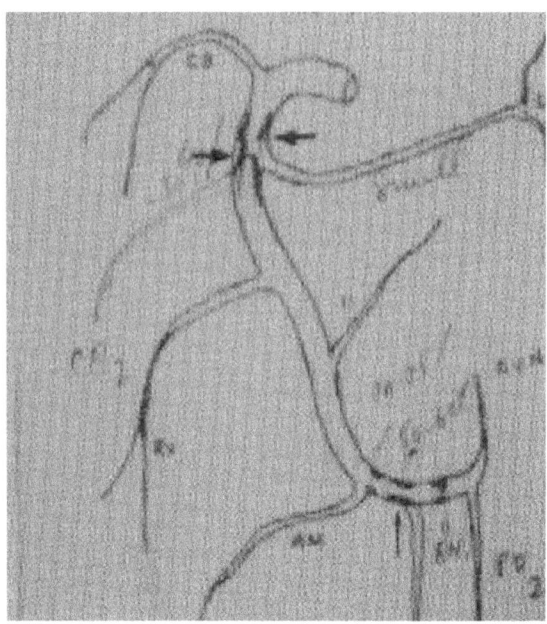

*Figure 6:7–*Big arrow showing 40–50% of the proximal portion of the right coronary artery in a person. Small arrow showing 70–75% occlusion of the distal right coronary artery. This right coronary artery has diffused atherosclerotic changes in other areas.

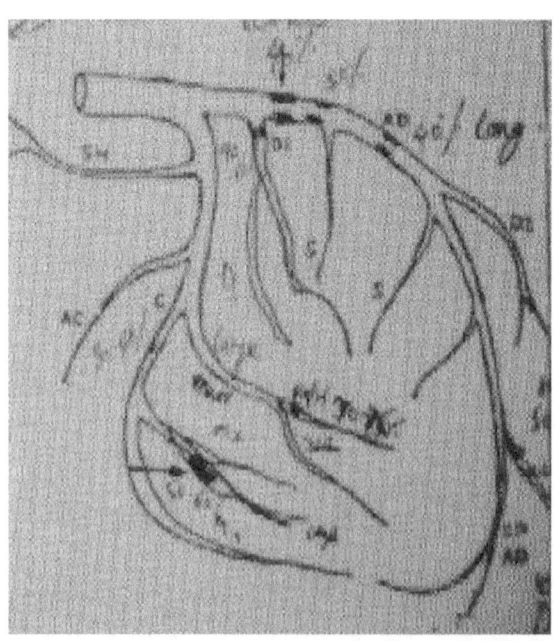

*Figure 6:8–*Small arrow shows 40% occlusion of the proximal left anterior descending artery. There is a 30% occlusion of the LAD in its proximal portion just before the first major septal artery and there is a 40% occlusion in the mid-portion of the LAD. Big arrow shows 50–60% occlusion of the epical diagonal branch of the left coronary artery. There are several areas of diffused atherosclerotic changes involving this left coronary artery. Occlusive changes of coronary arteries in a patient with hypertension and high cholesterol who smokes.

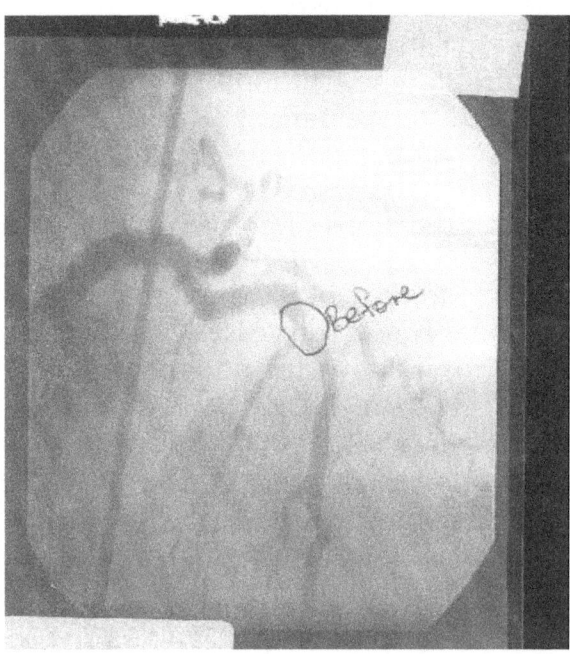

Figure 6:9–Stent placement of narrowed LAD (before) in a patient.

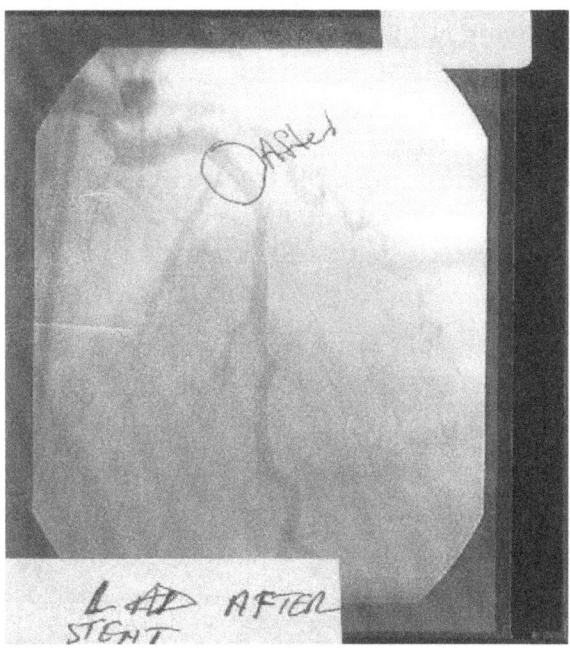

Figure 6:10–Showing how stent placement opens the LAD (after) in a patient.

Based on the findings of the cardiac catheterization just mentioned, recommendations are made as to what course of action to follow. If, for example, the coronary arteries are found to have plaques in them, then the following possibilities exist:

1. The patient can be offered angioplasty.
2. The patient can be offered cardiac bypass.
3. The patient can be offered medications assuming that the disease cannot be approached surgically and/or the patient refuses to have the angioplasty or cardiac catheterization.

There are sometimes contraindications to both angioplasty and cardiac bypass.

Angioplasty is simpler than coronary bypass, but it also has a higher rate of recurrence of disease. The very act of going through the vessels to push aside the plaques can damage the inside of the vessels, creating an area for new plaque formation. Sometimes a stent is placed inside a vessel to try to keep it open, which decreases the possibility of new plaque formation. These patients are frequently placed on anti-platelet medications such as Ticlid or Plavix in conjunction with aspirin to prevent platelet aggregation and closure of the coronary artery. Angioplasty is done in the cardiac catheterization lab and the same cardiologist who performs the cardiac catheterization usually performs it.

On the other hand, coronary bypass requires open-heart surgery which is performed by a heart surgeon. It is considered major surgery; the hospital stay is longer and it costs more money. The success of coronary artery bypass surgery is quite good, though some might say, in the aggregate, that coronary bypass relieves symptoms, but does not prolong life compared to medical management. It has been reported that some people suffer some degree of dementia after coronary bypass surgery, and it is believed that micro-particles that break off from the coronary plaques during surgery lodge into the brain and may be responsible for the dementia.

It is important to stress that after angioplasty or coronary bypass, heart medications are continued for life. The list of medications used in cardiovascular disease is very long. The following is a partial list of different heart medications that are presently in use:

1. Aspirin.
2. Ticlid.
3. Plavix
4. Nitroglycerin
5. Beta-blockers
6. Calcium channel blockers
7. Alpha channel blockers
8. Digitalis
9. Diuretics
10. Aldosterone
11. Angiotesin converting enzyme inhibitor (ACE)
12. Angiotensin ll receptor blocker (ABR)
13. Calcium channel blockers
14. Beta pace

15. Antiarrhythmic such as Lidocaine, Quinidine, Procainamide, Amiodarone IV Vasotec, IV Verapamil, IV Cardizem, Adenosine, etc.
16. Pacemakers also play a major role in the management of patients with heart disease.
17. Sometimes, a pacemaker is used in the setting of an acute myocardial infarction, and sometimes it is used to treat heart blockage of different types to treat sinus disease, or bundle branch blocks.
18. There are special pacemakers that are used to treat arrhythmias of different types and severity. These pacemakers can, on demand, shock the heart to eliminate rhythm abnormalities as they occur, without the patient being aware of what is happening. Moreover, these special pacemakers keep a record for the cardiologist to print out and evaluate management of patients. It is very important for people who are having unexplained cardiac arrhythmias to undergo electrophysiological studies to determine both the source and the cause of the arrhythmia, so that specific and appropriate anti-arrhythmic treatments can be prescribed for the affected patients.

How do these medications work to treat coronary heart disease?

Aspirin, Ticlid, and Plavix work to treat heart disease because these three medications are able to prevent clot formation within the lumen of the vessels around the heart. They do so by preventing platelet clumping, and in so doing they prevent aggregation of platelets, which is necessary for clots to form. Aspirin works both in the prevention of coronary artery disease and in the acute treatment of coronary artery disease.

When a patient presents to the hospital in the process of having a heart attack, if the patient is given two aspirins to chew and swallow, and, added to that, heparin, that patient frequently can lessen the amount of damage that is done to the heart. On top of that, if tPA is injected into the patient within the first hour or so while the patient is about to have a heart attack, a great deal of heart muscle can be spared.

Beta-blockers are a group of medications that are very useful in the treatment of cardiovascular heart disease of different types. Among the most commonly used beta-blockers are the following:

1. Inderal
2. Lopressor
3. Tenormin
4. Toprol XL
5. Coreg
6. Bystolic
7. Betapace etc.

Beta-blockers work to improve the function of the heart via different mechanisms. Beta-blockers have their main effect on the sympathetic system of the body to decrease stimulation of the heart. They also decrease the forcefulness of the pumping of the heart, thereby sparing the need for greater oxygen delivery. Beta-blockers are also anti-arrhythmic and they prevent arrhythmia from occurring. The long-acting beta-blockers in the Lopressor-type family actually cut down on the amount of adrenalin that the body can secrete, and this decreases the incidence of death from myocardial infarction.

This is the reason that long-acting beta blockers are used to protect the heart when a person is sleeping, so that in the early morning hours of the day, when the adrenalin is being secreted in large amounts to prepare the body for the upcoming day's work, protection will continue. By cutting down on the amount of adrenalin that is being secreted, the heart is spared the stimulation from the excess adrenalin, thereby cutting down on the incidence of sudden death.

The harder the heart pumps, the more blood and oxygen are needed to keep up with the needs of the heart muscle and if the vessels around the heart are narrowed by plaques, then that demand cannot be met. So it is in that manner that beta-blockers are effective in the treatment of angina pectoris, also known as chest pain. Beta-blockers also work in another way in the treatment of heart disease; that is, they slow the heart rate or make the heart beat in a regular fashion, thereby preventing what are called cardiac arrhythmias from occurring.

These arrhythmias are frequently the reason that the heart stops after a heart attack or as a result of a complex abnormal rhythm which prevents proper pumping activities of the heart that are needed for sustaining life. In fact, using long-acting beta blockers as just mentioned, especially a dose that has a 24-hour effect on the heart, not only can prevent these abnormalities, but also may in fact prevent heart attacks that frequently occur in the early hours of the morning.

Another group of medications that are frequently used in coronary disease is the nitrates. Nitroglycerin, which is a well-known medication, is in the family of nitrates. Nitrates come in different forms, from sublingual nitroglycerin to nitroglycerin capsules, nitroglycerin patches, nitroglycerin paste, to nitroglycerin liquid that can be used intravenously. Nitroglycerin works to relieve symptoms of angina pectoris by dilating the smooth muscles inside the coronary arteries, allowing for better blood and oxygen flow to go around the heart.

Calcium channel blockers are excellent medications that have multiple uses in the treatment of cardiovascular disease. Calcium channel blockers, such as Nifedipine, Cardizem, Verapamil, Norvasc etc; work to relieve some symptoms associated with coronary artery disease by blocking the effects of calcium to the smooth muscle inside the coronary arteries around the heart.

Calcium is needed for muscle contraction to occur at the cellular level. Muscle contraction is associated with vasoconstriction.

Vasoconstriction means that the inside of the blood vessel becomes narrowed. The narrowing of the blood vessel prevents proper circulation of blood and thereby prevents proper delivery of oxygen to the heart muscles. When oxygen fails to reach the heart muscle in sufficient amount, the result is chest pain. Another important function of calcium channel blockers is to decrease blood pressure. Increase in blood pressure is a major cause of cardiovascular disease.

Calcium channel blockers work to decrease blood pressure by blocking the effect of calcium on the muscle, resulting in relaxation of smooth muscle and that relaxation of smooth muscle causes the blood pressure to come down. In blacks, these medications must be used in combination with diuretics, assuming that the person is not in renal failure, for effective control of blood pressure.

Calcium channel blockers are frequently used to treat cardiac arrhythmias and they are very effective. In particular, Verapamil IV or Cardizem IV is used extensively in the emergency room setting to treat different types of ventricular cardiac dysrhythmias.

CHAPTER 7

CONGESTIVE HEART FAILURE IN AFRICAN AMERICAN MEN

Six million or 2% of people in the U.S. have congestive heart failure.

"African Americans have the highest risk of developing congestive heart failure, followed by Hispanics, Whites, and Chinese Americans (4.6,3.5,2.4 and 1.0 person -years, respectively)." Source: JAMA November 20, 2013 Volume 310, Number 19

"Early onset heart failure before age 50 years was more common among African Americans. Additionally, African Americans with congestive heart failure have a greater 5- year case fatality rate than do whites (51.8%, vs. 41.2% in men and 46.1% vs. 35.8% in women.

Less than 25% of African Americans with congestive heart failure receive guideline-recommended therapy for this disease." Source: JAMA November 20, 2013 Volume 310, Number 19.

Diuretics are very important medications in the treatment of cardiovascular disease. When the heart has been damaged, it frequently fails, and heart failure causes fluid to be accumulated in the lungs, the abdomen, the legs, and the ankles.

The so-called loop diuretics, such as Lasix, Bumex, etc are used to remove the fluid from the body, thereby improving heart function and relieving the symptoms of fluid overload from the body.

Salt plays a major role in causing fluid accumulation in the body; therefore the intake of salt must be curtailed significantly in the treatment of heart failure. Any person, who has chronic congestive heart failure, by definition, has a total body salt that is elevated. The daily salt intake ought not to exceed 1.5 grams per day. By genetics, blacks and Asians retain more salt in their bodies than any other racial groups.

Heart failure can occur because of acute damage to the heart. Heart failure can complicate heart attack and it frequently does. However, heart failure most frequently occurs because of damage that has occurred to the heart due to longstanding hypertension that was either not properly treated or left untreated. Because the muscles of the heart have been stretched to the limit, the heart enlarges and becomes incapable of pumping properly.

Once the heart loses its proper pumping ability then fluid backs up in the body, causing the person to be unable to breathe properly and unable to lie down flat. This person must use several pillows to sleep. Heart failure can also occur because of chronic damage that has occurred to the heart because of multiple previous heart attacks, whereby heart muscles have been damaged, and the scarred muscles lose their ability to pump properly. A combination of an enlarged heart, a condition referred to as Cardiomegaly, and hypertrophy of the muscles of the heart, can result in heart failure.

People with cardiomyopathy and congestive heart failure who eat too much salt in their foods can cause their heart failure to be worse. It is very important to make the point that in the process of using these diuretics to remove fluids from the body, a proper level of potassium must be maintained in order to prevent potassium deficiency, which can cause serious complications to develop.

Potassium must be given by mouth for those who are able to take it by mouth in an outpatient setting and it can be given intravenously when necessary for those who are in the hospital and cannot take it by mouth because they are acutely sick.

The incidence of heart failure is much higher in blacks compared to whites.

Three percent of blacks have congestive heart failure compared to two per cent of whites. In addition, heart failure occurs earlier in blacks compared to whites.

"One in 100 African-American men and women developed heart failure at an average age of 39, 20 times the rate in Caucasians." Source: New England Journal of Medicine Vol 360, March 19, 2009, Number 12.

The higher rate of congestive heart failure seen in blacks is not related to past heart attacks, but is related to the higher incidence of hypertension and diabetes mellitus seen in this sub-group according to an article in the Archive of Internal Medicine, 2008, 168(19):2138-2145.

The death rate from congestive heart failure is also higher in blacks compared to whites. Of the individuals who develop heart failure, 10% die within one year and 50% die within five years. The yearly cost of congestive heart failure, direct and indirect, was 37.2 billion dollars in 2008. Source: 2009 Update, American Heart Association Scientific American Session.

What are the causes of chronic congestive heart failure?

The causes of chronic congestive heart failure include:

1. Hypertension
2. Ischemic heart disease
3. Cardiomyopathy
4. Anemia
5. Myocardial infarction
6. Cardiac arrhythmias

7. Valvular heart disease
8. Bacterial endocarditis
9. Myocarditis
10. Hyperthyroidism (Thyrotoxicosis)
11. Pulmonary embolism
12. Acute intracranial hemorrhage with intracranial pressure
13. Infection with high fever, fast heart rate superimposed on a sick heart
14. Low vitamin D in the body
15. Hypothyroidism

Low vitamin causes congestive heart failure because it allows the Renin Angiotensin Aldosterone System to become activated thereby causing the retention of salt and water resulting in congestive heart failure. Source: Cleveland Clinic Journal of Medicine Volume 77, Number 5, and May 2010.

What are the symptoms of congestive heart failure?

The symptoms of congestive heart failure include:

1. Shortness of breath (dyspnea and orthopnea) left sided heart failure
2. Orthopnea or paroxysmal nocturnal dyspnea (right sided heart failure)
3. Lassitude
4. Irritability
5. Insomnia
6. Chest pain
7. Head ache
8. Restlessness
9. Tiredness
10. Weakness
11. Abdominal pain due to swollen liver
12. Nausea
13. Anorexia
14. Poor memory due to poor blood flow to the brain
15. Head ache

What are the clinical signs of congestive heart failure?

1. Rapid respiration
2. Labored respiration
3. Rapid pulse rate
4. Bulging neck veins
5. Rapid or irregular heart
6. Swollen ankles
7. Swollen legs
8. Swollen abdomen

9. Palpable liver
10. Tender liver to palpation
11. Swollen face
12. Third and fourth heart sounds when listening to the heart with the Stethoscope
13. Rales heard when listening to the lung with the stethoscope
14. Weight gain
15. Using several pillows under the chest to sleep (nocturnal Dyspnea)
16. Raising the head of the bed in order to sleep
17. Jaundice
18. Renal insufficiency (abnormal kidney function)

What is Acute Congestive heart failure? (Pulmonary edema)

Pulmonary edema is an accumulation of fluid in the lungs because of failure of the left side of the heart. As this happens, more blood enters into the pulmonary circulation than can be removed.

What are the causes of cardiac pulmonary edema?

The causes of pulmonary edema include:

1. Acute myocardial infarction (heart attack) resulting in severe muscle damage with heart losing significant pumping ability, thereby causing fluid to back up into the lungs;
2. Acute ischemic episode (angina pectoris) superimposed on an already sick heart;
3. Decompensated chronic congestive heart failure due to too much salt in the diet and/or failure to take prescribed diuretic;
4. Sinus tachycardia (rapid heart rate);
5. Cardiac arrhythmias;
6. Heart blocks;
7. Pulmonary embolism;
8. Acute bacterial endocarditis;
9. Acute rupture of a heart valve;
10. Acute intracranial hemorrhage, etc.

What are the symptoms of pulmonary edema?

The symptoms of pulmonary edema include:

1. Severe dyspnea
2. Severe tachypnea
3. Severe wheezing
4. Diaphoresis - sweating
5. Tachycardia
6. A feeling of doom
7. Cold feeling over the body etc.

What are the clinical and physical signs of pulmonary edema?

The clinical signs of pulmonary edema include:

1. Severe dyspnea (marked shortness of breath)
2. Severe tachypnea (very rapid respiration)
3. Severe diaphoresis (Severe sweating)
4. Marked inability to lie flat
5. Distended neck veins
6. Rapid heart rates or rapid an irregular heart rates
7. Rales and wheezings in both lungs
8. Swollen ankles, legs, abdominal walls and scrotum or groins
9. Chest X-ray evidence of pulmonary edema involving both lungs with fluid in them
10. EKG evidence of acute myocardial infarction
11. EKG evidence of acute ischemia of the heart
12. EKG evidence of complete heart block
13. EKG evidence of rapid atrial fibrillation or other cardiac arrhythmias etc.

Recommended methods of treating pulmonary edema include the following:

1. IV Lasix
2. 100% oxygen via re-breather mask
3. IV digitalis if there is no bradycardia or significant AV heart block
4. Application of nitro paste to chest wall or IV nitroglycerin (if the blood pressure is normal)
5. Administer Dobutrex or Dopamine in drip form if the patient is hypotensive
6. Administer IV Lopressor if the patient's pulse is not too low or there is no significant AV heart block
7. Administer IV Vasotec or an ARBs if the blood pressure is not to low
8. Administer IV nitroglycerine if the patient is having chest pain
9. Adminsiter IV morphine
10. Insert a Foley catheter to monitor urine output
11. Monitor oxygen saturation
12. Monitor serial portable chest x-ray
13. Continue treatment as per chronic congestive heart failure once the acute pulmonary edema is brought under control

How do physicians diagnose chronic congestive heart failure?

To diagnose congestive heart failure, conduct the following examinations:

1. History of shortness of breath by the patient
2. History of swollen ankles by the patient
3. History of needing several pillows to sleep
4. History of recurrent coughing when lying down

5. History of difficulty breathing when walking upstairs
6. Enlarged heart seen on chest x-ray with the presence of fluid in the lungs
7. Abnormal left ventricular function seen on Echocardiogram
8. Low Ejection Fraction on Echocardiogram, Rest Muga or Nuclear stress test
9. The presence of S3, S4 gallop on listening to heart using the stethoscope
10. Rales heard on listening to the lungs using the stethoscope
11. Elevated Beta naturatic peptide BNP
12. Swollen ankles
13. Swollen abdomen
14. Swollen abdomen
15. CBC
16. Complete metabolic blood chemistry profile
17. T4
18. TSH
19. EKG
20. Troponin 1
21. CPK
22. ABG
23. Chest-xray
24. Echocardiogram etc.

How to treat congestive heart failure

1. Lasix IV or by mouth
2. Bumex IV
3. Aldactone
4. Beta Blocker such as Coreg, Lopressor, Toprol XL, Tenormin etc;
5. Nitro paste on the chest wall or IV nitroglycerin
6. Digitalis IV or by mouth if the heart is enlarged
7. Nasal oxygen
8. Low salt diet
9. Daily weight when in the hospital
10. Isosorbide
11. Hydralazine
12. BiDil is said to be effective in the treatment of congestive heart failure in blacks This is a controversial issue because although this medication works to treat congestive heart failure, it is a good medication in all-racial groups to treat heart failure. The research was to done on this medication only in Negroes/Blacks. No white, no Asians, and no Hispanic patients were included and treated with BiDil during the research. However, BiDil works very well in both men and women and in all racial groups.

The two most important medications in BiDil namely hypresoline and isosorbide have been used in the treatment of patients with congestive heart failure for many years individually and in combination in some settings.

How does BiDil work to treat congestive heart failure?

BiDil works to treat congestive heart failure by Isosorbide one of the two medications in BiDil is a vasodilator, which on the venous system causes venous dilation and it also causes the release of nitric oxide which in turn activates guanylyl cyclase resulting in relaxation of the vascular smooth muscle.

Hydralazine, the other medication in BiDil is an arterial smooth muscle dilator; it also prevents the degradation of nitric oxide. It is saitd that blacks have lower level of nitric oxide than whites do. BiDil works to treat congestive heart failure in all patients with congestive heart failure, without regards to race. Medications that cause vasodilatation help to ease the load off the heart and help to perfuse the kidneys allowing for increase urine excretion, which is essential in the treatment of congestive heart failure.

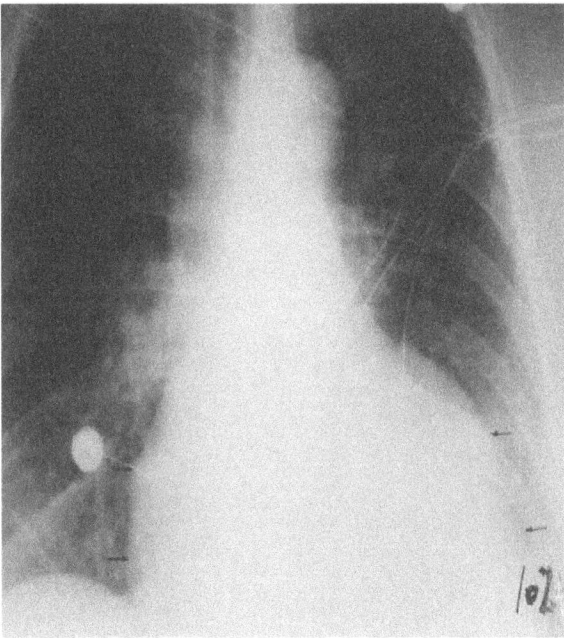

Figure 7:1 Chest x-ray of a patient with ischemic myocardial disease with associated congestive heart failure.

Digitalis is a medication that has been around for many years and it still is a very effective medication in the treatment of cardiovascular disease. If the heart is enlarged, the ejection fraction is low, and the person has congestive heart failure, digitalis is quite effective in helping the heart to pump well and thereby relieving the symptoms of congestive heart failure.

If the rhythm of the heart is irregular, such as in atrial fibrillation, digitalis is the drugs that can be used to regulate the heart rhythm. Digitalis has other uses also in the treatment of coronary heart disease, such as in the treatment of paroxysmal atrial tachycardia, and it is quite effective when used for that particular condition.

Other medications that are very important in the treatment of congestive heart failure include Betablockers, Angiotensin converting enzyme inhibitors, Angiotensin ll receptor blockers, Aldactone, Lasix, Bumex etc.

Medications in use to treat congestive heart failure are:

Lasix
Bumex
Torsemide
Aldactone
Cozaar
Diovan
Avapro
Atacand
Benicar
Micardis
Entresto (sacubitril/Valsartan 40mg/15 PO BID up to 97mg/103mg)
Teveten
Zestril
Capoten
Vasotec
Altace
Lopressor
Coreg
Toprol XL
Bystolic
Sectral
Tenormin
Kerlone
Zebetal
Brevibloc
Hydralazine
Nitropaste
Isosorbide
Nitro-Dur etc.

Cardiovascular diseases require a multitude of different medications, frequently used in combination in order to make the heart function properly.

Another common technique that is frequently used to help the heart to function better is the insertion of a pacemaker. Pacemakers are inserted for different reasons. Clinically when a man has sick sinus disease, that is when the area of the heart where the electrical system is located has become degenerated and a person develops heart block, a pacemaker has to be inserted in order to take over the proper electrical functioning of the heart. Heart block occurs usually in the aged or because of an acute myocardial infarction. Pacemakers are used in different sets of circumstances in different age groups for different reasons.

Some of the reasons for which a pace maker may be inserted are

1. Third degree AV block
2. Symptomatic left ventricular block
3. Symptomatic Right ventricular
4. Symptomatic bifascicular block

It is important to realize that the pacemaker, once inserted, must be tested periodically to assure that it is functioning properly. The pacemaker can be tested, even if the man in whose heart the pacemaker is inserted is away in a foreign country. It can be tested using a telephone. It is very important to realize that these things are being modified frequently and the technology has improved remarkably in the last few years. Pacemakers can do wonders to keep people alive who have different types of cardiovascular disease. Insertion of a mechanical pump is being frequently used in the treatment of medications resistant congestive heart failure with great success.

CHAPTER 8

CARDIAC ARRHYTHMIAS IN AFRICAN AMERICAN MEN

Another common problem that individuals with cardiovascular disease have to deal with is cardiac arrhythmias.

Some of the most common cardiac arrhythmias are:

1. Sinus tachycardia
2. Atrial fibrillation ("There are 35.5 million cases of atrial fibrillation globally and the annual incidence of AF is 5 million per year" and 2.5 million cases of AF in the U.S. every year. AF is the most common arrhythmia.
3. Atrial flutter
4. Premature ventricular contraction (VPC's)
5. Premature atrial contraction (APC's)
6. Paroxysmal supraventricular tachycardia
7. Ventricular tachycardia (V Tach)
8. Ventricular fibrillation

What are the most common causes of cardiac arrhythmias?
The most common causes of cardiac arrhythmias are

1. Atherosclerotic heart disease
2. Myocardial infarction
3. Cardiomyopathy
4. Congestive heart failure
5. Ischemic valvular heart disease
6. Congenital heart disease
7. Pulmonary embolism
8. Hyperthyroidism etc.

How to diagnose cardiac arrhythmias?

1. Patient's history of irregular heart beats
2. Examination of the heart using the stethoscope
3. 12 lead EKG

4. 24 hour Holter monitor
5. Monitoring the patient's heart rhythm on telemetry in the hospital
6. Echocardiogram
7. Nuclear cardiac stress test
8. Thyroid blood tests etc.

How to treat cardiac arrhythmias?

Each arrhythmia is treated differently and according to the underline heart disease

The different medications used to treat cardiac arrhythmias are:

1. Lidocaine
2. Tocainide
3. Digitalis
4. Quinidine
5. Procainamide
6. Amiodarone
7. Dronedarone (Multag)
8. Beta -blockers
9. Adenosine
10. Verapamil
11. Diltiazem
12. Vasotec
13. Aspirin
14. Coumadin
15. Heparin
16. Lovenox
17. Pradaxa
18. Elequis
19. Xarelto
20. Plavix etc;

Severe and life threatening ventricular arrhythmias are treated with implantable cardio ventricular defibrillation (ICD) Atrial fibrillation must be treated with Coumadin, Lovenox, Pradaxa, or aspirin long term to prevent the development of stroke.

Another aspect of cardiovascular disease, which ought to be mentioned, is heart valve replacement. The different valves of the heart can get damaged because of infection and because of the aging process. The heart valves can also get damaged because of congenital problems. In any event, cardiac valve replacement is being done all over the country and all over the world.

Cardiovascular surgeons are using different materials; some of them are prosthetic materials to replace heart valves to make the heart function better. Sometimes, acutely, in the process of a heart attack, a man's heart valve can become damaged and the result can be acute heart failure.

The acute heart muscle damage that occurs when a man suffers a heart attack can also cause acute congestive heart failure to develop. Cardiac catheterization can be done to document which coronary artery vessel or vessels is or occluded to have caused the heart attack and which heart valve if any is damaged by the acute myocardial infarction.

Following cardiac catheterization, angioplasty, bypass surgery with or without valve replacement may be carried out, depending on the particular clinical situation. The chordae tendineae are little strands cordlike structures that keep the heart valves together. They can become ischemic resulting in damages. They can also get damaged because of a heart attack, the aging process. When the chordae tendineae are ruptured, frequently acute heart failure develops.

One of the most common symptoms of sick sinus disease is dizziness, tiredness and a general feeling of unwellness and, fainting spells. A person may at times, actually lose consciousness. That happens because the person's pulse has become too slow, sometimes less than 30 beats per minute, so that the heart cannot pump enough blood to the brain, resulting in the loss of consciousness or blackout spells.

On EKG, different degrees of heart block can be seen to explain the person's symptoms. Third-degree heart block is the heart block most associated with the symptom complex just outlined. In the acute setting, the cardiologist can insert a temporary pacemaker to try to get the patient through the acute period. Sometimes, these patients will need a permanent pacemaker and sometimes they will not. As their hearts recover, the problem that causes the slow pulse may resolve itself and then the pacemaker may not be needed.

That usually occurs as part of an acute heart attack. In the setting of sick sinus disease and third-degree heart block, a permanent pacemaker is inserted by a chest surgeon. Sometimes, in an acute setting, the so-called bundle branch block can occur, and that bundle branch block can necessitate the insertion of a permanent pacemaker.

Be that as it may, if a person has a slow heart rate, a condition referred to as bradycardia, and the heart cannot pump well enough to perfuse the brain, it is very important that a temporary pacemaker be put in, in order to allow for better cardiovascular function.

Another common cause of severe bradycardia is elderly people on Beta-Blocker containing eye drops for the treatment of glaucoma. These medications can slow their heart rates. Beta-Blockers are used to treat various medical conditions. This combination of medications frequently leads to life threatening bradycardia that can cause congestive heart failure and syncope, because of the inability of the heart to pump forcefully to prevent fluid accumulation in the lungs.

CHAPTER 9

INFECTIONS OF THE HEART IN AFRICAN AMERICAN MEN

A problem that affects the heart quite often is infection:

The different infections that can affect the heart are

1. Infective endocarditis
2. Myocarditis
3. Pericarditis

What is endocarditis?

Endocarditis is when a heart valve becomes infected with a microorganism.

1. There are three different types of infective endocarditis.
2. Native valve endocarditis
3. Prosthetic valve endocarditis
4. Intravenous drug addicts endocarditis

The most bacteria that cause endocarditis in native valve endocarditis are Streptococci, Enterococci, Staphylococci, and many gram negative, as well as different fungi. The different types of native heart valves that that become infected in endocarditis are

1. Normal heart valve
2. Congenital heart valve
3. Degenerative heart valve
4. Rheumatic heart valve

The mechanism through which endocarditis develops is different in different heart valves and in different clinical settings. In an individual with normal heart vale, infective endocarditis can occur, and if the individual becomes either bacteremic or septic (bacteria circulating in the blood stream) and the bacteria settle on the heart valve leading to either sub-acute or acute bacterial endocarditis.

In congenital bacterial endocarditis the same situation exists as above, except that in this instance, the abnormal valve makes it easier for bacteria that are circulating in the blood to get trapped on causing endocarditis. The same situation occurs in degenerative heart valve and rheumatic heart valve.

Prosthetic valve endocarditis is responsible for about 20% of all cases of infectious endocarditis. Most of the individuals in this category are patients 60 years of age or older.

The different microorganisms that cause prosthetic endocarditis are Staphylococci epidermidis, Staphylococcus Aureus, gram-negative bacteria, and fungi.

Prosthetic endocarditis can develop 1 year, 2 years or many years after the prosthetic valves were placed. Bacterial endocarditis in intravenous drug addicts occurs usually on normal heart valves most of the time and in young adults.

The skin is the usual site of entry and the valves most frequently affected are tricuspid valve 52% of the time, the aortic is involved 25% of the time, the mitral valve is involved 20% of the time and 3% of the time, multiple valves are involved.

The microorganisms most often involved in causing infectious endocarditis are Staphylococci, Streptococci, Enterococci, Gram -negative bacteria, and fungi such as Candida and aspergillus.

The symptoms and clinical signs of endocarditis are:

1. Fever
2. Chills
3. Joints pain
4. Muscle pain
5. Heart murmur
6. Enlarged Spleen
7. Headache
8. Weakness

Skin lesions such as Janeway lesions, Roth's spots and Osier's nodes, splinter hemorrhages that can be seen in endocarditis.

Abnormal blood tests findings frequently seen in infectious endocarditis are:

1. Elevated white blood cell count
2. Low red blood cell count
3. Low platelets count
4. The Prothrombin time may be high which may indicate Desseminated intravascular coagulopathy (DIC)
5. There maybe red blood cells in the urine, due to emboli to the kidneys from the heart valves

6. There is protein in the urine
7. The erythrocyte sedimentation rate is quite high
8. The blood cultures are positive growing the responsible bacteria
9. The serum BUN and creatinine are usually high due to emboli and immune complexes to the kidneys
10. The rheumatoid factor is frequently positive
11. There may be circulating immune complexes
12. Serum Complement is usually is decreased
13. Elevated C-reactive protein

The cardiology tests that may be abnormal in infectious are:

1. Echocardiogram may show vegetation on heart valve or abscesses in the heart muscle
2. In addition, cardiac arrhythmias may develop
3. Myocarditis and pericarditis may develop
4. 24 hour Holter monitor
5. Cardiac Telemetry monitoring
6. Echocardiogram
7. Transesophageal echocardiogram (TEE)
8. Transthoracic echocardiogram (TTE)

The following are the different antibiotics that used to treat bacterial endocarditis

1. Penicillin G
2. Vancomycin
3. Cubicin
4. Ceftriaxone
5. Nafcillin
6. Gentamicin
7. Ceftazidime
8. Piperacillin
9. Cefotaxime
10. Levaquin
11. Ciprofloxacin
12. Erythromycin
13. Zoszyn
14. Xyvox etc;

These different antibiotics are used in different dosages based on the patient's sizes, ages and renal function and clinical settings for 6-8weeks IV.

Individuals who are at risks to develop endocarditis because of valvular heart diseases or heart murmurs of different types and in individuals who have received prosthetic implants such as heart valves and hip prostheses etc, of one kind or an other, the following antibiotics are used prophylactically when invasive procedures are being done in the body of the affected person.

The invasive procedures that require prophylactic antibiotics are:

1. **Intra-vaginal and intra-pelvis surgical procedures**
2. **Any intra-abdominal surgical procedures**
3. **Intraoral procedures of any kind**
4. **Any serious skin infection**
5. **Before colonoscopy etc;**

Antibiotic prophylaxis is recommended for before invasive procedure and the following antibiotics are recommended.

Erythromycin by mouth or IV
Amoxicillin by mouth or IV
Ceftriaxone IM or IV
Vancomycin IV
Cleocin by moth or IV

If acute bacterial endocarditis develops, a cardiothoracic surgeon must be brought to take the patient to operating room to replace the damaged heart vale. In addition, if it is discovered that on either TEE or echocardiogram that there is vegetation on the heart vale or abscesses on the heart muscle, a cardiothoracic surgeon must be brought in to surgically remove the infected part of the heart vale or muscle to save the patient's life and to prevent infected emboli from being thrown to multiple organs in the body.

Two other significant infectious conditions frequently affect the human heart and they are:

Infectious myocarditis
Infectious pericarditis.

Infectious myocarditis develops when a microorganism infects the muscles of the heart. The most common bacteria are Staphylococcus aureus, Streptococcus and Enterococcus, Staph epedipermidis, Pseudomonas, Proteus, E Coli, Klebsellia pneumonia, etc.

The most common viruses that cause infection of the myocardium is coxsackieviruses, Influenza virus, the AIDS virus can also cause myocarditis. Lyme disease can also affect the myocardium of the heart causing myocarditis etc.

The symptoms of myocarditis are:

1. Chest pain
2. Shortness of breath
3. Irregular heart beats
4. Tiredness etc.
5. Although the physical examination is frequently normal, signs of CHF and irregular Cardiac rhythm can be heard
6. Heart murmur

The EKG findings may be similar to that seen when the person is having an acute myocardial infarction.

The cardiac enzymes such as the CPK, LDH, and SGOT might be elevated as well. The erythrocytes sedimentation rate is usually elevated.

The test that are used to diagnose myocarditis are:

1. **CBC**
2. **SMA 20 and cardiac enzymes**
3. **ERS**
4. **ANA, rheumatoid factor, double stranded DNA to rule out collagen vascular diseases such as Lupus or Rheumatoid arthritis as a possible cause of the myocarditis**
5. **Blood cultures**
6. **Urine analysis**
7. **Viral titers for coxsackievirus B**
8. **Lyme disease blood tests**
9. **HIV blood test**
10. **Chest x-ray**
11. **EKG**
12. **24 hour cardiac monitoring**
13. **Echocardiogram**
14. **Myocardial biopsy when appropriate**

The treatment of myocarditis is based on the clinical profile and presentation of the affected individual and the best judgment of the treating physician.

At presentation, the patient ought to be treated with broadspectrum antibiotics that cover both for gram positive and gram negative bacteria. When bacterial myocarditis is ruled out, then other treatment modality may be considered based on viral titers or collagen vascular test results, such as the ANA, or Rheumatoid factor or other blood tests for Lupus etc. Supportive care with bed rest, nasal oxygen, pain medication, and antipyretics to control fever needs to be provided.

Infectious pericarditis is a condition that occurs when the pericardium becomes infected by microorganism such as bacteria, virus, or a fungus.

Although any microorganism can cause infection in the pericardial sac of the heart if it were to find its way there, the most common bacteria that cause acute infectious pericarditis are:

1. **Streptococcus**
2. **Pneumococcus**
3. **Staphylococcus**
4. **Tuberculous etc.**

The most common viruses that cause acute pericarditis are:

1. **Coxsackievirus A**
2. **Coxsackievirus B**
3. **Adenovirus**
4. **Hepatitis viruses**
5. **HIV /AIDS etc.**

The most common fungi that cause acute pericarditis are:

1. **Candida**
2. **Histoplasma**
3. **Blastoplasma**
4. **Coccidiomycosis**

The most common symptoms of acute infectious peircarditis are:

1. **Chest pain that is made worst by coughing**
2. **Chest pain that is made worst by lying in a supine position**
3. **Chest pain that is made worst by taking a deep breath**
4. **Chest pain that is relieved by leaning forward**
5. **Chest pain that is relieved by sitting up**

The clinical findings of pericarditis on physical examination are:

1. **Distant heart sounds**
2. **Pericardial friction rub**
3. **Irregular heart sounds may be heard secondary to different rhythm abnormalities that may develop because of the infection.**

Many .different abnormal findings may be seen on EKG, chest x-ray, in blood tests and echocardiogram in infectious pericarditis.

The most common tests done to diagnose infectious pericarditis are:

1. CBC and blood cultures
2. ESR
3. SMA20
4. Cardiac enzymes
5. Viral titers for Coxsackieviruses A and B
6. Adenovirus titer
7. Hepatitis A, B, and C
8. HIV virus blood test
9. Histoplasma titer
10. Blastoplasma titer
11. Coccidiomycosis titer

12. Blood for Candida culture
13. Pericardial tap and biopsy to obtain specimens for these different cultures including gram stain and AFB stain and culture for mycobacterium tuberculosis
14. Blood test for syphilis (VDRL)
15. EKG
16. Echocardiogram
17. Cardiac Telemetry monitoring
18. Chest x-ray etc.
19. A complete collagen vascular blood profile must always be drawn and sent to the laboratory such as ANA, Rheumatoid factor, double stranded DNA and Blood for Angiotensin -1-Coverting Enzyme ought to be sent to the laboratory as well to rule out the possibility of sarcoidosis as the cause of the pericarditis.

The treatments of infectious pericarditis include:

1. Broad spectrum antibiotics covering for both gram negative and gram positive bacteria pending the results of blood cultures, pericardia fluid, and pericardial biopsy if one was done.
2. Anti fungal IV Amphotericin B if there is a strong suspicion of fungal infection and or if the patient is immunosuppressed.
3. Nasal oxygen
4. Antipyretics to control fever
5. Bed rest and general supportive care

In infectious percarditis, pericardial fluid can build up inside the pericardial sac resulting in pericardiac temponade. If pericardial temponade develops in a patient, if it can cause sudden death.

The best way to diagnose pericardial is physical examination and echocardiogram; the best way to treat pericardial temponade is surgical intervention by a cardiothoracic surgeon.

Infectious pericarditis can develop into chronic as well as constrictive pericarditis, which can be markedly debilitating to affected individuals.

Pericarditis can be caused by:

1. Trauma
2. Acute myocardial infarction,
3. Lupus,
4. Rheumatoid
5. Arthritis
6. Cancer
7. Kidney failure
8. Hypothyroidism with myxedema and many more.

The following measures can help to lessen the incidence of cardiovascular heart disease in blacks:

1. Eat a low-fat, low-carbohydrate, low-salt, and high-protein diet to prevent weight gain.
2. Exercise regularly.
3. Visit the doctor frequently to have the blood pressure checked, so that hypertension can be detected and properly treated.
4. Take chest pain seriously and have it evaluated with an EKG and a stress test.
5. Stop smoking.
6. Don't abuse alcohol.
7. If diabetic, lose weight and control the blood sugar tightly.

If a person has family members who suffer from heart disease, it is very important that he or she mentions that to his or her physician, so that that fact can be entered into the clinical equation to ensure that he is properly evaluated to detect the existence of heart disease.

The incidence of coronary heart disease in and the incidence of deaths from coronary heart diseases in blacks are several times higher in blacks than in whites. The reasons for this blatant health disparity in blacks in the U.S. have its root cause in racial discrimination. Racism against blacks in the U.S. leads to wide spread poor education, low economic status, poverty, and poor education.

In addition, racism causes minorities to experience stress, poor diet, obesity, hypertension, diabetes mellitus, coronary heart disease, stroke, kidney failure, AIDS, depression, alcoholism, high infant mortality, high prenatal maternal death rates, drug addiction, high crime rates, high homicide rates in black Americans against black Americans, high suicide rates, low self esteem and over all poor health, and lower life expectancy.

America is the greatest country in the world, and if a cure can be found for the disease of racism against blacks and other minorities, millions of unproductive black American and other minority citizens can be put to work and the general economic situations of black Americans and other minorities would improve almost over night and in the process, the overall U.S. economy would improve as well.

The billion of dollars being spent by the Federal government and states governments every year to pay for Medicaid, food stamps and a multitude of other programs would no longer be necessary because poor folks who are receiving these benefits would be fully employed and paying taxes which would help to solve their economic problems in the U.S. and in the world.

Understanding these facts and paying close attention to them, would help poor folks to turn around their negative experiences brought on in part by racial discrimination and become positive about themselves.

The negative effects of racism against blacks and other minorities can be turned around in a positive direction if white people and other ethnic groups would make the necessary efforts to get to know black people other minorities and their cultures. This would be a motivating experience for blacks and other minorities to become successful human beings and in so doing, the high incidence and death rates from coronary heart disease and other deadly diseases that they are suffering from would decrease accordingly.

CHAPTER 10

CANCER IN AFRICAN AMERICAN MEN

As of 2017, there are 324,310,011 people in the U.S. population and according to the Census bureau.

In 2017, the total U.S. is 326,474, 013

There are 256.0 millions Whites, 45,8 millions Blacks, 57, 5 milloins Hispanics, 21.4 millions Asians, 6.7 and millions Native Americans/Alaska Navites and Native Hawaiian and other Pacific Islanders 1.5 million in the U.S, in 2017 Source: U.S. Census Bureau 2017

The world population in 2017 is 7,484,325, 476

In 2017, there are 1,688,780 new cancers cases in the U.S. and about 14 million people are diagnosed with cancer annually in the world. Sources: ACS Facts and Figures 2017 and WHO

In 2017, 600,920 people are expected to die of cancer in the U.S. and 8.2 million people are expected to die from caner in the world. Sources: ACS, Facts and Figures 2017 and WHO.

The number of cancer survivors in the United States, currently estimated to be 15.5 million would grow to almost 20 million in 2026." Source: ACS cancer facts and statistics 2017.

The leading cancers that kill people in the world are:

Lung 1.59 million deaths
Liver 745, 000 deaths (due to hepatitis B and C)
Stomach 723,000 deaths
Colorectal 694,000 deaths
Breast 521,000
Esophageal cancer 400,000 deaths Source: WHO

The incidence of cancer worldwide will rise by 57% in 20 years. 1 in 5 men and 1 in 6 women will have cancer in the world. Source: WHO

"Racial disparities in lung cancer rates still exist in the U.S." According to the CDC, "The highest incidence rates of lung cancer diagnosis annually were observed among blacks

76.1 Among blacks
69.7 Among whites
48.4 Among American Indians or Alaska Natives
38.4 Among Asians or Pacific Islanders
37.3 Among Hispanics
71.9 Among non-Hispanics "(Source: HemOnc today: December 10, 2010)

The most common cancers in males in the U.S. in 2016 were:

Prostate 161,360 (19%)
Lung & broncus 116,990 (14%)
Colorectal 71,420 (9%)
Kidney & renal pelvis 40,610 (5%)
Urinary bladder 60,490 (7%)
Pancreas 27,970
Liver & intrahepatic bileb duct 29,200 (3%)
Head and neck 35,720 (4%)
Non-Hodgkin lymphoma Non-Hodgkin lymphoma 40,080 (5%)
Leukemia 36,290 (4%)
Melanoma of skin 52,170 (6%)
All sites 836,150 ACS Cancer Facts & figures 2017

The most common cancers in Black males in the U.S. in 2016 were:

Prostate 29,530 (31%)
Lung & bronchus 13,720 (15%)
Colorectal 8,690 (9%)
Kidney and renal pwelvis 4,830 (5%)
Liver & intrahepatic 4, 250 (5%)
Non-Hodgkin lymphoma 3,230 (3%)
Pancreas 3,210 (3%)
Myeloma 3,070 (3%)
Urinary bladder 2,910 (3%)
Leukemia 2,840 (3%)
All sites 93,990
ACS Facts and Figures 2017

The most common cancer deaths in males in the U.S. in 2016 were:

Lung & bronchus 84,590 (27%)
Colrectal 27,150 (9%)
Prostate 26,730 (8%)
Pancreas 22,300 (7%)
Liver & liver intrahepatic bile duct 19,610 (6%)
Leukemia 14,300 (4%)
Esophagus 12,720 (4%)

Urinary bladder 12,240 (4%)
Non-Hodgkin lymphoma11, 450 (4%)
Brain & other nervous system 9,620 (3%)
All sites 318,420 ACS Facts and Figures 2017

The most common cancer deaths in Black males in the U.S. in 2016 were:

Lung and bronchus 9,710 (27%)
Prostate 4,450 (12%)
Colonrectal 3,800 (11%)
Liver & intrahepatic bile duct 2,880 (8%)
Pancreas 2,390 (7%)
Stomach 1,160 (3%)
Leukemia 1,110 (3%)
Myeloma 1,040 (3%)
Esophgus 920 (3%)
Kidney & renal pelvis 860 (2%)
All sites 35,660 ACS Facts and Figures 2017

Although the overall cancer deaths have gone down in the U.S., the cancer death rates in Blacks in the U.S. have going up to 15% according to some reports.

Significant disparity exists in both the rate of cancer in black men in the U.S. and deaths from cancer in the U.S.

At the core of these disparities in both the development of cancer and the death rates in black males VS whites are racial discrimination, which leads to poverty, ecocomic inequality, poor education, poor diet, obesity, lack of health insurance and poor medical care, all of which result higher incidence of colon cancer, prostate cancer, cancer of the pancreas, head and neck cancer, cancer of the esophagus, multiple myeloma, leukemia and higher deaths from these cancers

Overall, according to figures published by the American Cancer Society, the death rate for cancer of all types is 33% higher in black males and 16% higher in black females as compared to white males and females in the U.S. These astonishingly high figures further demonstrate the large health disparity that exists among blacks vs. whites in both diagnosis and treatments of cancer in the U.S. Cancer is the second leading cause of deaths in the United States next to cardiovascular heart diseases.

What is cancer?

Cancer develops when a cell loses its ability to grow and multiply in a normal growth pattern. A good example of this is contact inhibition. When a normal cell is placed in contact with a hard surface in a Petri dish, the normal cell stops growing.

However, in the case of an abnormal cell, it continues to grow because it has lost its contact inhibition ability, which allows it to grow uncontrollably, developing into a cancer growth.

The cancer cells fail in the process of cell-to-cell interactions. The development of cancer is a multi-step and multi-factorial process. In the multi-step and multi-factorial processes, there is normally a balance between growth-promoting genes (proteins) and growth-suppressive genes (proteins). Once mutation occurs for one reason or another, the growth-promoting genes (oncogenes) stop the suppressive effects of the suppressor genes.

The growth-promoting genes take control and promote abnormal cell growth, resulting in the formation of a cancerous clone of cells, resulting in cancer, as it is known. This is an out-of-control process of cell growth whose ultimate goal is to take over the body in which it is growing and destroys it.

The first step in the genesis of cancer is the process of oncogene. Oncogenes can be brought about by a hereditary or familial transmission of a protein from parent or parents to fetus at the time of conception. This protein (oncogene or oncogenes) can then enter over many years into a multi-step process, interactions, and reactions that can cause a cell or group of cells to mutate. Once this mutation occurs, then the cell or group of cells loses their ability to grow and multiply normally. The abnormal growth of cells then becomes a cancer mass. Many causative effects can bring about the damage that occurs to the cell or cells that cause this mutation to occur.

According to a recent report "Many cases of cancer are caused by bad luck". This bad luck comes in the form of random genetic mistakes, or mutations, that happen when healthy cells divide."The research suggests that random mutations may account for two-thirds of the risk of getting many types of cancer, leaving the usual suspects-hereditary and environmental factors- to account for only one-third."

"The cancers that could be explained with biological bad luck included pancreatic, leukemia, bone, testicular, ovarian and brain cancer."

All of the following can damage the DNA/RNA materials inside a cell, resulting in malignant mutations: The different risks for cancer are:

1. Transmission of a hereditary cancer oncogene
2. Exposure to oncogenic viruses such as Epstein bar virus, which can cause nasopharyngeal carcinoma
3. Exposure to human papilloma virus, causing cervical cancer
4. Exposure to either hepatitis B or C virus, causing cancer of the liver
5. Exposure to HTLV-I and HTLV-II, causing T cell leukemia/lymphoma
6. Sun exposure causing basal cell carcinoma of the skin
7. Exposure to carcinogens such as tobacco smoking, causing lung cancer, cancer of the mouth, throat, head and neck, etc.
8. Exposure to ionizing radiation, causing leukemia, lymphoma and other cancers
9. Exposure to toxic chemicals such as benzene, etc., causing malignancies of different types.

10. Consumption of excessive alcohol, resulting in cancer of the mouth, throat, and esophagus.
11. Exposure to estrogen, causing increased incidence of breast cancer and uterine cancer in women
12. Consumption of too much red meats, resulting in increased incidence of breast, uterine and colon cancer
13. Alcohol abuse and tobacco smoking, associated with increase incidence of cancer of the esophagus.
14. 14. Long-term exposure to toxic pollutants and chemical solvents in the work place, resulting in the development of different types of cancer
15. HIV-I and II causing AIDS with its high propensity to cause lymphoma and Kaposi's sarcoma
16. Non-acquired immunodeficiency and its propensity to cause malignancy of different types
17. A newly discovered risk for cancer is chronically elevated white blood cells count. Elevated white blood cells count causes increase development of colon cancer, endometrial cancer, breast cancer and lung cancer in post menopausal women. Source: Archive of Internal Medicine Vol. 167 NO, 17 Sep 24, 2007

Cancer genetics

Following are examples of cancers that develop because of oncogene activation:

Multiple endocrine neoplastic (MEN) type 2a and type 2b. MEN 2a include medullary carcinoma of the thyroid, pheochromocytoma and hyperparathyroidism.

MEN 2b include medullary carcinoma of the thyroid, pheochromocytoma, mucosal neuromas and bony abnormalities. Other cancers that occur as a result of damaged DNA and failure of DNA repair include:

Hereditary no polyposis colon cancer (HNPCC). This abnormality is responsible for about 10– 15% of colon cancers and is associated with ovarian, endometrial and urinary tract cancers.

Other genetically associated cancers include neurofibromatosis 1 and 2, hereditary Wilm's tumor, Li-Fraumeni syndrome, and familial adenomatous polyposis of the colon. The percentage of colon cancer in familial adenomatous polyposis is 100%. Treatment usually requires the affected individual to undergo total removal of the colon by 20 to 30 years of age.

Immunotherapy/Monoclonal antibodies in the treatments of different cancers. The body's immune system consisting in part of T cells is very efficient in fighting these cancers.

Lung Cancer:

In the U.S. in 2017, 116,990 men had lung cancer and 86,930 men died of lung cancer.

In 2017, 13,720 black men were diagnosed with lung cancer and 4,450 black men died of lung cancer in the U.S. Source: ACS Facts & Figures 2017

The number one reason that causes people to develop lung cancer is tobacco smoking. "An estimated 443000 deaths occur in the United States each year from tobacco-related diseases." Forty million Americans smoke in the U.S.

Blacks and other minorities have the third highest rate of touchback smoking in the U.S. and the tobacco companies target blacks and other minorities by putting mentol in the cigarettes because they know that minorities like the taste of mentol.

Tobacco related diseases cost $ 150 billion per year in the U.S.

Other risk factors for lung cancer include:

Genetic predisposition to cancer
Industrial exposure to toxic fumes
Asbestosis
Scar from pulmonary tuberculosis
HIV/AIDS
Chronic fungal infection/ other inflammatory diseases of the lung
Exposure to coal in the mines, (black lung disease) arsenic, air pollution
Second hand smoke etc;

Some of the symptoms of lung cancer include:

1.Chronic cough
2.Coughing with streaks of blood
3.Coughing up blood
4.Chest pain
5.Shortness of breath
6.Weight loss, etc.
7.Recurrent pneumonia and/or pneumonia that fail to respond to treatment over a long period of time etc.

Sometimes lung cancer is discovered on a chest x-ray without any symptoms. Early detection is crucial in order to increase the chance of curing lung cancer; a chest x-ray is the first test in the diagnosis of lung cancer. The chest x-ray is done either as part of a routine examination or because the patient presents with symptoms such as those described earlier here.

Things that can be seen on the chest x-ray or CT when a person has lung cancer include:

1. A mass
2. Effusion (fluid in the lung)
3. An infiltrate and in some cases, calcification mass (mesothelioma due to exposure to asbestos)

There are two broad types of lung cancer, large-cell lung cancer and small-cell lung cancer. Large-cell lung cancer may consist of adenocarcinoma of the lung, squamous cell carcinoma of the lung, or scar carcinoma of the lung.

Mesothelioma is a form of lung cancer associated with asbestos exposure. Another name for small-cell carcinoma is oat cell carcinoma.

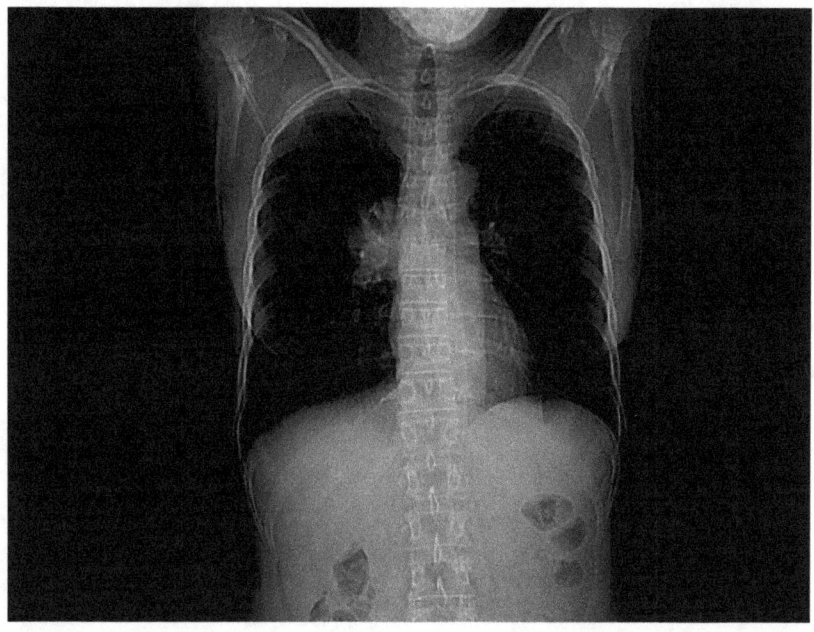

Figure 10:1 Cancerous mass on chest x-ray

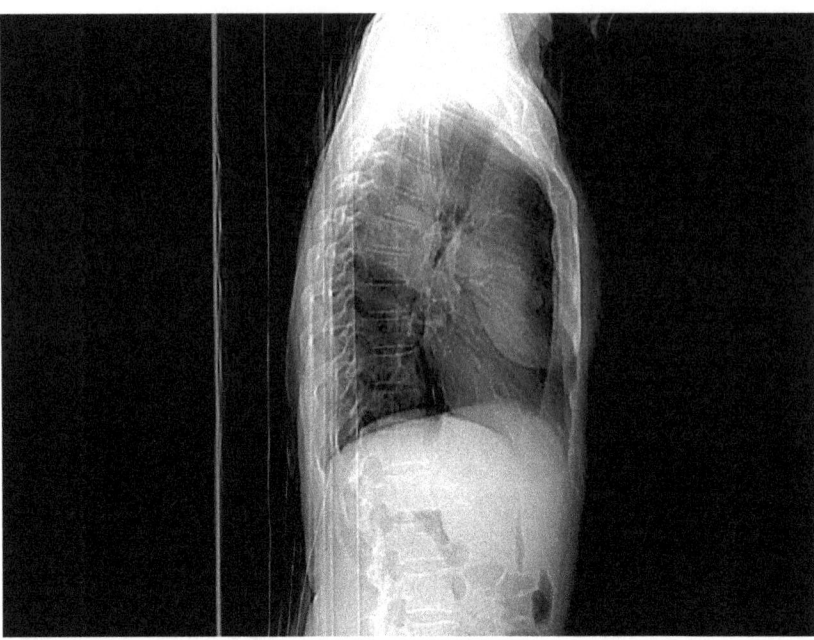

Figure 10:2 -Cancerous mass on chest x-ray

Once cancer of the lung is suspected on chest x-ray, the next test to be done is a CT scan of the chest.

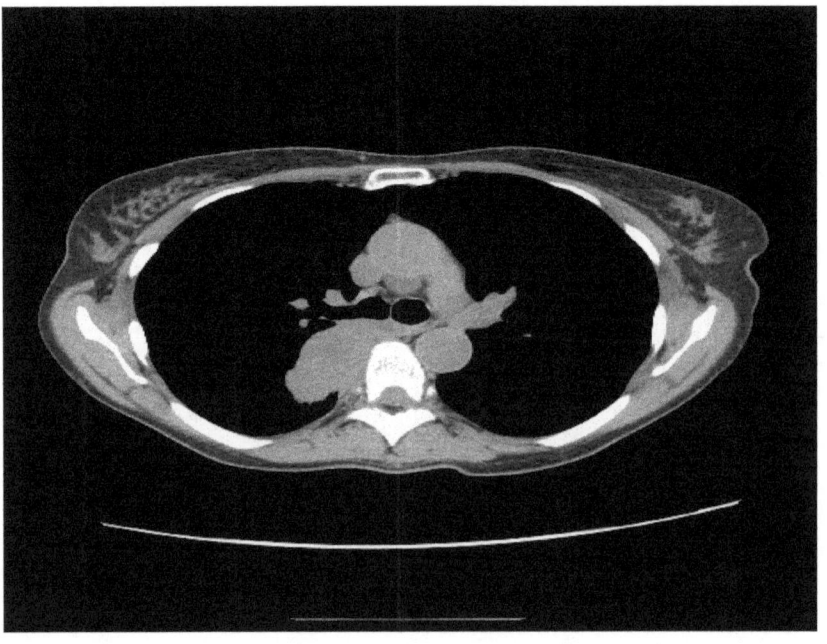

Figure 10:3 -CT Scan of the chest showing lesion in inferior segment of the lower lobe of the lung.

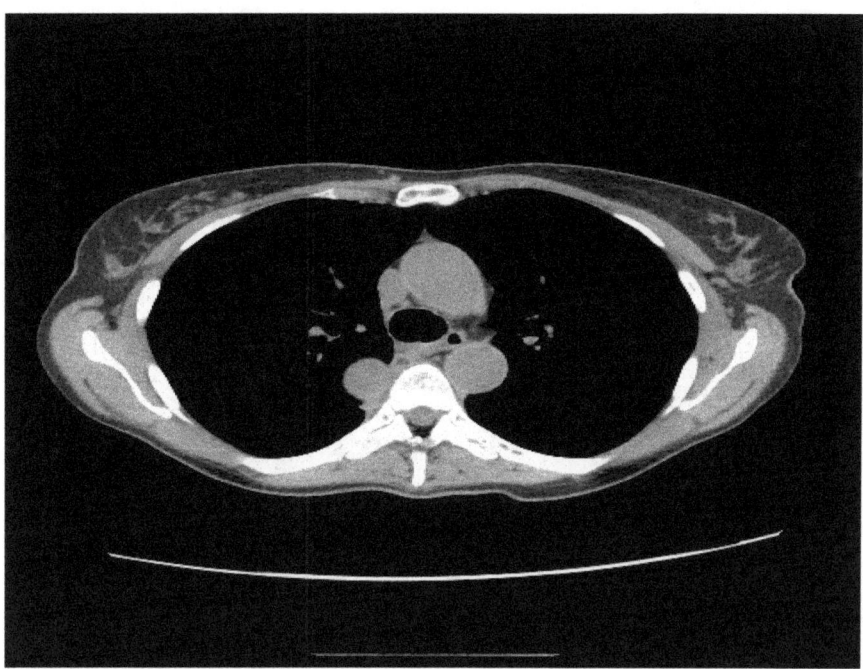

Figure 10:4 -*CT Scan of lung showing a lesion in the lung*

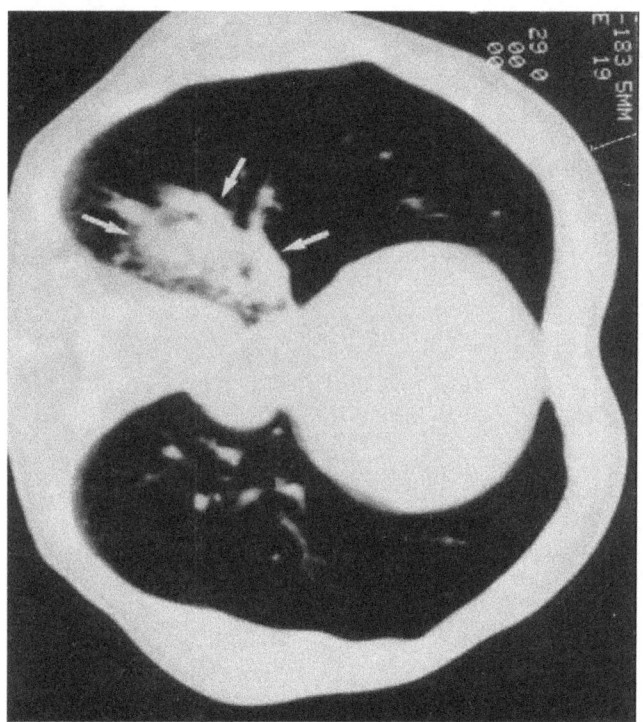

Figure 10:5–See CT Scan of the chest showing lobulated mass (cancer)
in the right upper lung in a patient who smokes.

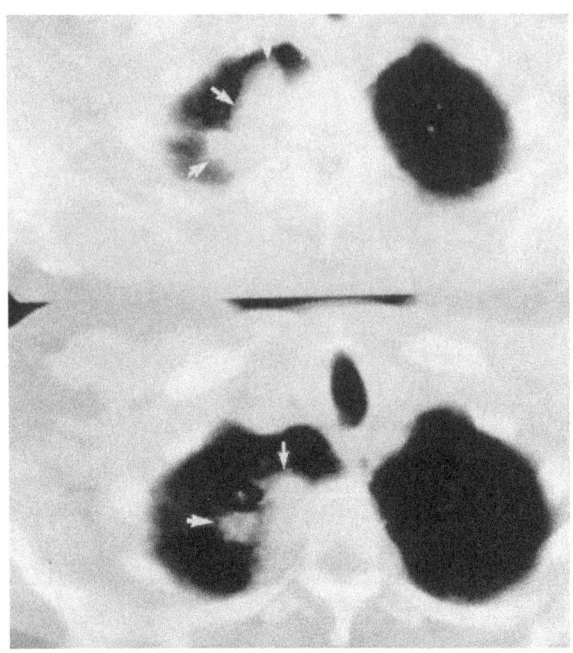

Figure 10:6 -Lung cancer mass

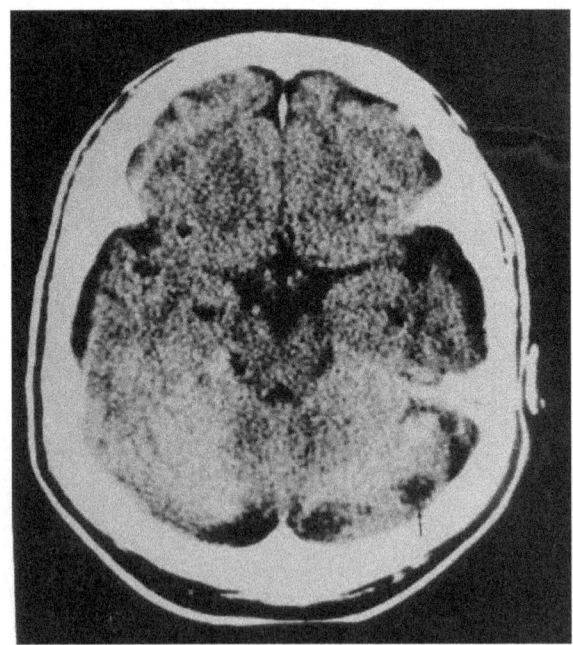

Figure 10:7–CT scan of brain: Hypodense mass left cerebellar hemisphere Metastatic cancer to the brain from a lung primary cancer in a smoker (arrow).

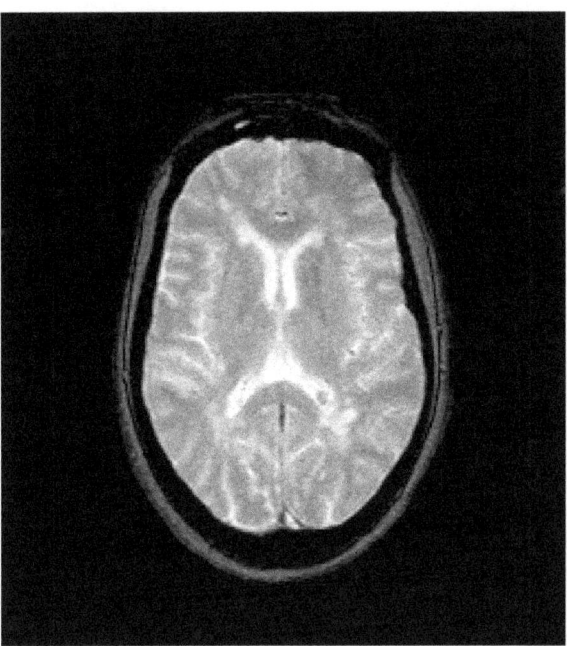

Figure 10:8 -Brain lesion from lung cancer.

Following the CT scan of the lung, the next step is to refer the patient to a pulmonary specialist for a bronchoscopic examination. Another approach is to refer the patient to a chest surgeon based on the location of the mass. Some masses of the lung are located so peripherally that it cannot be reached via bronchoscopy.

The bronchoscopic examination is a procedure during which an instrument is introduced into the lung after spraying the throat with an anesthetic. During the bronchoscopy, either a biopsy or washing is taken from the mass in the lung and send to the pathology lab for examination.

If it is cancer, then the chest surgeon may proceed to remove the segment of the lung that contains the cancer. During the procedure, several lymph nodes are taken out from the surrounding area to check if any of them has cancer.

Another method that is frequently used to diagnose lung cancer is CAT- or sonogram-guided needle biopsy to obtain tissue for diagnosis. An invasive radiologist with great precision carries out this procedure and it frequently saves the patient a bronchoscopy or an open-chest surgical procedure.

It is very important to know in advance what is the cell type of lung cancer the patient has in order to know how to proceed with further treatment. As just stated, there are essentially two different categories of lung cancer, large cell carcinoma, and small cell carcinoma. It is important to know whether a person has small cell lung cancer, or large cell lung cancer. Small-cell cancer or oat-cell lung cancer usually has already spread by the time a mass is seen on the chest x-ray regardless of how small the mass is.

That being the case, the entire approach to the evaluation and treatment of small-cell cancer is different from any other lung cancer. In fact, it is almost a given that by the time a coin-size lesion is found in the lung of a patient that turns out to be oat cell, the cancer probably has already spread to the brain and possibly the liver and other organs as well. Frequently, once the cell type is known to be oat cell because of biopsy, the question as to whether the cancer should or should not be resected becomes a major clinical decision because the prognosis is poor.

On the other hand, once a tissue diagnosis is made that the cancer in the lung is of the large-cell type, and if the cancer is deemed respectable, based on the size, location, and overall physical status of the patient, the decision usually is to resect the cancer because the chances of cure are better. Though it must be remembered that 20–25% of people with large-cell-type lung cancer frequently present with metastasis to the brain at the time of diagnosis.

Evaluation of lung cancer includes:

1. History and physical examination
2. Chest x-ray
3. Chest CT Scan
4. Sputum for cytology
5. Lung biopsy
6. Abdominal CT scan to look at the liver
7. Bone scan to be sure that the cancer has not spread to the bone
8. Brain CT scan with contrast because a brain CT without contrast will likely miss metastatic disease of the brain if its there or brain MRI can also be done.
9. In certain difficult cases a PET scan can be done.
10. Brain CT Scan with contrast because a brain CAT without contrast will likely miss metastatic disease of the brain if it is there, or, brain MRI can also be done.
11. PET Scan

Treatment of lung cancer includes:

1. Surgical resection of the cancerous mass
2. Adjuvant radiation therapy, after surgical resection
3. Adjuvant chemotherapy

Some frequently used chemotherapeutic agents in large-cell lung cancer include:

Cytoxan
Doxorubicin
Cisplatin
Etoposide
Taxol
Docetaxel
Carboplatin
Gemcitabine

Vinorelbine
Irinotecan
These are used in different combinations.

Some of the commonly used chemotherapeutic agents in small-cell lung cancer care consist of:

Cyclophosphamide
Doxorubicin
Vincristine
Etoposide
Cisplatin
Methotrexate
Carboplatin
Irinotecan
Topotecan
Docetaxel
Placlitaxel

These drugs are used in different combinations.

Some of the side effects of these chemotherapeutic agents have been outlined earlier under the treatment of breast cancer. The side effects of Vincristine include double vision, drooping eyelids, headache, jaw pain, tingling of the finger and toes with numbness (peripheral neuropathy), and constipation.

Some of the side effects of Cisplatin include nausea; vomiting; numbness of feet, fingers, and toes; blurry vision; possible kidney damage; and bone marrow suppression, resulting in pancytopenia.

Some of the side effects of Etoposide (VP 16) include bone marrow depression with low white blood cells, low red blood cells, low platelets; sores in the mouth; numbness in feet, fingers, and toes with tingling; loss of hair; nausea; vomiting; and alopecia.

To decrease the incidence of nausea and vomiting, different anti-emetic medications, such as Zofran or Kytril, in combination with Ativan, Benadryl, and Decadron, can be used.

"The FDA approved Pembrolizumab and nivolumab monoclonal antibodies to treat patients with metastatic non-small cell lung cancer that has progressed after treatment with other agents"

Colorectal Cancer:

In 2017, there were 71,420, cases of colorectal cancer diagnosed in men in the U.S. and 27,150 men died of this cancer during that year in the U.S.

8,690 black men were diagnosed with colorectal cancer in 2017 and 3,800 black men died of colorectal cancer in 2017 in the U.S. Source: ACS Facts & Figures 2017

Minorities in general have higher incidence of colorectal cancer and have higher rates of deaths from colorectal cancer than do whites.

" Disparities between black and white persons in risk for interval CRC are of particular concern because black persons have the highest incidence of and mortality rates from CRC of any race or ethnic group in the United States, with incidence rates 22% to 27% higher than white persons. Approxmately 40% of these disparities in CRC incidence are attributable to lower utilization of srceening among black persons."

"In this population-based study of elderly Medicare enrollees, risk for interval CRC was 31% higher among black persons yhan white persons, whereas the risk among Asian persons was lower than white persons." Source: Annals of Internal Medicine Vol. 166 No.12 20 June 2017

Risk factors for colorectal cancer include:

Genetic predisposition (family history of colon cancer)
History of prostate cancer
History of ovarian cancer
History of breast cancer
Physical inactivity
Obesity
Increase consumption of processed meat
Exposure to pesticide
Increase consumption of red meat
Colorectal polyps
Inflammatory bowel disease
Familial polyposis etc;

Colorectal cancer is a curable disease when diagnosed early and surgically removed. Common symptoms and signs of colorectal cancer:

1. Blood in the stools
2. Constipation
3. Diarrhea
4. Abdominal pain
5. Weight loss
6. Poor appetite
7. Hemorrhoids
8. Sudden development of inguinal hernia in a person in the cancer-age group (40 years old and older)
9. Anemia
10. Passing pencil-size stool
11. A combination of these signs and symptoms

How to diagnose colorectal cancer

To diagnose colorectal cancer, a complete history, and physical examination needs to be carried out. As part of this examination, a digital rectal examination needs to be done and the stool tested for occult blood. Sometimes, a person goes to the physician and states that he or she sees blood in the stool or on the toilet paper. Sometimes, a person might say that he or she has had hemorrhoids for a long time and suddenly the hemorrhoids have come out and are now bleeding. At times, a person in his or her 40s, or older, might come to see the doctor and reports that he or she has just developed an inguinal hernia with no known precipitating reason.

In all these instances, a complete lower bowel evaluation needs to be done to make sure that these signs and symptoms are not due to colon cancer. The stool needs to be tested for occult blood, unless gross blood is seen. It is important that the person being tested stays away from taking aspirin or NSAIDS for 7–10 days in the case of aspirin, and in the case of NSAIDS 12 to 24 hours.

It is also important that the person does not eat red meat for three days prior to testing the stool for blood. The person must not take Vitamin C in pill form for one week before having his or her stool the tested for occult blood. In addition, the person must not eat horseradish for several days before testing the stool for blood.

Aspirin and NSAIDS will cause the stool hem occult test to be positive because of the irritating effects on the lining of the stomach.

Red meat will cause the stool to be positive for blood because red meat has blood in it. Vitamin C causes the hemoccult test of the stool to be falsely negative for occult blood because Vitamin C is a reducing agent and the chemical reaction that is used in the test is an oxidation reaction.

So, adding a reducing agent to an oxidation reaction neutralizes the reaction, rendering it falsely negative. Eating horseradish can cause a person's stool to become black when it is exposed to the solution that is used to test the stool for blood. Taking Pepto-Bismol also causes the stool to become black, confusing it with bleeding from the stomach.

The tests most effective in evaluation of colorectal cancer consist of:

1. Digital rectal examination
2. Testing of the stool using the hemoccult test
3. Fecal Immunochemical Test (FIT)
4. DNA stool test
5. Checking the serum ferritin
6. Checking the red cell distribution width (RDW) during a complete blood count
7. Testing for the soluble serum transferrin receptor level. (If elevated, it proves that the patient has iron deficiency anemia. This test is better than bone marrow iron stain test, the serum ferritin and the RDW.)

8. Barium enema
9. Colonoscopy
10. Flexible sigmoidoscopy
11. Rigid sigmoidoscopy
12. Virtual colonoscopy
13. FDA just approved Cologuard to screen stools for blood cells and DNA mutations to dectect colon cancer and precancerous growths.
14. A new rapid new stool test "M2–PK Quick, a rapid pointy-of care test that detects the oncoprotein M2 pyruvate konase, provided a higly accurate diagnosis of colorectal cancer, according to recent study data."

According to the recent literature, flexible sigmoidoscopy is said to be as effective as colonoscopy detect cancer of the colon. Barium enema is an x-ray test during which the bowel is cleansed with cathartics, barium is put in the bowel from the rectum using a tube, and then x-rays are used to visualize the bowel, looking for abnormalities, such as cancerous growth.

Cancer of the colon begins at around age forty in blacks and other minorities. In addition there are several limitations with the barium enema.

Among the limitations:

1. Retained stool in the bowel.
2. 2.Barium enema is not able to diagnose colorectal if the cancer is located between 15 and 30 cm in the lower bowel from the entrance of the anus. This is so because the tube that is used to put the barium in the colon occupies that space, making it impossible to visualize a cancer that may be located in that space. Cancer is best discovered in that area by sigmoidoscopy or colonoscopy. In addition, another limitation of the barium enema is that if a mass or polyp is found it cannot be biopsied.

Colonoscopy is the best way to evaluate the colon because not only can the gastroenterologist or colorectal surgeon sees the entire lower bowel, but he or she can also biopsy any lesion or polyp that is there.

Once a biopsy is taken from either a polyp or mass, the specimen is sent to the pathology laboratory for histological evaluation.

Colorectal cancer begins to develop; blacks seem to produce more polyps and lager polyps than do whites. Blacks have more right-sided cancer of the colon, and right-sided colon cancer can be missed during colonoscopy than do left-sided colon cancer.

The followings are examples of colon cancer seen during colonoscopy.

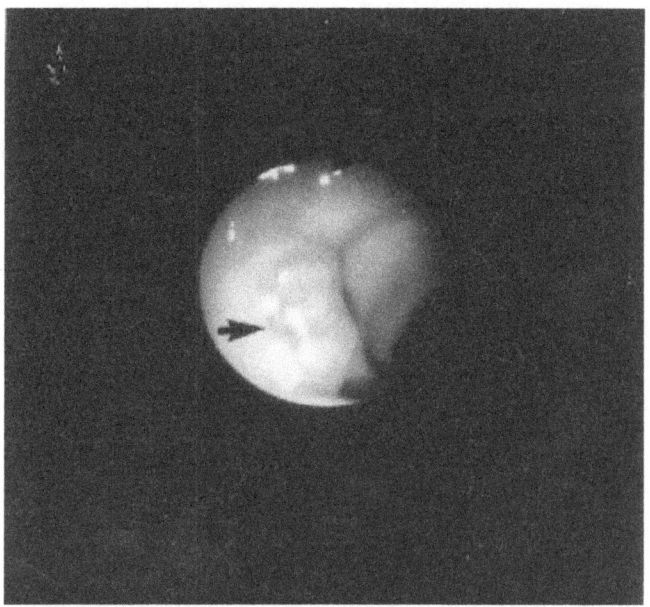

Figure 10:13- Colon cancer: sessile lesion of the colon (arrow)

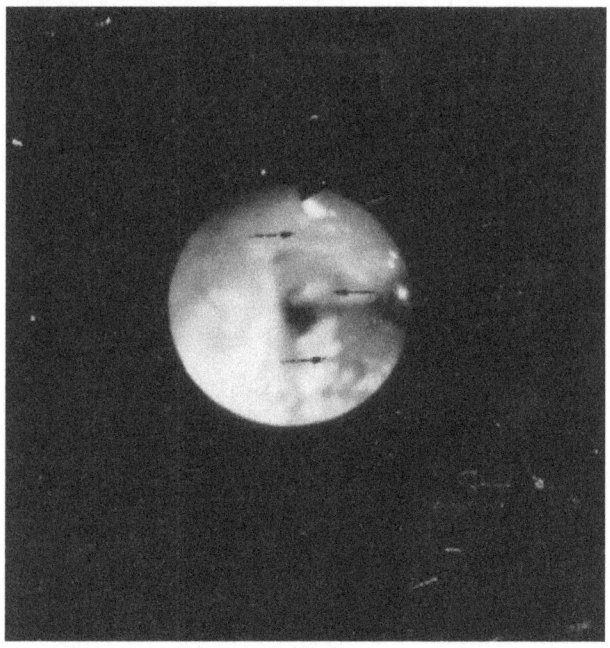

Figure 10:14–Large obstructing colon cancer with bleeding (arrows.

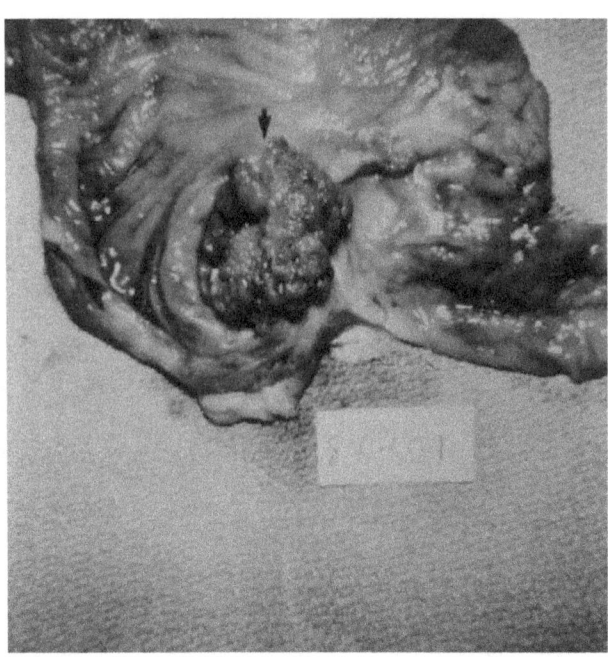

Figure 10:15–*Carcinoma in papillary adenoma of cecum (arrow).*

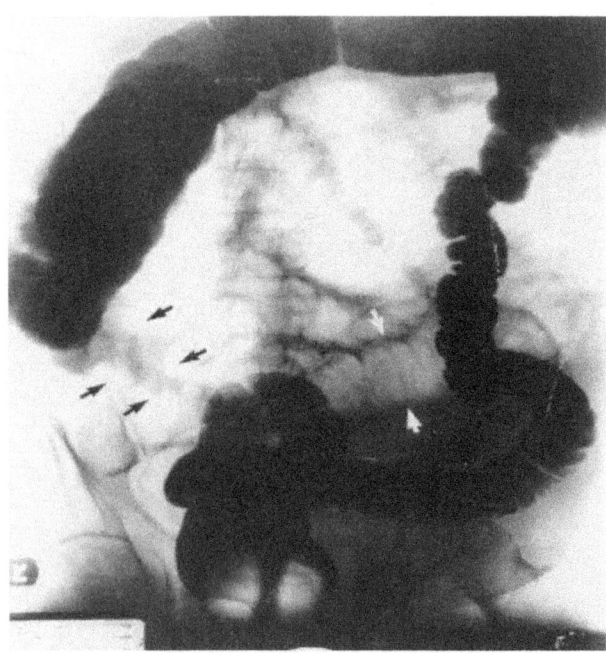

Figure 10:16–*Barium enema: Apple core lesion of the cecum (white arrows) with small bowel obstruction (white arrows).*

If the pathology report comes back that the polyp or polyps removed is or are negative for cancer, then in about two years the individual should have another colonoscopic examination. Some people have the propensity to develop polyps in their colon. It takes about 3-5 years for a precancerous polyp to develop into cancer. Some individuals who form a lot of polyps need surveillance colonoscopy every year for 2-3 years so that a polyp that has the potential to become cancerous can be removed before it becomes cancer. If the colonoscopy is negative, it can be repeated in 5 years.

The FDA has recently approved Celebrex to be used in people who have the propensity to form polyps in their colon. Celebrex, a Cox 2 inhibitor is used to treat arthritis. The enzyme cyclooxygenase is needed to mediate inflammation inside the colon and inflammation is a key component in the formation of colorectal polyps.

Using aspirin, NSAIDs and COX2 like Celebrex block the development of inflammation, thereby decreases polyps' formation.

It is very important to test frequently the stool of people who have the hereditary predisposition to colon cancer for blood, frequently using the hemoccult. It is also very important to begin to do surveillance colonoscopy for those people starting at age 35 and to clinically monitor them by doing:

1. Digital rectal examination
2. Testing of the stool using the hemoccult test
3. Checking the serum ferritin
4. Checking the red cell distribution width (RDW) during a complete blood count
5. Testing for the serum transferrin receptor level. (If elevated, it proves that the patient has iron deficiency amenia.)

In a person without hemoglobinopathy, or who is not hemolyzing, and does not have either B12 or folate deficiency, has elevated RDW (15 or greater), that means he or she is probably losing blood slowly and losing storage iron with it. In the routine setting, the elevated RDW is the earliest sign of slow blood loss. This occurs from the time that the precancerous polyp starts oozing blood, 2-3 years before real cancer develops.

Therefore, it is crucial that the treating physician understands and knows how to interpret the RDW. The RDW is given as part of the CBC report by most reporting laboratories that do blood counts.

The third very important test that indicates blood loss and iron loss is the serum ferritin. The ferritin is the storage iron that humans have in their bone marrow, muscles, liver, spleen, the reticuloendothelial system, the brain, and other tissues in the body. A normal size man has 3.5 grams of iron in his body, 2.5 grams are in the circulation and 1.5 grams are in the store.

Each milliliter of blood has 0.5 mg of iron in it, it is easy to calculate how much iron an individual has lost when he or she becomes anemic by working backwards, and calculating how much her serum ferritin is.

One unit of blood, which is 500 cc, has 250 mg of iron in it. The normal serum ferritin in a man is 22-322 ug/L. The serum ferritin is a range and as such it takes several years of slow and chronic bleeding from whatever source to deplete the ferritin down. It is also important and crucial to understand that an individual must deplete his or her serum ferritin totally before he or she starts using the iron in the circulation.

When a person is bleeding occultly, iron is being lost slowly and in stages.
The first stage of iron lost is called, pre-latent or iron deficient erythropoiesis.
The second stage of iron lost is called latent or iron deficient state.
The third stage is called late latent stage or frank iron deficiency anemia.

In pre-latent stage of iron deficiency, the hematocrit is normal, the level of serum ferritin is starting to go down, and the RDW is high. In the latent stage of iron deficiency, the hematocrit is low normal, the level of serum ferritin has fallen lower, and the RDW is high. In the late latent stage of iron deficiency, the serum ferritin is low, the hematocrit is low, the RDW is high and mean corpuscular volume or MCV is low, and the reticulocyte count is low. In late latent stage of iron deficiency, frank iron deficiency anemia exists.

Understanding how iron is lost in occult gastro-intestinal bleeding, and, using this information to think back when evaluating patient at high risk or no obvious risk for colon cancer can help physicians to resect pre-cancerous polyps and in so doing prevents many people from dying from colon cancer.

When a person is bleeding slowly and chronically, as is the case in cancer of the large bowel, rectum, small bowel, esophagus and stomach the first iron that is being lost is the iron in the store (the ferritin). Knowing that to be the case then, once it is noted that the range of the serum ferritin is starting to go down (being depleted) it is the crucial time to start evaluating the gastrointestinal tract to look for the reason or reasons for the blood loss.

In other words, if an evaluation is undertaken at this juncture, a respectable and curable precancerous polyp can be removed and cancer of the gastrointestinal tract, no matter where it is located, can be cured, in particular, if the cancer is located in the large bowel. The only cancer that may be difficult to cure surgically even if discovered and resected early is cancer of the esophagus.

If a mass is found during colonoscopy and biopsied and the pathology shows cancer, then a metastatic evaluation is carried out to determine if the cancer has or has not spread, before deciding to go ahead with surgical resection of the mass.

The metastatic evaluation for colon cancer includes:

1. Complete blood count
2. Liver function tests such as SGOT, SGPT, alkaline phosphatase, LDH
3. CEA (carcinoembryogenic antigen)
4. Abdominal CT to look at the liver and the retroperitoneal area etc., or abdominal sonogram

5. Chest x-ray or CT Scan of the chest and bone scan
6. PET Scan

If all these tests are normal, then the assumption can be made that the cancer has not spread to these organs; the patient can be scheduled for surgical resection of the cancerous mass.

The resected polypoid mass is sent to the pathology lab department for gross and histological evaluations. To know the extent of the spread of the colon cancer, a system of staging called Duke's staging is adhered to: Duke's A, Duke's B, Duke's C, and Duke's D.

or
Stage 1
Stage 2
Stage 3
Stage 4

Duke's A is when the cancer penetrates into the wall of the bowel, but not through it. Duke's B is when the cancer penetrates through the wall of the bowel. Duke's C is when the cancer penetrates through the wall of the bowel and spreads to the surrounding lymph nodes. There exists more refinement of the Duke's staging, which defines Duke's B, B2, Duke's C and Duke's C2. Duke's D is widespread distant metastasis.

The Duke's staging of colon cancer is very important in that it dictates the type of treatment modalities that are provided for the patient with colon cancer. It is also important in outlining the prognosis of the individual who has colon cancer.

Duke's A and B colon cancer are surgically curable cancers. Duke's B2 oftentimes requires surgical resection with 6 months of adjuvant 5FU. Duke's C colon cancer is less likely to be surgically curable.

After surgical resection, the best adjuvant chemotherapeutic treatment for Duke's C colon cancer is Levamisole 150 mg every 8 hours for 3 days every 3 weeks with 5FU 450 mg/m2 weeks for 52 weeks.

At times surgical resection may be necessary in Duke's D lesion if a large cancer mass is found and is deemed to be potentially about to obstruct the colon.

To avoid this problem, the surgeon then may decide to resect the cancer mass.

Otherwise, the treatment of Duke's D 5FU 500 mg/m2 IV bolus, Camptosar 125 mg /m2 IV over 90 minutes and Leucovorin 20 mg/m2 IV bolus on day 1, 8, 15 and 22 and 1 week off every month for 1 year.

Another frequently used regimen to treat Duke's or Stage 4 colon cancer is Oxaliplatin on Day 1, 85 mg/m2 IV over 2 hours, Leucovorin 200 mg/m2 over 2 hours IV, 5FU 400 mg/ m2 IV bolus and 5FU 600 mg/m2 as a continuous infusion over 22 hours. On day 2 Leucovorin 200 mg/ m2 IV over 2 hours 5FU 400 mg/m2 IV bolus, and 5FU 600 mg/m2 as a continuous infusion over 22 hours. This is repeated every 2 weeks. There have been good results seen using both these two regimens. Adding Avastin to different chemotherapeutic protocol has been effective at times. However, Avastin is a very expensive drug.

Other drugs used in cancer of the colon include:

1. Oxaliplatin
2. Irinotecan
3. Bevacizumab
4. Capecitabine
5. Cetuximab
6. Cisplatinum, 5FU, Mitomycin C for rectal cancer
7. Avastin
8. Radiation therapy is also used to treat cancer of the rectum either before or after.

Surgical removal of isolated liver mass from colon cancer has been done and is said to be at times successful.

The FDA has approved Lonsurf to treat refractory metastatic colorectal cancer.

Megace is at times added to the 5FU to increase the appetite of the patient with colon cancer and it helps with weight gain. Megace can cause clots to develop in the legs with serious clinical consequences. Oxandrin is also used to improve appetite in people with advanced colon cancer. The side effects are similar to Megace. Marinol is also quite effective in improving some cancer patients's appetite.

Another form of cancer that oftentimes develops in the large bowel is carcinoid tumor. The preoperative evaluation is the same, except that if the treating physician suspects carcinoid tumor, then serum serotonin or a 24-hour urine for (5HIAA) 5 hydroxyindoleacetic acid can be obtained as a baseline and to help firm up the diagnosis. These tests are helpful in the subsequent management of the patient with carcinoid tumor.

Non-Hodgkin's lymphoma of the large bowel does occur. The treatment approach is the same. First, surgical resection followed either by radiation therapy or by chemotherapy, depending on the histology and the extent of disease found at surgery.

Colorectal cancer is curable when found early. Therefore, yearly rectal examination and testing of the stool for blood once or twice per year and doing a complete blood count with RDW, serum ferritin and the serum-transferring receptors level together, can prevent colon cancer from ever killing anyone. It is very important for physicians to use the soluble serum transferrin level when evaluating black patients who may be suffering from sickle cell disease/ other abnormal hemoglobins that cause them to very high serum Ferritin/ RDW/ low MCV and yet may be bleeding from their GI track from pre-cancerous polyps or GI cancer.

The FDA has approved Lonsurf, which is a combination of trifluridine and tipiracil to treat metastatic colorectal cancer in people who no longer respond to chemotherapy.

If the treating physician does these tests and follow up on the results, pre-cancerous/ cancerous lesions of the colon, rectum, small bowel, and stomach and esophagus can be discovered early and treated appropriately.

Cancer of the esophagus:

In 2017, 13,360 men were diagnosed with cancer of the esophagus in the U.S. and 12,720 men died of cancer of the esophagus.

Cancer of the esophagus is the eight leading cause of cancer deaths in the world. Cancer of the esophagus is 50% more common in blacks compared to whites. Esophageal cancer is always diagnosed when it has already in an advanced stage.

Alcohol abuse and tobacco smoking are risk factors in the development of cancer of the esophagus.

Other risks include:

Barrett's esophagus
Achalasia
Plummmer-Vinson syndrome
Celiac disease
Consumption of too red meat
HPV infection of the throat from HPV types 16 and 18
Lye strictures of the esophagus etc;

The symptoms and signs of esophageal cancer include:

1. Difficulty swallowing
2. Upper stomach pain
3. Chest pain
4. Anemia
5. Weight loss etc.

The best ways to evaluate cancer of esophagus are:

CT Scan
MRI
Esophagram
Endoscopy
Esophageal biopsy
CBC
Serum ferritin
CEA
Chemistry profile

Treatments of cancer of the esophagus include:

1. Surgical resection
2. Radiation therapy
3. Chemotherapy such as:
4. 5FU, Cisplatin
   or
5. Epirubicin
6. Cisplatin
7. 5FU
   or
8. Epirubicin
9. Oxaliplatin
10. Capecitabine
    or
11. Irinotecan
12. Cisplatin
    or
13. Vinorelbine
14. The FDA has just approved Cyramza for advanced gastro-esophageal junction cancer.

The 5-year survival for cancer of the esophagus is 11% for blacks and 18% for whites.

Cancer of the stomach:

In 2017, 17, 500 men in the U.S. were diagnosed with cancer of the stomach and 6,720 men died of cancer of the stomach.

Cancer of the stomach is 2-3 times more common in blacks as compared to whites and the death rates are similarly higher for blacks as compared to whites. In addition,

H pylori infection of the stomach can cause lymphoma in certain percentage of individuals.

Risk factors for stomach cancer include:

Genetic
Environmental
Smoked fish
Pickles
Processed foods
H pylori infection
Smoking
Alcohol abuse
Obesity etc;

Symptoms and signs of stomach cancer include:

1. Recurrent indigestion
2. Hyperacidity/Heart burn
3. Nausea and vomiting
4. Diarrhea and constipation
5. Bloating
6. Upper stomach pain
7. Weight loss
8. Anemia
9. Poor appetite
10. Fatigue
11. Vomiting blood
12. Black tarry stools etc;

The best ways to evaluate cancer of the stomach include:

1. Endoscopic examination with biopsy when necessary
2. Upper GI series
3. H. Pylori examination
4. CBC
5. Serum ferritin
6. Stool hemoccult
7. CEA etc;

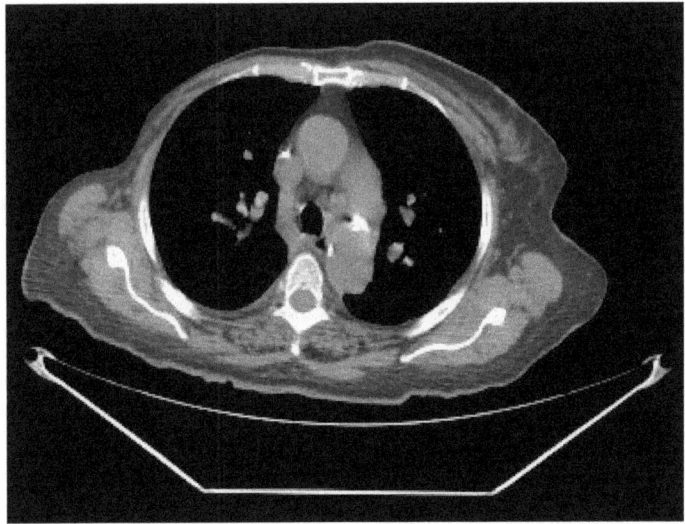

Figure 10:17- CT Scan of cancer of the stomach

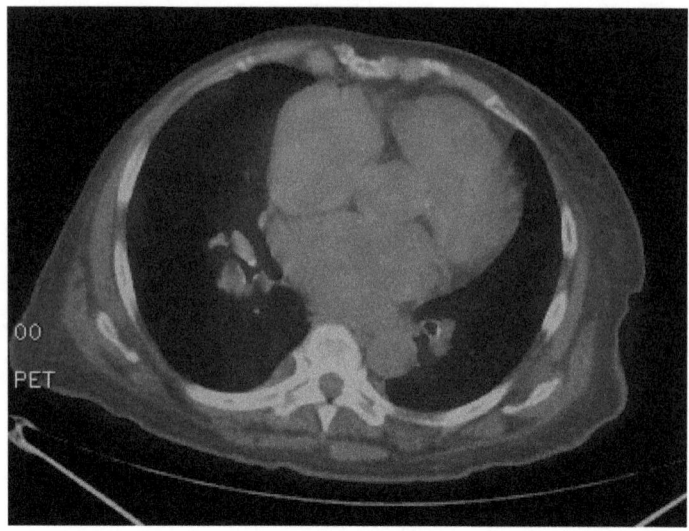

Figure 10: 18 -PET Scan in a person with cancer of the stomach

Treatments of stomach cancer include:

1. Surgical resection
2. Chemotherapy drugs such as
3. Epirubicin
4. Cisplatin
5. 5FU
    or
6. Docetaxel
7. Cisplatin
8. 5FU in combination
    or
9. Epirubicin
10. Oxaliplatin
11. Capecitabine in combination
    or
12. Irinotecan
13. Cisplatin in combination
14. The FDA has just approved Cyramza for advanced cancer of the stomach.

Cancer of the small bowel:

In 2017, 5,380 men in the U.S. were diagnosed with cancer of the small bowel and 7,70 men died from cancer of the small bowel. Cancer of the small intestine is a very rare form of cancer worldwide.

The death rate for cancer of the small intestine is higher in blacks as compared to whites.

Risk factors for cancer of the small bowel include:

Crohn's disease
Intestinal polyposis
Celiac disease
AIDS
Puetz-Jegher's syndrome

Symptoms and signs of small bowel cancer include:

1. Abdominal pain
2. Bloating
3. Palpable abdominal mass
4. Weight loss
5. Blood in the stools
6. Iron deficiency anemia
7. Constipation
8. Small bowel obstruction etc.

The best ways to evaluate cancer of the small bowel include:

1. Complete history and physical examination
2. Abdominal CT scan
3. Capsule scoping of the small
4. CBC
5. Serum ferritin
6. CEA
7. Small bowel biopsy

The best treatments for cancer of the small bowel include:

1. Surgical resection
2. Chemotherapy such as
3. Docetaxel
4. Cisplatin
5. 5FU
   or
6. 5FU
7. Cisplatin
   or
8. Epirubicin
9. Oxaliplatin
10. Capecitabine
    or
11. Irinotecan
12. Cisplatin

The mother cells that give rise to the stomach and the small bowel are the same, as a result, chemotherapy drugs in the treatment of stomach and small bowel cancer are the same. Chemotherapy for stomach and small bowel cancer are not very effective.

Cancer of the Liver and intrahepatic bile duct:

In 2014, 745,000 people in the world had cancer of the liver. Cancer of the liver is the fifth most common cancer in the world. Each year 8,000, people die worldwide from hepatocellular carcinoma/cancer of the liver in 2014. WHO

Liver cancer is the fifth most common cancer in men " Source: New England journal of medicine 365; 12 September 22, 2011 in the U.S.

In 2017, 29,200 men in the U.S. had cancer of the liver and 19,610 men died of cancer of the liver in the U.S.

In 2017, 4,250 black men were diagnosed with cancer of liver and intrahepatic duct and 2,880 died of cancer of the liver and intrahepatic duct in the U.S.

Cancer of the liver and intrahepatic bile duct is more common in blacks and other minorities as compared to whites. In 2005, 13.2 black males and 8.2 white males per 100, 000 had cancer of the liver Intrahepatic duct in the U.S.

In 2010, 6,316 whites, 3,022 Asians, 2,230, Hispanics and 1,397 had liver cancer. The median survival for liver cancer was 15 months for Asians, 10 months for whites, Hispanics, and 8 months for blacks.

The death rates for cancer of liver intrahepatic duct are higher in blacks as compared to whites. In 2005, 10.3 black males and 6.7 white males per 100,000

Risk factors for cancer of the liver include:

1. Hepatitis B
2. Hepatitis C
3. Alcoholism
4. Hemochromatosis
5. Alflatoxin B1
6. Cirrhosis
7. Anabolic steroid
8. Diabetes mellitus
9. Obesity
10. Alcohol abuse
11. Exposure to industrial toxins
12. Liver fluke
13. Vinyl chloride exposure
14. Arsenic exposure

15. Thorium dioxide exposure
16. Wilson's disease

The best ways to evaluate cancer of the liver include:

1. Complete history and physical examination
2. Abdominal ultrasound
3. Abdominal CT scan
4. CT guided liver biopsy
5. Alpha fetoprotein
6. CEA
7. CBC
8. SMA20
9. PT and INR
10. PTT
11. Cytology of abdominal fluid
12. Cell count of abdominal fluid
13. Gram stain of abdominal fluid
14. Culture of abdominal fluid
15. Protein and glucose analysis of abdominal fluid
16. Chest x-ray
17. Serum ferritin
18. C282Y in white patients
19. Serum hepcidin level
20. Serum ferroportin level

Signs and symptoms of cancer of the liver:

1. General weakness
2. Lassitude
3. Tiredness
4. Weight loss
5. Tiredness
6. Headache
7. Nausea/Vomiting
8. Needle marks from drug addicts
9. Alcoholism
10. Cirrhosis of the liver
11. Jaundice
12. Itching
13. Enlargement of the liver
14. Enlargement of the spleen
15. Portal hypertension
16. Esophageal varices
17. Vomiting blood /Hematemesis

18. Ascites
19. Abdominal mass
20. Hemorrhoid
21. Rectal bleeding
22. Anemia
23. Possible positive hepatitis B or C
24. Possible HIV/AIDS
25. Iron overload
26. Leukopenia
27. Thrombocytopenia
28. Coagulopathy (high PT and PTT)
29. Disseminated intravascular coagulopathy (DIC)
30. Abnormal liver function tests
31. Tissue confirmation of cancer of the liver
32. High serum ferritin
33. Hemolytic anemia
34. Iron deficiency anemia
35. Anemia of inflammatory diseases
36. Gynecomastia in men
37. Testicular atrophy
38. Plantar erythema
39. Spider angiomata
40. Recurrent vaginal bleeding
41. Secondary polycythemia

Treatments of liver cancer include:

Surgical resection
Radiation therapy
Chemotherapy treatment is not very effective in primary cancer of the liver (Hepatoma)
Some of the drugs in use to treat cancer of the liver include:
Doxorubicin
Cisplatinum
Capecitabine
Liver transplant as treatment modality is commonly carried out.
Blacks and other minorities are 36% less likely than whites to receive liver transplant.

Cancer of the gall bladder

In 2017, 5,320 men were diagnosed with cancer of the gall bladder in the U.S. and 1,630 men died of cancer of the bladder.

Worldwide 38,309 people had cancer of the gall bladder in 2013 and the 5 years survival is only 20 percent. Sources: ACS Facts and Figures 2014 and WHO.

Risks for gallbladder cancer include:

Obesity
Gallstones
Family history
Genetic (In the U.S. gallbladder cancer is most common in Native Americans)

Signs and symptoms of cancer of the gallbladder include:

Weight loss
Abdominal pain
Abdominal bloating
Chest pain
Appetite loss
Nausea
Vomiting
Yellowness of eyes
Yellowness of skin (jaundice)
Itching etc;

Evaluations of cancer of the gallbladder include:

History and physical examination
Abdominal ultrasound
Abdominal CAT scan with contrast by mouth and with IV contrast
Chest x-ray
CBC
Complete chemistry profile
CEA
GGTP
PT/INR
PTT
Urinalysis
Gastrointestinal consultation
Surgery consultation

Treatments of gallbladder cancer include:

Surgical removal of the gallbladder
Radiation therapy

Chemotherapy drugs to treat gallbladder cancer include:

5FU
Cisplatinum
Oxaliplatin
Gemzar
Xoleda

These chemotherapy drugs are frequently used in combination.

Cancer of the Pancreas:

In 2017, 27,970 men were diagnosed with cancer of the pancreas in the U.S. and 22,300 men died of cancer of the pancreas.

In 2017, 3,210 black men were diagnosed with cancer of the pancreas and 2,390 of black men died of cancer of the pancreas.

Worldwide 250,000 people have pancreatic cancer every year and more than 250,000 people die yearly from pancreatic cancer in the world. WHO

The incidence of cancer of pancreas and the death rates of cancer pancreas are both higher in blacks and other minorities than in whites. In 2008, 17.1 black males and 14.8 black females per 100,000 had cancer of the pancreas and 10.7 white females and 13.5 white males per 100,000 had cancer of the pancreas in the U.S.

In 2007, 15.4 black males and 12.2 white males per 100,000 died of cancer of the pancreas and 12.4 black females and 9.1 white females per 100,000 died of cancer of the pancreas.

Signs and symptoms of cancer of the pancreas usually occur when it is too late to do much to save the patient. If the cancer is located near the head of the pancreas, it might cause the common bile duct to become obstructed, causing the patient to become jaundiced with no pain.

However, if the cancer is located at either the body or the tail of the pancreas, jaundice may occur due to metastasis to the liver.

Therefore, early development of jaundice due to cancer of the head of the pancreas may in some instances lead to the person seeking medical help. This could result in a positive outcome because of early surgical intervention. Left–sided, mid-abdominal pain in association with weight loss and poor appetite may also be signs of and symptoms of cancer of the pancreas.

Signs and symptoms of cancer of the pancreas include:

Weight lost
Poor appetite
Abdominal pain
Fever
Jaundice
Itching
Nausea
Vomiting
Elevated liver function tests
CEA

Elevated CA19-9
Anemia
Palpable left sided mid abdominal mass

Risks for cancer of the pancreas include:

1. Tobacco smoking
2. Chronic pancreatitis
3. Diabetes mellitus
4. High fat diet
5. Cirrhosis of the liver.
6. Alcoholism
7. Obesity
8. Genetic predisposition
9. Eating too much red meat etc;

The best ways to diagnose cancer of the pancreas include:

1. Taking a good history
2. Physical Examination
3. Abdominal sonogram
4. Abdominal CT Scan
5. Abdominal MRI
6. ERCP
7. PET Scan
8. CT guided biopsy

During the ERCP or endoscopic ERCP if a mass is present, it can be seen and material can be obtained for diagnosis. In addition, a stent can be placed to relieve the obstruction of the common bile duct to relieve the jaundice etc.

Cancer of the pancreas is very difficult to cure, but if found early, surgical resection is the preferred treatment, but this cancer is hardly ever found early.

There are many gastrointestinal procedures available to relieve the many symptoms and complications of pancreatic cancer, but none is curable.

The most effective chemotherapeutic agents include:

Gemzar
Taxotere
Irinotecan
Oxaliplatin
Cisplatinum
Capecitabine
Tarceva
Afrinitor

These drugs are used in combination, but they are not curative most of the time and surgical removal and radiotherapy as modalities for pancreatic cancer have a role, but they are not curative.

Other modalities of treatment in pancreatic cancer include:

Surgical resection
Radiation therapy

Cancer of the Brain

In 2017, 13,450 men were diagnosed with cancer of the brain in the U.S. and 9,620 men died of brain cancer. The incidence of brain cancer is twice higher in whites as compared to blacks. However, the death rates for cancer of the brain is much higher for blacks and other minorities as compared to whites. This is so, because blacks and other minorities received inferior medical care for their brain cancer as compared to whites.

Symptoms and signs of brain cancer include:

1. Headache
2. Nausea
3. Vomiting
4. Blurry vision
5. Depression
6. Psychosis
7. Insomnia
8. Irritability
9. Weight loss
10. Dementia
11. Seizure
12. Weakness in arms
13. Weakness in legs
14. Difficulty talking
15. Difficulty with bowel function
16. Difficulty with urinary function etc.

Some of the most common brain cancers include:

1. Glioma
2. Astrocytoma
3. Meningioma
4. Acoustic neuroma
5. Oligodendroglioma
6. Glioblastoma multiforme
7. Medulloblastoma
8. Metastatic cancer to the brain etc.

Some of the most common cancers that can metastasize to brain include:

1. Lung cancer
2. Breast cancer
3. Colon cancer
4. Prostate cancer
5. Melanoma
6. Lymphomas
7. Leukemias
8. Head and neck cancer
9. Thyroid cancer
10. Cancer of the kidney
11. Sarcoma
12. Ovarian cancer
13. Cervical cancer
14. Uterine cancer
15. Testicular cancer etc;

The best ways to evaluate brain cancer include:

1. Complete history and physical examination
2. Brain CT Scan with IV contrast
3. Brain MRI with IV contrast
4. Brain biopsy
5. Chest x- ray
6. CBC
7. SMA20
8. Possible lumbar puncture if metastatic cancer to the brain is suspected, using
9. a small fine needle
10. Cytology of spinal fluid
11. Glucose of spinal fluid
12. Protein of spinal fluid
13. Gram stain of spinal fluid
14. Cell count of Spinal fluid
15. Culture of spinal flui

Treatments of brain cancer include:

1. Surgical resection
2. Radiation therapy
3. Chemotherapy such as:
4. Irinotecan
5. Carmustine
6. 6-Thioguanine
7. Procarbazine

8. Lomustine
9. Vicristine
10. Temozolomidine
11. 13-cis-Retinoic acid
12. BCNU etc;

Metastatic cancer to the brain is treated according to the primary tumor with chemotherapy plus radiation.

Cancer of the prostate:

In 2017, 161,360 men had cancer of the prostate in the U.S. and 26, 730 men died of prostate cancer. Prospate cancer accounts for 31% of all cancer in African American men.

In 2017, 29,530 black men were diagnosed with prostate cancer and 4,450 black men died of prostate cancer.

Worldwide 899,000 men had prostate cancer and worldwide 238,000 men died of prostate cancer. WHO

Prostate cancer is much more common in Negroe/Black and other minority men compared to white men. Asians have a low incidence of prostate cancer because Asians eat a diet that is not rich in fat, and Asians are less obese than other men. According to the American cancer society, "the average annual prostate cancer rate "between" 2001-2005 was 59% higher in black men than in white men". The death rate from prostate cancer is 2.4 times higher in black men than in white men according to the ACS. 5 of every 100 African American men are expected to die of prostate cancer.

In addition, prostate cancer occurs at an earlier age in Negroes/Blacks and other minority men than in white men.

Prostate cancer begins to occur at around age thirty five-forty in black men and at around age 50 in white men. The two groups of black men in the world that have the highest rates of prostate cancer is African American men and black men from the Jamaica West Indies

The incidence of prostate cancer in Jamaicans is 51.1 per 100,000.

Risks for prostate cancer in Negroe/Black men include:

Being a black man
Age
High fat diet
Obesity
Caribbean born (specially Jamaicans)
Genetics
Recurrent prostate infection

Tobacco smoking

A difference in the activity of the gene PRDM9

Oncotype DX test evaluates which subgroup of prostate cancer is aggressive and more likely to spread and thus more deadly.

Symptoms of prostate cancer are divided in early symptoms and late symptoms.

Early symptoms of prostate cancer include:

Urge to urinate frequently

Difficulty to pass urine

Pain on urination etc

Many men have early prostate cancer with no symptoms and their cancers are picked up during routine physical examinations.

The symptoms of advanced prostate cancer include all the symptoms listed above plus:

Blood in the urine

Urinary retention

Lower abdominal pain

Urinary tract infection etc

The ways to diagnose prostate cancer include:

Complete history

Complete physical examination

Digital rectal examination

Prostatic specific antigen (PSA)

Ultrasound of the prostate

Biopsy of the prostate

The PSA is crucial in establishing the diagnosis of prostate cancer. In prostate cancer the PSA is elevated. In obese men, the PSA may be abnormally lower because the higher blood volume the obesity creates. This fact must be taken into consideration when evaluating obese men for prostate cancer.

This is particularly important in evaluating Black, Hispanics and Native American men because of the high percentage of obesity that exists in these groups of men.

Another important and indispensable part of the evaluation of prostate cancer is the digital rectal examination. During the digital rectal examination, the physician can tell if the prostate gland is enlarged, and if so, how enlarged. In addition, the physician can tell if the gland is nodular or if the gland is tender. There have been times when the PSA was normal and a cancerous nodule was palpated.

The medical conditions that cause an elevated PSA include:

Prostate cancer
Benign prostatic hypertrophy (BPH)
Prostatitis
Urinary tract infection
Rectal examination
Ejaculation

The different types of PSA are:

Total PSA
Free PSA
PSA velocity
Aged-adjusted PSA

The normal PSA is 0-4ng/ml

The prostate ultrasound is mandatory in the evaluation prostate cancer. During this test, suspicious calcification and other abnormalities can be seen. However, the prostate biopsy is the definitive procedure that can tell for sure if cancer exists in the prostate gland. This biopsy is carried out in urologist office under the guidance of ultrasound. The biopsy is done using a special needle that is inserted inside the rectum.

The ultrasound guides the urologist to the different parts of the prostate gland to biopsy. The tissue is sent to the pathology laboratory for the pathologist to prepare and evaluate under the microscope. Waiting for the result of the prostate biopsy can be nerve racking for men.

Once the biopsy is done and the pathology result is back showing cancer in the prostate. The next step is for the urologist to meet with the patient and his wife, or girl friend or other love interest to discuss the treatment options.
The key point in this discussion is the stage of the cancer.

The most common staging system for prostate cancer in use in the U.S. is:

"T stages (primary tumor)
N stages (Regional Lymph Nodes)
M stages (Distant Metastasis)
T stages (primary tumor)

In the T stages, the cancer is localized in the prostate gland surrounding areas.

Clinical staging:

TX- Primary tumor cannot be assessed
T0- No evidence of primary tumor
T1- cannot detect tumor with imaging tests
T1a -Less than 5 percent of the prostate is affected by the tumor
T1b-More than 5 percent of the prostate is affected by the tumor
T1c-Tumor identified by needle biopsy, PSA elevated
T2- Tumor confined within prostate
T2a-Tumor affects one-half of one lobe or less
T2b-Tumor affects more than one-half of one lobe, but not both lobes
T2c-Tumor affects both lobes
T3- Tumor extends through the prostate capsule
T3a-Tumor extends beyond the prostate capsule
T3b-Tumor invades seminal vesicle(s)
T4- Tumor is fixed or invades surrounding areas, such as the bladder neck,
External sphincter, rectum, levator muscle, and/or pelvic wall

Pathological staging:

PT2- Tumor confined to the prostate
PT2a-Tumor affects one-half of one lobe or less
PT2b-Tumor affects more than one- half of one lobe, but not both lobes
Patch- Tumor affects both lobes
PT3- Tumor extends beyond the prostate
PT3b-Tumor invades seminal vesicle (s)
pT4- Tumor invades the bladder, rectum

N stages (Regional Lymph Nodes)
A N0 stage indicates the cancer has not spread to the lymph nodes.
N1 indicates the cancer has spread to one or more pelvic nodes.

Clinical:

NX-Regional lymph nodes were not assessed
N0- Tumor has not spread to regional lymph nodes
N1- Tumor has spread to regional nodes

Pathological:

pNX-Regional lymph nodes were not assessed
pN0- Regional lymph nodes not affected by tumor
pN1- Regional lymph nodes affected by tumor

M stages (Distant Metastasis)

A M0 stages indicates the cancer has not metastasized beyond the local lymph nodes. While M1 indicates the cancer has metastasized to distant lymph nodes and/or to other organs.

MX-Distant metastasis cannot be assessed

M0-No distant metastasis

M1-Distant metastasis

M1a-Non-regional lymph nodes affected by tumor

M1b-Bones affected by tumor

M1c-Other sites affected by tumor with or without bone disease"

Sources: National Cancer Institute/American Cancer Society

Treatment options for prostate cancer include:

Stage 1:

Radical prostatectomy (Using conventional surgical technic or DA Vinci/Robotic surgical technic inimically invasive)

or

External beam radiation

or

Seeds implantation

or

Watchful waiting

Stage II Prostate cancer:

Radical prostatectomy as stage I plus radiation

or

External beam radiation

or

Seeds implantation

Chemotherapy

Stage III Prostate cancer includes:

Radical prostatectomy as per stage I

or

External beam radiation

or

Hormonal therapy

or

Chemotherapy

Stage IV Prostate cancer:

External beam radiation
Hormonal therapy
Chemotherapy

The hormonal medications in use to treat prostate cancer include:

Lupron
Casodex
Zoladex
Eulexin

The chemotherapy medications in use to treat prostate cancer include:

Taxol
Etoposide
Estramustine
Doxorubicin
Mitoxantrone
"DNA-Repair Defects and Olaparib in Metastatic Prostate Cancer."
These drugs are used in advanced metastatic prostate cancer.

All treatments used to treat prostate cancer have side effects, Proastatectomy as a treatment modality while effective can cause serious side effects.

Among these side effects include:

Bleeding
Urinary incontinence
Urinary tract infection
Sexual impotence

Hormonal treatment is an integral part of the overall treatments of prostate cancer.

However, hormonal side effects of the medications can be significant. Among these side effects include:

Hot flashes
Enlargement of the breasts
No sexual desire
Sexual impotence

Chemotherapy drugs play a major and significant role in the treatments in prostate cancer. Among these side effects are:

Nausea
Vomiting
Low white blood cells
Low red blood cells
Low platelets
Sores in the mouth
Loss of hair
Diarrhea
General weakness
Numbness in the feet etc;

Some of the medications in use to treat sexual impotence after prostatectomy, radiation, and seeds implantation include:

Viagra
Cialis
Levitra

Radiation and Seeds implantation both play major roles in the treatment of prostate cancer.

Some of the side effects of radiation as a treatment modality for prostate cancer include:

Nausea
Vomiting
Weakness
Low white blood cells
Low red blood cells
Low platelets
Sexual impotence
Radiation proctitis
Rectal bleeding due to radiation proctitis

Some of the side effects of seeds implantation as a treatment modality for prostate cancer Include:

Nausea
Vomiting
General weakness
Sexual impotence etc;

Prostate cancer is a curable cancer if diagnosed early. Men ought to seek medical evaluation for prostate health starting at age 35 year if they are African Americans or

Jamaicans and all other black men ought to seek medical evaluation for prostate health beginning at age 40.

All men whose fathers have had or have prostate cancer should seek medical evaluation for prostate health at age 35. Caucasian, Asian, and men of other ethnic ancestries should seek medical evaluation for prostate health beginning at age 50.

Cancer head and neck:

In 2017, 35,720 men in the U.S. were diagnosed with head and neck cancer and 7,000 men died of head and neck cancer in the U.S.

Worldwide there are 600,000 cases of head and cancer annually and 320,000 people die from head and neck cancer. WHO

Head and neck cancer is 50 percent more common blacks and other minorities as compared to whites. The death rates are higher among blacks and other minorities with head and neck cancer than they are in whites.

Risk factors for head and neck cancer include:

Tobacco smoking
Alcohol abuse
HPV infection
Genetic transmission
Radiation to neck area during childhood

Some signs and symptoms of head and neck cancer include:

1. A sore that bleeds often and easily and fails to heal
2. Persistent hoarseness
3. Palpable mass in the neck
4. Pain on swallowing
5. Difficulty swallowing
6. Persistent sore throat etc.

Methods in use to diagnose o head and neck cancer include:

History
Physical examination
Fiberoptic Laryngoscopic examination
Chest x ray
CT Scan of the neck
MRI of the neck
Biopsy of any lesion seen under general anesthesia

The best treatment for head and neck cancers is radiation therapy given 5 days per week for 6 weeks together with Cis-Platinum 100mg/m2 given on day #1, day #22 and day# 43. The response rate for radiation and chemotherapy for stages 1, 2, and 3, head and neck cancers is in the range of 75% worldwide. The response rate for surgical resection of head and neck cancers with adjuvant radiation/ chemotherapy parallels the response rate of radiation and chemotherapy without surgical resection.

Frequently surgical resection of head and neck cancers requires the removal of the voice box with a permanent tracheostomy.

Other drugs used to treat head and neck cancer is:

1. Paclitaxel
2. Docetaxel
3. Carboplatin
4. Ifosfamide
5. Methotrexate

In evaluating the throat using the fiberoptic laryngoscope, it is mandatory that the physician doing the scoping passes the laryngoscope through both nasal passages so as not to miss cancer and other lesions that may be located in the upper right or upper left of the nasal anatom.

Some of the side effects of chemotherapy medications used to treat head and neck cancer include:

Nausea
Vomiting
Diarrhea
Loss of appetite
Weight loss
Sores in the mouth
Sores in the throat
Pain on swallowing
Low white blood cells
Low red blood cells
Low platelets
Fever
Infection
Dehydration
Severe pain in the mouth and throat
Numbness in feet etc

Some of the side effects radiation treatment used to treat head and neck cancer include:

Nausea
Vomiting

General weakness
Sore in the mouth
Sore in the throat
Severe damage to the upper esophagus with esophagitis
Dehydration
Low white blood cells
Low red blood cells
Low platelets
Infection
Severe damage to the salivary glands
Severe zerostomia (dry mouth)
Damage to teeth and gums with marked long term tooth decays
Severe damage to the skin around the neck with hyperpigmentation
Longterm tiredness etc;

Cancer of the Urinary Bladder:

In 2017, 60,490 men were diagnosed with cancer of the urinary bladder in the U.S. and 12,240 men died urinary bladder cancer.

In 2017, 2,910 black men were diagnosed with urinary bladder cancer.

Worldwide in 2013, there were 382,500 people that were diagnosed with cancer of the urinary bladder and 187,000 people die of cancer of the urinary bladder annually. WHO

In 2008, 21.6 black males and 40.6 white males per 100,000 had cancer of the urinary bladder in the U.S. Over all cancer of the urinary bladder is more common in men than women and it usually develops between the ages of 50 to 70.

In 2007, 7.9 white males and 5.4 black males per 100,000 died of cancer of the urinary bladder in the U.S.

Urinary bladder cancer is twice more common in whites than blacks and other minorities, but the death rate is higher in blacks and other minorities than whites. In addition, the death rate for this cancer is higher in women than men.

Some of the risk factors for urinary cancer include:

Smoking
Exposure to industrial dyes
Exposure to industrial rubbers
Exposure to industrial leathers
Schistosomiosis heamatobium infection
Genetic inheritance

Symptoms of urinary bladder cancer include:

Urinary frequency
Urinary incontinence
Recurrent urinary infection
Blood in the urine (gross)
Microscopic hematuria
Urinary retention
Low back pain
Abdominal pain
Hydronephrosis
Weight loss
Poor appetite etc;

The way to evaluate patients for possible urinary bladder cancer includes:

1. History
2. Physical examination
3. Urinalysis
4. Urine cytology
5. Ultrasound of the urinary bladder
6. IVP
7. CT of the urinary bladder
8. Cystoscopy with biopsy of suspected lesions

Surgery is frequently in the diagnosis and treatments of urinary bladder cancer.

Drugs in use to treat bladder cancer are:

1. Methotrexate
2. Vinblastin
3. Doxorubicin Cisplatinum
4. Gemcitabine
5. Isfosfamine
6. Mesna
7. Placlitaxel
8. Inmmunotherapy with BCG installation in the urinary bladder.
9. Photodynamic therapy

The chemotherapy drugs are used in different combinations.

Kidney Cancer & renal pelvis:

In 2017, 40,610 men were diagnosed with kidney and renal pelvis in the U.S. and 9, 470 died of kidney and renal pelvis cancer.

In 2017, 4,830 black men were diagnosed with kidney and renal pelvis cancer and 860 black men died of kidney and renal pelvis cancer.

Worldwide in 2013, 208,500 cancers of the kidney/renal pelvis were diagnosed and each year more 102,000 people died of cancer of kidney/renal pelvis. WHO

Cancer of the kidney is more common in blacks and other minorities than in whites.

In 2005, 21.3 black males per 100,000 were diagnosed with cancer of the kidney in the U.S. and 18.8 white males per 100,000 were diagnosed with cancer of the kidney.

During that same time, 6.1 black males per 100,000 died of cancer of the kidney and 6.2 white males per 100,000 died of cancer of the kidney.

Some of the risk factors for cancer of the kidney include:

1. Being a man
2. Smoking
3. Exposure to asbestos
4. Exposure to cadium
5. Genetic inheritance
6. Being black
7. Von Hipple –Lindau syndrome
8. Hypertension etc.

Signs and symptoms of cancer of the kidney include:

Hematuria (gross)
Hematuria (microscopic)
Low back pain
Palpable flank mass in lower abdomen
Unexplained and recurrent fevers
Weight loss
Poor appetite
Fatigue
Anemia
Secondary Polycythemia due (hypernephroma) etc;

Evaluating patients for possible cancer of the kidney includes:

1. History
2. Physical examination
3. Urinalysis
4. Urine cytology
5. Ultra sound of the kidney
6. CT of the kidneys

7. MRI
8. PET scan
9. Chest x-ray
10. CBC
11. Complete metabolic profile

Treatments of cancer of the kidney include:

Surgery to remove the cancerous kidney
Possible radiation therapy
Possible chemotherapy

Chemotherapy medications in used to treat cancer of the kidney include:

Interferon-alpha
Bevacizumab
Interleukin-2
Sunitinib
Sorafenib
Temsirolimus

Testicular cancer:

In 2017, 8,850 men were diagnosed with testicular cancer in the U.S. and 380 men died of testicular.

Worldwide in 2013, 36,000 are diagnosed with testicular cancer annually and 1 in 5000 men die of testicular. WHO

Testicular cancer is much more common in white men than in black and other minority men. In 2005, 1.4 black men and 6.3 white men per 100,000 were diagnosed with testicular cancer.

Risks for testicular cancer include:

Undescended testis
Family history of testicular cancer
Congenital abnormalities of the genitourinary tract

Signs and symptoms of testicular cancer include:

A painless lump of the testicle
Pain in the testicle
Pain in the groin
Lower abdominal pain
Low back pain

How is testicular cancer diagnosed?

Examination of the testicles
Ultrasound of the testicle
Abdominal CT Scan
Alpha Feto protein
Beta HCG
LDH
Biopsy of the testicular mass
Chest x ray
PET Scan

How is testicular cancer treated?

Surgical removal of the affected testis (Orchiectomy)
Radiation therapy and or chemotherapy
The chemotherapy medications in use to treat stage II testicular include
Bleomycin
Cisplatinum
Etoposide

These drugs are used in combination every 28 days

Drugs in use to treat advanced stage testicular cancer include:

Cisplatinum
Vinblastine
Ifosfamide
Mesna
Or
Cisplatinum
Paclitaxel
Ifosfamide
Mesna

It is extremely important for men to examine their testicles frequently.

Testicular cancer is extremely sensitive to both radiation therapy and chemotherapy with a very high cure rate.

Leukemias:

In 2017, 36,290 men were diagnosed with leukemia in the U.S. and 14,300 men died leukemia in the U.S.

In 2017, 2,840 black men were diagnosed with leukemia in the U.S. and 1,110 black men died of leukemia in the U.S. Source: ACS Facts and Figures 2017

The different types of leukemias are:

1. Acute lymphocytic leukemia
2. Chronic lymphocytic leukemia (CLL represents 35% of all leukemias in the world) and annually 75,000 people in the die of CLL in the world.
3. Acute myelogenic leukemia
4. Chronic myelogenic leukemia
5. Monocytic leukemia
6. Myelodysplastic syndrome
7. Acute megakaryocytic leukemia
8. T-cell leukemia/lymphoma due to HTLVI and II.

The risks for leukemia include:

Down's syndrome,
AIDS,
Exposure to ionizing radiation
Exposure to chemicals like benzene and other toxic chemicals
Genetic etc.

Evaluations of leukemia include:

History and physical examination
CBC with differential
Complete chemistry profile
Urinalysis
LDH
LAP
ESR
HIV/AIDS blood test
Bone marrow aspiration
Bone marrow biopsy
Cell surface marker studies
Cytogenetic studies
Abdominal CT with contrast by mouth
Chest x-ray
Chest CT
EKG
Echocardiogram
Rest MUGA

Sings and symptoms of Leukemia include:

Fatigue
Weight loss
Easy bruising
Nosebleed
Frequent infections
Enlarged liver
Enlarged spleen
Anemia
Elevated white blood cells
Low platelets
Abnormal peripheral blood smear
Abnormal bone marrow aspiration and bone marrow biopsy
Abnormal differential cells count on blood smear
Cytogenetics studies of chromosomal
Abnormal BCR/ABL Gene, QN, PCR (in CML)
Elevated LDH
Low leukocyte alkaline phosphatase (LAP)
Lymphocytes cell surface marker studies (CD5, CD 19, CD 20, and CD 23)

Different types of leukemias are treated with different chemotherapeutic regimens and bone marrow transplantation.

Induction therapy:

In 2017, 3, 350 men were diagnosed with acute lymphocytic leukemia in the U.S. and 800 died of ALL in the U.S.

Acute lymphocytic leukemia (ALL) is treated with:

Daunorubicin 50 mg/m2 IV every 24 hours on day 1-3
Vincristine 2 mg IV on days 1, 8, 15, and 22
Prednisone 60 mg/m2 daily on days 1-28
L-Asparaginase 6,000 U/m2 on days 17-28
There are Consolidation protocols and maintenance protocols available to treat ALL.
CNS prophylaxis is
Cranial irradiation is given with 1,800 rad in 10 fractions over 12-14 days
Plus Methotrexate 12 mg intra-thecally every week for 6 weeks
Newer medications in use to treat ALL are
Imatinib 600 mg by mouth every day
or
Dastinib 70 mg by mouth twice per day
or
Clofarabine 52mg/m2 IV for 5 days

In 2017, 11, 960 people were diagnosed with acute myelogenous leukemia in the U.S. and 6,110 men died of AML.

Acute Myelogenous leukemia (AML) is treated with:

Cytarabrine 100 mg/m2/day IV continuous infusion days 1-7
Daunorubicin 45 mg/m2 IV days 1-7
or
Cytabrine 100mg/m2/day IV continuous infusion days 1-7
Doxorubicin 12mg/m2 days 2, 4, 6, and 8
There are several more protocols and single agents available to treat AML

In 2017, 12,310 men were diagnosed with chronic lymphocytic leukemia in the U.S. and 2,880 men died of CLL.

Chronic lymphocytic leukemia (CLL) is treated with:

Cytoxan 400 mg/m2 days 1-5
Vincristine 1-4 mg/m2 IV day (maximum dose 2mg)
Prednisone 100mg/m2 by mouth days1-5
or
Fludaradine 25 mg/m2 IV days 1-5
Retuxan 375 mg/m2 IV days 1, and 4on cycle 1 and on day 1 there after
or
Fludarabine 25 mg/m2 IV days 1-3
Cytoxan 250 mg/m2 IV days 1-3
or
Retuxan 375 mg/m2 IV every week for 4 weeks
Imbruvica (Ibrutinid) just approved by the FDA is now also available to treat CLL in patients who were previously treated.
There are several more protocols and single agents' drugs in use to treat CLL.

In 2017, 5,230 men were diagnosed with chronic myelogenous leukemia in the U.S. and 610 men died of CML.

Chronic Myelogenous leukemia is treated with:

Imatinib 400 mg/day by mouth or 600 mg/day
Dasatinib 70 mg twice per day
Imatimid 400mg daily plus peginterferon alfa-2a 90ug weekly is said to be superior to Imatimid alone

Acute Promyelocytic leukemia is treated with:

All-trans-Reteinoic Acid 45mg mg/m2/day by mouth in 2 divided doses until remission
Idarubicin 12 mg/m2/day IV on days 1-5

Hairy cell Leukemia is treated with:

Cladribine 0.09 mg/kg/day IV as a continuous infusion days 1-7
Pentostatin 4 mg/m2 IV day 1
Repeat every 14 days for 6 cycles.

Lymphoma:

In 2017, 44,730 men were diagnosed with lymphoma in the U.S. that included 40,080 non-Hodgkin lymphoma and 4,650 Hodgkin lymphoma and 11, 450 men died of Non-Hodgkin lymphoma 1,070 died of Hodgkin lymphoma in 2017 in the U.S.

In 2017, 3,230 blacks were diagnosed with Non-Hodgkin lyphoma.

The incidence of lymphoma is higher in Caucasians than in Blacks and other minorities. In 2005, 2.9 black males and 2.3 black females per 100,000 were diagnosed with Hodgkin lymphoma and in comparison, 3.3 white males and 2.7 white females per 100,000 were diagnosed with Hodgkin lymphoma. During that time, 18.4 black males and 12.2 black females per 100.000 were diagnosed with Non-Hodgkin lymphoma and in comparison, 24.3 white males and 17.1 white females per 100,000 were diagnosed with Non-Hodgkin lymphoma.

The death rates for lymphoma are higher in whites compared to blacks and other minorities. In 2005, 0.5 black males and 0.3 black females per 100,000 died of Hodgkin lymphoma as compared to 0.6 white males and 0.4 white females per 100,000 died of Hodgkin lymphoma. During that time, 6.4 black males and 4.2 black females per 100,000 died of Non-Hodgkin lymphoma as compared to 9.7 white males and 6.2 white females per 100,000 died of Non-Hodgkin lymphoma.

Risks for lymphoma Hodgkin/Non-Hodgkin include:

History of Infectious mononucleosis
Epstein -Barr infection (50% of Hodgkin lymphoma is associated with Epstein-Barr infection)
HIV/AIDS infection
HLTV 1 infection (this infection is most commonly seen in the Caribbean, southern island of Japan, Northeastern South America, Central America, and New Guinea.
Non-acquired immunodeficiency disease
H pylori infection of the stomach
Being a male
Being highly educated
Exposure to chemical
Genetic inheritance etc;

Some of the signs and symptoms of lymphoma include:

Fever
Night sweats
Loss of appetite
Weight loss
Enlarged lymph nodes
Diarrhea
Fever of unknown origin FUO
Enlarged spleen
Enlarged liver
Abdominal pain
Jaundice
Anemia etc;

The best ways to evaluate a person for the possibility of lymphoma include:

A complete history and physical examination
Chest ray
Chest CT Scan
Abdominal CT Scan
MRI of the chest/abdomen
PET Scan
CBC
Complete chemistry profile
LDH
ESR
Urinalysis
PT/PTT
Bone marrow aspiration
Bone marrow biopsy
Cytogenetic studies
Lymphocytes cell surface markers
Lymph node biopsy

The best treatments available to treat Hodgkin's disease as published in the literature are:

(ABVD)
Doxorubicin
Bleomycin
Vinblastine
Dacarbazine
(ChiVPP)
Chlorambucil
Vinblastine

Procarbazine
Prednisone
(Stanford V)
Doxorubicin
Vinblastine
Mechlorethamine
Vincristine
Bleomycin
Etoposide
(ASHAP)
Doxorubicin
Methylprednisolone
Cisplatin
Cytarabine
(CHOP)
Cyclophosphamide
Doxorubicin
Vincristine
Prednisone

Some of the drugs available to treat non-Hodgkin's lymphoma as published in the literature are:

(CHOP plus Rituximab)
Rituximab
Cyclophosphomide
Doxorubicin
Vincristine
Prednisone
(CHOP-14 every 2 weeks)
Cyclophosphomide
Doxorubicin
Vincristine
Prednisone
(CODOX-M)
Cyclophosphomide
Vincristine
Doxorubicin
Methotrexate
Leucovorin
GM-CSF
(IVAC)
Etoposide
Ifosfamide
Mesna

Cytarabine
Methotrexate
GM-CSF
(DHAP)
Dexamethasone
Cisplatin
Cytarabine
(EPOCH plus Rituximab)
Rituximab
Doxorubicin
Etoposide
Vincristine
Cyclophosphamide
Prednisone
Ibrutinib is approved by the FDA to be used in small lymphocytic lymphoma.

Radiation therapy is a major treatment modality in the treatments of lymphomas.

Multiple Myeloma:

In 2017, 17,490 men were diagnosed with multiple myeloma in the U.S. and 6,660 men died of multiple myeloma in the U.S.

In 2017, 3,070 black men were diagnosed with multiple myeloma in the U.S. and 1,040 black men died of multiple myeloma in the U.S.

Multiple myeloma is more than twice as common in blacks and other minorities as compared to whites and the death rate for multiple myeloma is more than twice in blacks as compared to whites.

Risk factors for multiple myeloma include:

Being a man (multiple myeloma is more common in men than women are)
Being black and other minorities
Being age 50 or older
Obesity
Hypertension
History of monoclonal gammopathy of undetermined significance (MGUS), each year 1 percent of people with MGUS develop multiple myeloma
Exposure to radiation, benzene and other industrial chemicals

Signs and symptoms of multiple myeloma include:

Low back pain
Rib cage pain
Weight loss

Bone pain anywhere in the body
Weakness
Fatigue
Anemia
Blurry vision
Fever

Evaluations of multiple myeloma include:

History and physical examination
CBC
Complete blood chemistry profile
ESR
Urinalysis
Serum protein electrophoresis
Immunoelectrophoresis
Serum IgG, IgM, IgA, IgD
Urine for Bence Jones protein
Serum free light chain
Chest X-ray
Skeletal survey
Urine immunoelectrophoresis
Bone marrow aspiration
Bone marrow biopsyet

Abnormal findings that can be seen in multiple myeloma include:

Bence Jones protein in the urine
Monoclonal M protein in the blood
Abnormal protein electrophoresis
Elevated IgG, IgM, IgA, or IgD in the blood
Low IgG, IgM, IgA, and IgD in the blood (seen in light chain myeloma)
High IgA in the urine (seen in IgA myeloma
Lytic lesions on bone x-rays.
Abnormal plasma cells level in bone marrow aspiration/biopsy
Elevated BUN
Elevated serum creatinine
Elevated serum calcium
Elevated ESR
Elevated LDH
High total protein
Low total protein (seen in light myeloma)
High serum calcium
High serum free light chain (seen in IgA myeloma)
Elevated Beta-2-microglobulin

Low or high white blood cells
Low red blood cells
Low platelets
Recurrent pneumonia
Recurrent urinary track infection
Sepsis (people with multiple myeloma are immunosuppresed and as such get infected frequently with bacteria, fungi, or viruses)
Hyperviscosity syndromeetc;

The different stages of myeloma:

Stage 1:

" No anemia (in other words, a normal red cell count)
A normal level of blood calcium
No bone damage or a solitary plasmacytoma
Low levels abnormal antibodies (immunoglobulin) in your blood or urine

Stage 2:

Includes anyone who does not fit exactly into 1 or stage
Therefore, you would be stage 2 if you had 2 areas of bone damage. You can also have stage 2A or 2B. As with stage 1, this depends on whether your kidneys have been damaged at all by the myeloma.

Stage 3:

This is if you have:
Anemia (low red cell count)
High levels of calcium in your blood
More than 3 sites of bone damage
High levels of abnormal paraproteins in your blood or urine

Stage 3 is also divided into stages 3A an 3B, with those in 3B, having a high creatinine level in their blood, indicating that they have some kidney damage from their myeloma."

Treatments of multiple myeloma include:

Melphalan 8-10mg/m2 days 1-4 by mouth
Prednisone 60 mg/m2 days 1-4 by mouth
Repeat cycle every 42 days

or
Melphalan 0.25 mg/kg/days 1-4 by mouth
Prednisone 2mg/kg//days 1-4 by mouth
Thalidomide 100-400 mg daily by mouth

Repeat cycle every 42 days

or
Vincristine 0.4 mg/day IV as a continuous infusion days 1-4
Doxorubicin 9 mg/m2/day IV as a continuous in fusion days 1-4
Dexamethasone 40 mg by mouth days 1-4, 9-12, and 17-20

or
Velcade 1.3mg/m2 on day 1, 4, 8 and 11 and Adriamycin 30mg/m2 on day 4 and
Dexamethasone 40mg IV or by mouth on day 1-4, 9-11 and 17-20 repeat cycle every
21 days
Radiation therapy
Stem cells transplant is an option for suitable patients etc;

There are numerous other protocols in use to treat multiple myeloma. Bone marrow transplant is being quite often to treat patients with multiple myeloma with varying degrees of success. The FDA has recently approved Carfilzomid for treatment of second line multiple myeloma. The FDA has approved daratumumab " for treating the incurable blood cancer multiple myeloma in patients who have failed prior therapies and have few options left."

Melanoma

The most serious and malignant form of skin cancer is melanoma and in 2017, 52,170 men were diagnosed with melanoma in the U.S. and 6, 380 men died of melanoma in the U.S.

Risks factors for the development of skin cancer include:

1. Ultraviolet rays (exposure to the sun)
2. Being of fair complexion
3. Exposure to arsenic compounds
4. Exposure to radium
5. Exposure to coal tar
6. Family history of skin cancer
7. History of multiple skin moles
8. BRAF gene carriers
9. Frequent unprotected sun bathing

Signs and symptoms of melanoma include:

A mole that a change in color, size, and bleeds over the trunk, legs, abdomen, chest, arms a large brownish spot with darker speckles over sun exposed areas of the body A lesion with irregular border and portions that is red, white, blue, or black over sun

Exposed areas of the body Dark/black lesions on palms, soles of feet, fingertips, toes, mucous membranes in Mouth, nose, anus, and vagina etc.

Evaluations of melanoma include:

History and physical examination
Close examination of the skin by a Dermatologist
CBC
Complete chemistry profile
ESR
Urinalysis
V600E test (newly approved by the FDA)
V600K test (newly approved by the FDA)
Chest x-ray
Chest CT
Abdominal CT
PET Scan
Skin biopsy

A dermatologist and appropriate biopsies taken when necessary should examine any all lesions of concern. The most effective treatments for melanoma are surgical resection with regional lymph node removal, radiation therapy, immunotherapy, and chemotherapy.

The chemotherapy drugs in use to treat malignant melanoma include:

Dacarbazide 220mg/m2 IV days 1-3
Carmustine 150 mg/m2 IV days 1
Cisplatinum 25 mg/m2 IV days 1-3

or
Temozolomide 75 mg/m2/day by mouth for 6 weeks
Thalidomide 200-400 mg/m2/day by mouth for 6 weeks

or
Interferon Alpha-2b 15 million IU/m2 IV days 1-5, 8-12, and 15-19
Interferon Alpha-2b 10 million IU/m2 SC 3 times weekly post induction
Dacarbazide 200 mg/m2 IV days 22-26
Repeat every 28 days

New drugs approved by the FDA to treat melanoma include:

Yervoy
Zelboraf
Tafinlar
Mekinist
Keytruda

"Dabrafenib plus trametinib, as compared with vemurafenib monotherapy, significantly improved overall survival in previously untreated patients with metastatic melanoma with

BRAF V600E or V600K mutations, without increased overall toxicity." N Engl J MED 372; January 1, 2015

The FDA has recently approved iplimumab and nivolumab for the treatment of advanced melanoma to be taken together. "Each drug is expected to cost $250,000 in their first year" on the market.

Thyroid Cancer:

In 2017, 14,400 men were diagnosed with thyroid cancer in the U.S. and 920 men died of thyroid cancer in the U.S.

There are three types of thyroid cancer:

The most common form of thyroid cancer is papillary carcinoma, which is 70% of thyroid cancers. Follicular carcinoma represents 15% of thyroid cancer, and anaplastic cancer of the thyroid occurs 5% of the time. The most malignant and aggressive type of thyroid cancer is the follicular type.

Thyroid cancer is almost twice more common in whites than blacks and other minorities and the death rates for thyroid cancer is almost twice in whites than in blacks and other minorities.

Risk factors for thyroid cancer include:

Exposure to high dose radiation
People who were treated with radiation to treat tonsils/adenoids as children many years ago
History of thyroid goiter
Family history of goiter
Genetic inheritance etc;

Signs and symptoms of thyroid cancer include:

A lump in the neck
Hoarseness
Problem swallowing
Enlarged lymph nodes around the neck etc;

How to evaluate a person for possible thyroid cancer:

History and physical examination
T4 and TSH blood tests
Thyroid ultrasound
Thyroid Scan
Fine needle aspiration of a cold thyroid nodule
Chest x-ray

Treatments of thyroid cancer include:

Surgery to remove the thyroid gland
Radioactive iodine treatment to kill any remaining cancer cells
Synthroid
This thyroid hormone is to replace the hormone, which the thyroid can no longer produce, and to suppress the ability of the pituitary gland from making TSH. People, who have had their thyroid glands removed surgically or destroyed by radiation treatment, must take synthroid for the rest of their lives.

Most thyroid nodules are not malignant.

There are two types of thyroid nodules, hot nodule and cold nodule. Hot nodules are usually benign and are not cancerous. Cold nodules are not always associated with cancer, but when local thyroid cancers develop, frequently, they arise from a cold nodule.

Because the thyroid gland is extremely vascular, a lot of blood passes through it, and consequently metastatic cancer of the thyroid from lung, breast, melanoma, and esophagus occur frequently. Lymphoma of the thyroid also occurs and represents about 5% of all thyroid cancers.

Among the risks for the development of thyroid cancer are being female and exposure to radiation. People who have had radiation treatment to their tonsils as a child have high incidence of thyroid cancer when they become adults.

Once biopsy documents that thyroid cancer is present, surgical removal of the thyroid gland must be carried out. The extent of the surgical incision depends on the cell type of the cancer.

Treatments of thyroid cancer include:

Following resection of the thyroid cancer, radioactive iodine must be administered to destroy all remaining thyroid tissues.

The other necessary treatment is Synthroid by mouth, both for suppression and treatment for life. There is no effective chemotherapy available for thyroid cancer except for VP16, which has shown some response. People with thyroid cancer must remain under the care of an endocrinologist for many years.

Recently the FDA approved Lenvatinib to treat Radioiodine refractory thyroid cancer.

Malignant thymoma:

Malignant Thymoma is a cancer that develops in 0.15 cases per 100,000 representing 0.2% to 1.5% of all cancers. It's usually between the ages of 40-60.

Most of the time thymoma is discovered incidentally on chest x-ray or CAT Scan of the chest. The usual anatomical location of the thymoma is the anterior mediastinum.

Thymoma can be associated many diseases including:

Rheumatoid arthritis
Systemic Lupus Erythematosus
Scleroderma
Sarcoidosis
Thyroiditis
Acute pancreatitis
Alopecia areata
Aplastic anemia
Hemolytic anemia etc;

Symptoms of thymoma include:

Chest pain
Cough
Upper airway congestion

Evaluations of Thymoma include:

History and physical examination
Chest x-ray
CAT Scan of the chest
EKG
CBC
Complete blood chemistry profile
ANA
Direct comb's test
ESR
T4
TSH
Angiotensin converting enzyme inhibitor etc;

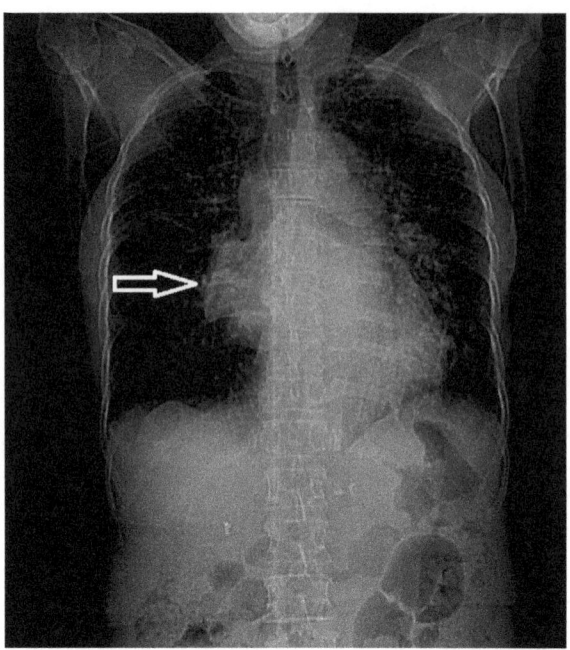

Figure 10:20 - Chest x-ray of a large right anterior mediastinal mass in a person with malignant thymoma.

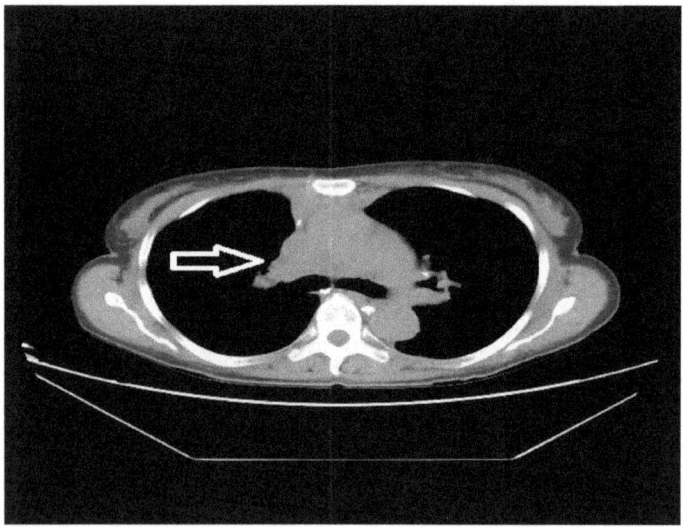

*Figure 10:21-*Chest CT of a large right anterior mediastinal mass in a person with malignant thymoma.

Treatments of malignant thymoma include:

Surgical resection of the thymoma
Radiation therapy
Chemotherapy

The most commonly used include:

" Cisplatin 50mg/m2 IV + Doxorubicin 50mg/m2 IV+ Cclophosphamide 500mg/m2 IV on day 1 Repeat every 21 days for 8 cycles.

or
Cyclophosphomide 500mg/m2 IV day1
Cisplatin 30mg/m2 IV days 1-3
Doxorubicin 2omg/m2 via 24-hour continuous IV infusion day 1-3
Prednisone 100mg PO days 1-5
Repeat every 3 weeks for 3 cycles

or
Cisplatin 50mg/m2 IV and doxorubicin 40mg/m2 IV day 1
Vincristine 0.6mg/m2IV on day 3
Cyclophosphomide 700mg/m2 IV day 4
Repeat every 3 weeks for 5 cycles."

Breast cancer in men:

In 2017 2,470 men were diagnosed with breast cancer and 460 men of different racial backgrounds died of breast cancer.

Evaluation of breast cancer in men include:

History and physical examination
Mammogram
Sonogram of the breast
MRI of the breast
Biopsy of breast mass
Estrogen/Progesterone
HER 2 testing of breast tissue
Chest-xray
CAT scans of chest and abdomen
PET Scan

Treatment of breast cancer include:

Lumpectomy
Mastectomy
Chemotherapy
Radiationtherapy
Hormonal therapy etc;

Much progress has been made in the detection and treatment of cancer and many cancers are curable when detected and treated early. However, much more needs to be done to understand the genetic transmission of cancer, the way cancer cells grow in the human body, so that genetic engineering can be used to prevent the growth of cancer cells in the human body. Society must do more to stop people from being exposed to cancer-causing agents and other toxic materials. Many men must stop their self-destructive habits such as cigarette smoking, alcohol abuse, and eating too many fat-rich foods; they must exercise more to lose weight to decrease their incidence of cancer.

The incidence of cancer and the death rates from cancer are much higher in Blacks and other minorities than Whites are. Higher rates of unemployment, lower level of education, high rates of uninsured and racism against Negroes/Blacks and other minorities all play a role in both the cancer rates and death rates being so much higher in Blacks and other minorities compared to Whites. Both government and the private sector must make available more money for cancer research and cancer treatments so that cancer can be eliminated once and for all. Source: ACS Cancer Facts & Figures 2017

CHAPTER 11

KIDNEY DISEASES IN
AFRICAN AMERICAN MEN

——◆◆——

There are more than 26 million people with kidney diseases in the U.S. and About 20 million more people are at risk for developing kidney diseases in the U.S.

Worldwide there are more than 141,503,782 people with kidney diseases:

"Country - # of People
China - 35,336,295
India - 28,976,185
USA – 26,000,000
Indonesia - 6,487,322
Brazil - 5,008,633
Pakistan - 4,331,076
Russia - 3,916,941
Bangladesh - 3,845,292
Japan - 3,464,206
Mexico - 2,855,518
Philippines - 2,346,281
Germany - 2,242,434
Egypt - 2,070,841
Ethiopia - 1,940,774
Turkey - 1,874,319
Iran - 1,836,484
France - 1,643,894
United Kingdom - 1,639,717
Congo Kinshasa - 1,586,566
Italy - 1,579,504
South Korea - 1,312,241
"South Africa - 1,209,259
Updated

Blacks and other minorities are at higher risk of developing kidney diseases and diseases of the urinary tract/bladder than whites and other ethnic groups.

Diseases of the kidney that frequently affect people include:

1. Infections UTI
2. Acute Pyelonephritis
3. Chronic Pyelonephritis
4. Hypertension
5. Diabetes mellitus
6. Hyperlipidemia
7. Kidney stone
8. Cancer of the kidney
9. Lupus (SLE)
10. Glomerulonephritis
11. Nephrotic syndrome
12. Papillary necrosis
13. HIV/AIDS
14. Thrombotic Thrombocytopenic Purpura (TTP)
15. Immune Thrombocytopenia (ITP)
16. Hemolytic uremic syndrome
17. Gastroenteritis
18. Polycystic kidney disease
19. Dehydration
20. Drug reaction
21. Azotemia-prerenal
22. Uremia (ESRD) etc.

Urinary tract infection is divided into lower tract urinary tract infection and upper tract urinary tract infection.

The most common symptoms of lower tract urinary tract infection include:

1. Urinary frequency
2. Burning on urination
3. Blood in the urine
4. Fever etc.

Among the problems that can affect people' kidneys and their urinary bladders are:

1. Urinary retention
2. Hematuria (bleeding from the urinary bladder and kidney)
3. Urinary tract infection
4. Cancer of the urinary bladder
5. Cancer of the kidney
6. Urinary incontinence
7. Prostate cancer
8. Sickle cell disease etc.

The most common causes of urinary retention include:

1. Diabetes mellitus
2. Stroke
3. Multiple sclerosis
4. Cancer of the bladder with bleeding and too much clots
5. Cancer of the kidney with bleeding and too much clots
6. Sickle cell disease with papillary necrosis, bleeding and too much clots
7. Urinary tract infection
8. Spinal cord injury
9. Benign prostatic hypertrophy
10. Prostate cancer

The most common causes of hematuria include:

1. Kidney stone
2. Urinary tract infection
3. Cancer of urinary bladder
4. Cancer of the kidney
5. Hemophilia
6. Von Willebran disease
7. Aspirin ingestion
8. Sickle cell anemia or sickle cell trait
9. Low platelets
10. Disseminated intravascular coagulopathy (DIC) etc.

The most common causes of urinary tract infection include:

1. Diabetes mellitus
2. Stroke
3. Insertion of Foley catheter in the bladder
4. Old age with poor toileting
5. Multiple sclerosis
6. Cancer of the urinary bladder
7. Kidney stones with hydronephrosis
8. Cancer of the urether with hydronephrosis
9. Sexual intercourse (women)
10. Frequent baths
11. Tampon use
12. BPH etc;

The most common causes of cancer of the urinary bladder include:

1. Genetic predisposition
2. Exposure to different dyes at work
3. Tobacco smoking
4. Schistosoma haematobium etc;

The best ways to evaluate hematuria include:

1. Renal ultra sound
2. Bladder ultra sound
3. CT scan of the kidney
4. CT scan of the bladder
5. MRI of the kidney/bladder
6. Urine cytology
7. Urinalysis
8. Urine culture
9. Hemoglobin electrophoresis
10. Ova and parasite
11. Serum antibody screen for Schistosoma haematobium
12. Cystoscopy etc.

The most common symptoms of lower tract urinary tract infection include:

1. Urinary frequency
2. Burning on urination
3. Urinary hesitancy
4. Nocturia
5. Urinary retention
6. Gross hematuria
7. Microscopic hematuria
8. Fever
9. Chills
10. Head ache
11. Lower abdominal pain
12. General weakness
13. Tiredness etc.

The most common symptoms of upper tract urinary tract infection include: all the above, plus flank pain, nausea and vomiting.

The best ways to evaluate UTI both lower tract UTI and upper tract UTI are:

1. Take good history from the patient
2. Do a complete physical examination
3. Do a urinalysis

4. Do a urine culture
5. Do 2 sets of blood culture
6. Do a complete CBC
7. Do SMA 20-chemistry profile
8. Renal ultra sound

If the person has UTI and is not febrile, he or she can be treated as an outpatient. If he or she is febrile, he or she should be admitted to the hospital for in hospital treatments. The most common bacteria responsible for UTI in blacks are gram negative enteric Bacteria such as E coli, Klebsiella, Pseudomonas, Proteus, Enterobacter, and gram positive bacteria such as Enterococcus, Staphphylococcus aureus etc.

The antibiotics that are available to treat UTI include:

1. Ampicillin
2. Keflex
3. Kefzol
4. Cipro
5. Levaquin
6. Ceftazidime
7. Cetriaxone
8. Bactrim DS
9. Gentamicin
10. Tobramycin
11. Vancomycin
12. Zosyn
13. Nitrofurantoin etc;

Upper tract UTI is also called pyelonephritis and must be treated with IV antibiotic for 14-21 days. Lower tract UTI in people who are febrile can be treated with antibiotic IV for 7-10 days if the blood cultures are negative. Sepsis due to UTI must be treated for 14-21 days with IV antibiotics.

Lower UTI in people who are afebrile can be treated with antibiotic by mouth for 3-4 days for first UTI or 7-10 days in those who have history of recurrent UTI.

Either people who have recurrent UTI lower tract or an urologist to find out the reason for the frequent UTI must evaluate upper tract. As part of the urological evaluation, the following tests must be done.

1. Urinalsiis and culture
2. Ultrasound of the bladder
3. Ultrasound of the Kidneys
4. CT scan of the kidneys and bladder with contrast
5. CT scan of the kidneys without contrast looking for kidney stones
6. Cystoscopy

7. Urinary cytology
8. Hemoglobin electrophoresis

Sexually active women frequently have UTI, which is associated with sexual intercourse. The way to prevent post coital UTI is for women to empty their bladder immediately after intercourse to prevent any bacteria that may have enter into the bladder during intercourse to be urinated thereby decreasing the incidence of UTI.

Kidney stones are quite common and this condition is quite painful. The most common stones are calcium oxalate and calcium phosphate. Calcium stones are most commonly seen.

The most common causes of kidney stones are:

1. Hyperuricosuria
2. Primary hyperparathyroidism
3. Intestinal hyperoxaluria
4. Hereditary hyperoxaluria
5. Hyperuricosuria
6. Gout
7. Lymphoma
8. Lymphocytic leukemia
9. Dehydration

The most common symptoms of kidney stones are:

1. Severe and excruciating lower back pain
2. Hematuria, (gross or microscopic)
3. Nausea
4. Vomiting

The best ways to evaluate people for kidney stones are:

1. Take a good history
2. Do a complete physical examination
3. Do a urinalysis to look for blood
4. Do a flat plate of the abdomen x-ray to look for a stone
5. Do a CT of the abdomen without contrast looking for a stone (Kidney stone protocol)
6. Strain the urine to look for stones
7. Do an SMA 20 chemistry profile
8. Do a serum uric acid
9. Do a CBC looking leukocytosis, lymphocytosis, elevated neutrophyls, elevated lymphocytes, blasts, or red blood cells (polycythemia

The best treatments available to treat kidney stones are:

1. Pain killer medication
2. Allopurinol
3. Thiazide diuretic
4. Diet
5. Surgical removal of kidney stones
6. External Shock Wave Lithotripsy (ESWL)

Hematuria can occur in individuals who have abnormal coagulation problems such as

1. Hemophilia A and B
2. Factor V deficiency
3. Factor VII deficiency
4. Factor X deficiency
5. Factor XI deficiency
6. Von Willebran disease
7. Disseminated intravascular coagulopathy (DIC)
8. Thrombocytopenia (low platelet) due infection, PPT, ITP, Cirrhosis of the liver
9. Aspirin/ nonsteroidal anti-inflammatory drugs.
10. Sickle cell trait and sickle cell anemia (the reason for the hematuria in sickle cell disease is papillary necrosis of the kidney)

Hypertension is the number one disease in blacks in the United States. One out of every tow black adults aged 55 and older are hypertensive and 1 out of every three white adults is hypertensive. However, since hypertension is the number one disease in blacks, it is safe to say many blacks aged 55 and older are at risk for kidney disease. The incidence of end-stage renal disease (ESRD) leading to renal failure is higher in blacks than in whites.

The reason that hypertension causes ESRD that ultimately results in the need for dialysis is that the kidneys have many vital structures within them that are essential for proper functions. Among those structures are the glomeruli, which are indispensable in the proper functioning of the kidneys. The elevated blood pressure causes plaques to develop inside the small vessels that carry blood and oxygen to the kidneys and the glomeruli within them.

Ordinarily, the inside of the blood vessels is smooth, and blood passes through them freely. When the blood pressure is high, as the blood passes through those vessels, the high pressure causes these vessels to lose their smoothness.

The high pressure therefore damages the first layer of the vessels within the kidneys, resulting in plaque depositions.

The deposition of plaques in turn causes the narrowing of these vessels. The narrowing of the small vessels that is necessary to carry blood and oxygen to the glomeruli of the kidneys results in ischemia of the tissues of the kidney, resulting in the deaths of the glomeruli. The deaths of these glomeruli and other vital structures result ultimately in end-stage renal disease.

Blacks, Hispanics, and other people with the slightest trace of immediate African heritage fall within the category of people with low renin by genetic predisposition. Asians also have low renin level in their blood for an entirely different genetic reason. Low-renin hypertension is referred to as high-volume hypertension.

However, as the kidneys fail, the renin level rises, resulting in greater elevation of the blood pressure, causing even more damage to the kidneys. Therefore, blacks who are hypertensive are at high risk of developing kidney disease from many years of uncontrolled or poorly controlled blood pressure. Diabetes mellitus also causes kidney disease that can lead to ESRD.

In order to determine if the kidneys are sick and are about to fail from long years of being affected by hypertension or diabetes, the physician needs to do a history and physical examination and several blood tests, urine tests and radiological evaluation of the kidneys.

During the history and physical examination, the physician can determine how high the blood pressure is and whether the patient has evidence of hypertensive retinopathy (inside the eyes is the only place a physician can see a naked blood vessel in the human body without cutting the patient).

By examining the vessels inside the eyes, the physician can tell if the damage has occurred in the vessels because of longstanding and either untreated or poorly treated hypertension and the degree of damage. The kidneys are referred to as end organs as are the eyes, heart and brain, and if any of these end organs are damaged by the chronic effect of hypertension, then the examining physician can have a very good idea as to how long the blood pressure has been uncontrolled.

Further, the physician, by taking a history and examining the patient, he or she can tell whether the patient has entered into the uremic stage.

The best way to evaluate the kidneys for chronic kidney disease is to measure the glomerular filtration rate (GFR) and the amount of albumin in the urine.

Chronic renal disease has 5 stages, 1-5.
Stage 1.is GFR 90 ml/minute/1.73m2
Stage 2. is GFR 60-89ml/minute/1.73m2
Stage 3. is GFR 30-59ml/minute/1.73m2
Stage 4 is GFR 15-29ml/minute/1.73m2
Stage 5. Is GFR less than 15ml/minute/1.73m2?

Alternatively, urine can be collected for 24 hours to evaluate creatinine clearance and protein.

In uremia, a patient may have sweet breath, may have flaky salty material over his or her skin, or the patient may have swollen abdomen, swollen legs, the patient may be confused, the patient may have seizures, etc. On laboratory examination of the urine of the patient whose kidneys are failing chronically, the urine may be un-concentrated with a very low specific gravity. Normal specific gravity is about 1.010–1.025. A chronically sick kidney can only concentrate the urine to about 1.002–1.005. The specific gravity is the measure of the ability of the kidneys to concentrate urine. The sicker the kidneys are, the lower the specific gravity.

A chronically sick kidney from hypertension filters out plenty of protein. So by testing the urine during a routine urinalysis for proteins, the physician can be alerted as to how sick the kidneys are.

On microscopic examination of the urinary sediment, certain cellular materials such as certain types of casts can be seen.

By examining the electrolytes, like sodium, in the urine of a patient with failing kidneys, the physician can tell whether the kidneys are failing acutely, a condition called acute tubular necrosis due to some sort of acute event such as heart attack with a drop in the blood, sepsis with shock, acute and heavy bleeding with hypotension. Slow and progressive chronic disease such as hypertension or diabetes with damage to the kidneys can also cause the kidneys to fail. The urinary sodium is easy to do. One needs only to get a few milliliters of urine from the patient and send it to the lab for urinary sodium testing.

In acute failure of the kidneys (acute renal failure), the urinary sodium is low. In chronic renal failure (the kidneys that have been failing for a long time), the urine sodium is high. This quick and easy test is of paramount importance in the treatment approach of a patient who shows up in the emergency room or the doctor's office with unexplained evidence of renal failure.

When the kidneys are failing acutely, they hold sodium in order to hold on to water to maintain the blood pressure to preserve the body and keep it alive.

On the other hand, chronic failing kidneys have lost their ability to hold on to sodium a long time ago, due to chronic damage that has occurred in the kidneys as a result of the insults of high blood pressure or diabetes to the kidneys; as a result, a large quantity of sodium is allowed to pass in the urine. Knowing this simple, but crucial fact allows the physician to know how to approach both the acute and chronic medical management of the patient with failing kidneys.

Another indispensable crucial test that is done in every patient with failing kidneys who can pass urine is the 24-hour creatinine clearance. This test allows the physician to know the ability of the kidneys to function. It allows the physician to know how much function is left in the kidneys. The normal range of creatinine clearance in is 125 milliliters per minute down to about 75 milliliters per minute; and as a person gets older, these numbers decrease accordingly.

In order to do this test, the serum creatinine must be measured and a complete collection of all urine passed by the patient in 24 hours must be obtained and placed in a plastic bottle and sent to the laboratory to be tested. This urine must be kept refrigerated.

The next series of tests that are essential in evaluating the status of the kidneys are:

Serum sodium
Potassium
Chloride
Bicarbonate
Creatinine
CBC

The reason why these tests are so important is that when the kidney is failing, it is unable to filter waste materials from the bloodstream properly, allowing these substances to accumulate in the body, and a reflection of this problem manifests itself with a rise in the BUN and serum creatinine first.

Then as the kidney failure progresses, the serum potassium rises while the serum bicarbonate decreases, resulting in a serious condition called hyperkalemic acidosis. Serum potassium of 6 or greater is a medical emergency that must be dealt with immediately because the high serum potassium can trigger cardiac arrhythmias, which can cause the death of the affected person with kidney failure.

Other serum chemistry tests that are important in evaluating a patient with kidney failure include the serum calcium, the serum phosphatase, the serum bilirubin, the LDH (lactic dehydrogenase), the CPK (creatinine phosphokinase), the total protein, and the serum albumin.

What role does an abnormality of each of these blood chemistry tests and CBC play in the evaluation of a patient with kidney failure? The blood tests to obtain in evaluating the kidney failure in patients include:

Serum sodium
Serum potassium
Serum bicarbonate
Serum chloride
Serum BUN
Serum creatinine
Serum phosphate
Serum calcium
Serum bilirubin
Serum protein
Serum albumin
Serum LDH
Serum CPK
CBC with differential

High serum sodium of 150–160, means that the kidney probably failed because of loss of volume (fluid) due to dehydration. Moreover, that rehydrating the patient with hypo-osmolar fluid such as water by mouth or water and sugar (D5W) intravenously will normalize the sodium, and depending on how long the dehydration state existed, the kidney function will probably return to normal.

High serum potassium is quite a bit more complex and complicated than that because there are other conditions that can cause the serum potassium to be high that has nothing to do with renal failure. Assuming that the high potassium is due to kidney failure, then this occurs because the kidneys are unable to get rid of the breakdown products of proteins, which contain potassium plus potassium ingested as foods or beverages.

This also occurs because of electrolyte abnormalities of different types that cause the kidneys either to reabsorb too much potassium or to be unable to excrete enough potassium to maintain good potassium tolerance. The potassium accumulates in the blood, risking severe cardiac arrhythmias with potential lethal consequences if not brought down with either medications or dialysis.

Low serum bicarbonate known as acidosis, though important, is less crucial because the human body is made to tolerate acidosis much better than alkalosis the reverse of acidosis meaning the serum bicarbonate is high.

When the serum bicarbonate is high, low potassium result, which is as serious as high potassium in causing cardiac arrhythmias that, can lead to sudden death. Medications and/ or dialysis can correct acidosis and high potassium.

The high serum BUN is a reflection of the inability of the kidneys to function well enough to get rid of the breakdown products of proteins. High BUN and creatinine are some of the indices of kidney failure.

Even though high BUN and creatinine are important indices of renal failure, by themselves, they do not represent a threat to the life of a patient. However, when the BUN and creatinine are high, the potassium is at the critical level of 6.5 or greater. If the phosphate is high, the serum calcium is low, the creatinine clearance is 10 ml per minute or less, and the patient looks and feels sick, then the time has arrived for dialysis to start.

High phosphatase is a very important abnormality that must be corrected quickly because as the phosphatase goes up, the serum calcium goes down and the low serum calcium is potentially deadly because low calcium can cause cardiac arrhythmias, seizures, tetany with muscle cramps and twitching. Examining the blood for possible elevation of both total and indirect bilirubins is important because in acute and severe hemolysis, the kidney can acutely fail due to the clogging effect of debris from red blood cells, damaging the tubules of the kidneys.

Testing the blood for serum albumin is very important in renal failure because as the kidneys fail they allow protein to pass into the urine, reducing the serum albumin. This, in turn, causes fluid to pass into the extravascular compartment of the body, resulting in swelling of the abdomen and lower extremities, etc. This set of problems is referred to as "nephrotic syndrome." In nephrotic syndrome, the patient passes three (3) grams of protein or greater in the urine over a 24-hour period.

Testing the blood for total protein is very important because there are conditions such as multiple myeloma and other types of plasma cell dyscrasias in which the total protein is elevated and when protein is elevated, many bad things can happen, including a condition called hyperviscosity syndrome. If viscosity syndrome develops, the patient may experience blurred vision, dizziness, unsteady gait, memory loss, etc. The acute treatment for hyperviscosity syndrome is plasma pheresis.

In multiple myeloma, renal failure occurs because light chain proteins filter out of the kidneys, resulting in severe damage to the kidney tubules, which causes renal insufficiency or renal failure to develop. There is a form of myeloma called light chain myeloma in which the total protein is typically low and this is so because the light chains are passing out in the urine in large quantities and not accumulating in the blood to be reflected as elevated total protein.

As the light chain proteins pass through the kidneys' tubules, the light chain proteins damage the kidneys.

In fact, light chain myeloma is more frequently associated with renal failure than multiple myeloma. Multiple myeloma is much more common in black and Hispanics than in whites and other racial groups. Therefore, it stands to reason that more blacks and Hispanics suffer from myeloma kidney than do whites are.

It is very important to test the blood for lactic dehydrogenase (LDH). For example, an elevated LDH may be seen in a patient who has an occult cancer that no one knows about yet.

Sometimes many routine blood tests and the physical examination are normal, but the LDH, BUN and serum creative are elevated.

This could be a case of lymphoma, because in lymphoma and other cancers, the cancer cells grow via the anaerobic pathway, meaning that these cells grow in the absence of oxygen.

When cells grow in the absence of oxygen, lactic acid is produced as the product of the anaerobic pathway and lactic acid leads to lactic dehydrogenase (LDH). Therefore, a unilateral elevation of LDH in association with acute renal failure can mean one of several things:

1. Acute lymphoma with rapid cancer cell turnover, resulting in large breakdown products of protein making it difficult for the kidneys to filter them out in the urine, and the result is acute renal failure.

2. When the LHD is unilaterally high, it could be acute hemolysis due to hemolytic anemia or any other number of medical problems that can cause red blood cells to hemolyze.

Once hemolysis occurs, the by-products of the red cells will clog up the kidney tubules, which can result in acute renal failure. Blacks and Hispanics as well have the propensity to hemolyze because of sickle cell disease, thalassemia and sickle thalassemia, etc., and if these hemolytic episodes are not handled in a proper clinical way, acute renal failure can be one of the results. Some women of Greek and Italian ethnic background also have the propensity to have hemolytic diseases such as the beta thalassemia.

Elevation of serum creatinine phosphokinase (CPK) can be very important in the development of acute renal failure. There are many medical conditions that cause the CPK to be elevated so high as to be threatening to the health of the kidneys.

Among these conditions are rhabdomyolysis, caused by severe muscle trauma, severe seizure with muscle damage, muscle trauma because of a long march with trauma to the feet. Trauma to muscle because of marathon bongo drum beating with hands; all these conditions and more can cause damage to the skeletal muscles, resulting in acute damage to the tubules of the kidneys, which, if not treated properly, can cause kidney failure.

Therefore, when a patient presents with unexplained acute failure, testing the serum for elevation of CPK is an important thing to do. Any one of the statin anti-cholesterol medications can, at times, cause muscle breakdown, which if not recognized and properly treated, can lead to acute renal failure.

Doing a complete blood count in a patient who presents with acute renal failure is extremely important. Three parts of the CBC that a physician caring for a patient with acute renal failure must be concerned with:

1. Renal failure. The white blood cell count (WBC)
2. The platelet count
3. The hematocrit

A WBC of greater than 100,000 with lymphocytosis represents evidence of lymphoproliferative disorder out of control.

The rapid cell turnover that occurs in this condition results in the production of a large amount of purine, a protein breakdown product that can clog the kidney tubules, resulting in acute.

If the platelet count is found to be very low, less than 40,000–50,000, in association with acute renal failure that could mean several things. Low platelets, low hematocrit and acute renal failure could be seen in DIC, TTP, sepsis, Evan's syndrome as seen in SLE, leukemia or lymphoma, red cell transfusion reaction, AIDS, etc. Low hematocrit and acute renal failure could mean acute hemolysis with debris from the break-up of red cells clogging the kidney tubules, resulting in acute renal failure such as what occurs in thrombotic thrombocytopenia purpura (TTP). 1, 200 individuals in the U.S. develop TTP every year.

TTP causes renal failure because it is a small vessels disease that causes platelets to aggregate forming clots inside small vessels inside the kidneys preventing and oxygen to go to the kidneys. Abnormality in the activity of ADAMTS13 enzyme is responsible for hereditary TTP by its adverse effects on Von Willebrand factor.

Acquired TTP can occur because of:

1. Cancer
2. Pregnancy
3. HIV/AIDS
4. Infection
5. Lupus
6. Some chemotherapy
7. Ticlopidine
8. Plavix
9. Cyclosporine A
10. Birth control pills and other estrogenic hormones etc;

TTP affects other organs beside the kidney, it also affects:

1. The Skin
2. The blood system
3. The brain
4. The heart

Symptoms and signs of TTP include:

1. Bleeding
2. Purpura (bleeding in the skin)
3. Thrombocytopenia (low platelets)
4. Anemia
5. Kidney failure
6. Stroke
7. Coma
8. Seizure
9. Cardiac arrhythmia etc;

The best ways to evaluate kidney failure due to TTP are:

1. Complete history physical examination
2. CBC
3. SMA20
4. Urinalysis

5. CPK
6. LDH
7. PT& INR
8. PPT
9. Glomerular filtration rate (GFR)
10. Plasma fibrinogen
11. Peripheral blood smear
12. Urinary sodium
13. Renal ultra sound
14. Chest -ray
15. EKG
16. Brain CT Scan with no contrast
17. Brain MRI with no contrast
18. EEG

The best treatments available to treat TTP associated kidney failure are:

Infusion of fresh frozen plasma, plasmapheresis, and aspirin by mouth or in suppository form if a patient is too sick to take it by mouth may be given.

Even though a patient may be bleeding because the platelet count is low, Aspirin is needed to disaggregate platelet on the one hand and to prevent further platelet aggregations on the other hand.

Dialysis is used to remove wastes from the body if the kidneys failed. Both acquired and hereditary TTP can have recurrent flare up 30-60 of the times necessitating treatments. The disease that is similar to TTP that can cause the kidney to fail is hemolytic uremic syndrome (HUS).

HUS is similar to TTP in that platelets aggregate inside small vessels in the body preventing blood and oxygen to freely flow to different organs in the body. The result are low platelets and hemolytic anemia. Hemolytic anemia occurs because as red blood cells try to pass through the vessels that are occluded with platelets and clots inside the small vessels, they get damaged resulting in microangiopathic hemolytic anemia.

The mechanism of platelets aggregation and clot formation occur in HUS because a substance such as endotoxin damages the inside small blood vessels, allowing platelets to get trapped which starts the platelets aggregation and clot forming process. The most common cause of HUS is food poisoning (acute gastroenteritis) secondary to E.Coli OH157:H7, which occurs as result of, contaminated hamburgers or other meat Products.

Other things that can cause HUS include:

1. Pneumonia cause by Streptococcus pneumonia bacteria
2. Tic lid
3. Quinine
4. AIDS etc;

Symptoms of HUS include:

1. Fever
2. Abdominal pain
3. Nausea
4. Vomiting
5. Diarrhea (sometimes blood)
6. Weakness
7. The best ways to evaluate HUS include:
8. Complete history and physical examination
9. CBC
10. Microscopic examination of peripheral blood smear, looking for schizothymes and helmet cells, if present, this establishes the diagnosis of HUS. Blood smear of patients with TTP,
11. Does not have schizothymes and helmet cells.
12. Reticulocytes count
13. Direct comb's test
14. SMA20
15. LDH
16. Urinalysis
17. Urine culture
18. Stools culture
19. Blood culture
20. Sputum culture and gram stain of sputum if there is a productive cough
21. Chest x ray
22. EKG
23. Abdominal ultrasound
24. Renal ultrasound

The following abnormalities are usually found in HUS:

1. Microangiopathic hemolytic anemia
2. Thrombocytopenia (low platelet count)
3. High reticulocyte count
4. High LDH
5. High indirect bilirubin
6. High alkaline phosphatase
7. High BUN
8. High serum creatinine
9. Low serum potassium (when the patient is vomiting and having diarrhea)
10. High serum potassium (when the kidneys failed)
11. High serum sodium
12. High serum bicarbonate (C02) (when the patient is vomiting and having diarrhea)
13. Low serum bicarbonate (C02) (when the kidneys failed)
14. Abnormal urinalysis with both protein and red blood cells found in the urine.
15. Sometimes anuria and kidney failure.

The treatments of HUS include:

IV fluid
Electrolyte replacement
Anti-fever medication (specifically (Tylenol by either mouth or suppository)
IV antibiotic to cover for both E. Coli OH157:H7 and for possible Streptococcus
Pneumonia
Folic acid
Anti -nausea medication
Anti- diarrhea medication
Pain medication
Plasmapherisis
Blood transfusion when the hemoglobin drops to less than 7 grams
Dialysis if renal failure develops.

In the pediatric age group, HUS is self -limiting and supportive care with IV fluid and electrolyte replacement may be all the treatments that are necessary. another significant differentiating point between HUS and TTP, beside the angiopathic hemolytic anemia is the fact; in HUS the brain is never affected.

To prevent the devastation of the kidneys that leads to kidney failure, hypertensive and diabetic women have to decrease the salt and simple carbohydrate in their diets by half. Rather than eating an average of 7–8 grams of sodium per day, they ought to eat 3–4 grams of sodium per day.

The decrease in sodium will decrease high blood pressure in women, which in turn will decrease their incidence of kidney failure.

Another common cause of kidney disease in Blacks, Hispanics and many other ethnic groups is sickle cell anemia. Sickle cell anemia damages the kidneys, because of both the occlusive and its inflammatory nature. Blood and oxygen flow to the glomeruli of the kidneys are both impaired, resulting ultimately in a significant percentage of people suffering with sickle cell disease developing end-stage renal failure requiring dialysis. Sickle cell trait often causes papillary necrosis, causing bleeding from the kidney, often the right kidney.

When hypertension, diabetes mellitus and sickle cell disease exist in the same person, the incidence of kidney failure increases. Blood pressure of 130/80 is normal in a person not suffering from sickle cell disease, but in someone with sickle cell anemia, this is hypertension.

1. The most effective treatments for renal failure are a low-salt and low-protein diet.
2. When the renal function deteriorates to the point that the BUN and the creatinine are excessively high, along with high serum potassium, high phosphatase, low calcium and a very low creatinine clearance combined with evidence of uremia, dialysis becomes necessary.

Two types of dialysis are in routine use:

1. Peritoneal dialysis
2. Hemodialysis.

In the U.S. more than 500,000 people undergo dialysis yearly and wordwide about 2 million people receive dialysis on a regular basis.

More than 50,000 people died of kidney disease every year in the U.S. and worldwide 57 million people die yearly from kidney disease. The annual cost of kidney disease in the U.S. is 60 billion dollars.

Different clinical situations along with the patient's preference will help to determine which type of dialysis will be used to treat the individual patient with end-stage renal failure. Kidney transplant is an available option for some patients, if a match can be found.

CHAPTER 12

KIDNEY STONES IN AFRICAN AMERICA MEN

Kidney stone is a very common disease. Five percent of the world population is affected by kidney stones. Eighty per cent of people who are affected by kidney stones are men.

White people are affected more by kidney stones than other racial groups. In the U.S. Whites suffer more from kidney stones follow by Mexican Americans and African Americans.

One of the many functions the kidney has to do is to remove waste materials from the body through the urine. Some of the wastes the kidney has to remove include uprates, calcium, xanthine, cysteine, oxalate and phosphate etc.

The most common kidney stones are:

1. Calcium oxalate stone
2. Cystine stone (occurs because of an autosomal disorder and has nothing to do with diet)
3. Struvite stone (occurs because of recurrent UTI) and change in urine PH.
4. Calcium phosphate stone (occurs because of too much calcium and phosphate in the urine and not enough citrate in the urine, resulting in alkaline PH that can be caused by UTI or renal tubular acidosis.
5. Uric acid stone (occurs because uric acid in the urine and or low PH)

When the state of dehydration exists resulting in the urine being too concentrated, these waste materials can crystallize resulting in the formation of stones.

In addition, there are several medical conditions that are associated with the development of kidney stones. Among these conditions are:

Gout
Lymphoma
Leukemia
Polycythemia
Hyperparathyroidism
Obesity

Gastric bypass surgery
Crohn's disease
Malabsorption
Gout
Low magnesium level
Renal tubular acidosis
Cystinuria
Dehydration
Being a man
High protein diet
High salt diet
High sugar diet
Age 40 and above
Certain medications used in HIV/AIDS like Bactrim can cause kidney stones
Some antacids
Chemotherapy medications
High animal protein
Grapefruit juice
Apple juice
Refine sugar
Fructose corn syrup
Calcium supplements
High vitamin D supplement
Low urine pH
Medullary sponge kidney
Dent's disease (X-linked recessive nephrolithiasis)
Urinary infection cause by Klebsiella, Serratia, Proteus Mirabilis Morganella to name a few

The percenate occurrence of different kidney stones is:

Calcium oxalate 74%
Calcium phosphate 5-10%
Uric acid 5-10%
Struvite 10-15%
Cystine 1-2%
Xanthine stone is rare

Symptoms of Kidney stones include:

Severe flank pain (renal colic)
Nausea
Vomiting
Urinary frequency
Hematuria-gross or microscopic

Evaluations of kidney stones include:

History and physical examinations
Urinalysis
Urine culture
CBC
Complete blood chemistry profile
Serum uric acid
Serum parathyroid hormone
24 hours urine calcium, magnesium, sodium, uric acid, citrate, phosphate and oxalate
Urine straining
Renal ultrasound
Non contrast abdominal CT

Treatments of kidney stones include:

Hydration IV or by mouth
Pain medication
NSAIDs
Allopurinol
Thiazide diuretic
Low animal protein diet
Low sodium intake
Decrease soft drink intake
Diamox to increase the pH of the urine
Urological consult
Extracorporal shock wave lithotripsy (ESWL)
Surgical consult
Surgical procedures to remove kidney stones

Complications of kidney stones include:

Urinary tract infection
Uro-sepsis
Hydronephrosis
Acute pyelonephritis
Chronic pyelonephritis
Kidney failure
Death

CHAPTER 13

PROSTATE DISEASES IN AFRICAN AMERICAN MEN

In 2017, 161,360 men in the U.S. are diagnosed with prostate cancer and 26,730 men are estimated to die of prostate cancer. The incidence of prostate cancer in black American men and black men from the island Jamaica West Indies is more than twice that of other black men, white men and men of other ethnic groups.

Worldwide in 2016, 1.688,780 million men were diagnosed with prostate cancer and 600,920 men died of prostate cancer in 2016.

"Men who get circumcised are slightly less likely to get prostate cancer."
"Men circumcised after age 35 were 45% less likely to develop prostate cancer."
"Meanwhile, men who were cut within a year of being born cut their risk by 14%."
Source: BJU International June 3rd 2014

"USPSTF Releases Draft Guidelines On PSA Testing.

The Washington Post 4/11 reports the US Preventive Services Task Force (USPSTF) "has dropped its controversial opposition to routine screening for prostate cancer, and now says that men between the ages of 55 and 69 should discuss the test's potential benefits and harms with their" physicians "and make decisions based on their own 'values and preferences.'" The group said in proposed new guidelines on Tuesday morning, "The decision about whether to be screened for prostate cancer should be an individual one."

The New York Times reports that the task force "continues to recommend that men 70 and older forgo screening altogether."

USA Today 4/11 reports that the USPSTF's "2012 advice against screening said there was little evidence that PSA screening was reducing deaths." Since that time, "PSA screening rates have declined by as much as 10%, and now fewer than one-third of US men get the tests." Meanwhile, "fewer men are being diagnosed with early-stage disease, when it is more treatable, while more are being diagnosed with more aggressive harder-to-treat cancer."

The AP 4/11 reports, "The draft prostate cancer recommendations, announced online in the Journal of the American Medical Association, are open for public comment...until May 8." "

Prostate cancer is entirely a different disease in Black men than men of other ethnic designations. Prostate cancer occurs at an earlier age in Black men and is always very aggressive. It occurs sometimes in Black men as young as age 35. Therefore the recommendation made by the USPSTF must be taken in context.

What is the prostate gland?

The prostate gland is a gland the size of two walnuts that seat on either side of the neck of the urinary bladder.

What is the function of the prostate gland?

The Prostate gland secretes a liquid that helps to liquefy semen that is ejaculated by men during sexual intercourse, which allows the sperm to swim easier towards female eggs. That is the only useful function that the prostate is known to have.

The prostate gland can cause many miseries for men. In fact, all men, if livelong enough will have one form of prostate problem or another.

The different problems that men are likely to suffer from with their prostate glands include:

1. Acute prostatitis (acute infection of the prostate gland)
2. Chronic prostatitis (chronic infection of the prostate)
3. Benign prostatic hypertrophy (enlargement of the prostate gland without the presence of cancer)
4. Urinary retention
5. Hematuria (blood in the urine)
6. Urinary track infection
7. Pyelonephritis
8. Sepsis
9. Prostate cancer

Which men who should worry about the development of prostate cancer?

All men have a high probability of developing prostate cancer, but the incidence of prostate cancer is higher in black men than it is in men of other ethnic background.

For example, the incidence of prostate cancer is 2-3 times higher in Black American men than their white counterparts. Black American men and Jamaican men have the highest percentage of prostate cancer among all black men in the world and among men in general.

Risk factors for prostate cancer include:

1. Heredity, that is if a man's father has prostate cancer; if his brother has prostate, colon, or breast cancer; if his uncle has prostate, colon, or breast cancer; if his mother has breast, colon, or ovarian cancer; if his aunt has breast, colon, or ovarian cancer. There is a 10% genetic crossover between prostate cancer, colon cancer, and ovarian cancer. In a certain mother is capable of transferring the gene for prostate cancer to her son. Once there is a cluster of cancer in the immediate family, any member of that immediate family has a higher likelihood of developing cancer of one kind or another, more so that the general population.
2. Obesity is associated of development of prostate cancer because the obese men have too much fat in their bodies, and therefore are able to use the cholesterol ring associated with fat to overproduce the male hormone-Androgen. The male hormone a man produces, the more he is able to stimulate the prostate gland, and the more the prostate gland is stimulated by the male hormone, the higher the incidence of developing prostate cancer.
3. Eating fat-reach diets – Eating too much fat leads to the production of too much male hormone-Androgen, which in turn results in over-stimulation of the prostate gland, resulting in a higher incidence of prostate cancer.
4. Frontal baldness is associated with a high incidence of prostate cancer, in particular frontal baldness.
5. Several genes have been identified that predispose Black men and other men to a higher incidence of prostate cancer. Among these genes are TMPRSS2:ETS gene fusion in prostate cancer and the RAF geneses;
6. It is believed that the fact that African-American men and Jamaican men eat a diet that is very rich in fat and that is why the incidence of prostate cancer is the highest in these two groups' men than other black men and other men in the world. I was the first person to have made that observation in 1994 in my first book "The Status of Health of Blacks in the United States – a Prescription for Improvement", published by Kendle Hunt Publishing Company. The medical community has now recognized this as scientific fact.
7. "Study links abnormal lipid levels with prostate cancer recurrence" Source: Cancer Epidemiology, Biomarkers & Prevention.
8. Prostsate cancer is the most common cancer in black men. 31% of black men are diagnosed with prostate cancer.

At what age should men begin to have themselves medically evaluated for prostate cancer?

Prostate cancer usually appears in black men at age 40. However, there are few cases known to have occurred as early as age 35. Prostate cancer usually appears in white males and males of other ethnicities at age 50, there are few cases known to have occurred as early as age 45 in them as well. 1 in 5 African American will be diagnosed with prostate cancer in their life times and prostate cancer is the second leading cause of cancer deaths in African American men.

What are the early symptoms of prostate cancer?

Usually there are no early symptoms.

What are the late symptoms of prostate cancer?

1. Blood in the urine.
2. Burning in urination.
3. Urinary frequency.
4. Hesitancy in urination.
5. Poor urinary stream.
6. Nocturia (getting up too many times at night to urinate).
7. Urinary retention.
8. Weakness.
9. Bone pain.
10. Constipation.
11. Paralysis from the waist down, due to spinal cord compression by the prostate cancer.

How can a man find out if he has prostate cancer?

To find out if a man has prostate cancer he must go to the doctor to have:

1. A digital rectal examination.
2. He must have a blood test done to examine the Prostatic Specific Antigen (PSA).

The rectal exam allows the physician to palpate the prostate gland to determine whether it is smooth, hard, or has a nodule, or whether the gland is 1+, 2+, 3+, or 4+ in size; 1+ being the smallest, 4+ being the largest.

The PSA is a blood test when elevated can mean that the man has prostate cancer. The normal PSA value is from 0 to 4.0, but is age-variable. In older men, PSA above four may not necessarily mean that prostate cancer is present. The normal value for PSA is set at a lower level for obese men than men of normal sizes.

The more obese a man, the more diluted the concentration of the PSA is in his blood stream, because his blood volume is higher. For example, a PSA of 2.0 in an obese man may in fact be 5.0

The PSA may be high in:

1. Acute prostatitis.
2. Chronic recurrent prostatitis.
3. Benign prostatic hypertrophy.
4. Post coital (a day after sexual intercourse).
5. Prostate cancer.

It is important to understand that a man may have a PSA of 1 and still has prostate cancer if he has a prostate nodule that is palpated during the rectal examination. In the same vain, a man may have a PSA of 1 in one year, and the next consecutive year the PSA is doubled to 2.0: that may indicate the presence of prostate cancer in that gland because of the doubling of the PSA value that occurs so rapidly.

It is also very important that close attention is paid to the difference that occurs in the PSA reading from year to year. If the PSA let us say was 1.8 in 1 year and the following year the PSA becomes 2.7, this is a PSA reflection of 0.9. This very important and may indicate the presence of cancer in the prostate gland. The accepted PSA Reflection is 0.7

It is not unusual, for a man to present to the doctor with a high PSA and it is due to infection of the prostate or an enlargement of the prostate and not cancer.

By the age of 35, it is a good idea for Black men to begin the process of having yearly digital rectal examination and yearly PSA done. This is even more important if prostate cancer is known to exist in his immediate family.

How to evaluate an asymptomatic elevated PSA?

The first thing to do is to refer the man to a urologist. The urologist will take a history from him, examine him, and most likely do one or two things:

1. Depending on history he/she may choose to treat the man with an appropriate antibiotic.
2. After the completion of the course of the antibiotic, the urologist will likely repeat the PSA.
3. If the PSA returns to normal, he/she may decide to observe the patient.
4. If the PSA fails to return to normal, or did not change at all after the antibiotic treatment, the urologist is likely to recommend a prostate biopsy.
5. Alternatively, the urologist may decide to immediately recommend a prostate biopsy.
6. If the PSA velocity is greater than 0.7 form the previous year's PSA that also calls for a prostate biopsy to done.

How is the prostate biopsy done?

The night before the biopsy, as well as the morning before the biopsy, the patient is given an antibiotic named Cipro to take. That prevents infections from developing. Then a special needle is used trough the rectum using sonographic technique as a guide and prostate tissue is taken from several parts of the prostate gland and placed in formalin and sent to the pathology laboratory for microscopic evaluation by a pathologist.

1. **What if the prostate biopsy comes back indicting that cancer is present in the prostate gland?**
2. **What then must the man do?**

The first thing is that the urologist is going to arrange for a meeting between the man and his wife, girl friend or significant other.

This meeting is extremely important because the man is going to hear this most unpleasant of all news in that he has prostate cancer. Any news telling anyone he/she has cancer is devastating to say the least, but telling a man that he has prostate cancer, and that his sexuality and life are both on the line is a matter of extraordinary emotional importance. For that reason, the man needs to have present during the discussion that is going to take place the one person that he trusts the most to help him handle the news of the moment.

Paramount in the discussion of the discovery of prostate cancer is what is the stage of the cancer? This is important because the stage of the cancer dictates what treatment alternatives the urologist can offer to the affected man.

A short synopsis of the staging system use to evaluate needle biopsy of the prostate is the Gleason stage system. The Gleason stages system rages from Gleason 1 to Gleason 10. The lower the Gleason stage, the more localized the cancer is and the better the prognosis. Conversely, the higher the Gleason stage, the more advanced the cancer is and the poorer the prognosis.

A Gleason stage up to 7 in most situations may lend itself to surgical intervention as a modality of treatment. A Gleason greater than 7 is less likely to be cured by surgery alone as a modality. A more detailed and thorough staging of prostate cancer is usually given after a pathological examination of the surgical specimen.

What are the different treatment modalities available to treat prostate cancer?

1. Nerve spearing - Radical prostatectomy for early stage prostate cancer.
2. Nerve-spearing Robotic prostatectomy
3. Radiation therapy.
4. Seeds placement.
5. Hormonal treatments for advanced prostate cancer.
6. Chemotherapy for metastatic prostate cancer.

Each one of these treatment modalities has their upsides and downsides.

The nerve spearing radical prostatectomy is offered as a curative treatment for early prostate cancer. It is a very extensive form of treatment during which the network of tubes within which sperm is produced is removed because frequently cancer cells are found hidden there. The nerves that are necessary to help a man to have an erection are evaluated and spared as best as possible to enable to have an erection some time in the future after surgery. Multiple nodes are removed and sent to the pathology lab to be evaluated for presence or absence of cancer. The valve that seats at the neck of the bladder is sacrificed to be sure that no cancer remains in that area.

Consequently the alternate valve which all men have and have never used before, is now used to attach the urether to enable the man to urinate once the Foley Catheter is removed several weeks postoperatively. The reason why it takes several weeks before the Foley Catheter can be removed is that it takes that long for the new valve to get accustom to function as a valve.

Radiation therapy is an excellent non-invasive modality to treat prostate cancer in men who for one reason or another are not good candidate for radical prostatectomy or their cancer's stage is not clinically appropriate for surgery.

The down side with radiation therapy for prostate cancer is that it is not always curative and it can cause proctitis, rectal bleeding and it can in significant percentage of cases cause erectile dysfunction.

Seeds Placement is superb alternative treatment for early prostate cancer for men who do not want surgery or who for medical reasons of one kind or another cannot have surgery. It too can cause erectile dysfunction in certain percentage of men.

In some men who have advanced prostate cancer seed placement can also be used as good treatment modality. In men, whose prostate gland is too large, hormone such as Leupron can be given intramuscularly to shrink the size of the prostate to allow for easier placement of the seeds. The seeds are radioactive materials that are placed inside the prostate gland to kill the cancer cells.

Hormonal treatments that commonly used to treat prostate cancer are:

1. Leupron (antitestosterone)
2. Flutamide (total Androgen Blockage)
3. Casodex
4. Zytiga
5. The FDA has just approved Xtandi to treat prostate cancer

These hormones block the production of the male hormone from the prostate gland. By blocking the production of Androgen from the prostate gland, the growth of cancer cells are slowed down and the level of PSA in the blood decreases. Androgen is needed for prostate cancer cells to grow.

The side effects of Hormonal treatments for prostate cancer are:

1. Erectal dysfunction
2. Gynecomastia (large breasts)
3. Feeling warm all the time (Hot flashes)
4. Sweating a lot

The most effective Chemotherapy presently to treat metastatic prostate cancer is TAXOL intravenously.

Another common problem that causes miseries for men is benign prostatic hypertrophy (BPH). BPH occurs when the prostate gland becomes enlarged and the enlargement impedes the free flow of urine. This results in frequent urination and sometime difficulty in urination.

The symptoms of BPH include:

Urinary frequency
Urinary urgency
Hesitancy on urination
Dribbling
Waking up at night multiple times to urinate
Weak urine stream
Leaking of urine
Burning on urination
Urinary tract infection
The diagnosis of BPH is established by the
History
Digital examination
Renal ultrasound
Cystoscopy

Treatments of BPH include:

Flomax 0.4mg by mouth daily
Avodart 0.5 mg by mouth daily
Terazosin 1mg, 2mg, 5mg, 10mg by mouth daily
Proscar 5mg by mouth daily

Minimally invasive procedures to treat BPH in use are:

Transurethral needle ablation
Transurethral microwave
High-intensity focused ultrasound

Surgical treatments to treat BPH include:

Transurethral surgery (TURP)
Laser surgery
Interstitial laser coagulation
Photoselective Vaporization"

The most common causes of urinary retention in men are:

1. Benign Prostatic Hypertrophy
2. Prostate cancer
3. Diabetes mellitus
4. Stroke
5. Multiple sclerosis etc;
6. Cancer of the bladder with bleeding and too much clots
7. Cancer of the kidney with bleeding and too much clots
8. Sickle cell disease with papillary necrosis, bleeding, and too much clots
9. Urinary tract infection
10. Spinal cord injury

The most common causes of urinary tract infection in men are:

1. Benign prostatic hypertrophy
2. Diabetes mellitus
3. Stroke
4. Insertion of foley catheter in the bladder
5. Old age with poor toileting
6. Multiple sclerosis
7. Cancer of the urinary bladder
8. Kidney stones
9. Cancer of the urether etc;

It is important that men understand the importance of having a digital rectal examination done every year from age 35 onward, which can save their lives. It is equally important that white males and men of other ethnic background do the same by age 40. It is important that men understand that having a PSA blood test every year from age 35-40 onward can save their lives.

In particular, Black American men, Jamaican men, other Black men and men in general, must be urged to modify their diet by removing the excessive amount of red meat, pork, fried foods, and replacing them with non-shellfishes fish, poultry, fruits, vegetables, beans, olive oil cooking oil and low simple carbohydrate foods, corn meal. In general, exercise along with a good diet program will help to decrease their total body fat and decrease their incidence of prostate cancer. All men no matter their racial make up ought to follow the advice of their physicians to decrease their incidence of prostate cancer.

A common problem that many men are suffer from is Erectil dysfunction (ED) Some of the causes of ED include:

Diabetes mellitus
Hypertension
Atherosclerosis

Cerebrovascular accident
Multiple sclerosis
Radical Prostatectomy
Seed implantation into the prostate gland (in certain percentage of patients)
Radiation therapy to the prostate gland (in certain percentage of patients)
Low testosterone
Depression and other psychiatric disorders
Medications side effects etc;

The most effective medications available to treat **ERECTIL DYSFUNCTION** include:

Viagra
Cialis
Levitra
Injection of prostaglandin into the Penis
Muse
Penal implant
Viagra and the other similar medications work to bring about penal erection by releasing Nitric Oxide in the penis, which relaxes smooth muscle, and dilating the blood vessels that carry blood to the Penis. These two things bring about erection in men in this setting. Men can have a multitude of problems affecting their urinary bladders
The FDA just approved Stendra (avanafil) to use 15 minutes before sex.

CHAPTER 14

PROSTATITIS IN AFRICAN AMERICAN MEN

—◄═◊═►—

Men frequently suffer from prostatitis.

In most sexually active younger men, prostatitis is usually due to exposure to either gonorrhea or Chlamydia during sexual intercourse. In the majority of older men, prostatitis is usually due to BPH or bladder infection. However, recent reports in the literature have documented significant increase in the incidence of STDs in elderly men.

The symptoms of prostatitis include:

Fever
Chills
Lower abdominal pain
Pain down the testicles
Low back pain
Pain in the groin
Dysuria
Frequent urination
Microscopic hematuria
Nausea
Vomiting
Headache

Evaluations of prostatitis include:

Taking a good history
Physical examination
Urinalysis
Urine culture
Urethral culture for gonorrhea and Chlamydia
RPR
HIV blood test
Prostate ultrasound

It is not always a prudent idea for the prostate gland to be palpated by a physician when the gland is acutely infected. Doing so may spread the infection in the blood stream causing sepsis.

The microorganisms that are frequently associated with the development of prostatitis include:

E.coli
Klebsiella
Proteus
Gonorrhea
Chlamydia

The medications in use to treat acute prostatitis include:

Levaquin
Cipro
Zithromax
Doxycycline
Teracycline
Floxin

Prostate infection can be very difficult to eradicate. The prostate gland sits inside a very thick capsule, which is very difficult for antibiotics to penetrate. Because of that, the infection frequently becomes chronic.

The symptoms of chronic prostatitis include:

Recurrent lower abdominal pain
Chronic and recurrent pain in the groin
Dysuria
Frequent urination
Fever- when there is an acute flare up
Chills when there is an acute flare up

Evaluation of chronic prostatitis includes:

History
Physical examination
Palpation of the prostate gland
Urinalysis
Urine culture
Urethral culture for gonorrhea and Chlamydia
RPR
HIV blood test
Prostate ultra sound

Treatments of chronic prostatitis include:

Massage of the prostate gland by a Urologist to remove the thick and pussy material from the prostate gland
Levaquin for 4 weeks by mouth
Cipro for 4 weeks by mouth
Zithromax by mouth for 4 weeks
Doxycycline by mouth for 4 weeks
Floxin by mouth for 4 weeks
Hematuria is a common sign seen in prostate diseases,

The most common causes of hematuria include:

Hemophilia A and B
Factor V deficiency
Factor VII deficiency
Factor X deficiency
Factor XI deficiency
Von Willebran disease
Disseminated intravascular coagulopathy (DIC)
Sickle cell disease etc;

Hamaturia can also occur because of platelet abnormalities such as

Thrombocytopenia (low platelet)
Thrombopathy (qualitative platelet Abnormality)

Kidney stone
Bladder cancer
Kidney cancer
UTI

Hematuria can also occur because ingestion of aspirin and nonsteroidal anti-inflammatory drugs. Heparin, Lovenox, Pradaxa, Xarelto and Coumadin etc.; can also cause hematuria.

The reason for the hematuria in sickle cell disease is papillary necrosis of the kidney.

All individuals with hematuria ought to be evaluated by a urologist.

CHAPTER 15

DISEASES OF THE URINARY BLADDER IN AFRICAN AMERICAN MEN

—⟨⟨⟨⟨⟨⟨⟩⟩⟩⟩⟩⟩—

Among the problems that can affect people and their urinary bladders are:

1. Urinary retention
2. Hematuria (bleeding from the bladder)
3. Urinary tract infection
4. Cancer of the urinary bladder etc;

The most common causes of hematuria are:

1. Prostate cancer
2. Kidney stone
3. Urinary tract infection
4. Cancer of urinary bladder
5. Cancer of the kidney
6. Benign prostatic hypertrophy
7. Hemophilia
8. Von Willebran disease
9. Aspirin ingestion
10. Sickle cell disease
11. Thrombocytopenia
12. Thrombotic thrombocytopenic purpura (TTP)
13. Disseminated intravascular coagulopathy (DIC)
14. Cytoxan;

The most common causes of cancer of the urinary bladder are:

1. Genetic predisposition
2. Exposure to different dyes at work
3. Tobacco smoking
4. Schistosoma haematobium etc;

The best ways to evaluate hematuria are:

1. Renal ultrasound
2. Bladder ultrasound
3. CT Scan of the kidney
4. CT Scan of the bladder
5. MRI of the bladder
6. MRI of the kidney
7. Urine cytology
8. Urinalysis
9. Urine culture
10. PSA
11. Hemoglobin electrophoresis
12. Ova and parasite
13. Serum antibody screen for Schistosoma haematobium
14. Cystoscopy etc.

Diseases of the kidney that frequently affect people include:

1. Urinary tract infection
2. Pyelonephritis
3. Kidney stone
4. Cancer of the kidney
5. End stage kidney disease
6. Glomerulonephritis
7. Nephrotic syndrome
8. Papillary necrosis
9. Polycystic kidney disease
10. Azotemia
11. Uremia etc;

The most common causes of urinary tract infection in are BPH, insertion of a foley catheter, kidney stones, sickle cell disease, aberrant urinary tract, prostate cancer, diabetes mellitus, stroke etc;

Urinary tract infection is divided into lower tract urinary tract infection and upper tract urinary tract infection.

The most common symptoms of lower tract urinary tract infection are:

1. Urinary frequency
2. Burning on urination
3. Urinary hesitancy
4. Nocturia
5. Urinary retention
6. Gross hematuria

7. Microscopic hematuria
8. Fever
9. Chills
10. Headache
11. Lower abdominal pain
12. Flank pain
13. General weakness
14. Tiredness
15. Nausea
16. Vomiting

The most common symptoms of upper tract urinary tract infection are: all the above, plus flank pain, nausea and vomiting.

The best ways to evaluate UTI both lower tract UTI and upper tract UTI are:

1. Take good history from the patient
2. Do a complete physical examination
3. Do a urinalysis
4. Do a urine culture
5. Do 2 sets of blood culture
6. Do a complete CBC
7. Do SMA 20-chemistry profile
8. Renal ultrasound

If a man who has UTI and is not febrile, he can be treated as anoutpatient.

If he is febrile, he should be admitted to the hospital for in hospital treatments.

The most common bacteria responsible for UTI are gram negative enteric bacteria such as E. coli, Proteus, Klebsellia pneumonia, pseudomonas etc;

Some of the most common antibiotics available to treat UTI are:

Ampicillin
Keflex
Kefzol
Cipro
Levaquin
Ceftazidime
Ceftriaxone
Bactrim DS
Gentamicin
Doripenem
Imipenem etc.

Upper tract UTI is also called pyelonephrytis and must be treated with IV antibiotic for 21 days. Lower tract UTI in men who are febrile can be treated with antibiotic IV for 10 days if the blood cultures are negative.

Lower UTI in men who are afebrile can be treated with antibiotic by mouth for 10 days. Levaquin by mouth is as effective as Levaquin IV.

People who have UTI in lower either tract or upper tract must be evaluated by a urologist to find out the reason for the UTI. As part of the urological evaluation, the following tests must be done.

1. Ultrasound of the prostate
2. Ultrasound of the bladder
3. Ultrasound of the Kidneys
4. CT scan of the kidneys and bladder with contrast
5. CT scan of the kidneys without contrast looking for kidney stones
6. Urinary cytology
7. Serum PSA (after the UTI is treated)
8. Hemoglobin electrophoresis
9. Cystoscopy
10. Pelvic ultrasound etc;

CHAPTER 16

GENITAL HERPES IN AFRICAN AMERICAN MEN

According to the WHO, Worldwide "two-third of the population under age 50 suffer from herpes simplex virus type 1, while an additional 417 million people between the ages 17 to 49 suffer from HSV-2, which causes genital herpes."

"In America 39 percent of men, are infectected with herpes simplex" According to the WHO.

Genital herpes is a very common sexually transmitted disease. 68 million individuals are infected with Herpes Viruses I and II in the United States of America and about 1 million people become infected every year with these Herpes Viruses. Herpes Simplex Type II causes about 90 percent of genital herpes infections and Herpes Simplex Type I causes about 10 percent. Genital herpes is most often transmitted during sexual intercourse or during oral sex with an infected partner.

The incidence of genital herpes is quite high in females and herpes infection of the genital spares no ethnic groups and socioeconomic status. Any man who is sexually active can become infected with the herpes virus and this is particularly so if he has sexual intercourse without the use of a condom.

The diagnosis of herpes infection of the genital area can be made by culture taken from the infected areas or by rupturing the vesicles and culturing the fluid within them with clean culturette, place the culturette in a special herpes liquid medium in a tube, and send the tube to the microbiology lab for processing.

Scraping the ulcerated area on a clean slide and send it to the lab for a Zanck stain

can also use to diagnose herpes. The culturing of the herpes infection is much more specific and definite evidence of the presence of the herpes infection if the culture is positive. Herpes infections tend to recur in the same area repeatedly. Stressful situations tend to cause the herpetic lesions to come back. Some of the stresses that can cause the recurrence of herpes infections are the common cold, and stress associated with taking school examinations, work related stress, indigestion etc.

These stressful situations increase the level of adrenalin which has a lowing effect on the immune system allowing the dormant herpes infection to wake up and proliferate, causing the recurrence of the disease.

Treatment of Herpes Infection:

If the genital herpes infection is more diffused and the patient is immunosuppressed the treatment is intravenous acyclovir. If the herpes infection is localized, the treatment is acyclovir by mouth or if the infection is localized and mild, acyclovir cream will help to relieve the symptoms, but medication by mouth is needed, in addition. The question is how long to treat. Primarily, Genital herpes should be treated with acyclovir 200 mg by mouth, 5 times a day for 10 days or Valtrex 1000 mg by mouth, 2 times per day for 10 days.

Treatment for recurrent genital herpes is Valtrex 500 mg by mouth, 2 times per day for 5 days or acyclovir 400 mg by mouth, 3 times per day or Famvir 250 mg by mouth, 2 times per day for 5 days. The treatment for suppression of chronic genital herpes is Famvir 250 mg by mouth, 2 times per day or Valtrex 500 mg by mouth daily or acyclovir 400 mg 2 times per day.

This virus is very difficult to treat because it is slow growing, has a thick capsule, has the ability to hide for a very long time in the human body, and flares up on and off causing miseries for those who are infected. Therefore, the treatment for recurrent flare up of herpes infection may be for life.

CHAPTER 17

GONNORHEA IN
AFRICAN AMERICAN MEN

Gonorrhea is second most commonly reported STD health departments in different localities in the US. In 2015, 395.216 cases of gonorrhea were reported.

Men, who are infected with Gonorrhea, become infected during sexual intercourse with women or men who are infected with Gonorrhea. Once infected, several things can happen to a man. Five days to a week after being exposed, the man may notice a foul smelling penal discharge with pain and irritation in the head of the penis. If he does not seek medical care right away, the symptoms will get worst.

How to Diagnose Gonorrhea in Men

The first thing to do is to take a good history as to the man's sexual habits and his symptoms, which are usually burning on urination, urinary frequency and seeing a discharge coming out of the penis.

Sometimes, there is no discharge to be seen coming out of the penis, in this case,a culture swab must be put inside the penis to collect specimen to send to the lab.

In many instances the man may not have any symptoms and yet he may beinfected with gonnohrea.

Part of the penis discharge can be placed on a clean glass slide and smeared. Once the slide is dried, it can be stained with gram stain. The gram stained slide can be examined under the microscope. A number of things can be seen on that smear, including evidence of a purulent infection if many white blood cells are seen.

The gonnorhea organism is an intracellular diploccocus gramnegative bacterium.

It is important to realize that sexually transmitted diseases rarely present as one infection. And the symptoms and physical findings are the same for gonorrhea as there are for Chlamydia. Blood must be sent to the lab to test for syphilis, (VDRL), and for HIV (with consent).

The approach to treatment of Gonorrheal and Chlamydia infections in men is guided by the clinical presentation.

How to treat Suspected or uncomplicated Gonorrhea in the office/outpatient Clinic:

The treatment is Ceftriaxone 250 mg IM in one dose with Doxycycline 100 mg 2 times per day for 14 days and Flagyl 250 mg by mouth twice per day for 4 days. Alternatively, the patient can be treated with Floxin 400 mg by mouth twice per day or Zithromax 500mg 2 tablets taken by mouth at the same time if Chlamydia is the suspected infection. If Gonorrhea is the suspected infection, then the same regimen can be used, except that the dose of Zithromax must be 1 gram by mouth taken at the same time.

Ceftriaxone is the best medication available to treat uncomplicated or suspected Gonorrhea intramuscularly in the office or in the clinic. Ceftriaxone, however, will not treat Chlamydia and since it is oftentimes impossible to tell Gonorrhea from Chlamydia, it is wise to treat for both by adding Doxycycline, Floxin or Zithromax. These three medications are efficacious against Chlamydia. Floxin and Zithromax are both effective against both Gonorrhea and Chlamydia.

For men who are allergic to Penicillin who therefore cannot be treated with Ceftriaxone, the regimen containing Floxin or Zithromax can be used.

If a joint is swollen and painful, it is critical to tap the joint fluid and send it to the lab for gram stain, cell count, and culture, glucose, and protein. Treatment of Gonorrheal arthritis must be started immediately to prevent the destruction of the affected joint or joints.

The different conditions that can cause abdominal pain in a man include:

1. Acute appendicitis
2. Urinary tract infection
3. Acute diverticulitis
4. Cancer of the colon
5. Ischemic colitis
6. If he has Polycythemia Vera or Essential Thrombocytopenia, he can have acute splenic vein thrombosis causing the abdominal pain.
7. Inflammatory bowel disease, either ulcerative colitis or Krohn's disease in the affected part of the bowel causing severe lower abdominal pain.
8. If he has congenital antithrombin 3 deficiency, factor V Leiden deficiency, protein C or protein S deficiency, elevated lipoprotein-a etc. he may become hypercoagulable and as a result, he may develop thrombosis of her intra abdominal vasculature which can cause severe lower abdominal pain, etc.
9. For the reasons just mentioned above, he may also develop pain in her lower leg because of Deep Vein Thrombophlebitis
10. He may also develop chest pain with shortness of breath because of pulmonary embolism associated with one of the thrombophilias outlined above etc.

Evaluations include:

History and physical examination
CBC with differential
Complete blood chemistry profile
Urinsalysis
Urine culture
VDRL
HIV 1&2 blood test
Comlpete abdominal ultrasound
Abdominal CT with PO contrast

In-Hospital Treatment of Gonorrhea

1. Ceftriaxone - 2 grams IV every 12 hours
2. Doxycycline - 100 mg PO or IV every 12 hours until the culture result is back from the laboratory.
3. Alternatively, Clindamycin - 900 mg IV every 8 hours in addition to Gentamycin 2 mg/KG IM or IV and once the patient is improved then add Doxycycline - 100 mg by mouth every 12 hours to complete a 14-day course. Add Flagyl 500 mg every 6 hours during the acute phase of the infection to cover for not only possible accompanying Trichomonas infection, but also anaerobic organisms that may be playing a role in the infectious process.
4. Patients who cannot tolerate Doxycycline or who are allergic to Penicillin can be treated with Norfloxin 400 mg IV every 12 hours.

Once the culture result and sensitivity are back from the laboratory, then specific antibiotics can be used to treat the infection.

Prevention of Gonorrhea Infection

1. Men ought not to engage in frivolous and irresponsible sexual intercourse.
2. They ought to strive to remain monogamous.
3. They ought to use condom to prevent being infected with gonorrhea and other STDs.

When people are high on drugs they inevitably become irresponsible, carefree and careless and the result is unprotected sexual intercourse and frequently with multiple sexual partners.

There are 19 million new cases of STD (not including AIDS) reported annually in the United States according to a recent report by the Institute of Medicine. One-fourth of these cases are among teenagers according to that report. 22 percent of people above the age of 15 are carrying the herpes infection. It costs taxpayers $16.4 billion per year to treat STD in the United States. By the 11th grade, 70 percent of teenagers have had sexual intercourse and 40 percent of them have had four or more sexual partners.

Complications of untreated Chlamydia infection in men include crhonic urethritis, chronic prostastitis and urethral fistula, infertility etc.

CHAPTER 18

CHLAMYDIA INFECTION IN AFRICAN AMERICAN MEN

There are 2.8 million cases of Chlamydia annually in the U.S. As such, Chlamydia is the most commonly reported bacterial STD in the United States (Accordingto the CDC). "Chlamydia rates in African Americans are eight times higher than in white Americans".

Men become infected with Chlamedia by having sexual intercourse with infected sexual partners, be it women or men.

Chlamydia trachomatis is the most nationally reported STD in the US. Men pass the infection to women in their ejaculates causing a mucopurulent endocervical discharge.

Symptoms of Chlamydia in men include burning on urination, urinary frequency, yellow discharge coming out of the penis, urethritits, urethral discharge, superpubic pain, prostatitis, and in men who have sex with men, rectal pain, rectal discharge, or some times no symptoms at all.

Diagnosis of Chlamydia is established by taking a historty, examination of the penis, examination of the rectum, examination of the prostate gland and getting specimen of the discharge either from the penis, retum of the prostate, and send that specimen the microbiology laboratory for gram stain and culture.

Treatment of Chlamydia can be started with Doxycycline 100 mg 2 times per day for 7 days or Floxin 300 mg 2 times per day for 7 days or Azithromycin 1 gram by mouth for 1day or Erythromycin 500 mg by mouth 4 times per day for 7 days. Other STDs such asGonorrhea, Syphilis infections, often accompany chlamydia infection. So the clinical thing to do is to test for Gonorrhea, draw blood for VDRL (syphilis test) and HIV, thentreat for Chlamydia Gonorrhea till the laborarory results come back.

Treatment of Suspected Uncomplicated Chlamydia Infection

1. Doxycycline 100 mg by mouth 2 times per day for 7 days.

    or

2. Floxin 800 mg once by mouth with Ceftriaxone 250 mg IM and Flagyl 250 mg 4 times by mouth per day for 4 day

    or

3. Zithromax 1 gram by mouth

Complications of untreated Chlamydia infection in men include crhonic urethritis, chronic prostastitis and urethral fistula, infertility etc.

CHAPTER 19

SYPHILIS IN AFRICAN AMERICAN MEN

The different stages of syphilis are:

Chancre
Primary syphilis
Secondary syphilis
Tertiary syphilis
Congenital syphilis
Neuro-syphilis

Syphilis has historically been one of the most common STDs to afflict mankind and has been in the new world since 1494 when Columbus and his men came to America. Syphilis is caused by the spirochete Treponema Pallidum.

"In the year 2015 number syphilis cases in the U.S. were 23,870 according to the CDC".

Syphilis is usually transmitted sexually, or from mother to baby. Once the organism is deposited into the human tissue it takes anywhere from 14 to 21 days for primary syphilis to develop.

The Oslo study was the first study done to see the effect of of untreated syphilis on the human dody. The sudy took place between 1891 and 1951. It included 2000 patients diagnosed clinically. The dark field test and Wasserman test were not yet in existence. Penicillin had not yet been discovered either so there was no effective way to treat these patients.

That study amply demonstrated the devastating effects of untreated syphilis on all parts of the human body, in particular, the brain, the aorta, the skeletal system, etc.

The second study is the infamous **Tuskegee study**, which took place from 1932 - 1974 in Tuskegee, Alabama under the control of the **United States Public Health Service**

The shameful reason given for **this cruel, inhumane, barbaric, and racist study** was to find the effects of untreated syphilis on the human body. There were no scientific justifications for this study in view of the fact that the Oslo study had already shown what untreated syphilis could do to the human body.

From 1932 to 1974, under the leadership of the United States Public Health Service, 431 (Negro men) black men were injected with live syphilis organisms for the sole purpose of seeing what effects syphilis would have on their bodies. These men did not sign consent for participating in the study. They did not know that they were being injected with live syphilis organisms.

In 2010, a report came out showing that some of the same American scientists involved in the infamous Tuskegee study also carried out experiment in Guatemala injecting syphilis in 696 men and women Guatemalan prisoners, people with mental illness, and prostitutes. The experiments were carried out to test the effects of penicillin on STDs during 1946 to 1948. A Wellesley College medical historian made this discovery. The U.S. Secretary of State Hillary Rodham Clinton and the Secretary of Health and Human Services Kathleen Sebelius apologized to the Guatemalan Government and the Guatemalan people for the actions of these American Scientists. Taxpayer's money through the National Institute of Health financed the Guatemalan syphilis study.

The present U.S Government has ordered an investigation to be carried out by a Presidential Commission and the Institute of Medicine to find out what happened in the Guatemalan syphilis experiment.

In the history of the world, many events have taken place to catalogue men's cruelty towards each other: **Slavery, the Holocaust, the Rwanda Massacre, and the Tuskegee Study** and the Guatemalan syphilis experiment are a few such examples. In the Tuskegee Study, 431 men were sacrificed for nothing other than racism and bigotry, while the U.S. government, organized medicine, some black and white physicians, some white and black hospital administrators and society, at large, stood by silently.

How shameful and how disgusting!!!

Evaluations of Syphillis include:

History and physical examination
VDRL
FTA-ABS
HIV 1&2 blood test
CBC
Complete blood chemistry profile
If there is a chancre, specimen must be taken from it and send to the microbiology laboratory for study.

Treatment for the Different Stages of Syphilis in men

1. Primary syphilis - chancre stage (not allergic to penicillin) 1.2 million units of Benzathine penicillin in each buttock, IM.
2. Secondary syphilis - (not allergic to penicillin) - 1.2 million units of Benzathine penicillin in each buttock IM weekly times three weeks in sequence.

3. Latent syphilis (not allergic to penicillin) - 1.2 million units of Benzathine in each buttock IM weekly times three weeks in sequence.

4. Tertiary syphilis - (not allergic to penicillin) - 1.2 million units of Benzathine penicillin in each buttock IM weekly times three weeks in sequence.

5. Neuro syphilis - (if not allergic to penicillin) - spinal tap ought to be done; send CSF for VDRL and FTA-ABS testing. If positive, admit patient to the hospital and treat with 12 to 24 million units per day of aqueous penicillin G IV for ten days or 600,000 units daily of procaine penicillin IM daily for 14 days. Either the IV or the IM treatment can be carried out on an outpatient basis.

Any man who is HIV positive, VDRL, and FTA positive must be assumed to have neurosyphilis. A spinal tap must be done and the CSF study for syphilis. It does not matter, in fact, whether the CSF is positive or not. Any HIV positive individual with positive VDRL and positive FTA-ABS must be treated in the same way as some one with documented neuro-syphilis as just outlined above, and additional weekly doses of Benzathine penicillin IM must be given for three weeks.

If a man is allergic to penicillin and has early stages of syphilis, the treatment of choice is Erythromycin or Tetracycline 500 mg by mouth, four times a day for 15 days. For more advanced stages of syphilis, including neuro- syphilis, the treatment of choice is Erythromycin or Tetracycline 500 mg by mouth four times a day for 30 days.

It is very important to do follow-up VDRL after treating a person for syphilis. Every three months a repeat VDRL ought to be done to show that the VDRL titer is going down. Sometimes, the VDRL remains high even though adequate treatment was given. This situation can be quite confusing because a person can get re-infected with syphilis. It's hard to tell sometimes whether a person has become reinfected or not. An increasing VDRL titer after treatment may mean that re-infection may have taken place.

All cases of Syphillis must be reported to the local Health Departments.

Complications of untreated syphilis include:
Brain damages
Heart damages
Neurological damages
Dmages to both abdominal and thoracic aortas
Psychiatric diseases
Liver diseases
Kidney diseases
Skin diseases
Eye diseases etc;
And death.

CHAPTER 20

HERPES ZOSTER IN AFRICAN AMERICAN MEN

Herpes Zoster/Shingles develops as a result of latent varicella virus that has remained in the human body following an episode of chickenpox. The varicella virus stays in the cells in the body causing no symptoms.

During stress or immunosuppression the varicella virus can come out from their nerve cells in the body and cause Herpes Zoster/Shingles to occur.

Herpes Zoster/Shingles causes a painful, red, skin rash with blisters. This rash usually develops over the chest wall, torso, around the neck, around eyes, under the breasts, over the abdomen, over the lower back, face, or anywhere over the body where the nerve roots contain the viral organisms is located.

Sometimes the Herpes zoster/Shingles can become disseminated throughout the body and goes to the brain, liver, bone marrow resulting in hepatitis, meningitis/encephalitis or bone marrow red blood cells failure.

One million cases of Herpes Zoster/Shingles occur every year in the U.S. and 1 in 3 people in the U.S. will have Herpes Zoster during his or her lifetime.

Worldwide 3-4 healthy individuals per 1000 develop Herpes Zoster/Shingles every year.

Risk factors for Herpes Zoster/Shingles include:

Previous exposure to Chickenpox
Immunosuppression state
Stress (causes over secretion of adrenalin, adrenalin is an immunosupressor)
HIV/AIDS
Non-acquired immunodeficiency diseases
Cancer
Chemotherapy
Radiotherapy
Chronic steroid treatment
Chronic use of Biologics

Sickle cell anemia
SLE
Rheumatoid arthritis etc
Signs and symptoms of Herpes Zoster/Shingles include:
Fever
Headache
Stiffed neck
Light sensitivity
Malaise
Itching
Burning pain
Hyperesthesia
Parasthesia
Tingling pain
Prickling pain
Throbbing pain
Aching pain
Numbness
Reddish rash
Blistering reddish rash
Exudates filled rash
The rash can become dark and crusted.

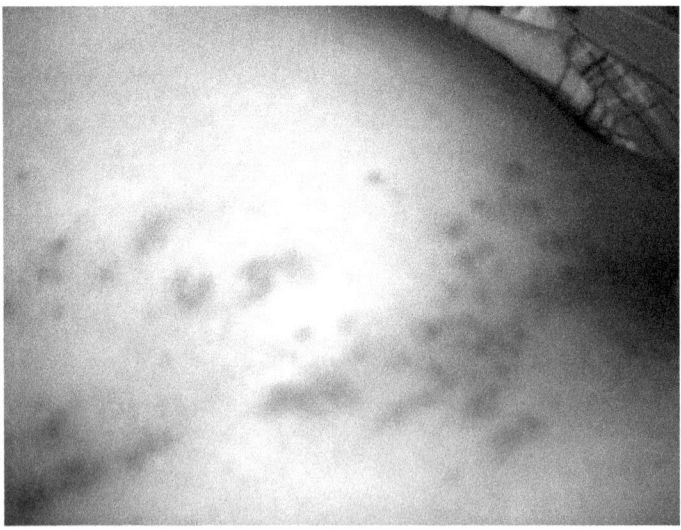

Figure 20:1 **Herpes Zoster/Shingles rash**

Evaluations of Herpes Zoster/Shingles infection include:

History and Physical examination
Herpes Zoster/Shingles titers
CBC
ESR
Complete metabolic chemistry profile
LDH
Serum IGG, IGM, IGA and IGD
Serum protein electrophoresis
Serum immuno-electrophoresis
PT/INR PTT
Urinalysis
Blood culture
RPR
HIV1 and 2
Chest-x-ray
Abdominal ultrasound
Abdominal CT
Brain CT for headache
Brain MRI for headache
Spinal Tap for headache, stiffed neck and light intolerance
White blood cell count in spinal fluid
Protein in spinal fluid
Sugar in spinal fluid
Gram stain of spinal fluid
Bacterial culture of spinal fluid
Viral culture of spinal fluid
Tzanck smear
PCR of spinal for Herpes Zoster/Shingles etc;

Treatments of Herpes Zoster/Shingles include:

Bed rest
Tylenol for fever
Analgesics
Neurontin
Aciclovir by mouth or IV
Famciclovir
Steroid
Aciclovir cream
Lidocaine cream

Complications of Herpes Zoster/Shingles include:

Postherpetcic neuralgia
Chronic weakness
Blindness
Hepatitis
Red cell aplasia
Meningitis
Seizure
Deaths (There are 96 deaths from Herpes Zoster/Shingles every year in the U.S.)

Prevention of herpes Zoster includes:

Zostavax vaccine
"It is recommended that individuals with primary or acquired immunodeficiency should not receive the Herpes Zoster/Shingles vaccine"

CHAPTER 21

HIV/AIDS IN AFRICAN AMERICAN MEN

In 2015, they were 36.7 million people in the world living with AIDS, and 1.8 million of them were children. Since AIDS was first reported in June of 1981, 78 million people have become infected with HIV and 35 million people have died of AIDS worldwide. Source: UNAIDS

"In 2015, 2.1 million individuals worldwide became newly infected with HIV, including 150,000 children."

"Currently only 60% of people with HIV know their status. The remaing 40% (over 14 million people still need to access HIV testing services." As of June 2016, 18.2 million people living with HIVwere accessing antiretroviral therapy (ART) globally. " Source UNAIDS

In 2013, 1.5 million people in the world died of AIDS about 40% fewer than in 2005. In 2014, 1.2 million people in the world died of AIDS. In 2013, "24.7 million Cases or 71% of HIV/AIDS are found in Sub-Sahara Africa 2.3 million Cases or 7% of HIV/AIDS are found in Western and Central Europe and 2.4 million North America. 4.8 million Cases or 14% of HIV/AIDS are found in Asia and the Pacific. 1.6 million Cases or 5% of HIV/AIDS are found in Latin America 250,000 Cases or <1% 1% of HIV/AIDS are found in the Caribbean. 1.1 million Cases or 3% of Cases HIV/AIDS are found in Eastern Europe and Central Asia. 230,000 Cases or <1% of HIV/AIDS are found in the Middle East and North Africa"

In 2016, there were 1.2 million people living with HIV/AIDS in the U.S. and every year there are 500,000 new cases of new HIV/AIDS infection in the U.S. and 1 in 8 of them don't known it.

Since the HIV/AIDS epidemic began in 1981 650,000 people in the U.S. have died from AIDS. The incidence of HIV/AIDS is much higher in blacks than other racial groups in the U.S. "In 2012-the most recent year in the analysis – the death rate per 1,000 HIV – infected people was 20.5 for blacks, 18 for whites and 14 for Hispanics, "and "8,165 blacks with HIV died, more than whites and Hispanics combined."

In 2015, 37 million people are living with HIV/AIDS in the world. In 2015, 2 million new people became infected with HIV/AIDS in the world. By the end of 2014, 1.2 million people died of HIV / AIDS in the world and since the AIDS epidemic began in 1981 about 36 million people have died worldwide from HIV/AIDS. Only 54% of people who are infected worldwide with HIV/AIDs are aware that there are infected according to the WHO.

"In 2013, there were 2.1 or 0.8% million new HIV/AIDS infection in the world 1.5 million or 4.7% infections occurred in Sub-Sahara Africa

350,000 or 0.2% infections occurred in Asia and the Pacific
94,000 or 0.4% infections occurred in Latin America
12,000 or 0.05% infections occurred in the Caribbean
88,000 or 0.3% infections occurred in Western and Central Europe and North America
110,000 or 0.6% infections occurred in Eastern Europe and Central Asia
25,000 or 0.1% infections occurred in the Middle East and North Africa."

"In 2013, 12.9 million living with HIV were receiving antiretroviral therapy (ART) Globally, of which 11.7 million were receiving ART in low –and middle –income countries." WHO

According to WHO, 16 million people got treated with ART worldwide in 2015. Male circumcision (Also known as Dr. Valiere Alcena AIDS vaccine) has proven to be the most effective way to prevent to prevent the transmission of HIV/AIDS and according to the WHO, by the end of 2015, more than 10 millions men in Africa have voluntarily been circumcised to prevent the transmission of HIV/AIDS to their sexual partners.

"HealthDay 7/18, 2017 reports that the CDC "report [pdf] found that nearly one in four adults with diabetes didn't even know they had the disease, and less than 12 percent with prediabetes knew they had that condition." CDC Director stated, "More than a third of US adults have prediabetes, and the majority don't know it." In a news release, Director added, "Now, more than ever, we must step up our efforts to reduce the burden of this serious disease."

"The AP 7/20, 2017 reports that "for the first time in the global AIDS epidemic...more than half of all those infected with HIV are on drugs to treat the virus, the United Nations said in a report released" yesterday. Additionally, "AIDS deaths are also now close to half of what they were in 2005...although those figures are based on estimates and not actual counts from countries." "

VALIERE ALCENA, M.D., M.A.C.P. was the first Physician in the world to have suggested/doing male circumcision to prevent sexual transmission of the AIDS virus in August of 1986 in an article he published in the NEW YORK STATE Journal of Medicine. (a copy of the original article can be seen below in this chapter).

To date more than 70 million male cirmcumsicions have done throughout the world, mostly in Africa according to the WHO.

WHAT IS AIDS? AIDS STANDS for Acquired Immune Deficiency Syndrome (as opposed to Inborn Immune Deficiency Syndrome). AIDS is referred to as Acquired Immune Deficiency Syndrome because the virus, the HIV Type I or Type 2, a retrovirus, enters the human body and attacks and kills the T helper lymphocyte (T4 or CD4), causing a decrease in their numbers, resulting in immunodeficiency of the body and in turn causing vulnerability to a multitude of diseases.

Some of these diseases are caused by the HIV viruses themselves and some of the diseases are caused by different opportunistic organisms that enter into the body at different times in the course of the HIV/AIDS syndrome. The T4 helper lymphocytes are in the body to help the body to be healthy, while the T8 suppressor lymphocytes are in the body to cause it to be sick when their numbers increase.

Therefore, in HIV/AIDS, the number of T helper lymphocytes is lower than the number of the T suppressor lymphocytes, thereby inverting the T helper–to-T suppressor ratio. How does the AIDS virus cause immunosuppression? Answer:

The AIDS virus enters the bloodstream of the person being infected and quickly enters into the T cell CD4 lymphocytes. Once inside these lymphocytes, the virus multiplies by making copies of itself. Sometimes the virus can copy itself in numbers as large as a billion copies or several billion copies per day, until the body gradually becomes more and more immunosuppressed, stage by stage, leading ultimately to full-blown AIDS and all its associated problems and complications which, without treatment, or if the treatment fails, causes death of the affected person.

AIDS a historical perspective

The first reported cases of AIDS appeared in an article published in June 1981 in *The New England Journal of Medicine*, in which a group of homosexual men was found to be sick with Pneumocystis carinii pneumonia.

Further evaluation of these problems revealed that they were immunosuppressed and that the immunosuppressive state that they were suffering from had predisposed them to the development of Pneumocystis carinii pneumonia (PCP).

From that point on the AIDS epidemic was underway. Subsequently it was published that a young man who was retarded and who lived in the streets of St. Louis, Missouri, who was a vagrant in the street of that city and who had frequent contacts with homosexual men, became very sick with an unknown disease associated with fever, weight loss, and pulmonary infection. He went on to die in the early 1960s from complications of the disease.

After his death, an autopsy was performed on him and the pathologist wisely froze tissues and plasma that were taken from his body. In the 1980s after the AIDS epidemic was already underway, this pathologist evaluated these specimens that he had frozen and tested them for the AIDS virus and found that these specimens were teeming with the AIDS virus, which documented that this young man in fact had died of AIDS.

Therefore, in retrospect, the AIDS virus had been around in the United States, since the early 1960s, as documented by this case. Many of us, including this author who, while in training in the inner city of New York City, saw many drug addicts presented to the hospital with febrile illness associated with large lymph nodes, etc., and had no idea what they had. When these lymph nodes were biopsied and the pathologists would report them to us as lymphocytic hyperplasia.

We used to think that the different materials that were used to cut the cocaine or heroin that these drug addicts were using were responsible for the so-called lymphocytic hyperplasia. Little did we know that most probably these people had AIDS that killed them? We simply did not know of the existence of the disease at that time. Therefore, one does not have to go to Africa or to Haiti and other Third World countries to look for a scapegoat for the origin of the AIDS virus.

The AIDS virus was in the inner cities of the world, long before 1981 when the first cases of AIDS were published. According to the literature, the virus that muted into the HIV1 virus may have originated in certain specie of monkey indigenous in Africa.

Be that as it may, blame passing aside, scapegoating aside, name calling and finger pointing aside, AIDS is now worldwide and it knows no racial boundaries; it spares no social classes, spares no sexes and it affects people of all ethnic backgrounds and religious beliefs. AIDS is the largest epidemic that mankind has ever known.

Every few seconds a new person in the world is being infected with the AIDS virus and those infections are mainly being transmitted through sexual intercourse. As of the end of December 2001 there were 40 million cases of HIV/AIDS in the world and 28.1 million people in Sub-Saharan Africa live with the HIV virus (Source: UNAIDS/WHO, Dec. 2001). Source: UNAIDS

Why is AIDS so much more prevalent among blacks in the U.S., as compared to whites.

HIV/AIDS in African American men:

"There are 1.2 million people living with HIV/AIDS in the U.S. and more than 500,000 of them are Blacks" "Black represents about 14% of the U.S. populations and about 2% of them are HIV positive and African American males had 8 times the rate of AIDS as whites in 2007". Source: The office of Minority Health U.S. Department of Health and Human Services. 44% of the 1.2 million Americans that are positive for HIV are Blacks.

The reason more blacks are infected with the AIDS virus than whites is because more blacks are using intravenous drugs than whites are. Once these blacks become infected with the AIDS virus, they quickly pass it on to their sexual partners.

Many black women get infected with the AIDS virus although they are not using IV drugs, but their drug-using sexual partners pass the virus on to them during unprotected sexual intercourse.

AIDS is causing a great deal of suffering in all communities, in all ethnic groups, all social standing, all economic status and in all genders. Since the HIV/AIDS began, 230,000

African Americans have died of AIDS representing 40% of the total deaths from AIDS in the U.S.

Sixty seven percent 67% of the HIV/AIDS cases in women in the U.S. is found among black women as compared to 19% in white women. 1 in 16 African American man is expected to be diagnosed with HIV, and 1 in 30 African American women are expected to be diagnosed with HIV. About 50% of HIV/AIDS in the U.S. are found in blacks. Blacks represent 14% of the U.S. population.

Over all the incidence of HIV/AIDS in the U.S. is on the rise. In the recent 12 month periods, it is reported that 63,000 individuals became infected with the HIV/AIDS virus. The rate of new HIV/AIDS infection has gone down across the world and the death rate From HIV/AIDS has also gone down in 2007.

There are several reasons why both the rate of new HIV/AIDS infection and the deaths from HIV/AIDS have gone down.

" "NYTimes Highlights Hidden HIV Epidemic Among Gay And Bisexual Black Men in the US In a 8,700-word article in its Magazine, the New York Times (6/6 2017, Subscription Publication) reports that there is a hidden HIV/AIDS epidemic in the US among gay and bisexual black men, especially in Southern states. The Times reports that the HIV infection rate among this group is higher than any country in the world. The article explores in depth the history of the HIV/AIDS epidemic in the US and how a combination of policies and cultural perceptions have contributed to the higher infection rate among the group. The director of the Centers for Disease Control and Prevention's National Center for HIV/AIDS, Viral Hepatitis, STD and TB Prevention, said, "It's deeply troubling when 50 percent of African-American gay men are expected to get H.I.V. during their lifetime, but it's also been a clarion call for all of us to improve on what we're doing." "

First and most important is the fact the program of male circumcision that has been implemented in several African countries is working to prevent to prevent the transmission of HIV/AIDS infections in Africa where both rate infection and deaths are most numerous. Second, the wide spread distribution of condoms in several African countries is working.

Third, sex education programs, which have been implemented with an emphasis on abstinence, seem to be making a difference.

As just mentioned above more than 10 millions men in Africa have voluntarily been circumcised resulting in several millions less HIV infections and deaths.
Source : WHO

Male circumcision has done more than anything else in reducing HIV/AIDS around the world.

Fourth, the programs, which have been implemented to treat some HIV/AIDS individuals with HAART medications, are making a difference to keep some of these infected people alive.

The author is credited, as being the first person in the world to have proposed the idea that male circumcision would decrease the transmission of the HIV/AIDS by Eliminating balanitis, phimosis, paraphphimosis, and other mini-ulcerations of the foreskin of the penis.

These conditions represent an entry point for the HIV/AIDS virus to enter the blood stream of men while engaging in intra-vaginal or intra-anal sexual intercourse.

1. "AIDS in Third World Countries"
NEW YORK STATE JOURNAL OF MEDICINE, Vol. 86 August 1986
By: VALIERE ALCENA, M.D., F.A.C.P.
"That male circumcision might reduce risk of HIV acquisition was first proposed in 1986" Alcena V. AIDS in third world countries. NY State J Med 1986; 86 446. MEDLINE
2. The Lancet, Volume 369, Number 9562, February 2007

This idea is being acclaimed as one of the most important contributions made since the HIV/AIDS epidemic began in 1981. It has already prevented the transmission of millions of HIV/AIDS infections and undoubtedly million of lives in Africa. According to the World Health Organization, seventy percent of men in the world are not circumcised. If a program of circumcision were carried out worldwide, 3 million of HIV/AIDS infections could be prevented and millions lives could be saved says the WHO.

On December 2, 2014, the CDC recommends voluntary elective male circumcision to prevent HIV and other sexually transmitted diseases. According to the CDC the benefit of male circumcision outweighs the risks.

New HIV Diagnoses in the United States for the Most-Affected Subpopulations, 2015

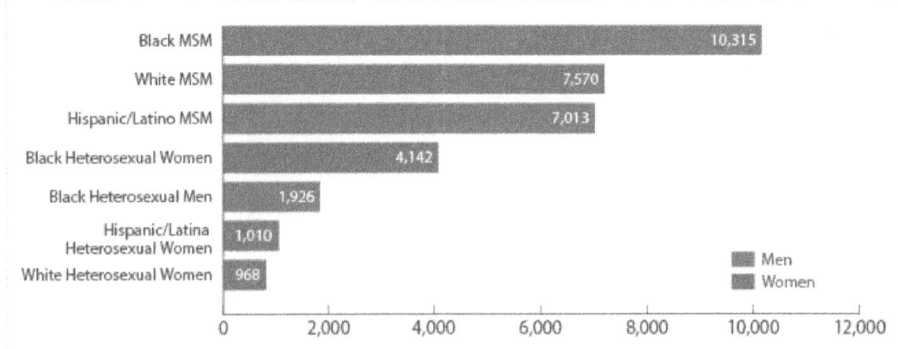

Source: CDC. Diagnoses of HIV infection in the United States and dependent areas, 2015. *HIV Surveillance Report* **2016;27. Subpopulations representing 2% or less of HIV diagnoses are not reflected in this chart. Abbreviation: MSM, men who have sex with men.**

Male circumcision can prevent STDs such as herpes simplex, syphilis, and gonorrhea, Chlamydia, HPV. Male circumcision will also decrease the incidence of cervical cancer. Source: Valiere Alcena, M.D., and M.A.C.P.

The different ways in which a man can get infected with the AIDS virus include:

Sexual intercourse:

1. Black men who have sex with black men
2. Black men who have sexual intercourse with both men and women
3. Black men or women who are injected with IV drugs
4. Black men who have sexual intercourse with men who use IV drugs
5. Black men who have sexual intercourse with bisexual men
6. Black men who receive blood or blood products contaminated with the HIV virus
7. Black men who use IV drugs
8. Black men health workers who get stuck with needles contaminated with the HIV virus
9. Black men bitten by an AIDS-infected person
10. Using the same toothbrush as that used by an AIDS-infected person
11. Engaging in passionate kissing with an AIDS-infected person
12. Engaging in oral sex with an AIDS-infected person

What are some of the high-risk behaviors that can lead to the transmission of the AIDS virus from one person to another?

1. Anal intercourse, men with men
2. Intravenous drug use
3. Male prostitution
4. Male promiscuity
5. Having unprotected sexual intercourse with strangers

In order for a person to become infected with the AIDS virus, the virus must enter the bloodstream of the person at risk.

What happens when the HIV virus first enters into a person's bloodstream?

When the HIV virus enters the blood, the virus goes into the T helper lymphocytes, also known as CD4. Inside the CD4 lymphocytes that are in the circulation, the HIV virus multiplies into millions at first then into billions of HIV virus copies per day. Within two to four weeks of the entry of the HIV virus into the bloodstream, the newly infected person often develops a flu-like syndrome with fever, general aches, chills, runny nose, and even a cough, simulating acute rhinovirus or influenza infection. These symptoms quickly disappear and the person feels fine.

The HIV viruses continue to multiply in the bloodstream and within the nodes of the person's body where they have entered. This represents the HIV stage 1 infection. During ten days to two weeks the P24 antigen level becomes elevated.

However, the HIV RNA PCR becomes elevated within about a week of someone becoming infected with the HIV virus, making it the earliest test and the most sensitive test that becomes positive, indicating the presence of HIV infection.

The ELISA test becomes positive after the window period, which is from 6 to 12 weeks after infection. During the window period the ELISA for the HIV, the P24 antigen, and the HIV RNA PCR all will be positive, if the person is infected with the AIDS virus.

As the HIV viruses continue to multiply, the number of T4 lymphocytes decreases while the number of the T8 or T suppressor lymphocytes increases.

This situation is what triggers the immunosuppressive states that occur in AIDS. As the infection progresses the disease moves into different stages.

First the HIV infection moves from the HIV-infected stage to ARC (AIDS-related complex) stage and then to the AIDS stage.

The HIV stage may be completely silent, except for some patients who may develop thrombocytopenia (low platelet count) with or without enlarged nodes.

The second stage is ARC. In this stage the person will start to lose weight with diffuse lymph node enlargement, thrush in the mouth, diarrhea, fever, headache, oral hair leukoplakia, shingles, thrombocytopenia, molluscum contagiosum, recurrent herpes simplex, aphthous ulcer, condyloma etc.

Some individuals take many years to progress from these stages to full-blown AIDS, 8 to 10 years, and still other individuals go quickly from these early stages to full-blown AIDS in 4 to 6 years. How fast the infected person becomes infected.

The mode of infection and the stage of HIV infection that the person who is doing the infecting has play a role on how quickly a person develops fullblown AIDS.

There is a discussion in the literature regarding chemokine receptors CCR5 and CX4 that seem to play a role in when certain individuals who are infected with the HIV virus progresses to full-blown AIDS. For that matter, certain individuals who have some of these chemokine receptors may be resistant to the HIV infection. This is a new concept yet to be fully elucidated, but it would appear that there are different effects of the CCR2 and the CCR5 variants on HIV disease.

This new concept will be further evaluated and elucidated in the future.

One of the important factors is the overall makeup of the infected individual, in terms of his or her immune strength, his or her ability to pay for medical care, to pay for anti-retroviral medication, his or her ability to afford good nutrition etc. All these factors interplay on how well the AIDS-affected person does.

In order to say that a person has AIDS, clinically established criteria have to be met, as defined by the CDC. For example, a person with HIV infection whose CD4 count drops below 200 can be said to meet one of the criteria to have AIDS.

The list of AIDS-defining illnesses includes the following:

Diseases diagnosed definitively without confirmation of HIV infection in patients without other causes of immunodeficiency

Candidiasis of the esophagus, trachea, bronchi, or lungs
Cryptococcuses, extra pulmonary
Cryptosporidiosis > 1 month's duration
Cytomegalovirus infection of any organ except the liver, spleen,
Or lymph nodes in patients > 1 month old
Herpes simplex infection, mucocutaneous (> 1 month's duration) or
of the bronchi, lungs, or esophagus in patients of 1 month's
duration Kaposi's sarcoma in patients < 60 years old
Primary CNS lymphoma in patients < 60 years old
Lymphoid interstitial pneumonitis (LIP) and/or
pulmonary lymphoid hyperplasia (PLH) in patients < 13 years old
Mycobacterium avium complex of Mycobacterium kansasii disseminated
Pneumocystis carinii pneumonia
Progressive multifocal leukoencephalopathy
Toxoplasmosis of the brain in patients > 1 month old

Diseases diagnosed definitively with confirmation of HIV infection

Multiple or recurrent pyogenic bacterial infections in patients
< 13 years old
Coccidioidomycosis, disseminated
Histoplasmosis, disseminated
Isosporiasis > 1 month duration
Kaposi's sarcoma, any age
Primary CNS lymphoma, any age
Non-Hodgkin's lymphoma (small, noncleaved lymphoma;
Burkitt or non-Burkitt type; or immunoblastic sarcoma)
Mycobacterial disease other than *Mycobacterium tuberculosis*, disseminated
M. Tuberculosis, extra pulmonary *Salmonella* septicemia.

Diseases diagnosed presumptively with confirmation of HIV *infection*

Candidiasis of the esophagus
CMV retinitis
Kaposi's sarcoma
LIP/PLH in patients < 13 years old
disseminated mycobacterial disease (not cultured)
P. Carinii pneumonia Toxoplasmosis of the brain in patients > 1 month old HIV
encephalopathy HIV wasting syndrome

CDC definition of AIDS

To diagnose AIDS in a patient, the first blood test that is often done is the screening test called ELISA. If the ELISA test is positive, then the Western Blot Test is done to confirm whether the ELISA test is truly positive.

The Western Blot Test is an actual electrophoresis of the protein contained within the body of the virus itself. The problem with the ELISA test is that it does not become positive until about 8 to 12 weeks and it can be falsely positive.

Another problem is that during this so-called window period, the HIV test could be falsely negative. To deal with this problem, the P24 antigen test can be done because it becomes positive within a minimum of 10 days after the virus enters into the human body. In addition, the HIV DNA PCR test can be done to determine whether the HIV test is truly positive or not.

Among the tests that are available to diagnose AIDS are the following:

1. ELISA Test
2. Western Blot Test
3. HIV1 DNA PCR test
4. HIV1 RNA PCR test
5. P24
6. "The FDA approves HIV infection assay
   The Bioplex 2200 HIV Ag-Ab asay is intended for use in adults, children aged 2 years and older and pregnant women. It can be used to screen organ donors for HIV-1 and HIV-2."

AIDS is a multi-systems disease in that it affects all systems in the body in one form or another or to one degree or another, leading eventually to certain death of the infected individual. The first system that is affected with the AIDS virus is the immune system, resulting in immunosuppression.

The immune system has three parts to it:

1. Cell-mediated
2. Humoral-mediated
3. The complement system

As outlined in the book **AIDS,** *The Expanding Epidemic: What the Public Needs to Know A Multicultural Overview,* by V. Alcena, MD, 1994

Cell-mediated immunity, this system is dominated mainly by T-lymphocytes. Macrophages also play a role in this system. There are different types of T lymphocytes such as CD4 or T helper lymphocytes, CD8 or T-suppressor lymphocytes. Delayed-type hypersensitivity plays a major role in the immune system CD4 or T helper lymphocytes and macrophages are necessary for the antigen specific part of this system.

Delayed -type's hypersensitivity is crucial in vaccination. CD4 or T helper lymphocyte is necessary to help the body maintain a normally functioning immune system.

A decrease in the total T helper lymphocytes leads to immune deficiency state maybe congenital or acquired. When the level of CD4 goes down, the level of CD8 or T suppressor goes up, leading to further suppression of the immune system. The humoral-mediated immune system is dominated by B-lymphocytes.

These B-lymphocytes give rise to plasma cells, which then produce antibodies. These antibodies are known as immunoglobulins IgG, IgM, IgA, IgD and IgE. These antibodies have many functions, but paramount amongst them is to protect the human body from infections.

When the level of antibody-producing B-lymphocytes goes down, as occurs in AIDS, then all sorts of infections can occur in the human body.

The third immune system that plays a major role in the fight against infection in the human body is the complement system. The complement system is divided into the classical pathway and the alternate pathway.

These complement systems have many components and these components work in concert with other immunoglobulins to lyse microorganisms, such as bacteria, viruses, fungi, parasites and protozoa to kill them, thereby preventing them from killing the human organism.

When there is a decrease in the level of complement in the human body, this can lead to a state of immunodeficiency that, if not corrected, can lead to different infections such as bacterial, viral, fungal, and parasitic infections, leading to many problems for the human organism and ultimately its death, if appropriate treatments are not provided.

Several more sophisticated systems that are known to play different roles in the immune system, but the three outlined above are the major ones that are responsible to fight infections and maintain good health.

Normal Immune Competence Profile in a person

Normal Values

% T cells (60.1–88.1%)
% B cells (3–20.8%)
% Helper cells (34 –67%)
% suppress T cells (10–41.9%)
Lymphocytes (0.66–4.60 THO/UL)
T cells (644–2201 CELLS/UL)
B cells (82–392 CELLS/UL)
Helper cells (493–1191 CELLS/UL)
Suppressor cell (182–785 CELLS/UL)
H/S ratio 1

Abnormal Immune Competence Profile in a person infected with HIV

T- and B-Cell Surface Markers:
T-Helper/T-Suppressor

Lymphocyte Ratio, Blood		Patient's	Normal
% T Cells		75%	60.1–88.1
% Helper Cells	L	16%	34–67
% Suppressor T Cell	H	60%	10–41.9
% B Cells		6%	3–20.8
Lymphocytes		3.0 thou/UL	0.66–4.60
T Cells	H	2250 cells/UL	644–2201
Helper Cells	L	480 cells/UL	493–1191
Suppressor Cells	H	1800 cells/UL	182–785
B Cells		180 cells/UL	82–392
H/S Ratio	L	0.27	1 or greater

The second most frequently affected system in HIV infection is the hematopoietic system (the blood). The routine blood system includes the white blood cells, the red blood cells, the platelets, and the coagulation system. The two earliest affected cells are the white blood cells and the platelets. Frequently, the first indication that someone is HIV infected is a low platelet count, known as thrombocytopenia. In this situation, the HIV virus directly infects the megakaryocytes, the cells that produce the platelets, which result in thrombocytopenia. Thrombocytopenia can also occur in AIDS because of idiopathic thrombocytopenia (ITP) or thrombotic thrombocytopenic purpura (TTP).

The mechanisms of idiopathic thrombocytopenic purpura, or thrombotic thrombocytopenic purpura as seen in HIV/AIDS, are most likely autoimmune in nature, in particular, the ITP.

Leukopenia, low white cell count, is due to a combination of HIV infection plus the different medications that people with HIV infection are treated.

The red blood cells are low (anemia) due to different reasons. One reason is that the HIV virus enters into the earliest red cells (erythroblasts), infect them, thereby preventing them from maturing, resulting in anemia.

Another reason is that the HIV infection is frequently associated with parvovirus B#19. The parvovirus enters into the early red blood cells, resulting in pure red cells aplasia, resulting in anemia. Still another cause of anemia in HIV-infected individuals (AIDS) is low levels of erythropoietin. Erythropoietin is a protein made by the kidneys whose job is to stimulate the production of red blood cells. AIDS patients with an erythropoietin less than 500 usually respond to erythropoietin injections to correct the anemia, usually in association with AZT.

Another reason HIV-infected individuals become anemic is chronic gastrointestinal blood loss, fungal gastritis, esophagitis, viral and other infections of the GI tract, resulting in chronic anemia. Patients with AIDS frequently have folate deficiency, and at times B12 deficiency, resulting in anemia. A condition called red cells aplasia can occur due to the HIV/AIDS infection.

The poor nutritional state of these patients can cause a low protein anemia. Further, the chronic infection state of these patients causes a cytokines-associated anemia of chronic diseases. The pulmonary system is commonly affected by different infections in patients with AIDS. Pneumocystis caranii pneumonia (PCP) is prominent among these infections of the lungs.

Other pulmonary infections seen in AIDS patients are pneumococcal infections, H. Influenza infections, pseudomonas infections, etc. Fungal infections of the lung are also quite common in AIDS patients.

Still other pulmonary infections seen frequently in AIDS patients are mycobacterium tuberculosis (MTB), mycobacterium avium intracellulare (MAI). Both MTB and MAI can be diffuse, affecting multiple organs in the body. About 80% to 90% of patients with full-blown AIDS who die are found at autopsy to have MAI.

People with AIDS are frequently infected with viruses of different types. Among these viruses that infect AIDS patients most frequently are herpes simplex, Herpes Zoster, Epstein-Barr virus, and cytomegalovirus (CMV). All of these viruses can infect different organs, resulting in severe morbidity and mortality.

A multitude of fungi can cause infections in AIDS patients. The most common ones are Candida histoplasma and cryptococcus. The brain, quite frequently, becomes infected with different microorganisms (see tables below).

AIDS patients frequently become infected with protozoal organisms, such as, Pneumocystis carinii and toxoplasma, etc. (Source: *AIDS, The Expanding Epidemic: A Multicultural Overview*, 1994, by Valiere Alcena, MD, FACP). Valiere Alcena, M.D., F.A.C.P.

The different infections seen in AIDS patients and how they are treated.

Infecting Agent	Manifestations	Treatment	Prophylaxis	Drug Toxicities	Comment
Pneumocystis carinii			TMP/SMX 1 DS tablet daily or 3x/wk, or	Rash, fever, neutropenia	Begin once CD4+T cell count <200/uL or CD4%<15
				Bronchospasm	
			Aerosolized pentamidine 300 mg/month, or Dapsone 50 mg/d PO+	Methemoglobinemia, neutropenia	Contraindicated in patients with G6PD deficiency
	Mild to moderate pneumonia (Pao2 ≥ 70 mmHg and (A-a)dO2 ≤ 35 mmHg}	TMP/SMX 15-20 mg/kg/d PO	Pyrimethamine 50 mg/wk PO + Folinic acid 25 mg/wk PO	Rash, fever, neutropenia Methemoglobinemia C. *Difficile* colitis	Treat for 21 d if possible; no less than 14 d
	Severe pneumonia [Pao2 < 70 mmHG or (A-a)dO2> 35 mmHG]	TMP 20 mg/kg/d PO qd+ Dapsone 100 mg PO qd Clindamycin 600 mg PO q6h+ Primaquine 15 mg PO qd IV Pentamidine 3-4 mg/kg/d Atovaquone, 750 mg, PO, tid for 21 d Aerosolized penta-midine 300 mg/d TMP/SMX 15-20 mg/kg/d IV initially (total course 14-21 d) Pentamidine 3-4 mg/kg/d IV for 14-21 d Clindamycin 900 mg IV q 8h then 450 mg PO q6h+		Rash, Neutropenia, nephritis, pancreatitis, hypoglycemia, diabetes Bronchospasm Rash, fever, leukopenia, thrombocytopenia, hepatitis, nephritis, pancreatitis, hypoglycemia, diabetes, C. *Difficile* colitis Rash, neutropenia Rash, neutropenia	Contraindicated in patients with G6D deficiency Contraindicated in patients with G6D deficiency Provides no systemic effects. Not recommended , , ,,but an option for multidrug-allergic patient with mild pneumonia Prednisone, 40 mg bid for 2 d, then 40 mg/d for 5 d, then 20 mg/d to the end of therapy (21 d total) added to specific antimicrobial ASAP and no later than 36 h after diagnosis
	Disseminated disease	Primaquine 30 mg PO qd for total of 14-21 d Trimetrexate 45 mg/m2 IV (over 60-90 min) qd x 21 d + Leucovorin 20 mg/m2 IV q6h x 24 d Eflornithine (DFMO) 100 mg/kg IV q6h for 14 d followed by 75 mg/kg PO q6h for 4-6 wk Any of the systemic therapies outlined above		Thrombocytopenia	Contraindicated in patients with G6D deficiency For patients intolerant of other regimens. Less effective than standard therapy. Bone marrow-suppressive effects blunted by use of leucovorin Call 1-800-TRIALSA for information

Toxoplasma tondii			TMP/SMX 1 DS tablet qd	Rash, fever, neutropenia	Alternative is dapsone, 50 mg PO qd.+ pyrimethamine, 50 mg, PO weekly + folinic acid, 25 mg, PO weekly Treatment is generally for life.
	Encephalitis, brain abscess, chorioretinitis, myocarditis	Sulfadiazine 1-2 g PO q6h + Pyrimethamine 25 - 100 mg qd + Folinic acid 10-20 mg PO qd Clindamycin initially 200-400 mg IV q6h		Crystalluria, rash	
				Rash, fever, neutropenia, C.difficile colitis	Leucovorin to minimize bone marrow suppression
Toxoplasma gondii - (continued)		Pyrimethamine 25-100 mg qd + Folinic acid 100-20 mg qd followed by Clindamycin 300-900 mg PO q8h+ Pyrimethamine 25-100 mg qd Atovaquone 250 mg PO tid+ Pyrimethamine 25-100 mg qe + Folinic acid 10-20 mg qd Macrolides (clarithromycin or azithromycin) + Pyrimethamine		Rash, fever, neutropenia	Leucovorin to minimize bone marrow suppression
				Rash, fever, neutropenia	
					Leucovorin to minimize bone marrow suppression Early results disappointing
Ttospora Belli	Diarrhea	TMP/SMX 1 DS tablet PO qid for 10 d then bid for 3 weeks		Rash, fever, neutropenia	TMP/SMX 1 DS tablet PO 3x/week for maintenance NTZ;
Cryptosporidia Microsporidia	Diarrhea	No known specific therapy; supportive measures include parenteral nutrition			NTZ; bovine colostrum in trials
Mycobacterium avium complex			Clarithromycin 500 mg PO bid or Azithromycin 1200 mg weekly or Rifa , , ,,butin 300 mg PO qd		Begin prophylaxis once CD4+T cell count <100/ uL or <50/uL. Treatment is generally for life. Macrolides + rifa , , ,,butin may be more effective; however, mor toxic and costly
	Disseminated disease that may involve lung, bone marrow liver	Etham , , ,,butol 15 mg/ kg qd+ Rifa , , ,,butin 600 mg/ qd + Clarithromycin 100 mg PO bid		Hepatitis, neuropathy (peripheral/optic)	
Mycobacterium tuberculosis	Asymptomatic, PPD test positive	Isoniazid 15 mg/kg up to 900 mg PO twice a week or 300 mg daily		Hepatitis	
	Active disease	for 1 y+ Pyridoxine 50 mg/d Isoniazid, 300 mg PO qd x 1y + Rifampin 600 mg PO qd x 1y + Pyrazinamide 30 mg/ kg/d in 2 doses		Hepatitis	Treat with 3 drugs for 2 mo. If isolate is sensitive to Isoniazid and rifampin, then switch to 2 drugs. Treat a minimum of 9 mo and at least 6 mo after third negative culture. Quinolones may also be considered as a fifth drug
				Hepatitis	
				Hepatitis	
	Active disease in a setting where there is a possibility of multidrug resistance			Neuropathy (peripheral/ optic) Nephrotoxicity, hearing loss	
		Add etham , , ,,butol 15-25 mg/kg/d and Streptomycin or Amikacin			
Candida Albicans	Thrush, vaginitis	Clotrimazole troches, Nystatin prn Fluconazole 200 mg PO qd for 7-14 d Amphotericin B 0.25 mg/kg/d IV for 7-10 d	Fluconazole 200 mg PO qd (optional)	Hepatotoxicity Hepatotoxicity Nephrotoxicity, fever/ chills	Primary prophylaxis generally not indicated. Treatment is generally prn

Cryptococcus neoformans	Meningitis, brain abscess, pneumonia, disseminated disease	Amphotericin B 0.3 mg/kg/d IV + Flucytosine 150 mg/kg/d PO for 6 wk followed by Fluconazole 100-200 mg PO qd indefinitely	Fluconazole 200 mg PO qd (Optional)	Hepatotoxicity Nephrotoxicity, fever/ chills, bone marrow suppression Hepatotoxicity	Begin prophylaxis if CD4+ T cell count <50/uL (optional; depending on risk). Approximately 50% will need to have flucytosine held during therapy due to neutropenia. An alternative is amphotericin B alone at a dose of 0.8 mg/kg/d
Histoplasma capsulatum	Disseminated disease, pneumonia	Amphotericin B 0.6-1 mg/kg/d to a total 1 g then Itraconazole 200 mg qd indefinitely		Nephrotoxicity, fever/ chills	
Bartonella henselae (quintana)	Nodular skin lesions, peliosis hepatitis, trench fever	Erythromycin 500 g PO or IV qd for 2 months			
Penicillium marneffei	Disseminated disease, umbilicated skin lesions	Amphotericin G, 0.6-1 mg/kg/d to a total of 1 g then Itraconazole 200 mg qd indefinitely		Neurotoxicity, fever, chills, hepatitis	
Cytomegalovirus	Retinitis, esophagitis, colitis, and pneumonia	Ganciclovir 5 mg/kg q 12h for 14 d followed by 5 mg/kg qd IV indefinitely Foscarnet 90 mg/kg q 12h for 14 d followed by 90-120 mg/kg qd IV indefinitely	Ganciclovir 1.0 g PO tid with food (optional)	Neutropenia Intestinal nephritis, seizure, hypocalcemia	Expensive, marginal efficacy. Neutropenia may be ameliorated by colony-stimulating factors Retinitis may also be treated with ocular implant Oral ganciclovir, 1 g PO tid with food may be used for maintenance Should be preceded by saline infusion to minimize nephrotoxicity
Herpes simplex virus	Recurrent perioral, perirectal, or genital ulcers	Acyclovir 200-400 mg PO 5id as needed			Foscarnet 60 mg/kg q8h x 14 d for patients with acyclovir-resistant herpes simplex or zoster
	Esophagitis; acute retinal necrosis	Acyclovir 5 mg/kg IV q8h for 10-14 c			
Varicella-Zoster virus	Cutaneous (local or disseminated);retinal necrosis	Acyclovir 800 mg PO 5id or 10 mg/kg IV q8h for 10-14 d or longer			Famciclovir 500 mg PO q8h x 7 d is an alternative
Treponema pallidum	Early syphilis	Benzathine penicillin G 2.4 million units IM weekly for 3 wk			Approximately 20% relapse, need retreatment. Immunologic abnormalities may cause inaccurate serology
	Late or neurosyphilis	Aqueous penicillin G 12-24 million units IV daily for 10-14 d + probenecid 500 mg PO qid Ceftriaxone 1-2 g IM or IV aq 10-14 d			

Source: *AIDS, the Expanding Epidemic: A Multi-Cultural Overview*, 1994 by Valiere Alcena, MD, FACP
Different diseases of the brain in AIDS Patients

Opportunistic infections
Toxoplasmosis
Cryptococcosis
Progressive multifocal leukoencephalopathy

Cytomegalovirus
Syphilis
Mycobacterium tuberculosis
HTLV-1 infection
Neoplasms (cancers)
Primary CNS lymphoma
Kaposi's sarcoma
Result of HIV-1 infection
Aseptic meningitis
AIDS dementia complex (HIV encephalopathy)
Myelopathy
Vacuolar myelopathy
Pure sensory ataxia
Paresthesia/dysesthesia
Peripheral neuropathy
Acute demyelinating polyneuropathy
Mononeuritis multiplex
Distal symmetric polyneuropathy
Myopathy

Disease	Clinical Features	Characteristic CSF Findings	Characteristic Radiologic Findings
HIV encephalopathy (AIDS dementia complex)	Personality changes, dementia, unsteady gait, seizures	Nonspecific increases in cells and protein	Cortical atrophy, ventricular dilation, bright spots on T2-wieghted MRI
Toxoplasmosis	Fever, headache, focal neurologic deficits, seizures, + antibodies in 95%	Nonspecific	Single or multiple ring-enhancing lesions in multiple locations
Cryptococcal meningitis	Fever, nausea, vomiting, confusion, headache	Elevated protein, low glucose, positive cryptococcal antigen or culture	Nonspecific
Progressive multifocal leukoencephalopathy	Multiple focal deficits without changes in level of consciousness	Nonspecific	Multiple white matter lesions on T2-weighted MRI images
Neurosyphilis	Meningitis, neuroretinitis, deafness, focal neurologic deficits	Positive VDRL, elevated protein, increase in cells	Nonspecific
Lymphoma	Seizure, focal neurologic deficits, headache	Nonspecific in primary CNS lymphoma; malignant cells in systemic lymphoma	Single or few ring-enhancing lesions
Tuberculosis meningitis	Fever, headache, confusion, meningitis, cough	Elevated protein, low glucose, pleocytosis, positive smear/culture for acid-fast bacilli (AFB)	Mass lesions in approximately 50%, abnormal chest x-ray

Source: AIDS, The Expanding Epidemic: What the Public Needs to Know — A Multi-Cultural Overview, 1994 by Valiere Alcena, MD, FACP

Clinical management of HIV stage infection

The decision as to when to start treatment in a person who becomes HIV positive is quite controversial. Most clinicians, however, start patients who are HIV positive on AZT and, to prevent resistance, frequently add 3TC (Epivir) to that regimen. This thinking, however, has changed in recent years. Up to now, in most cases, treatment is being withheld till the CD4 count reaches the range of 300, at which point, HAART (Highly Active Antiretroviral Treatment) or Combivir medication is started. In addition, Bactrim DS, 1 tablet per day, is started as prophylaxis against PCP (Source: Joel E. Gallant, et al., *HIV Forefront*, Vol. 2, No. 1, April 2000). If the CD4 is 200, even if the patient is asymptomatic, HAART must be started (Source: *Report of the Panel on Clinical Priorities, Department of Health and Human Services,* and Feb. 2001).

Now in 2013, WHO recommends starting anti-retroviral medications (HAART) at CD4 of 500 cells/mcl.

A recent report came out that shows that treating HIV stage disease early decreases transmission of HIV to a person's sexual partner. Source: CDC

A new report just came out that shows that starting "ART treatment for the HIV stage when the CDC cell counts reaches 350 cells/mcl and 499 cells/mcl was associated with slower disease progression compared with a deferral strategy" Source: ARCHIVE of Internal Medicine 2011; 171:1560-1569

November, 2015 WHO Updates HIV Treatments and Prevention Guideline.

"Individuals from all populations and age groups who are infected with HIV should begin antiretroviral (ART) immediately after diagnosis, regardless of CD4 cell count, according to updated treatment and prevention recommendations for HIV issued in September by the World Health Organization."

Seizure is a common problem seen in patients with AIDS, due to either fungal infection of the brain, lymphoma of the brain, or possibly PML. After appropriate evaluation with brain CT scan or brain MRI, followed by lumbar puncture with evaluation of the cerebrospinal fluid, chemically and bacteriologically, the doctor looks for microorganisms and, in the case of lymphoma, looks for cancer cells. Once these things are done then appropriate treatments are given for the specific problems discovered or empirically for whatever the treating physician feels clinically appropriate for the particular circumstances.

Toward the end of full-blown AIDS, the wastage stage usually sets in. Few people, if any, ever recover from this stage of AIDS, in spite of expensive nutrition and androgenic steroid treatments. Megace in high doses works well to increase AIDS patients' appetite.

However, using Megace in treatment of full-blown AIDS patients is risky because many of these patients have nephrotic syndrome through which they lose Protein C and Protein S and anti Thrombin III in their urine, resulting in a hypercongealable state, which, by its very nature, can lead to clot formation and thrombosis. Even in those patients who have no evidence of renal disease, a loss of Protein S in the urine is known to occur, resulting potentially in the same syndrome as just described.

It is a known fact that Megace and other estrogenic-like hormones can cause a hypercoagulable state through the loss of anti-thrombin III.

Therefore, it is prudent to use Megace in AIDS patients or any patient very carefully and when necessary to avoid the development of deep vein thrombosis (DVT) and its possible associated complications, which can result in morbidity and mortality.

While there is no cure and no vaccine available for people infected with HIV Type I or Type II and full-blown AIDS, there are many medications available. The first category of medications made to treat AIDS patients was the reverse transcriptase inhibitors.

Examples of reverse transcriptase inhibitors are Zidovudine (AZT), didanosine (ddI), zalcitabine (ddC) and stavudine (D4T).

AZT, ddI and ddC can be used both as combination therapy and as mono therapy in early HIV disease. D4T is best used in people with advanced AIDS who are not able to tolerate the other medications.

These reverse transcriptase inhibitors work to prevent the multiplication of the HIV virus by blocking the production of the enzyme reverse transcriptase, thereby preventing the synthesis of RNA and DNA and in so doing preventing viral multiplications. Lamivudine (Epivir, 3TC) is used in combination with AZT to treat HIV infections.

The importance of this combination is that HIV virus becomes resistant to AZT reasonably quickly in many individuals who are treated with the AZT alone. When 3CT is added to the AZT, the DDI, or the DDC it enhances the sensitivity of the reverse transcriptase that is used along with it to kill the HIV virus. 3TC by itself has very little effect against the HIV virus.

A new drug for the treatment of HIV was just approved by the FDA. It is a combination of AZT and 3TC and it is named Combivir. It has the advantage of being used two times per day.

The newest invention in the treatment of AIDS that has shown the most promise in the last few years is triple therapy, HAART. The key component of the triple therapy is the addition of a protease inhibitor. The protease inhibitors in use are Saquinavir, Ritonavir, Indinavir, and Nelfinavir. The so-called AIDS cocktail is usually made of a reverse transcriptase inhibitor, such as AZT, with 3TC and a protease inhibitor such as Indinavir.

Once it becomes clear that the patient has gone into the full-blown AIDS stage, and then the whole way of clinically managing the patient is dictated by the particular AIDS-defining signs, symptoms, and disease that affect the patient. If the patient has PCP, she is to be treated for PCP using PCP-effective medications. If the patient has MAI, she is to be treated for MAI using MAI-effective medications.

If the patient has gastroenteritis, diarrhea, she is to be evaluated and treated for the diarrhea based on the clinical and laboratory findings. If the patient has blurry vision and

CMV retinitis is suspected, then an evaluation must be carried out by an ophthalmologist, to document whether this is so or not. Ganciclovir is used IV to treat CMV retinitis.

If the patient has herpes simplex infection, appropriate culture ought to be taken and sent to the lab, and treatment with Zovirax IV or PO is to be started, depending on the severity of the herpes infection and which organ system is affected. If the patient has community-acquired pneumonia, treatment with IV antibiotics must be given. If the patient is severely anemic, transfusion of red blood cells must be given.

Epogen or Procrit is very effective in treating anemia in AIDS patients if the serum erythropoietin level is low. If the patient has fungal infections of either the GI tract or the brain, antifungal treatment must be given using either Ketoconazole or Amphotericin B IV.

The most recently recommended HAART medications to treat HIV/AIDS are
Efavirenz + tenofovir + emtricitabine
Ritonavir-booster atazanavir + tenofovir + emtricitabine
Ritinovir-boosted darunavir + tenofovir + emtricitabine
Raltegravir + tenofovir +emtricitabine

The most recently recommended combinations of antiretroviral medications for patients with known HIV infection are as follows:

1. Indinavir + Stavudine + Lamivudine
2. Efavirenz + Stavudine + Didanosine
3. Nelfinavir + Zidovudine + Didanosine
4. Ritonavir + Indinavir + Zidovudine
5. Ritonavir + Saquinavir + Zidovudine
6. Ritonavir +Lopinavir + Zidovudine
7. Viracept (Nelfinavir Mesylate)

Different Suggested Dosages of Anti-Viral Medications
Nucleoside Reverse Transcriptase Inhibitors

Zidovudine (AZT) — 200 mg 3 times a day
Combivir (300 Mg. ZDV and 150 mg. Epivir) — 1 tablet twice a day
Didanosine (ddI) — 250 mg. twice a day
Zalcitabine (ddC) — 0.75 mg. three times a day
Epivir — 150 mg. twice a day
Abacavir (ABC) — 300 mg. twice a day (or Trizivir — ZDV 300 mg, Epivir 150 mg., Abacavir 300 Mg.)
Stavudine (Zerit) — 40 mg. twice a day
Non-nucleoside Reverse Transcriptase Inhibitors
Nevirapine (Viramune) — 200 mg. by mouth daily for 14 days, then 200 mg. by mouth twice a day, thereafter
Delavirdine (Rescriptor) — 400 mg. 3 times a day

Efavirenz (Sustiva) — 600 mg. by mouth at bed time
Protease Inhibitors
Indinavir (Crixivan) — 800 mg. every 8 hours
Ritonavir (Norvir) — 600 mg. every 12 hours
Nelfinavir (Viracept) — 750 mg. 3 times per day or 1250 Mg. twice a day
Saquinavir (Invirase) — 400 mg. twice a day
Fortovase — 1200 mg. 3 times a day
Amprenavir (Agenerase) — 1400 mg. twice a day
Lopinavir + Ritonavir (Kaletra) Lopinavir 400mg/day and. Ritonavir 100mg twice a day
Atazanavir 400mg/day with AZT 100mg and Epivir 150mg twice per day.
Efavirenz 600mg/day with AZT 100mg and Epivir 150mg twice per day.

Atripla, which is a combination of efavirenz, emtricitabine and tenofovir, is the world top selling AIDS medication. The FDA has just approved Tivicay to be used in combination with other AIDS medications.

New NRTI in use include:

Emtriva
Entecavir
Epzicom
Retrovir
Truvada
Zerit
Ziagen
Viread
Videx
Videx EC

Recently approved AIDS medications by the FDA include:

Prezcobix
Triumeq
Trizivir
Evotaz
Genvoya
Stribild
Odefsey
Descovey
PrEP Truvada (emtricitabine and Tenovir disoproxil fumarate) is in use
as prophylaxis to prevent HIV infection in individuals who are at high
risk of being infected.

The newest NNRTIs include:

Rescriptor
Edurant

Sustiva
Intelence
Viramune
Viramune XR

Newest Protease Inhibitors include:

Kaletra
Lexiva
Viracept
Aptivus
Prezcobix
Evotaz
Olysio
Victrelis
Viekira
Integrase Inhibitos
Trivicay
Vitekta
Isentress

Different antiretroviral medications have different side effects and must be used under different types of clinical circumstances using physician's advice. There are many more combinations of treatment of antiretroviral medications available, but the ones just listed are the most commonly used. Valiere Alcena, M.D., MACP.

As outlined by the CDC, HIV-infected pregnant women give birth to about 60% of infants who are born infected with HIV virus. However, when these pregnant women are treated during pregnancy with AZT, most of these women give birth to HIV-negative infants. AZT is the only one of the reverse transcriptase inhibitors that is safe to use during pregnancy. The protocol for treating women who are pregnant and infected with the AIDS virus is as follows:

Start treatment with Zidovudine at 14–34 weeks of pregnancy and the treatment must be continued throughout the pregnancy. The Zidovudine can be given 100 mg.5 times per day or 200 mg. 3 times per day or 300 mg. 2 times per day. During labor the Zidovudine must be given at 2 mg. per kg intravenously over 1 hour followed by a continuing infusion of 1 Ml per kg until the baby is delivered. After delivery, Zidovudine, also known as AZT, is given to the newborn in syrup form at 2 Ml per kg every six hours for the first 6 weeks of life. The medication must be started 8–12 hours after birth.

Health professionals who get stuck with needles contaminated with blood from AIDS patients are treated with triple therapy of AZT, 3TC and Indinovir. Once the injury occurs, the wound must be cleansed and antiseptic applied immediately. These individuals usually get their blood taken for baseline HIV and hepatitis B, C and VDRL. In 4–6 weeks they must get tested again using the ELISA/Western Blot blood tests or, better still, using the

HIV RNA PCR test. The incident must be reported to the appropriate authorities where the person works and then the person must be seen by the employee health physician to be examined and treated.

Two blood tests are used to evaluate the status of HIV patients. They are the CD4 and the HIV viral load. Ideally, one looks for CD4 of 500 or greater and a viral load of less than 500 copies. A sign of HIV disease progression is a CD4 count of less than 200 and a plasma HIV RNA level of greater than 20,000 copies. HIV-infected patients with a viral load of 100,000 copies have a tenfold greater risk of progressing into full-blown AIDS than patients with 10,000 copies of viral load per ml. Although a CD4 count of less than 200 is usually seen in patients with full-blown AIDS, the viral load test is much more sensitive in evaluating the status of HIV infections.

If the viral load is 20,000, even if the CD4 is in the normal range, it is recommended that HAART treatment be started. The addition of a protease inhibitor to the regimen of AZT or any of the other reverse transcriptase inhibitors and 3TC frequently can lead to an undetectable level of HIV in the blood of the infected person. This does not mean that HIV infection has gone. It just means that the level is low, but the infected individual still has the infection and can still transmit it to an uninfected person, thereby giving him or her AIDS.

The turnover of the HIV virus in an infected person is tremendous. On any one day about 10 billion viral particles can be produced and cleared from the HIV-infected person. About 2 billion CD4 lymphocytes are produced and destroyed from the HIV-infected person daily.

Cancer is one of the multitudes of complications that can afflict the HIV-infected person. Among the cancers that AIDS-infected people would have to contend with is Kaposi's sarcoma is said to be caused by herpes virus #8.

Another common form of cancer seen in AIDS patients is large cell lymphoma.

Blacks and other minorities are at higher risk to become infected with HIV than other racial groups in the United States and around the world because more blacks and other are using IV drugs, thereby exposing themselves to a higher risk of contracting the HIV infection through sharing dirty needles.

Further, since most blacks and other minority women have sexual intercourse with black men and other minority men, and since black men and other minority men have the highest incidence of HIV infection, many blacks and other minority women get infected with HIV by having sexual intercourse with their HIV-infected black and other minority men sexual partners.

The take-home lesson for all people is not to involve themselves in high-risk behaviors, such as, using IV drugs, having sexual intercourse with multiple sexual partners without the protection of a condom, and having sex with men or women whom they have just met, without a condom, etc. These changes in behavior will decrease the incidence of HIV infection in all individuals.

"AIDS in third world Countries:

The notion that the AIDS virus had its genesis from Africa is a controversial topic. In my opinion, the data are not at all convincing as to where the virus originated.

It is my opinion that because the majority of men from Central Africa and Haiti are not circumcised, they constantly develop balanitis as a result of the heat and other problems, leading to breakage of the skin. This leads to chronic infections such as phimosis and paraphimosis. In this setting, there is frequent mini-ulceration of the foreskin of the penis. This represents an easy portal of entry for the virus during coitus with, let us say, an infected prostitute. Another possibility arises because the women in that part of the world do not shave the pubis. Thus there is the possibility of mini-lacerations occurring during coitus as the foreskin comes into contact with pubic hair. This is another possible portal of entry for the virus. This, to me, seems a more plausible explanation for female-to-male transmission in Central Africa and Haiti.

By
Valiere Alcena M.D.F.A.C.P.
N.Y. State J Med 1986: 86. 446"

Male circumcision and HIV/AIDS

Dear Editor:

I have been reading with interest the recent spate of articles on findings that link circumcision of men in certain African countries with the incidence of the HIV/AIDS virus. One reporter in *The New York Times Magazine* has even described male circumcision as possibly the best method of eliminating the AIDS virus – superior even to an AIDS vaccine, which may still be several years in development.

You may be interested in knowing that in August 1986, in a letter to the editor of *The New York State Journal of Medicine*, Vol. 86, page 446, I first discussed the significance of male circumcision in lowering the incidence of the HIV/AIDS virus in Africa, Haiti and other developing countries. In my published letter, I wrote in part:

"It is my opinion that because the majority of men from Central Africa and Haiti are not circumcised, they constantly develop balanitis as a result of the heat and other problems, leading to breakage of the skin. This leads to chronic infections such as phimosis and paraphimosis. In this setting, there is frequent mini-ulceration of the foreskin of the penis. This represents an easy portal of entry for the virus during coitus with, let us say, an infected prostitute. Another possibility arises because the women in that part of the world do not shave the pubis. Thus, there is the possibility of mini-lacerations occurring during coitus as the foreskin comes in contact with the pubic hair. This is another possible portal of entry of the virus. This, to me, seems a more plausible explanation for female-to-male transmission in Central Africa and Haiti."

Later, I repeated my theory in my two books that were published in 1992, "The Status of Health of Blacks in the United States of America: A Perspective for Improvement" and "The African American Health Book." I again described the significance of male circumcision in possibly eliminating the HIV/AIDS virus altogether in a subsequent book that was published in 1994 entitled "AIDS: The Expanding Epidemic: What the Public Needs to Know: A Multi-Cultural Overview."

I would be happy to discuss with the researchers for these most recent articles this most exciting subject in the future if needed.

Valiere Alcena, MD, FACP

WHITE PLAINS, NY

I am grateful to Dr. Alcena for his letter. He purports therein to be the first to suggest that male circumcision might somehow play a role in reducing the risk of heterosexual transmission of HIV, then known as HTLV-III. A brief search on PubMed suggests that he may indeed be correct; other authors made such suggestions several years later, in 1988 and thereafter. Thus, the spate of publications in recent years offering proof of that hypothesis represents solid support of his earlier thinking.

Source:

Infectious Disease News
Vol; 20, number 3
March, 2007

That Male circumcision might reduce risk of HIV acquisition was first proposed in 1986. 3
Reference 3
Alcena,V AIDS in third world countries. NJ State J of Med 1986; 86: 446

Male circumcision for HIV prevention in young men
In Kisumu, Kenya: a randomized controlled trial
The Lancet 2007, 369:643-656
24 February 2007

WHO, UNAIDS recommend male circumcision world-wide to decrease the incidence HIV/AIDS transmition by 60% and save 3 million lives. WHO, UNAIDS estimate that worldwide only 30% men are circumcised

According to the WHO, 70% of men in the world are not circumcised. The vast majority of black men in the developing world and largely in the developed world are not circumcised. Male circumcision to reduce the spread of HIV/AIDs first suggested By Dr Valiere Alcena on August of 1986 has made the biggest difference so far in controlling the AIDS epidemic and preventing deaths from AIDS.

When an uncircumcised man has sexual intercourse with HIV an infected individual, be it a female or a male sexual partner, the foreskin of the penis is frequently the entry point for the HIV virus to enter the blood stream.

Circumcision of male babies and men in the world and in particular in the developing world will continue to decrease the incidence of HIV/AIDS and deaths from this terribly deadly disease.

As mentioned above, the CDC after 13 years of evaluation, on December 4th, 2014 recommends male circumcision in the U.S. to prevent HIV and other STDs infections. Finally, the U.S. through the action of the CDC has joined the WHO and the rest of the world by recommending male circumcision to prevent HIV/AIDS infection and other STDs infections. Other than the ART medications, male circumcision, an idea I proposed in an article I published in August of 1986 has done and is doing the most to prevent the transmission of HIV/AIDS in the world, making it the most important thing that has so far occurred in the HIV/AIDS epidemic since it began officially in 1981. Before male circumcision began, the number of people living with HIV/AIDS in the was close to 40 million and today mostly because of male circumcision the total number of people living with HIV/AIDS is down to 35 million. The ART medications are making a difference as well, but it costs on an average $12,000-15,000 per year making very difficult for most people to get them.

ART can turn AIDS into a chronic disease by preventing its progression in people who have access to it.

By right, full credit belongs to me for proposing the idea of male circumcision to prevent the transmition of the HIV virus during sexual intercourse with an infectedw woman in 1986.

According to a study carried out by the Institute for Global Health and Infectious Diseases which began in April of 2005, funded by the National Institute of Allergy and Infectious Diseases, and reported in May 12, 2011. 1, 763 people (890 men, 873 women) were entered in the study. HIV infected sexual partners from Botswana, Brazil, India, Kenya, Malawi, South Africa, Thailand, the United States, and Zimbabwe participated in the study. The CD4+ T-cell levels were between 350 and 550 cells per cubic millimeter (mm2)

Eleven HIV drugs were used in various combinations to treat these people involved in the study including:

"atazanir 300 mg once daily
didanosine 400 mg once daily
efavirenz 600 mg once daily
Emtricitabine/tenofir disoproxil furmarate 200 mg emtricitabine/300 mg tenofovir mg twice daily (BID)
nevirapine 200 mg taken once daily for 14 days followed by 200 mg taken twice daily
ritonavir 100 mg once daily, used only to boost atazanavir
stavudine (weight dependent dosage)
senofovir disoproxil fumarate 300mg once daily
zodovudine/lamivudine (150 mg lamivudine/300 mg zidovudine taken orally twice daily)"

The risk of sexually transmitted HIV was reduced by 96% in the people in the study because of the anti-retrovirus drugs."

The AIDS epidemic which was officially first reported in The U.S in June of 1981 is 34 years old this year and yet no cure has been found. 60 million people have been infected with HIV since the epidemic was first recognized. 25 million people have died of AIDS world wide including 650,000 people in the U.S. 33 million people are in the world are living with HIV/AIDS. While some progress has been made by using anti-retrovirus (ART) drugs, this epidemic is still unfolding in the U.S. and worldwide. Source: Annals of Internal Medicine 7 June, Volume 154 Number 11

ART are very expensive and must be taken for life. On top of the list of preventive measures to take to protect one self from getting infected with HIV 1&2 is male circumcision. It might as well be called the "AIDS vaccine" or better still the "Dr Valiere Alcena AIDS vaccine" Male circumcision is Dr Valiere Alcena's AIDS vaccine. According to the New York Times.

Dr Valiere Alcena first proposed using male circumcision to prevent HIV/AIDS
In August of 1986 as described in this chapter above. Male circumcision has decreased the total HIV/AIDS infection in the world from 42 millions before male circumcision to 37 at the end of 2014 million and has brought the yearly death rates from AIDS down by more than 1 million per year. No other idea, concept, scientific research has made such a big difference in the prevention of HIV transmission and deaths from AIDS in the world than male circumcision. No physician or physicians in the world other than Valiere Alcena, M.D., M.A.C.P. has made such a major contribution in the prevention and deaths from HIV/AIDS.

CHAPTER 22

GASTROINTESTINAL DISEASES IN AFRICAN AMERICAN MEN

DISEASES OF THE GASTROINTESTINAL TRACT are among the most common diseases that people suffer from.

More than 1 billion people in the world have no access to health care. 36 million people die every year in the world because of non-communicable diseases such as:

CVD
Cancer
Diabetes
Chronic lung diseases etc;
All together, 56 million people die every year in the world because of diseases of on kind or another including gastrointestinal diseases. WHO

The most frequent GI symptoms that people go to see the doctor for consist of:

1. Heartburn
2. Bitter taste in the mouth
3. Indigestion
4. Bloating
5. Gaseousness
6. Increased flatus
7. Nausea
8. Vomiting
9. Loss of appetite
10. Easy filling of the stomach when eating (dysphasia)
11. Pain on swallowing food
12. Pain in the stomach area
13. Pain in the abdomen
14. Recurrent diarrhea
15. Rectal bleeding
16. Pain on defecation
17. Hemorrhoids
18. Burning pain in the chest
19. Hematemesis (vomiting blood) etc.

The reasons for these symptoms include:

1. Hiatal hernia
2. Reflux esophagitis
3. Slow motility of the esophagus
4. Esophagitis due to fungal infection of the esophagus
5. Cancer of the esophagus, etc.
6. Gastroesophageal reflux disease (GERD)
7. Duodonal ulcer
8. Cancer of the stomach
9. Crohn's disease
10. Gastric ulcer
11. Mallory Weiss tears
12. Esophageal varices
13. Ulcerative colitis

"There are two different types of hiatal hernia: the sliding type and the para-esophageal type" Both types cause significant symptoms such as heartburn, regurgitation, and bitter taste in the mouth, and chest pain. In hiatal hernia, acid backs up toward the throat, causing the symptoms just outlined. As the acid bathes the part of the esophagus that dips into the stomach, the symptoms develop. Bleeding due to hiatal hernia occurs frequently because of erosion that the acid causes in the wall of the part of the esophagus affected by the acid.

More bleeding occurs in para esophageal hernia than in sliding hernia. The reason why more bleeding occurs in para esophageal hernia than in the sliding type is because in the para esophageal type of hiatal hernia, the part of the esophagus that is involved is stuck in one place. In the sliding type of hiatal hernia the affected part slides up and down into the area containing the acid, exposing the esophageal tissues much less to acid and thus reducing the incidence of bleeding.

Chronic coughing and throat irritation are frequent symptoms of GERD. Another important and serious condition that affects the esophagus is *achalasia*. People who have AIDS frequently suffer with *esophagitis* due to fungal infection, viral infection such as cytomegalovirus, or herpes viral infection resulting in severe pain on swallowing.

The incidence of smoking and alcohol abuse is quite high among blacks and, as a result, their incidence of cancer of the esophagus is higher than among black men who do not drink alcohol and do not smoke tobacco.

One of the most common complaints that the physician sees in his or her office is stomach pain. The reasons for the stomach complaints are many and wide-ranging in characteristics. A frequent contributor to stomach problems is the ingestion of contaminated foods resulting in indigestion and/or acute gastroenteritis with nausea and vomiting.

Another common reason for acute gastroenteritis is viral infection affecting the stomach, resulting in stomach pain, stomach cramps, nausea, vomiting, and fever. Because most blacks are poorer than their white counterparts are, they eat foods that are of a lower quality and frequently these foods become contaminated resulting in infectious gastroenteritis from bacteria such as Staphylococci bacteria, E. Coli, Salmonella, Shigella, Campylobacter, etc.

Another common and frequent complaint of the stomach problems in blacks is stomach pain due to ulcers. The reason why stomach ulcers are so much more common in blacks as compared to whites is that blacks face racial discrimination every day. As a person faces racial bigotry, the person first becomes intensely angry, followed with intense fear. Both anger and fear cause the stomach to produce an excessive amount of acid and the increased level of acid in the stomach causes a burning pain, indigestion, and, eventually, ulcer of the stomach. In order to cope with the daily pressure and stress of racial discrimination, blacks frequently resort to alcohol abuse and cigarette and other tobacco smoking, both of which, via different mechanisms, can cause severe stomach problems including peptic ulcers.

Smoking cigarettes places a large amount of nicotine in the bloodstream, causing marked acid secretion, which increases symptoms of peptic dysfunction and increases the incidence of peptic ulcer disease. Therefore, people who smoke have more ulcers of the stomach.

Peptic dysfunction is one of the common symptoms of alcohol abuse. Some of these symptoms include nausea, vomiting, retching, stomach pain, gastritis, hematemesis (vomiting of blood), and Mallory-Weiss, as a result of forceful and persistent vomiting due to the adverse effects of alcohol on the stomach and the junction into the stomach. (Mallory-Weiss tear is a tear that occurs at the junction where the esophagus enters into the stomach- Gastro-Esophageal Junction, this tear can occur as a result of forceful and prolonged vomiting/wretching from any cause, but it is seen most frequently in alcoholics.)

A Mallory-Weiss tear causes severe upper gastrointestinal bleeding, occurring because of forceful vomiting and retching, resulting in a tear at the junction where the esophagus meets the stomach. Mallory-Weiss tears occur most frequently in alcoholics.

One of the most serious upper gastrointestinal complications of chronic alcohol abuse is esophageal varices. Varices are small superficial blood vessels that develop on the surface of the esophagus because of portal hypertension, which is the result of occlusion of the small vessels within the liver. The occlusions of these vessels cause the spleen to become enlarged, which in turn causes the development of portal hypertension. Because the esophageal varices are superficial, they bleed easily, frequently and profusely. It is almost impossible to stop the bleeding from esophageal varices.

All the different treatments that have been tried have very little effectiveness. Bleeding from gastritis is an extremely common occurrence. Alcohol is quite irritating to the lining of the stomach, and because of this irritation, bleeding occurs. This bleeding can be quite profuse at times.

Attached to the lower part of the stomach and to the beginning of the large bowel is the organ called the small intestine.

The most common abnormalities that affect the small intestine are:

1. Malabsorption.
2. Inflammatory bowel disease (Crohn's disease).
3. Cancer of the small bowel.
4. Aterial-venous (AV) malformation
5. Lymphoma of the small intestine
6. Cancer of the small intestine
7. Bacterial infection of the small intestine
8. Viral infection of the small intestine
9. AIDS of the small intestine
10. Tuberculosis of the small intestine
11. Scleroderma of the small intestine
12. Parasitic infestation of the small intestine
13. Chronic pancreatitis etc.
14. Many other conditions affect the small intestine.

Malabsorption can occur because of

Tropical sprue
Non-tropical sprue
Gluten enteropathy
Scleroderma
Chronic pancreatitis
AIDS etc.

Patients suffering from these conditions, frequently develop severe diarrhea with massive loss of fluid, minerals, electrolytes, and vitamins. Malabsorption results in general weakness, overall worsening the patient's condition.

Sprue – tropical type, the cause of which is not known, but is probably due to some form of microorganism, which releases a toxin into the small bowel, resulting in malabsorption of iron, folic acid, vitamin B12 and a multitude of minerals and electrolytes. Weight loss, anorexia, diarrhea, and anemia are some consequences of tropical sprue.

Nontropical sprue is another abnormality of the small bowel. This form of sprue is due to intolerance to gluten, which is a protein found in wheat and its products.

It is believed that this form of sprue is inherited via a dominant gene of incomplete penetrance. The result of this type of sprue is diarrhea, malabsorption, weight loss, and anorexia.

One of the common symptoms of small bowel disease is pain around the umbilicus. Another frequent symptom of small bowel disease is diarrhea. Still another common symptom of small bowel disease is rectal bleeding.

The rectal bleeding can be due to angiodysplasia or AVM, ischemic colitis, Crohn's disease, Meckel's diverticulum, polyps and cancer, etc. The lower part of the small bowel is attached to the large bowel and the large bowel is afflicted with the most devastating disease of the gastrointestinal tract, namely cancer.

In the year 2009, 16,890 blacks were diagnosed with colon rectal cancer in the United States and 7,120 blacks died of colon rectal cancer. Another common cause of colon-rectal bleeding is polyps of the colon. Polyps of the colon can bleed, but can also give rise to cancer of the colon. Still another frequent cause of colon and rectal bleeding is diverticulosis of the colon.

Diverticular disease of the colon is more common in the blacks who live in developed countries as compared to the blacks who live in the third world. Blacks who live in the third world have more meager diets that contain more roughage, more fibers, and less fat, which allow for more regular and more bulky bowel movements. The lack of roughage, and the lack of fibers and too much fat lead to constipation, which is associated with increase in the incidence of diverticular disease of the colon and colon cancer.

Diverticular bleeding is most often painless. Painful diverticular bleeding may be associated with diverticulitis. Diverticulitis is a condition that results from an infected diverticulum. Diverticulum is an outpouching from the inside wall of the bowel. Every now and then erosion occurs in these diverticuli due to actions of the stool on them. The result is acute diverticulitis, which causes abdominal pain, fever, chills, and malaise. Diverticulitis is a very serious condition, which can cause abscesses and sometimes perforation of the large bowel, resulting in peritonitis and death of the affected person if left untreated.

Another frequent cause of bleeding from the lower GI tract is AVM. Bleeding associated with AVM (arteriovenous malformation) is not only common, but at times, very difficult to diagnose and even more difficult to treat. Ulcerative colitis and Crohn's disease are common in blacks and the most common problems associated with these conditions are anemia and rectal bleeding.

Ischemic colitis is seen in elderly individuals who suffer from diabetes mellitus and arteriosclerotic disease and is associated with rectal bleeding and abdominal pain, fever chills, and elevated white blood cell count. Bloody diarrhea is seen frequently in AIDS patients because of enterocolitis due to fungi, viruses, bacteria, protozoa and parasites.

Enterocolitis is a serious problem in anyone who is afflicted by it, but it is particularly devastating in AIDS patients because of their already weakened condition.

Constipation is a common problem and one of the reasons women frequently seeks medical advice. Constipation can be due to many different things. Poor dietary habits can lead to constipation.

A diet deficient in roughage, fiber, and bulk can cause constipation. An underlying condition such as hypothyroidism can cause constipation. Taking medications such as calcium channel blockers to treat hypertension or to treat angina pectoris can cause constipation because the calcium channel blocker relaxes the smooth muscle of the colon, preventing contraction of smooth muscles, which is necessary for the colon to excrete its contents, namely the stool.

Taking too many laxatives is a frequent cause of constipation. When an individual uses laxatives too frequently, the colon becomes lazy, and loses its ability to contract properly and will not work without help to excrete stool. This condition is called cathartic colon. The treatment for this is to retrain the person as to the proper bowel habits to help him or her to refrain from using cathartics to bring about a bowel movement.

Constipation must always be brought to the attention of the physician because frequently constipation can be the first sign noticed in cancer of the large bowel.

The same can be said of diarrhea as it is related to cancer of the colon. Any significant changes of bowel habits ought to be brought to the attention of a physician because major pathologies can be the reason of the change in bowel habits.

Another frequent ailment is hemorrhoids. Hemorrhoids are found on the very end of the lower GI tract, namely the anus. Hemorrhoids have many causes, but the most frequent ones consist of:

1. Straining at stool due to impatience
2. Constipation causing a person to strain at stool
3. Obesity resulting in too much pressure being placed on the anal area
4. Too much weight gain during pregnancy resulting in too much pressure on the anal area
5. Occupational hazards such as driving long distances over long periods of time
6. Standing for long periods of time over many years
7. Obstructive colonic polyps or cancer of the colon resulting in straining at stool.

If a person suddenly protrudes a hemorrhoid while at the same time passing pencil-thin stool, that usually means there is something obstructing the normal passage of the stool resulting in acute protrusion of a hemorrhoid and that person needs immediate medical attention to evaluate the large bowel by colonoscopic examination to seek out the problem. One of the frequent symptoms associated with the anal area is bleeding. Bleeding from the rectum is always serious and must always be evaluated medically.

It is necessary to bring it to the attention of a physician anytime blood is seen coming from the rectum. Self-diagnosis of rectal bleeding, assumed to be due to hemorrhoids, leads frequently to the missing of early diagnosis of colon and rectal cancer.

Some black men have a tendency to be bashful to seek medical help when they see blood in their stools. This is a most dangerous habit, which can cause a person to delay the diagnosing of serious problems such as colon or rectal cancer.

In addition to hemorrhoids, there are other conditions that can cause bleeding in the part of the perirectal area; among these conditions are anal fissures and inflammation-associated colitis, both of which can cause rectal bleeding.

How to evaluate gastrointestinal complaints

The first thing a physician must do is to take a careful history. The next step is to carry out a careful physical examination. Having done these two things, the doctor should next try medications along with diet modifications. Depending on the severity of the symptoms and /or the physical findings, intervention by way of blood tests, x-ray tests, or endoscopy/ colonoscopy/sigmoidoscopy/examinations might be carried out in an attempt to establish a diagnosis. If the patient's complaint is inability to swallow liquid or solid foods, then a CBC, SMA 20 chemistry profile, and serum ferritin are the necessary and appropriate blood tests to do.

Doing an upper GI series, with an esaphogram, or doing an endoscopy of the upper GI tract is the appropriate and necessary x-ray or endoscopic examination. These examinations are capable of discovering all abnormalities that cause symptoms and diseases of the upper and lower GI tracts.

If a patient's complaint is pain in the stomach, heartburn, hyperacidity, vomiting blood or bleeding from the stomach, then doing a CBC, serum ferritin, upper GI series, endoscopic examination, and abdominal sonogram are sufficient to discover most of the problems associated with the upper GI tract, the gall bladder and the pancreas.

Frequently, an abdominal CT scan is needed to help evaluate the pancreas to be certain pancreatic cancer is not causing the patient's abdominal pain. Abdominal sonogram is the choice test to diagnose stones in the gall bladder, while the abdominal CT is good to evaluate cancer of the gall bladder and the liver.

To evaluate the small intestine, one needs to do an upper GI series with a small bowel follow-through. It is not routine to do endoscopic examination of the small bowel. To evaluate the large intestine, one can do a barium enema, which is putting barium in the intestine through the rectum into a rubber tube, and once the barium is in the large bowel then x-ray pictures are taken in different positions.

They are gastroenterologists who are trained to scope the small intestine. In addition, a special capsule study can be done to evaluate the small intestine.

An instrument called a sigmoidoscope can be used to look inside the lower bowel. There are two different types of sigmoidoscopes, a rigid one, and a flexible one. The rigid scope can be passed up to 30 cm, and the flexible scope can be passed up to 60 cm. Different complaints and different circumstances dictate which procedure is done.

There is an instrument called a colonoscope, which is a long, flexible, and hollow instrument that allows the gastroenterologist to examine the entire large bowel, looking for abnormalities. Biopsies can be taken during these procedures and lesions such as polyps can be removed entirely, and cancerous mass can be biopsied.

According to the recent literature, flexible sigmoidoscopic examination missed up to 34% of cancer of the colon. Therefore, since the bowel preparation is the same for both colonoscopy and flexible sigmoidoscopy, it is preferable to do a colonoscopy instead of flexible sigmoidoscopy. When necessary, an anoscope can be used to look inside the rectum to evaluate local problems in that part of the bowel.

How can people prevent the development of some of these gastrointestinal ailments?

Starting with the esophagus, people will decrease their incidence of esophageal cancer by stopping cigarette smoking and alcohol abuse. Both of these bad habits cause a predisposition to the development of cancer of the esophagus. Esophageal varices are associated, most frequently, with alcohol abuse and alcoholic liver disease.

If people would abstain from alcohol abuse, their incidence of alcohol-associated esophageal problems would likely disappear.

Hiatal hernia is a frequent problem and it can be quite troublesome, at times resulting in heartburn and sometimes in iron deficiency anemia because of slow, but chronic bleeding from the hiatal hernia. People can help themselves by losing weight and in so doing they can either prevent and/ or decrease the incidence of hiatal hernia. About 51% of blacks in the United States are obese/overweight, and 80% of black women are obese/overweight. Obesity plays a significant role in the development of hiatal hernia and the worsening of its symptoms.

Symptoms associated with diseases of the stomach are more common in black and other minorities as compared to whites and the reasons are many.

To start with, the foods that most black and other minorities like to eat have too much fat, salt, and spices in them. When the combination of a diet of fatty, salty, and spicy foods, cigarette smoking, and alcohol abuse are considered and added to the day-to-day stress that poor minority people have to deal with, it is easy to see why the incidence of stomach ailments of all sorts is so much higher in them than in whites

According to the recent literature, a microorganism lives in the stomach of many individuals who have chronic peptic ulcer disease of the stomach.

This organism is called Helicobacter pylori. H. pylori is said to play a major role in the causation of peptic ulcer. It is also said that if left untreated this organism can ultimately cause cancer (lymphoma) of the stomach to occur.

To diagnose this infection, gastric material is taken from the stomach and tested for the presence of the organism.

A blood test is also available for the presence of H. pylori antibody. The CLO test can also be done by getting a sample of gastric juice and adding a chemical solution to it. If the solution turns yellow to orange color, the test is positive. There is also a breath test available to test for the presence of H pylori as well. A stool test is also available to diagnose H pylori.

Obesity is very highly connected with gallstones formation and gall bladder diseases. Further, many Blacks and other minorities suffer with hemolytic diseases such as sickle cell anemia and sickle thalassemia and thalassemias that predispose them to gall bladder stone disease. Minorities who suffer from these hemolytic anemias produce a substance called indirect bilirubin, which is a pigment that comes from the breakdown products of the hemolyzed red cells. The bilirubin pigment forms bilirubin stones in the gall bladder.

However, most of the gallstones seen in obese people are cholesterol stones. Symptoms of gall bladder stones, which include nausea, vomiting, right-sided abdominal pain which can at times be referred to the left side of the upper abdomen, can easily be confused with diseases of the stomach such as peptic ulcer or hiatal hernia with reflux. Symptoms of gall bladder disease can also be confused with diseases of the pancreas. Both acute and chronic pancreatitis can have symptoms that are similar to gall bladder disease. Frequently, a person would present to the doctor with jaundice and no pain.

Then the question becomes is it due to gallstones occluding the common bile duct, resulting in backing up of bile into the bloodstream, or is it due to a tumor (usually cancer at the head of the pancreas pressing on the common bile duct), causing the jaundice to occur. This condition is called painless jaundice.

Many other serious conditions that can affect the gall bladder, such as ascending cholangeitis, cancer of the gall bladder, gangrene of the gall bladder, etc. Another common cause of abdominal pain is disease of the pancreas. In women, the most common disease of the pancreas is acute pancreatitis. Gallstones are the second most common cause of pancreatitis. Gall bladder and gallstones diseases are quite high in incidence in American Indians and Eskimos.

Gallstones cause pancreatitis by blocking some of the tubes that carry enzymes out of the pancreas, resulting in back flow of enzymes into the pancreas, and causing inflammation of the pancreas. This pancreatitic inflammation starts the process of acute pancreatitis.

The most common reason why people suffer from pancreatitis is alcoholism, although the incidence of alcohol abuse is high in whites than it is in blacks and other minorities. Alcohol is very toxic to the pancreas, resulting in acute inflammation causing acute pancreatitis.

Acute pancreatitis causes abdominal pain, nausea, vomiting, fever, dehydration, electrolyte imbalance and high serum or urine amylase.

When pancreatitis occurs along with other tissue damage, resulting in chronic pancreatitis, pseudocyst of the pancreas and pancreatic abscess can also occur. The symptoms of chronic pancreatitis include the symptoms outlined in acute pancreatitis, plus severe diarrhea, malabsorption, weight loss, and diabetes mellitus, etc.

The reason why malabsorption and diarrhea occur in chronic pancreatitis is that the pancreas, having been destroyed by the effect of alcohol, is not able to produce the different enzymes that are necessary for proper digestion of foods. In particular, fatty foods cannot be digested, resulting in oily diarrhea. The reason that diabetes mellitus occurs in chronic pancreatitis is that the cells that produce insulin are located in the pancreas, and once the pancreas is destroyed then insulin cannot be made. The result is high blood sugar in the blood and all of its consequences.

Many more conditions affect the small bowel and large bowel that can cause pain, and among them are ulcerative colitis and Crohn's disease. Some of the first signs are rectal bleeding, cramps, diarrhea, pain, iron deficiency anemia, etc. No one knows what causes Crohn's disease and ulcerative colitis. To diagnose inflammatory bowel diseases, both barium studies and colonoscopic examinations are used.

To diagnose inflammatory bowel of the small bowel, barium study is needed. Diagnosis of inflammatory bowel disease of the large intestine can be made by both barium studies and colonoscopic examinations. In inflammatory bowel disease, the inner surface of the bowel is swollen and inflamed and bleeds easily.

The cause or causes of these changes are not known in spite of many years of research. In addition to abdominal pain, diarrhea, and rectal bleeding, there is an increased incidence of colorectal cancer in people suffering with inflammatory bowel disease.

How to evaluate diseases of the gastrointestinal tract

The beginning of the GI tract is the mouth, and the best way to evaluate the mouth is by the naked eye. To evaluate the throat, sometimes an instrument like the laryngoscope may be used.

To evaluate the esophagus, either barium swallows followed by x-ray or endoscopy can be used.

To evaluate the stomach, the best two ways are upper GI series with barium swallow or endoscopic examination, during which the different parts of the stomach can be directly visualized and, when necessary, biopsies can be done. It is important to understand that if a gastric ulcer is detected during the upper GI series, then endoscopic examination must be carried out so that it can be biopsied to rule out cancer.

Gastric ulcers have a high propensity to be cancerous and must always be biopsied when discovered. There are multitudes of other abnormalities that can be found in the upper GI tract during the endoscopic examination.

The best way available to evaluate the small bowel is using barium swallow with small bowel follow-through. Some of the diseases found in the small bowel are Crohn's disease, cancer, malabsorption, Meckel's diverticulum, arteriovenous malformation, polyps, cancer etc.

To evaluate the large bowel (colon or intestine), barium enema, colonoscopy, rigid or flexible sigmoidoscopic examination is used. Using these examinations, the physician can evaluate the entire large bowel from the anus up to the area where the large bowel is joined with the small bowel. Conditions such as cancer, polyps, diverticulosis, ulcerative colitis, ischemic colitis, arteriovenous malformations, hemorrhoids, anal fissures, etc., can be discovered and, when necessary, biopsies can be taken to determine the true nature of some of these diseases, to allow for appropriate treatments," whether surgical or medical treatments".

How to best treat the different diseases of the gastrointestinal tract

One of the common complaints that bring patients to the physician's office is heartburn. Heartburn is due to hiatal hernia with reflux esophagitis. Women suffer a lot from this condition because of the fact that a large percentage of women are obese and obesity has a close association with hiatal hernia and heartburn. The best treatments consist of:

1. Weight loss
2. Low-fat diet
3. Decrease of caffeine intake
4. Decrease of alcohol consumption
5. Sleeping with head of the bed up, or placing 2–3 pillows under one's head when sleeping, to prevent the free flow of acid to reflux up towards the throat
6. Reglan 10 mg, 15 minutes before meals, three times a day and at bedtime.
7. H2 blockers like Zantac, Axid, Pepcid, and Tagamet etc.
8. Protein pump inhibitors (PPI's) like Nexium, Prilosec, Prevacid, Protonic, and AcipHex

Reglan works to propel the foods down the stomach with more ease, preventing too much acid production. When food sits in the stomach too long, too much acid is produced. It backs up toward the upper chest, causing hyperacidity, heartburn, and bad taste in the mouth, bad breathe and, frequently, severe chest pain simulating cardiac chest pain and, at times, a chronic cough. Whenever the stomach detects food it sends a signal to the lining of the stomach where the acid-producing cells are located to secrete more acid to digest the food.

The idea then is to help move the food along so that less acid is produced, thereby decreasing the symptoms of heartburn. H^2 blockers such as Tagamet, Axid, Zantac, and Pepcid are used also in hiatal hernia with reflux with very good success because these medications block the production of excess acid, preventing the formation of ulcerations around the esophagogastric junction, thereby decreasing the symptoms of heartburn. Protein pump inhibitors such as Prilosec, Prevacid, Nexium and Protonic, AcipHex are also very effective in medical management of GERD (gastroesophageal reflux disease).

There is no definite surgical procedure available to repair hiatal hernia in common use, though there have been some recent claims being made that hiatal hernia can be repaired using laser. However, GERD is being treated laparoscopically using a wraparound surgical technique that seems to be enjoying some degree of success.

Antacids such as Mylanta, Maalox, Rolaids, etc. are also helpful in relieving symptoms of heartburn and hyperacidity associated with hiatal hernia with reflux.

The most common disease of the stomach is ulcer. Other diseases of the stomach that are frequently seen are cancer, lymphoma, gastritis associated with aspirin ingestion or alcohol abuse and H. Pylori infection, etc.

The best treatment available to treat stomach ulcers is the H2 blockers, such as Tagamet, Axid, Zantac, Pepcid and more powerful acid blockers, namely protein pump inhibitors like Prilosec, Prevacid, Nexium, Protonix, AcipHex etc. These medications are commonly used for two months to treat ulcers that are proven by upper GI series or endoscopic examination. After two months, a repeat upper GI series or endoscopic examination is done. If the ulcer is healed, then based on symptoms, the physician may choose whether to continue treatment for a few more weeks or not.

If the ulcer is only partially healed, then treatment with H2 blockers can continue for two more months. If the last two months of treatment trial of the ulcer still fails to heal it fully or not at all, then at this point a biopsy via endoscopic examination becomes mandatory to rule out cancer. It is now accepted practice to test for H. pylori at the time of endoscopic examination, using gastric tissue via biopsy to test for the presence or absence of this microorganism. (See above for a discussion regarding other tests available to diagnose H pylori) H. pylori is believed to play a major role in the causation of peptic ulcer disease and malignancy of the stomach, such as lymphoma, as stated above. H. pylori is the most common nosocomial infection in the world.

About 50% of the world population is infected with H. pylori. About 75% of the population of New York City it is said carries the H. pylori organism in their stomach because of migration of people from different parts of the world who live there. Countrywide in the U.S., the incidence of H. pylori is 30%.

Chronic peptic ulcer disease is associated with H. pylori, the latter being tagged as a causative reason for the development of the ulcer. (See chapter on H. pylori below) There are several protocols available to treat H. pylori, but Prevpac is a frequently used one. It is used for either 10 days or 14 days. H. pylori get into the body through the" oral /fecal" route. It is important to understand that diagnosing peptic ulcer using the upper GI series is only 65%–70% accurate, while diagnosing peptic ulcer using endoscopy is about 95%–100% accurate.

Surgical treatment is still used for treating ulcers of the stomach under specific circumstances. When an ulcer of the stomach fails to stop bleeding in spite of all medical treatments and in particular when the patient who is bleeding receives too much blood; a gastrectomy is usually carried out to stop the bleeding and save the patient's life. Another situation that requires gastrectomy is when a biopsy of the stomach reveals the presence of cancer, a gastrectomy is usually undertaken to remove the cancerous part of the stomach. More often than not, other treatments such as chemotherapy and/or radiotherapy are used as additional treatments when cancer of the stomach is surgically removed.

The small intestine is frequently affected by Crohn's disease, and the most frequent treatment for Crohn's disease is steroids with Azulfidine steroid enemas with added folic acid to prevent the folic acid deficiency that the Azulfidine causes. Surgical resection of part of the small intestine is also frequently carried out as part of the treatment for small bowel Crohn's disease. (See chapter on Crohn's disease below) Another common disease of the small bowel is cancer. The cancer seen in the small bowel can vary from solid tumor like adenocarcinoma, lymphoma, carcinoid tumor, and different types of metastatic cancer to the small bowel. Another frequent disease of the small bowel is sprue, both tropical sprue and non-tropical sprue. The treatment of choice for tropical sprue is antibiotics such as Tetracycline and the treatment for non-tropical sprue is a gluten-free diet.

Many other serious medical problems can affect the small intestine such as arteriovenous malformation causing severe bleeding, Meckel's diverticulum with severe bleeding and severe malabsorption due to chronic pancreatitis and a multitude of other causes.

The different treatments for these different diseases of the small intestine are handled individually as each disease situation warrants.

The large bowel is the site for a multitude of diseases, some very serious and some less serious, but nevertheless, they afflict many people.

Some of the most frequent diseases and conditions of the colon include:

1. Diarrhea
2. Constipation
3. Diarrhea alternating with constipation
4. Abdominal cramps
5. Flatulence
6. Abdominal pain
7. Rectal bleeding
8. Ulcerative colitis
9. Crohn's disease of the colon
10. Diverticulosis
11. Diverticulitis
12. Bacterial overgrowth
13. Lactose intolerance
14. Acute infectious gastroenteritis
15. Parasitism
16. Ischemic colitis
17. Intestinal obstruction

18. Colon cancer
19. Rectal cancer
20. Rectal fissures
21. Hemorrhoids
22. Inguinal hernias
23. Familial polyposis
24. HIV/AIDS
25. Lymphoma
26. Blind loop syndrome etc.

Diarrhea occurs fo.r a multitude of reasons in humans, resulting in serious discomfort and inconveniences. Cancer of the colon is frequently presented with diarrhea as an initial complaint. Sometimes the diarrhea occurs because there is a mass obstructing the colon, but watery stool is able to pass around it, expressing itself as diarrhea. Sometimes diarrhea occurs because of other cancers such as carcinoid tumor, mucus-producing adenocarcinoma of the colon, etc. Diarrhea is frequently seen in people who are suffering from ulcerative colitis or Crohn's disease of the colon. (See chapter on ulcerative colitis below)

Diarrhea is seen in both acute and chronic pancreatitis. Diarrhea is frequently seen in individuals suffering from sprue. Diarrhea is seen frequently in people suffering from irritable bowel syndrome. Parasitic infestations such as giardiasis are frequently manifested with diarrhea and there are multitudes of other parasitic infestations which cause diarrhea. Many individuals abuse cathartics and come to the physician with a complaint of chronic diarrhea when in fact the diarrhea is self-afflicted.

Lactose intolerance is quite common in blacks. About 65% of blacks suffer from this condition and develop the disease to one degree or another at some point in their lives. In addition to abdominal cramps, flatulence, nausea, gaseousness, lactose intolerance causes diarrhea. There is an enzyme called lactase, which is produced by certain cells in the lining of the intestine, and the role of this enzyme is to break down lactose into glucose and galactose.

If a person lacks lactase completely or has a diminished quantity of this enzyme, when that person ingests dairy products such as milk, cheeses, butter etc., he or she develops symptoms of lactose intolerance as just outlined. The ingested lactose becomes almost like a cathartic, resulting in bowel discomfort. Lactose intolerance is hereditary, but oftentimes it gets worse as a person gets older.

Avoiding dairy products is the mainstay of treatment. Some individuals with a mild to moderate form of this condition may benefit from taking a pill called LactAid or drinking milk containing LactAid. Blacks suffer from lactose intolerance in combination with lack sun of exposure, plus the fact the darker the skin, the harder it is for the sun's rays to penetrate and stimulate vitamin D production are the reasons why vitamin D deficiency is so high in blacks and other people with dark skin. (See the chapter on osteoporosis for a more detailed discussion about vitamin D deficiency).

AIDS is one of the most prevalent diseases that causes diarrhea. The causes of the diarrhea seen in AIDS patients are due to a multitude of different microbial, viral, fungal, and parasitic organisms, and in some cases cancer, such as rectal cancer or Kaposi's sarcoma, lymphoma can also cause rectal bleeding and diarrhea. CMV-associated enterocolitis is quite common in AIDS patients. Herpes simplex gastroenteritis with diarrhea is common in AIDS patients. Other well known microorgisms that can cause diarrhea in AIDS patients include Giardiasis, amoebiasis, candidiasis, cryptosporidium, isospora belli, salmonella, shigella, etc.

Lymphoma of the GI tract with diarrhea is reasonably common. Another common cause of diarrhea is acute infectious gastroenteritis with diarrhea due to contaminated foods. The foods, water, raw vegetables, poultry, and meats can become contaminated with fecal-associated bacteria including salmonella, shigella, E. coli, campylobacter (usually seen in red meat/ground meat), Listeria, typhoid, and cholera organisms etc. These foods also can become contaminated with staphylococci resulting in severe abdominal pain, nausea, vomiting, diarrhea, and fever, sometimes resulting in dehydration, electrolyte imbalance, rectal bleeding and, at times, death of the affected individuals.

Poorly cooked meats are a good source of E. coli contamination. In the case of staphylococcus food poisoning, the endotoxin that this organism produces is actually ingested by the individual being contaminated, resulting in symptoms 6–8 hours later.

This happens quickly because the bacterial organisms do not have to multiply in the intestine in order to produce the endotoxin that is produced by the staphylococcal organism. In other situations, the bacteria need time to multiply in the colon to bring about the symptoms. Therefore, a person may get sick 1 day, 1 ½ days, or 2 days later. Diarrhea is clearly a very common medical problem and must be dealt with seriously when it develops. Self-diagnosis can be very dangerous.

It is a good idea to let your physician know if you are troubled with diarrhea so that appropriate steps can be taken to evaluate the cause or causes of the diarrhea and the proper treatments can be prescribed. Viral gastroenteritis includes Rotavirus, Norwalk virus, enteroviruses, reoviruses etc.

Clostridium difficile is a very common cause of diarrhea in and out of the hospital. When it occurs inside the hospital, it is usually due to nosocomial transmission (from a person to another). When it occurs outside the hospital, it is most frequently due to exposure to antibiotics. Antibiotic exposure can cause it to occur inside the hospital as well. 1 out of 10 people with C. difficile die. Other causes of diarrhea include hyperthyroidism, irritable bowel syndrome, lactose intolerance, chronic pancreatitis, short loop syndrome, etc.

Constipation is an extremely common complaint. Constipation is found in all ethnic groups. Blacks living in the third world suffer less with constipation because their diets have more grains and roughage, resulting in more normal bowel movements. Constipation, as a condition, can be due to numerous things, and prominent among these are the following:

1. Stress
2. Poor eating habits
3. Hypothyroidism
4. Taking laxatives too often, resulting in a condition called cathartic colon—that is to say, the colon has lost its ability to contract properly because the individual is compulsively abusing laxatives to bring about daily bowel movements. It is not necessary to have a bowel movement every day. A bowel movement every other day is perfectly fine.
5. Constipation due to medications. Good examples of medications that can cause constipation are the calcium channel blockers. The very reason why these medications work to bring down blood pressure is by relaxing the smooth muscles within the vessel in the people taking them. The intestines have smooth muscles in them and once these smooth muscles are relaxed, the bowel is likely to lose its contractile force, resulting in constipation. Fortunately, these very important medications don't cause this problem in everybody who takes them.
6. Irritable bowel syndrome, a condition associated with spasm of the bowel is frequently associated with abdominal cramps and constipation.
7. The most feared condition sometimes seen in people who are constipated is cancer of the large bowel.

Cancer of the large bowel causes constipation by mechanically preventing stool from passing through the area where the cancer is, resulting in pencil-sized stools and straining during defecation.

Before prescribing treatments for any of these conditions, thorough evaluations must be carried out to be sure of the cause or causes of these symptoms.

In the case of constipation, it most probably plays a major role in the causation of cancer of the large intestine. This happens because the foods and fluids we consume in the developed world contain a lot of cancer-causing materials. These materials are either outright carcinogens or cancer promoters.

Some of these cancer promoters are things produced by the human body itself. For instance, when a person eats a lot of fat containing foods such as red meat, the body via the biliary system produces a lot of bile acids in order to digest fats contained in these red meats. These bile acids are very harsh and irritating to the tissue of the large intestine. The long-term effects of the constant irritation of the tissues of the colon result in the development of colon cancer.

Constipation is bad, because not only is it uncomfortable, but it also can predispose the colon to the development of many serious medical conditions, and colon cancer is among them.

Abdominal cramps are a very common complaint and it can be due to things such as constipation, diverticulitis, lactose intolerance, irritable bowel syndrome, acute and chronic infections, parasitic infestation, ulcerative colitis, Crohn's disease, enterocolitis, acute and chronic pancreatitis, cancer of the stomach, cancer of the gall bladder, cancer of the pancreas, cancer of the colon, and stress, etc.

Flatulence is a condition that manifests itself by excessive passing of gas from the rectum. It is a normal biological function to pass gas from the rectum. The gas that is formed and expelled from the rectum is essentially methane. It is, however, abnormal when the gas a person passes is malodorous (smells bad) and when the frequency of passing gas is excessive and when the amount of gas one is passing is excessive. When a person passes large amounts of malodorous gas from the rectum too frequently, clearly this situation requires medical evaluation.

There are many conditions that affect the GI tract that can cause a person to produce too much and malodorous gas from the rectum, but the most common reasons are lactose intolerance and eating too much gas-producing foods such as green bananas, cabbage, peas, beans and dairy products when one is lactose intolerant.

Abdominal pain can be due to many things, including acute appendicitis, acute peritonitis due to conditions such as intra-abdominal abscess of different types, ischemic colitis, ulcerative colitis, cancer, peptic ulcer, perforated peptic ulcer, gall bladder disease, acute and chronic pancreatic diverticulitis, kidney stones.

Other common causes of abdominal pain are acute gastroenteritis due to viral, bacterial, fungal, and parasitic and protozoal infections. One of the severest and most common abdominal pains is due to menstruation.

Rectal bleeding is a frequent complaint for which people seek help from a doctor. Most people think they have hemorrhoids when they see blood in their stools. While hemorrhoids are frequently responsible for rectal bleeding, it is wrong to assume that if blood is coming from one's rectum, it must be due to hemorrhoids that are bleeding. Yes, hemorrhoids can bleed, but so can rectal cancer, colon cancer, small bowel cancer, cancer of the stomach, colon polyps, diverticulosis of the colon, ischemic colitis, Meckel's diverticulum, angiodysplasia of the GI tract, and anal fissures etc.

In fact, a person with no previous history of hemorrhoids who suddenly develops hemorrhoids either with or without bleeding would be wise to seek medical help because an obstructing polyp or cancer of the colon or rectum can cause that person to be straining during defecation, resulting in the development of hemorrhoids. That is not to say that every time someone develops a hemorrhoid he or she necessarily has colon or rectal cancer, but that possibility exists if the person is in the cancer age group of 45 years or older.

If a person bleeds from the rectum, regardless of age, he or she requires a lower gastrointestinal evaluation by colonoscopy to determine the cause. In point of fact, a person in the cancer age group with known hemorrhoids, which have been quiescent, that suddenly comes out and starts to bleed ought to also seek medical care to be certain that he or she does not have other reason or reasons to explain the sudden aggravation of the heretofore-quiescent hemorrhoids.

Blacks and other minorities seem to have a higher predilection to the development of hemorrhoids because they eat a poor diet with lots of fat, less grain, less vegetables and overall use less bulk, resulting in more constipation, which in turn leads to more hemorrhoids due to more straining during defecation. Another obvious reason that blacks have more hemorrhoids than do whites is that blacks tend to be more obese and obesity places a great deal of stress on the lower end of the GI tract, namely the anal area, resulting in hemorrhoids and their associated pain and bleeding symptoms.

Bleeding from the rectum is always abnormal and ought to be evaluated by a physician. The treatments for hemorrhoids are many and each person's case may be different from another person, because the cause or causes can differ. Conservative treatments, such as anal suppositories containing steroids, along with Sits baths or surgical removal of hemorrhoids, either the conventional way or with laser, are being used. Stool softeners, weight loss, and diet modifications are all approaches that can work for different people. It is best really to see your physician who can evaluate you and tailor a treatment program that is suitable for you.

Inflammatory bowel disease, which represents in the aggregate ulcerative colitis and Crohn's disease, are diseases of unknown cause, which cause different degrees of inflammations of the gastrointestinal tract, resulting in bleeding from the rectum, abdominal pain, and sometimes fever, weight loss, diarrhea, iron deficiency anemia, etc.

Sometimes, people suffering from inflammatory bowel disease can develop acute abdominal pain, megacolon, perforated viscous, intestinal obstruction, intestinal abscess, peritonitis, requiring emergency surgical intervention. Inflammatory bowel disease cuts across racial lines and oftentimes starts in the pediatric age group. Inflammatory bowel disease imposes a major burden on the individuals suffering from it and frequently these individuals develop significant psychological problems such as depression and the like.

No cure has been found for inflammatory bowel disease, but significant progress has been made with different forms of steroid medications either in pill form, intravenously, or in enema form. Medications such as Azulfidine as well as Asocal have made a big difference in the majority of people suffering from inflammatory bowel disease. There is a higher incidence of colon cancer in people suffering from inflammatory bowel disease. The reason is not altogether clear, but certainly the repeated inflammatory reactions and scarring that the bowel is exposed to for sure play a major role in the genesis of the development of bowel cancer in these individuals.

Polyps of the colon are quite common in modern society. It is believed that this is so because those who live in the modern worlds eat poorly. That is to say, people in the developed world eat poorly because they eat too much fats, carbohydrates and salt and not enough grains, roughage, and vegetables and fruits. Some of the vegetables and fruits that people eat in the developed world are contaminated with insecticides placed there by some food growers to prevent insects from destroying their crops, hence maximizing their profit margins at the expense of the consumers. It is believed that the interplay of all these factors plus genetic predisposition facilitates the development of colonic polyps, which in time three to five years may become cancerous. People in the third world develop only a fraction of the colon cancer that people in the modern world suffer from.

Blacks in Africa and other third world countries suffer only a fraction of the colon cancer that American Blacks and other minorities suffer from. Dietary habits have a lot to do with blacks' health problems.

They eat too much red meat, too much bacon, too many eggs and too much fat and too little of grains, fruits and vegetables. The "soul food" tastes good, but it's not healthy food.

The inability to pay for the healthy foods remains a serious problem among poor blacks, and this economic problem is getting worse instead of better. As the economic situation of black people in this country worsens, the health of blacks will continue to get worse. The incidence of colon cancer is going to get worse as black people's diet gets poorer in the United States and the poorer diet is a direct reflection of the poor economic status of blacks as compared to whites.

Another condition that predisposes to the development of colon cancer is familial polyposis. Familial polyposis is a hereditary condition that parents who carries this gene pass on to their children. The children who inherit this gene develop multiple polyps in their colons and, unfortunately, develop colon cancer arising from these polyps.

Once a diagnosis of familial polyposis is established, surgical treatment is advised to remove the colon via total colostomy and prevent colonic cancer from developing.

Diverticulosis of the colon is another common condition seen in the developed world. This is related to the dietary habits of people who live in the developed world.

A diet that is deficient in bulk and roughage predisposes to the development of diverticulosis. Diverticula are small outpouchings from the wall of the large bowel.

Every so often, the walls of some of these diverticula erode resulting in vascular breakdown, which in turn results in bleeding.

Sometimes this bleeding can be severe and life threatening and the bleeding is usually painless and recurrent. Frequently, the only real treatment that is available is surgical removal of the part of the bowel that is bleeding in order to stop the bleeding when all other conservative treatments have failed.

Diverticulitis occurs when a diverticulum or many diverticula become infected. Sometimes diverticular abscesses can develop. Diverticulitis occurs because the outpouching membrane from the wall of the bowel is bathed with fecal materials and fecal materials contain many bacteria. When the membrane of the diverticulum becomes inflamed and infected, the result is the development of diverticulitis. The symptoms of diverticulitis are abdominal cramps and pain, usually in lower abdominal area, fever, chills; sometimes diarrhea with or without blood and increased white blood cell count (leukocytosis) can occur.

Treatments of diverticulitis include antibiotics by mouth with low-residue diet, for low-grade diverticulitis. For moderate-grade diverticulitis, patients should be admitted to the hospital and keep NPO (no foods by mouth); treatment is given through IV fluids and IV antibiotics. Patients with high-grade diverticulitis with possible diverticular abscesses also need to be hospitalized keep NPO and treated with IV antibiotics.

Hyperalimentation may be given to sustain the patient off all foods. Sometimes, if peritonitis is deemed to exist because of perforation of the bowel resulting from diverticulitis, surgical resection of the affected part of the bowel may be necessary.

Bacterial overgrowth or blind-loop syndrome occurs when a situation exists that allows bacteria to grow in a part or parts of the bowel where a piece of bowel is left in a pouch-like manner due to surgical repair or due to multiple diverticuli.

One of the consequences of blind loop syndrome is low B12 level and all its consequences. A good indication that blind loop syndrome may exist is a very high folic acid level in the blood in conjunction with a low serum B12 level.

The approach to make this diagnosis is to try to correct the problem if possible, by treating the condition with antibiotics to eradicate the bacteria that are causing the overgrowth, and then replenish the B12 level with B12 injections.

The enzyme lactase is found in cells that are located in the walls of the intestine to facilitate breakdown of lactase into glucose and galactose; both are sugars found in milk. When the amount of lactase is too low or completely absent, this breakdown process (metabolism) is impaired. The result is abdominal cramps, bloating, nausea, flatulence, and, frequently, diarrhea.

In children, this is particularly troublesome because infants need the calcium and other nutrients that milk contains for proper growth. In infants the treatment is milk substitutes. In adults, the treatments include abstinence from milk and other dairy products or lactase containing milk or taking LactAid when eating or drinking dairy products.

Acute bacterial gastroenteritis can be very serious and sometimes fatal, as well as moderate-to-mild. This usually occurs because of eating contaminated foods, usually with fecal material from food handlers who don't wash their hands after using the bathroom. The fecal contamination can also occur in the plants where the meat or poultry products are prepared for shipping to supermarkets or a variety of other ways in the chain of events that the foods pass through before they get to the consumer's table.

Improperly cooked and contaminated foods in fast food places is a common situation that can result in acute staphylococcus or E. coli gastroenteritis or any number of other causative bacterial gastroenteritis. Microorganisms including E. coli, salmonella, shigella, staphylococcus, campylobacter, cholera, and viruses of different types can cause gastroenteritis. Salmonella or shigella gastroenteritis is a common form of gastrointestinal infection that can cause misery for travelers.

Acute infectious gastroenteritis causes fever, headache, nausea, abdominal pain, and vomiting, severe diarrhea, which can result in marked dehydration, bacteremia with sepsis and sometimes death if not treated in time and properly. When traveling abroad in certain countries, it is prudent to avoid drinking the water. Use only bottled water even to wash the mouth or to brush one's teeth.

Do not eat raw or rare meat. Eat meat or fish that is well cooked. Eat only hard-boiled eggs. Do not eat uncooked vegetables of any kind.

Before leaving to go away, make sure you check with your physician to get you a supply of Cipro 750 mg tablets or 500 mg. to be taken one tablet twice per day in the event you get sick with diarrhea. Levaquin 500 mg once per day is just as effective to treat infectious gastroenteritis. Erythromycin 500 mg 4 times per day is the treatment of choice for infectious gastroenteritis that is caused by campylobacter.

Anti-diarrhea medications such as Lomotil, Imodium, and Kaopectate suspension are important to have on hand to treat the diarrhea. Compazine 10 mg tablets to be taken 3 times per day for nausea or vomiting or Zofran 4 mg once per day also are important to treat the symptoms of acute gastroenteritis. Pepto-Bismol taken one tablespoon 4 times per day helps to ease some of the crampy symptoms of acute gastroenteritis

Do not be alarmed if your stool becomes black when taking Pepto-Bismol, it is not blood; the bismuth in the Pepto-Bismol that becomes black because of bacterial actions on it. Tarry-black stool, called melena, smells distinctly like old blood, and is a terrible smell.

Pepto-Bismol associated black stool smells like regular stool, except it is black. When not sure, check with your physician.

Frequently, acute infectious gastroenteritis requires treatment in the hospital with IV fluid, electrolyte replacement IV and IV antibiotics. The IV fluid must contain dextrose with sodium chloride of different concentrations. The purpose of the dextrose is to maintain the affected patients in an anabolic state to hasten recovery. In this setting, even a diabetic patient can be given dextrose with added regular insulin. More commonly, the affected patient can be treated at home with medications by mouth.

Acute gastroenteritis can also be due to viruses. Viral gastroenteritis is quite common and can be very severe if not treated promptly and properly and can lead to a multitude of complications such as electrolyte imbalance, cardiac arrhythmia, renal failure, and DIC, depending on different underlying chronic medical problems and the age of the individuals affected, and death can result.

Treatments of viral gastroenteritis are fluid IV or by mouth to prevent dehydration and electrolyte replacement by mouth by ways of soups, sodas, juices or IV. Antipyretics such as Advil and Tylenol are important to bring fevers down. Anti-diarrhea and anti-nausea medications such as just described are very important in dealing with these conditions.

Differentiating bacterial, viral, fungal, or parasitic gastroenteritis is left to the judgment and clinical experience of the examining physician. He or she can usually arrive at the proper diagnosis with a high degree of certainty.

Ischemic colitis usually occurs in the elderly with multiple medical problems such as diabetes mellitus, arteriosclerotic heart disease, etc. Ischemia colitis occurs when the blood flow to the affected bowel is impeded either because the patient's blood pressure falls for one reason or another, preventing blood to flow properly to perfuse the bowel. Lack of blood flow causes a segment of the bowel to become ischemic, resulting in abdominal pain.

Sometimes, the circulation of blood is occluded by a clot that is thrown to that area from an embolus, usually from the heart, resulting in occlusion of blood causing ischemia of that part of the bowel, which means, if not diagnosed quickly, the affected bowel will die resulting in a multitude of complications with possible death as a final result.

Surgical resection is frequently carried out to treat ischemic colitis. Once ischemic colitis becomes a serious consideration in the differential diagnosis of abdominal pain in an elderly person who presents to the doctor with abdominal pain, a flat plate of the abdomen must be done. A sign called finger printing can sometimes be seen on that x-ray film and if seen, ischemic colitis is highly possibly present. However, even if that is seen or not seen, angiogram is necessary to confirm the presence of ischemic colitis. The most frequently used treatment of ischemia colitis is surgical resection of the ischemic bowel.

Intestinal obstruction is an extremely common medical problem, which brings patients to physicians complaining of nausea, vomiting, and abdominal pain, and feeling generally sick. The list of things that can cause both small and the large intestine to be obstructed is quite long. Things such as:

1. Adhesions resulting from previous abdominal surgical procedures
2. Fecal impaction
3. Tumor of different types
4. In the third world and to some degree in rural south of the United States, where parasitic infestations are common, certain parasites such as ascaris can cause obstruction of the bowel.

Many inflammatory conditions such as ulcerative colitis or Crohn's disease that can destroy and cause narrowing of the lumen of the bowel, causing fistula to develop, resulting in intestinal obstruction. At the other extreme, these inflammatory bowel diseases can at times present with a condition called megacolon, whereby the lumen of the bowel becomes markedly enlarged, representing a surgical emergency.

Megacolon is best diagnosed by obtaining a simple x-ray of the abdomen called flat plate of the abdomen. Many things or conditions that can cause the intestine to become mechanically obstructed or to lose its ability to contract, resulting in the backing up of intestinal contents, resulting in nausea, vomiting, abdominal pain, etc.

Colorectal cancers are common in all groups in the United States. These cancers are more common in minority men as compared to white men. This is due to many reasons, and prominent among these reasons are the fat-rich diet that many blacks eat and the fact that so many blacks are obese/over weight and the fact that blacks, as a rule, go less frequently to physicians to be examined. By the time a black person develops symptoms such as abdominal pain, nausea, vomiting, diarrhea, rectal bleeding because of colorectal cancer, often the cancer is already in an advanced stage.

If the person is lucky, the rectal bleeding might be due to a precancerous polyp or some other nonmalignant lesion.

Intestinal obstruction is treated with a Cantor tube that is passed through the nose into the bowel. This tube has a little bag at the end of it filled with mercury to pull it down into the bowel slowly, forcing the area of obstruction to open.

Every day an x-ray of the abdomen is obtained to see the progress of the tube and to see if the obstruction has opened up.

The tube is attached to a machine called the Gomco machine to suction gastrointestinal contents, relieving the nausea, vomiting and abdominal pain. During this period, the patient is fed with intravenous fluid containing saline, glucose, and potassium chloride. Suctioning GI contents in this fashion causes the loss of a large amount of potassium chloride and it is crucial that potassium be replaced to prevent severe hypokalemia, which can cause serious cardiac complications.

Rectal fissures are lesions of the rectum, which represent cracks in the rectal tissue. They can bleed and are quite painful. Rectal fissures are treated with Sitz baths and different ointments made specifically for treating superficial rectal ailments.

Hemorrhoids are tissue protrusions that occur immediately inside the rectum (internal hemorrhoids) or immediately outside the rectum (external hemorrhoids). Hemorrhoids may at times be associated with obesity, causing undue pressure to the anal area, resulting in weight gain and pressure to the anal area. Obesity is more common in black and other minority men than in white men.

Conditions such as constipation commonly lead to the development of hemorrhoids. Colorectal cancer can at times result in the development of hemorrhoids or the aggravation of pre-existing hemorrhoids. If pre-existing hemorrhoids suddenly got worse, either by bleeding or by coming out, causing pain, this may be the result of an obstructing lesion above in the colon or the rectal area, causing straining at stooling. The high pressure generated during straining causes the development of hemorrhoids and the aggravation of pre-existing hemorrhoids.

It is therefore always necessary to pay close attention to the complaints of rectal bleeding or worsening of pre-existing hemorrhoids by undertaking a lower

Inguinal hernia can be associated with colorectal cancer. An obstructing mass within the large bowel inevitably causes the person harboring the mass to generate a great deal of pressure in the muscle of the lower abdomen. This set of interactions can result in the spontaneous development of inguinal hernia. Therefore it is very important to investigate black men who are in the cancer age group, age 45 and older, who spontaneously develops an inguinal hernia.

Any person who fits this profile ought to have a lower GI evaluation with either a barium enema or a colonoscopy before she undergoes an inguinal hernia repair.

Many gastrointestinal diseases are seen commonly in blacks; therefore it is crucial that blacks pay close attention to the multitude of factors outlined in this chapter to help them from falling victims of these diseases.

CHAPTER 23

DIARRHEAL DISEASES/FOOD POISONING IN AFRICAN AMERICAN MEN

Diarrheal diseases are very common and every year there are 5 billion episodes of diarrheal diseases worldwide. Every year 2 million people die from diarrheal diseases in the world and 1.5 million of these deaths occur in children under the ages of two years. In addition, a diarrheal disease is the number one cause of malnutrition of children in the world. Source: WHO.

Every year there are 211 million cases of diarrheal diseases in the U.S. And 1 in 6 people in the U.S. get gastroenteritis every year. Source: CDC

Each year 76 million people get sick from food poisoning in the world and food poisoning causes 1.8 million deaths per year. Every year 48 million people in the U.S. get sick from food poisoning and 325,000 are hospitalized from food poisoning. Every year food poisoning kills 5,000 people in the U.S. The medical Cost of food poisoning per year in the U.S. is $152 billion. : Sources CDC and WHO:

According to the CDC the most common sources of food borne illnesses are leafy vegetables such as spinach, kale and lettuces 23% and dairy products 14% and they also found that dairy products were responsible for 16% of hospitalizations, leafy vegetables 14% and poultry 12%. Other sources of food poisoning include poultry, meat, fish, shellfish, and contaminated water etc.;

There are two types of diarrheal disease:

The noninflammatory and the inflammatory types, example of the noninflammatory type include Cholera and Giardia and example of inflammatory type include microbes like Shigella and Entamoeba histolytica.

Cholera and Giardia cause diarrhea by interfering with intestinal fluid absorption causing massive watery diarrhea, abdominal cramps, fever, and dehydration. Shigella, Entamoeba histolytica viruses, bacteria, cause diarrhea, abdominal pain, nausea, vomiting, and fever.

Diarrheal /food poisoning diseases are transmitted from person to person and via fecal contaminated foods to the oral route.

Risk factors for diarrheal/food posoning dieases include:

Residing in countries where diarrheal diseases are prevalent
Traveling to countries where diarrheal diseases are prevalent
Residing in hospitals
Residing in nursing homes
Children in day care centers
Living in overcrowding houses
Having type O blood type
Eating contaminating foods
Drinking contaminated water
Eating contaminating fruits
Eating contaminating vegetables
Eating contaminating eggs
Eating contaminating hamburger meats
Eating contaminating meats
Eating contaminating chickens
Eating contaminating shell fish
Eating contaminating fish
Using bath rooms without washing one's hands
AIDS
Anal sex (HIV, Giardia, and Entamoeba histolytica can be transmitted via this route)
Eating in restaurants with unsanitary conditions
Traveling on cruise ships
Cancer
Radiation therapy
Chemotherapy
Non-acquired immunodeficiency diseases etc;

Bacterial organisms that can cause diarrheal disease/food poisoning diseases include:

Staphylococcus aureus
Escherichia coli (E. coli O157:H7)
Shigella species
Campylobacter
Salmonella
Vibrio vulnificus
Yersinia
Listeria
Clostridium botulism
Clostridium perfringes
Clostridium Difficile

Viruses that can cause diarrheal diseases include:

Adenovirus
Rotavirus Norvovirus
Calcivirus

Protozoa organisms that can cause diarrheal diseases include:

Entamoeba histolytica
Giardia lamblia
Cryptosporidium

Symptoms of diarrheal diseases include:

NauseaVomiting
Abdominal pain
Diarrhea
Bloody diarrhea
Fever
Sepsis
Weakness
Fatigue
Headache
Joints pain
Muscle cramps
Thirst
Dehydration
Hypotension
Kidney failure
Confusion
Disseminated intravascular coagulopathy (DIC)
Anemia
Deaths in many cases

Evaluations of diarrheal diseases include:

History and physical examination
Vital signs
Stool culture
Stool Gram stain
Stool leukocytes
Stool ova and parasites examination
Toxin and antigen assays of stool
"Xtag GPP (Gastrointestinal Pathogen Panel) stool test (this test was approved by the FDA in January 2013, it can detect 7 bacterial pathogens-Clostridium Difficile toxin A and B, Campylobacter, E.coli O157,

E. coli Lt/ST, Salmonella, Shigella, and Shigella-like toxin producing E. coli stx 1/stx 2
2 viruses- N Rotavirus and Noroviruses, 2 parasites Cryptosporidium and Giardia"
CBC
Complete metabolic –chemistry profile
T4, T3, and TSH
Blood culture
RPR blood test
HIV blood test
Serum IgA (Giagia lambia diarrheal disease can be seen in people who have IgA deficiency)
Serum titer for antamoeba histolytica
EKG
Chest X-ray
Abdominal CT Scan

Individual microorganisms that cause gastroenteritis include:

Staphylococcus aureus
Campylobacter Jajuni
Clostridium botulinum
Clostridium perfringes
Shigella
E.coli
Salmonrlla
Salmonela typhi
Vibrio vulnificus
Cryposporidium
Entomoeba histolytica
Giardia lamblia
Listeria
Hepatitis A
Hepatitis E
Noroviruses
Rotavirus etc;

CHAPTER 24

STAPHYLOCOCCUS GASTROENTERITIS IN AFRICAN AMERICAN MEN

Treatments of diarrheal diseases are different for different causative organisms. The most frequent food born diarrheal infection is staphylococcus aureus associated infection. Staphylococcus food infection is the result poorly refrigerated foods, in particular diary products containing foods such as milk, cheese, cream, ice cream, and other foods such as rice, grits, meats, chicken, fish that left outside too long. Staphylococcus is everywhere, on the hands, nostrils, mouth, the skin, kitchen counters etc.

Staphylococcus aureus develops the fastest because the bacterium produces an endotoxin in the food that is being infected. The person being infected actually swallows the already made endotoxin in the contaminated food making them sick in 1 to 6 hours. The endotoxin causes the swelling and inflammation in the colon that results in the symptoms complex that is responsible for the diarrheal disease manifested in staphylococcus aureus gastroenteritis/enterocolitis.

Outpatient treatments for staphylococcus aureus gastroenteritis include:

Compozine 10mg by mouth every 6 hours
                          or
Zofran 4 mg by mouth every 8 hours
Cipro 500 mg by mouth every 12 hours for 7 days
Lomotil or Imodium may be given to ease the diarrhea
Pepto-Bismol 15cc 4 times per day as needed
Tylenol may be given for fever

If patient is unable to drink and eat, to avoid dehydration, the patient ought to be hospitalized.

Patients with staphylococcus aureus who present to the emergency room with high fever, chills, abdominal pain, vomiting, diarrhea, should be admitted into the hospital. These patients need abdominal CT scan, Chest x-ray, EKG, blood cultures stool culture, stool gram stain, stool leukocytes count, stool ova and parasites, CBC, Complete chemistry metabolic profile, Clostridium Difficile toxin, Cipro 500mg IV every 12 hours or Cefriaxone 1 gram IV every 12 hours, Zofran 8 mg IV every 8 hours Tylenol 650mg by mouth every 4 hours for fever, D5 normal saline, and 20MEQ of potassium at150cc per hour Lacted Ringer's at 150cc per hour Infectious disease and gastroenterology consults.

CHAPTER 25

E. COLI GASTROENTERITIS IN AFRICAN AMERICAN MEN

Escherichia Coli O 157: H7 infection is a very common infection. People who come in contact with it by eating foods contaminated with it or feces from infected humans or animals like cows can become infected. It is most frequently transmitted by contaminated meat, chicken, unpasteurized milk, fruits, unpasteurized apple cider, vegetables such as lettuce, alfalfa sprouts, unpasteurized juices, and contaminated water. The most virulent E. coli that causes intestinal infection is E. coli O157:H7. It gets people sick whiten 1-8 days.

The most frequent symptoms of E. coli gastroenteritis include:

Nausea
Vomiting
Abdominal cramps/pain
Bloody diarrhea
Fever
Weakness
Thrombocytopenia
Hemolytic anemia
Bruising of the skin due to low platelets
Hemolytic uremic syndrome
Sepsis
Dehydration
Kidney failure

Evaluations of E. coli gastroenteritis include:

Complete history and physical examination
Vital signs
Stool culture
Stool Gram stain
Stool leukocytes test
Stool ova and parasites
Stool for C. Difficile toxin A and B
Xtag GPP stool test

Blood culture
CBC
Complete chemistry-metabolic profile
PT/INR
PTT
Reticulocyte count
Close review of peripheral blood smears
Serum LDH
HIV blood test
Urinalysis
Chest x-ray
EKG
24 hours urine creatinine clearance
24 hours urine protein
Glomerular filtration rate (GFR)
Renal ultrasound
Abdominal CT Scan

Treatments of E. coli O157:H7 gastroenteritis includes:

Hospital admission
IV fluid with D5 Normal saline with 20MEQ of potassium at 150cc per hour
Lacted Ringer's 150cc per hours
Tylenol 650mg by mouth every 4 hours for fever
Antibiotics, aspirin, NSAID, and Lomotil ought to be avoided in gastroenteritis due to O157:H7 as these might make the disease worst.
Traveler's diarrhea can be treated with Cipro 500mg by mouth twice per day for 1 week or Azithromycin 500mg by mouth

If Hemolytic uremic syndrome develops, a hematologist needs to take over the management of this problem. If kidney failure develops, a nephrologist needs to take over the management of the kidney failure. Dialysis can be carried out on people who require it.

The best way to prevent O157:H7 E. coli gastroenteritis is adhere to personal hygiene and cook foods to a temperature of 160 degrees and avoids eating contaminated foods.

When traveling to underdeveloped countries don't drink the water. Don't eat uncooked foods and avoid eating uncooked vegetables. In addition, it is a good idea to carry Cipro, Zithromax, Compozine, and zofran with you to take at the first sign of symptoms. Infectious disease and gastroenterology consultations;

CHAPTER 26

SHIGELLA GASTROENTERITIS IN AFRICAN AMERICAN MEN

Shigella gastroenteritis is very serious infection. World wide 166 million people get infected with the shigella bacterium and 1 million people die from the infection. Source: WHO. In the U.S., 14, 000 people get infected with Shigella and 1 percent of those infected with Shigella die annually in developed countries like the U.S.

Shigella gastroenteritis occurs by fecal contamination from person to person and in particular those living in crowded dwellings and food handlers. It is transmitted from contaminated seafoods, water and ready to eat food products. People become sick 24 to 48 hours after eating contaminated foods.

The symptoms of Shigella gastroenteritis include:

Fever
Nausea
Vomiting
Watery diarrhea
Mucoid diarrhea
Bloody diarrhea
Abdominal cramps
Abdominal pain
Anorexia
Malaise
Dehydration etc.

Evaluations of Shigella gastroenteritis include:

History and Physical examination
Vital signs
Chest x-ray
Abdominal ultrasound
Abdominal CT scan
EKG
CBC

Complete chemistry-metabolic profile
Blood culture
Stool culture
Stool ova and parasites
Stool leukocytes
Stool Gram stain
Xtag GPP stool test
Blood HIV test
T4 and TSH

Treaments for Shigella gastroenteritis include:

Water by mouth
Fruit juices
Diluted tea
No foods by mouth
Intravenous fluid with Normal saline with 20 MEQ of potassium per liter
Intravenous fluid with Normal saline and glucose with 20 MEQ of potassium per liter
Lacted Ringer's at 150cc per hour
After a few days of putting the stomach to rest start with bananas, rice, applesauce and toast
Zofran 4 mg by mouth every 4 hours for nausea and vomiting
Zofran 8 mg IV every 8 hours for nausea and vomiting
Reglan 10 by mouth every 6 hours as needed for nausea and vomiting
Compozine 10 mg by mouth every 6 hours as needed for nausea and vomiting
Cipro 500mg IV every 12 hours
                    or
Cipro 500mg by mouth every 12 hours
                    or
Ceftriaxone 1 gram IV every 12 hours
                    or
Azithromax 500mg by mouth every 12 hours
                    or
Azithromax 500mg IV every 12 hours
                    or
Bactrim DS 1 tablet twice per day
Infectious disease and gastroenterolgy consultations.

CHAPTER 27

CAMPYLOBACTER JEJUNI GASTROENTERITIS IN AFRICAN AMERICAN MEN

Campylobacter Jejuni food poisoning/diarrheal illness is the most common food born gastroenteritis in the world. 2.4 million People in world get sick every year from Campylobacter dirrheal illness/gastroenteritis. Source: WHO

In 2010, 845,000 individuals got sick from Campylobacter gastroenteritis in the U.S. Source: CDC All together, there are 17 different spices, and 6 subspices of Campylobacter bacteria, but C. Jejuni is the one that causes diarrheal disease/ gastroenteritis in humans.

Eating contaminated chicken, meat, water transmits Campylobacter Jejuni, and when cross contamination occurs with other foods. Campylobacter infection occurs usually as a result animal or human feces that come in contact with chicken, meat, water or unpasterized milk. Campylobacter infects more infants, children than adults and more common in men.

Each year 124 People die from Campylobacter gastroenteritis/diarrheal illness. Worldwide most People who get sick from Campylobacter jenuni don't die from it except infants, children, and those who have HIV/AIDS.

Sources of Campylobacter infection include:

Poultry
Pig
Cattle
Sheep
Shellfish
Cats
Dogs
Pets
Ostriches

Campylobacter Jejuni is transmitted through poorly cooked chicken, meat, unpasterized milk, water, anal sex, and coming in contact with all the above things when there are contaminated, plus cross contamination in kitchens.

Symptoms of Campylobacter begins from 2-5 days and sometime up to 10 days from the time of contamination.

The symptoms of Campylobacter include:

Nausea
Vomiting
Abdominal cramps
Abdominal pain
Diarrhea
Bloody diarrhea
Fever
Pain in joints
Weakness
Headache
Dizziness etc;

Complications of Campylobacter infection include:

Septic arthritis of joints
Endocarditis
Guillan-Barre syndrome (about 1 in every 100 cases of Campylobacter diarrheal infection results in Guillan Barre with general paralysis. This usually occurs several weeks after the onset of the C. infection.
Sepsis
Hepatitis
Pancreatitis
Appendicitis
Cholecystitis
Urinary tract infection etc;

Evaluations of Campylobacter diarrheal/gastroenteritis infection include:

History and physical examination
Vital signs
Stool culture
Stool ova and parasites
Stool toxin A B for C. Difficile
Xtag GPP stool test
Stool leukocytes
CBC
Complete chemistry-metabolic profile

Urinalysis
Urine culture
Blood culture
Erythrocyte sedimentation rate
HIV blood test
Acute hepatitis A, B and, profile
Abdominal ultrasound
Abdominal CAT Scan
Chest x-ray
EKG
Echocardiogram

IV fluid with Normal saline with 20 MEQ of potassium in each liter at 150cc per
                                              or
IV D5 normal saline with 20 MEQ of potassium in each liter at 150cc per hour
                                              or
Lasted Ringer's 150cc per hours
Zofran 8 mg IV every 8 hours for nausea and vomiting
                                              or
Zofran 4 mg by mouth every 8 hours for nausea or vomiting
                                              or
Compazine 10mg by mouth every 6 hours for nausea and vomiting
                                              or
Reglan 10 mg by mouth every 8 hours for nausea and vomiting
Pepto-Bismol 1 tablespoon every 6 hours as needed
The most frequent antibiotics in use to treat Campylobacter diarrhea/gastroenteritis
Are:
Erythromycin 500 mg IV or by mouth every 6 hours for 10-14 days
                                              or
Azythromycin 500mg IV or by mouth every 12 hours for 7-10 days
                                              or
Tetracycline 250mg by mouth every 6 hours for 10-14 days

If a person with Campylobacter diarrheal/gastroenteritis disease is septic, dehydrated with pancreatitis, hepatitis, cholecystitis, appendicitis, or Guilland Barre, he or she should be hospitalized for in hospital care.

The ways to prevent the transmission of Campylobacter include:

Wash hands with soap and water
Cook foods to temperature to 167 F
Drink only pasteurized milk
Animal and poultry handlers should use gloves when touching and while working with poulrty.

Food handlers should wash their hands with soap and water should ware gloves when handling foods.

When traveling to underdeveloped countries drink only bottle water or boil water Don't eat raw vegetables and fruits when traveling to areas where Campylobacter infection is prevalent don't let foods sit unrefrigerated for more than 2 hours and wash hands always after using bathrooms etc;

CHAPTER 28

SALMONELLA GASTROENTERITIS IN AFRICAN AMERICAN MEN

Salmonella is a very common cause of diarrheal disease/gastroenteritis. Worldwide 93.8 million cases of salmonella gastroenteritis are reported every year. The annual death rate due to Salmonella diarrheal disease is 155,000.

In the U.S. more than 1 million cases of Salmonella gastroenteritis were reported In 2011, 20,000 cases resulted in hospitalization and 378 people died. Source: CDC

Salmonella can cause three different kinds diseases:

Gastroenteritis
Typhoid fever
Bacteremia/Sepsis

Risk factors for Salmonella infection include:

Eating contaminated raw meat
Eating or drinking raw eggs
Eating undercooked meat, eggs, poultry, eggs products and unpasteurized milk
Contaminated knives, cutting surfaces
Infected food handlers
Owners of birds or reptiles
Living group homes
Traveling to countries where poor sanitary conditions exist
AIDS
Un-acquired immunodeficiency diseases
Chemotherapy treatment
Radiotherapy treatment
Sickle cell anemia
Longterm steroid treatment
Biological medications
Anti-rejection medications during organ transplants

Symptoms of Salmonella Diarrheal disease/gastroenteritis include:

Symptoms of salmonella develop between 1-3 days after exposure
Nausea
Vomiting
Fever
Abdominal cramps/pain
Diarrhea
Chills
Headache
Muscle pain/myalgia
Blood in stool

Evaluations of Salmonella diarrheal disease/gastroenteritis include:

History and physical examination
Blood pressure
Pulse
Temperature
Respiratory rate
Stool culture
Stool Gram stain
Stool leukocytes
Stool ova and parasites
Stool toxin for Clostridium Difficile
Xtag GPP stool test
CBC
Complete chemistry-metabolic profile
Blood culture
Urinalysis
RPR
HIV blood test
Hemoglobin electrophoresis
Malaria smear
Chest x-ray
Abdominal sonogram
Abdominal CT scan
Brain CT
Brain MRI
Lumbar puncture
Spinal fluid culture
Gram stain of spinal fluid
Spinal fluid glucose
Spinal fluid protein
EKG
Echocardiogram

Complications of salmonella gastroenteritis include:

Dehydration
Dry mouth
Dry tongue
Reduced urine output
Joints swelling
Joint pain
Sepsis
Septic arthritis
Endocarditis
Osteomyelitis
Meningitis
Seizure
Brain abscess etc;

Treatments of Salmonella diarrheal/gastroenteritis include:

Usually symptoms resolve in five to seven days requiring no treatments at all
Re-hydration with water by mouth to treat dehydration
Intravenous fluid with normal saline with 20 MEQ of potassium per liter at 150cc per hour

or

Intravenous normal saline and glucose (D5W) with 20 MEQ of potassium per liter at 150cc per hour

or

Lacted Ringers 150cc per hour
If the symptoms get worst, then antibiotics can be used to treat the infection.
Antibiotics in use to treat salmonella diarrheal disease/gastroenteritis include:
Ampicillin 1 gram IV every 4 hours for 7-14 days

or

Ceftriaxone 1 gram IV every 12 hours for 7-14 days

or

Cipro 500mg IV or by mouth every 12 hours for 7-14 days

or

Bactrim DS 1 tablet every 12 hours for 7-14 days
Pepto-Bismol 1 tablespoon every 6 hours by mouth
Compozine 10 mg by mouth every 6 hours for nausea and vomiting
Zofran 4 mg by mouth every 8 hours for nausea and vomiting

Prevention of Salmonella diarrheal disease/gastroenteritis includes:

Wash hands after using bathrooms
Cook chicken, turkey, red meat, and ground meat, eggs thoroughly up to a temperature to 167 degree F
Don't drink unpasteurized milk

Don't eat or drink raw eggs

Wash hands with soap and water after handling birds, reptiles

When traveling to developing countries don't drink water unless it is boiled and drink bottle water, don't eat uncooked vegetables, and don't eat uncooked fruits and avoid living in crowded housing etc;

CHAPTER 29

TYPHOID FEVER IN AFRICAN AMERICAN MEN

Typhoid fever is caused by Salmonella serotype typhi. After infection occurred, it takes from 5 to 21 days for symptoms to appear. Typhoid fever occurs because of contaminated food and water.

Worldwide 13 million people get typhoid fever every year and 500,000 people die every year. Each year about 400 people contracted typhoid fever in the U.S. These infections occur as a result U.S. Citizens traveling to developing countries.

The symptoms of typhoid fever include:

Headache
Sore throat
Cough
Diarrhea or constipation
Intestinal bleeding
Poor appetite
Abdominal pain
General aches and pain
Slow heart rate
Fever up to 104
Chills
Lethargy
Dehydration
Seizure in children

Evaluations of Typhoid fever include:

History
Physical examination
Temperature
Pulse
Blood pressure
Respiration rate

Oxygen saturation
Stool culture
Stool Gram stain
Stool leukocytes
Stool ova and parasites
Stool toxin A and B for C. Difficile
Xtag GPP stool test
CBC
Complete metabolic profile
Blood culture
Urinalysis
Urine culture
Chest x-ray
Abdominal CT Scan
Echocardiogram
EKG

Treatments of typhoid fever include:

Intravenous fluid with normal saline glucose and 20 MEQ of potassium at 150cc per hour
or
Normal saline and 20 MEQ of potassium at 150cc per hour
or
Ringer's lactate at 150cc per hour
Ampicillin 1 gram IV every 4 hours or Ampicillin 500mg by mouth every 6 hours
or
Cipro 500mg IV or by mouth every 12 hours
or
Amoxicillin 500mg by mouth every 8 hours
or
Ceftriaxone 1 gram IV or IM every 12 hours
or
Bactrim DS 1 tablet by mouth every 12 hours
or
Gentamicin 1.5 mg/kg IV every 8 hours

Zofran 4 mg IV or by mouth every 8 hours for nausea or vomiting
Compozine 10mg every 6 hours for nausea or vomiting
Tylenol 650mg by mouth every 4 hours for fever or Ibuprofen 400-600mg every 6 hours
Aspirin is not to be used in children to treat fever because it might cause Reye's syndrome.

Complications of Typhoid fever include:

Aspirin is contraindicated in typhoid fever because it might cause acute degranulation of mast cells resulting in hypotension and shock.

Bacteremia/Sepsis
Arthritis
Reiter's syndrome

The typhoid organism can remain in the gall bladder for a very long time while causing no immediate symptoms, while shedding salmonella taphi in the stool resulting in recurrent typhoid fever infection in a carrier of salmonella typhi.
Chronic carriers of salmonella typhi can transmit the infection to people.

CHAPTER 30

LISTERIA GASTROENTERITIS IN AFRICAN AMERICAN MEN

Listeria gastroenteritis develops within 9-48 hours after eating lunchmeats, hot dog, cheese, unpasteurized milk, eating unwashed raw food products, and exposure to contaminated soil and water. It may take as long as 2 months before symptoms appear sometimes.

About 2.500 people in the U.S. get sick every from Listeria and about 500 people die every year from Listeria in the U.S.

Risk factors for Listeria infection include:

HIV/AIDS
Chemotherapy
Radiation therapy
Cancer
Alcoholism
Cirrhosis of the liver
Organ transplants
Longterm treatment with steroid
Biological medications
Pregnancy

Symptoms of Listeria gastroenteritis include:

Nausea
Diarrhea
Abdominal cramps
Abdominal pain
Fever
Muscle aches
When the listeria organism enters into the blood stream, it can cause Sepsis, Meningitis, Headache, Stiff neck, Confusion, and Seizure

During pregnancy symptoms of listeria infection include:

Miscarriage
Stillbirth
Premature delivery
The infants may have irritability, fever, vomiting and may refuse feedings ;

Evaluations of listeria infection include:

History and physical examination
CBC
Complete chemistry profile
Blood culture
Urine culture
Lumbar puncture (brain CT or brain MRI should always be done before lumbar puncture)
CSF culture
Gram stain of CSF
Cells count of CSF
Protein level of CSF
Glucose level of CSF
LDH of CSF
Stool culture
Stool Xtag GPP
Brain CT
Brain MRI etc;

Treatments of listeria infection include:

Zofran 4mg IV or by mouth every 8 hours for nausea or vomiting
Tylenol 650mg every 4 hours for fever
NSAIDs for fever
Aspirin 650mg every 6 hours for fever
Lomotil 1tab every 6 hours for diarrhea
Imodium A-D 2mg every 6 hours for diarrhea
Kaopectate II caplets 1 tab qid for diarrhea
Pepto-Bismol 1 tablespoon 4 times per day for diarrhea
Ampicillin 1 gram IV every 6 hours
or
Amoxicillin 500mg by mouth every 8 hours
or
Bactrim DS 1 tab twice per day
or
Levaquin 500mg IV every 24 hours
or
Levaquin 500mg by mouth every 24 hours

D5 normal saline at 150cc per hour
                    or
D5 ½ normal saline at 150cc per hour
Ringer's lactate at 150cc per hour etc;

Prevention of listeria infection includes:

Wash hands with soap and water after using the bathroom
Heat hot dogs, lunchmeat, and deli meat well
Wash vegetables well before eating
Keep all foods well refrigerated
When traveling to developing countries, drink only bottle water, do not eat uncooked vegetables, do not eat uncooked foods of any kind etc;

Other bacterial gastroenteritis include:

Clostridium botilinum which causes gastroenteritis when people eat contaminated foods such as improperly home canned foods, salted fish, smoked fish, baked potatoes and foods that kept outside at warm temperature for long period of time.
Symptoms begin to develop between 12-72 hours.

Clostridium perfringens causes gastroenteritis when people eat contaminated foods such as meats, gravies and stews. Clostridium perfringes causes symptoms to appear between 8-16 hours after ingestion.

Vibrio vulnificus causes gastroenteritis when people eat contaminated raw oysters, poorly cooked muscles, clams and scallops. Symptoms begin between 1-7 days from ingesting these foods.

CHAPTER 31

GIARDIA LAMBLIA GASTROENTERITIS IN AFRICAN AMERICAN MEN

Giardia lamblia gastroenteritis is a parasitic infection that is very common and causes about 22,000 people in the U.S. to get gastroenteritis every year and about 200 million people around the world to get gastroenteritis every year.

The organism is transmitted via the fecal oral route primarily due to contaminated foods and water.

Risk factors for getting from giardia lamblia include:

Eating raw food products
Drinking contaminated water
Infected food handlers
Residing in institutions
Residing in nursing homes
Day-care workers
Traveling to developing countries
Failure to wash hands after using the bathroom
Anal sex
HIV/AIDS
Non-acquired immunodeficiency diseases
Sickle cell anemia
Chemotherapy
Radiotherapy
Longterm steroid treatment
Biological medications
Organ transplants etc.
A-splenetic (people who have no spleen)
Pregnancy
Symptoms of giardiasis can begin to develop 1-2 weeks after exposure.

Signs and symptoms of giardia gastroenteritis include:

Nausea
Loss of appetite
Vomiting
Diarrhea watery or loose stool
Cramps in the stomach
Cramps in the abdomen
Bloating
Burping
Malabsoprtion
Vitamin B12 deficiency
Blood in the urine (hematuria) etc;

Evaluation of giardia gastroenteritis includes:

History and physical examination
CBC
Complete chemistry profile
Serum IGA (people with IgA deficiency are at high risk for giardiasis)
Stool for ova and parasites
The entero-test
ELISA blood test (this test can detect giardiasis up to 90%)
Bladder sonogram
Urinalysis
Urine culture
Urine cytology
Urology consultation
Hemoglobin electrophoresis

Medications to treat giardia gastroenteritis include:

Metronidazole (Flagyl)
Albendazole
Tinidazole
The course of treatment usally lasts for 5-10 days
Compozine
Kytril
Zofran
Lomotil
Immodium
Kaopectate
Peptobismol etc;

CHAPTER 32

CRYPTOSPORIDIUM GASTROENTERITIS IN AFRICAN AMERICAN MEN

Every year there are 300,000 cases of cryptosporidium infection in the U.S. and worldwide there are 2.5 million cases of cryptosporidium gastroenteritis annually. Worldwide there are 100,000 deaths annually from cryptosporidium.

Cryptosporidium infection occurs mainly in children and in people with HIV/AIDS. When this infection occurs in healthy people, the infection is usually self-limited.

Risk factors for cryptosporidium gastroenteritis include:

Childcare workers
Children in day care centers
People who travel to developing countries
Swimmers who drink contaminated water in pools or lakes
Parents of infected children
Anal sex
Oral to anal sex
Hackers who drink contaminated water
Campers who drink contaminated water
Handlers of infected animals
Pregnancy
Chemotherapy treatments
Radiotherapy treatment
Long term steroid use
Biological medications
HIV/AIDS
Non-acquired immunodeficiency diseases etc.

Signs and symptoms of cryptosporidium gastroenteritis include:

Nausea
Vomiting
Watery diarrhea
Dehydration

Abdominal cramps
Abdominal pain
Fever etc;

Evaluations of cryptosporidium gastroenteritis include:

History and physical examination
CBC
Complete chemistry profile
PT/INR, PTT
Urinalysis
Serum B12
Stool culture
Xtag GPP stool test
Stool for ova and parasites
Stool for white cells
Abdominal ultrasound
Small bowel biopsy
HIV/AIDS 1 and 2 blood tests

Treatments of cryptosporidium include:

Nitazoxanide
Zithromax
Imodium A-D
Lomotil
D5 normal saline at 150cc per hour with 20-meq kcl
Lacted Ringer's at 150cc per
HAART for AIDS patients

Complications of cryptosporidium gastroenteritis include:

Dehydration
Weight loss
Acute cholecystitis (acute gall bladder infection)
Hepatitis
Acute pancreatitis
Infection of the small bowel
Headache
Joint pain
Fatigue
Dizzy spells
Pain in the eyes
Malabsorption
B12 deficiency
Deaths can occur in people with AIDS.

CHAPTER 33

ENTAMOEBA HISTOLYTICA GASTROENTERITIS IN AFRICAN AMERICAN MEN

Worldwide 50 million people have entamoeba histolytica gastroenteritis every year and about 100,000 people die in the world every year from this infection.

Entamoeba histolytica is a parasitic organism that is transmitted via the fecal oral route and is most common in developing countries. In the U.S. the prevalence E. histolytica is about 4% and most these cases are asymptomatic.

Risk factors for E. histolytica include:

Living in developing countries
Eating contaminated foods
Drinking contaminated water
HIV/AIDS
Anal sex
Anal/oral sex
Cancer
Longterm use of steroid
Biological medications
Chemotherapy treatment
Radiotherapy treatment
Non-acquired immunodeficiency diseases
Pregnancy
Children
Neonates
Malnutrition etc;

Signs and symptoms of entomoeba gastroenteritis include:

Nausea
Vomiting
Watery diarrhea

Bloody diarrhea
Rectal bleeding
Abdominal cramps
Abdominal pain
Fever
Weight loss
Anorexia etc;

Evaluations of E. histolytica include:

History and physical examination
CBC with differential
Complete chemistry profile
PT/INR, PTT
Stool for ova and parasites
Stool culture
Serologic testing
Polymerase chain reaction (PCR)
HIV/AIDS 1 and 2 blood tests
ESR
Chest x-ray
Abdominal sonogram
Adnominal CAT Scan with contrast both by mouth and IV
Abdominal MRI with IV contrast
Infectious disease consultation
GI consultation
Surgical consultation etc;

Complications of Amebiasis include:

Toxic megacolon
Fulminant colitis
Necrotizing colitis
Rectovaginal fistula
Amebic liver abscess
Brain abscess
Seizure
Bowel perforation
GI bleeding
Peritonitis
Sepsis
Intussusceptions
Empyema
Anemia
Leukocytosis

Eosinophilia
Elevated liver function tests
Elevated ESR
DIC
Malabsoption
B12 deficiency etc;

Treatments of entomoeba gastroenteritis/amebiasis include:

Flagyl
Paromomycin
Tinidazole
Iodoquinol
Broadspectrum IV antibiotics as indicated

For people who need to be admitted to the hospital, D5 and normal saline at 150cc per hour   or
Lactated Ringer's at 150cc per hour
Zofran 4mg IV of by mouth every 8 hours
Compozine 10mg by mouth every 6 hours
Lomotil 1 tablet every 6 hours as needed for diarrhea
Imodium A-D 1 tablet every 6 hours as needed for diarrhea
Tylenol 325mg 2 tablets every 4 hours for fever.

CHAPTER 34

YERSINIA ENTEROCOLITICA GASTROENTEROCOLITIS IN AFRICAN AMERICAN MEN

Yersinia enterocolitica is a Gram-negative coccobacillus. It causes disease both in humans and animals such as cattle, deer, birds and pigs. Most of these animals become Asymptomatic carriers. Once the organism enters into the human body through the mouth, it replicates in the ileum and invades Peyer's patches. From there it disseminates into the Mesenteric lymph nodes resulting in enlarged lymph nodes.

The pain on the right side of the abdomen is frequently confused with appendicitis. In immunosupressed individuals, the Yersinial organism can spread to the liver and spleen causing the development of abscesses.

Risk factors for Yersinia enterocolitica infection include:

Eating fecal contaminated foods
Eating raw pork
Eating undercooked pork
Eating chitterlings (pork intestine)
Drinking unpasteurized contaminated milk
Drinking contaminated water
Touching infected cattles, pigs and birds
Hemochromatosis

Symptoms of Yersinia enterocolitica include:

Nausea
Vomiting
Abdominal pain
Fever
Watery bloody diarrhea
Lymphadenopaty (enlarged nodes)
Joint pain
Skin rash (erythema nodosom) etc.

Evaluations of Yersinia enterocolitica include:

History and physical examination
Temperature
Blood pressure
Pulse
Respiratory rate
Oxygen Saturation
Stool culture
Stool leukocytes
Stool ova and parasites
Stool toxin
CBC
Complete metabolic-chemistry profile
Serum ferritin
Blood culture
HIV blood test
Erythrocyte sedimentation rate
ANA
Rheumatoid factor
PPD (TB test)
Abdominal CT scan
Abdominal sonogram
Chest x-ray
Gastroenterology consultation to a colonoscopy
Infectious disease consultation

Treatments of Yersinia enterocolitica include:

Intravenous fluid with Normal saline plus 20MEQ of potassium in each liter at 150cc per hour   or
Normal saline with D5W plus 20 MEQ of potassium in each liter at 150cc per hour
                                        or
Ringer's lactate at 150cc per hour
Zofran 4mg IV every 8 hours as needed for nausea and vomiting or Compozine 10mg every 6 hours as needed for nausea and vomiting
Ceftriaxone 1 gram IV every 12 hours or Levaquin 500mg IV or by mouth every 24 hours or Bactrim DS twice per day.

Prevention of Yersinia enterocolitica includes:

Wash hands with soap and water after using the bathroom
Don't eat undercooked meat
Don't drink unpasteurized milk
Wash hands with soap and water after touching raw meat
Wash hands with soap and water after handling pigs, cattles, and birds
Refrain from eating chitterlings.

CHAPTER 35

CLOSTRIDIUM DIFFICILE GASTROENTERITIS IN AFRICAN AMERICAN MEN

Clostridium Difficile diarrheal disease/gastroenteritis is a very common infection that results from taking some antibiotics and nosocomially. In addition the infection can also develop when a person is exposed to individuals carrying the bacterium in their bowels. There are 500,000 C. Difficile infections annually in the U.S.

The C. Difficille bacterium is found in the air, soil, water, human feces, animal feces and different food products and many contaminated materials and medical instruments. Once it enters the GI tract through the mouth it multiplies and replaces the natural bacterial flora of the person bowel. C. Difficile bacteria produce large quantity of toxin A an B into the bowel causing severe swelling of the bowel resulting in profuse diarrhea, abdominal and fever etc.

Three million or 25% C. Difficile infections occur in hospitals every year in the U.S. 20% of C. difficile infection occurs in nursing home and 20,000 or 55% C. Difficile infections occur in community settings in the U.S. every year. 14,000 people die from C. Difficile infection every year in the U.S.

Millions of people get infected with C. Difficile around the world every year and many thousands of them die as a result of C. Difficile diarrheal illness.

Many people both children and adults carry the C. Difficile organism in their colon as carriers and never get sick.

The facilitities where the C. Difficile organism is found include:

Hospitals
Extended care facilities
Nursing homes
Nurseries
Community centers
Neighborhood health centers
Living in the communities (about 32% of community based C. Difficile infection had

some contact with health care facilities in recen

The materials that are frequently contaminated with C. Difficile spores include:

Furnitures
Linens
Bedpans
Toilets seats
Floors
Hands
Telephones
Rings
Stethoscopes
Diaper pails etc.

The most common antibiotics that have been known to cause C. Diffficile diarrheal disease/gastroenteritis and pseudomembrenous colitis include:

Clindamycin
Amoxicillin
Ampicillin
Cephalosporins/Keflex
Bactrim
Cipro
Penicillin
Erytrhomycin
Levaquin etc; (all antibiotics can cause C. Difficile infection)

The majority of C. difficile infections that occur in the community occur because of the tremendous amount of antibiotics prescribed in communities in the U.S. Health care professionals prescribe 258 million courses of antibiotics every year in the U.S. outside hospitals every year and about half are unnecessary.

Other risk factors for C. Difficile colitis include Ulcerative colitis and Crohn's disease with no exposure to antibiotics. HIV/AIDS, non-acquired immunodeficiency diseases, Cancer, Radiotherapy, and chemotherapy.

Symptoms of C. Difficile diarrheal/gastroenteritis include:

Fever
Chills
Diarrhea
Constipation
Nausea
Loss of appetite
Weight loss

Abdominal cramps/pain
Dehydration
Electrolytes imbalance

Evaluations for C. Difficile diarrhea include:

History and physical examination
Temperature
Blood pressure
Pulse
Respiratory rate
Oxygen Saturation
Stool for C. Difficile toxin A an B
Stool culture
Xtag GPP stool test
Stool ova and parasites
Stool Gram stain
Stool leukocytes
Stool for enzyme immuno assay or
Stool for Polymerase chain reaction (PCR is the most sensitive test available to diagnose
C. Difficile infection). or
Stool for Cell cytotoxicity)
Blood culture
CBC
Complete metabolic /chemistry profile
Urinalysis
Urine culture
Chest x-ray
Abdominal CT scan
EKG
Flexible sigmoidoscopy
Colonoscopy etc;

A negative A and B toxin for C. Difficile does not rule out C. colitis therefore, it is necessary to sigmoidoscopy or colonoscopy to document colitis/pseudocolitis.

In addition, it is not necessary for some one to have diarrhea for the suspicion of C. Difficile infection to be arisen.

People can develop sepsis with high fever due C.difficile infection and be constipated. It is prudent always to check for C. Difficile infectionin anyone with unexplained fever in the hospital.

Treatments of C. Difficile colitis include:

Stop the antibiotic causing the colitis
Intravenous fluid with Dextrose and normal saline plus potassium at 150cc per hour
or
Normal saline plus potassium at 150cc per hour
Ringer's lactate at 150cc per hour
Tylenol 325mg 2 tablets every 4 hours to keep temperature below 100
Vancomycin 250mg by mouth four times per day in addition to Vancomycin 500mg in 100cc of normal saline via rectum every 6 hours as retention enema
or
Flagyl 500mg IV every 8 hours

Fidaxomicin is more effective to treat C. Diff because it is bacteriocidal as compared to Flagyl andVancomycin, that are Bacteriostatic. Recurrence of C. Difficile infection occurs less often in patients with non-NAP strains of C. Dificile bacterium.

The dose of Fidaxomicin is 200mg twice per day by mouth for 10 days. Fidaxomicin should be the antibiotic of first choice in C. Difficile colitis.

The FDA has approved Zinplava 10mg /kg IV over 1 hour to treat C. Diff colitis. Zinplava (bezlotoxumab is a monoclonal antibody.

Stool transplantation ("While the standard antibiotic treatment cured 27% of patients in the trial, fecal transplants cured 94 %") Source: Einstein connection; Issue 45, Jan 30, 2013.

Probiotics are extremely important in the treatment of C. Difficile infection VSL #3 1 cap three times per day or Florastor 250mg by mouth twice per day work to re-populate the bacteria flora of the bowel thereby improving the C. Difficile infection.

Complications of C. Difficile colitis include:

Dehydration
Low blood pressure
Electrolytes imbalance
Kidney failure
Disseminated intravascular coagulopathy
Megacolon
Perforation of the bowel
Peritonitis
Death

Prevention of C. Difficile colitis includes:

Wear mask, gown, and gloves to the rooms of patients with C. Difficille colitis
Disinfection of stethoscopes after examining patients with C. Dificille colitis is mandatory
Wash hands with soap and water
Use antibiotics only when necessary
Retest stools of people recently treated for documented C. Difficile for several months/
Avoid using the same toilets with people being treated for C. Difficile colitis or recently
treated for C. Difficile colitis. If at all possible avoid residing in adults home, nursing home
and all other crowded residential facilities.
Twenty percent of C. Difficile infection recurs and have to be retreated.

CHAPTER 36

VIRAL GASTROENTERITIS IN AFRICAN AMERICAN MEN

Viral diarrheal disease/stomach flu is quite common. The viruses that frequently cause diarrheal disease/Gastroenteritis include: Norvovirus (responsible for 50% to 70% of all gastroenteritis in adults and is the most common cause of gastroenteritis in the U.S.) Source CDC

Norvovirus (Norwalk virus)

Every year norvovirus cause 21 million cases of gastroenteritis in the U.S. Every year norvovirus causes 70,000 hospitalizations and 500 deaths in the U.S.

Worldwide there are 90 million cases of norvovirus gastroenteritis every year resulting in 218,000 deaths annually.

Rotavirus

Worldwide 133 million people develop rotavirus gastroenteritis every year and in the U.S. there 3 million cases of rotavirus gastroenteritis. In the U.S. rotavirus causes 60,000 hospitalizations, resulting in 40 deaths.

Rotavirus gastroenteritis kills 1.3 million people in the world every year. 500,000 of them are children.

Adenovirus
Calcivirus
Sapovirus

Viral gastroenteritis occurs through the oral fecal route, symptoms develop 1-3 days for Norvovirus and 1-3 days for Rotavirus.

Risk factors for viral diarrheal disease/gastroenteritis include:

Poor hand hygiene
Failure to wash hands with soap and water after using the bath room
Touching bath room door knob after using the bath room

Living in the same house with a person who has stomach flu
Living in crowded living facilities
Young children
School children
Day care workers
Children in day cares
Children living in developing countries
Adults living in developing countries
Being in the hospitals
Nursing homes residents
Dormitory residents
Being in cruise boats
Eating contaminated foods
Drinking contaminated water/fluids
Shaking hands
HIV/AIDS
Anal sex
Anal/ oral sex
Non-acquired immunodeficiency diseases
Cancer
Chemotherapy treatment
Radiotherapy treatment

Symptoms of viral gastroenteritis/stomach flu include:

Nausea
Vomiting
Abdominal cramps
Abdominal pain
Diarrhea
Fever
Chills
Headache
Muscles ache
Malaise
Weakness
Poor appetite
Dehydration etc.

Evaluations of viral gastroenteritis/stomach flu include:

History and physical examination
Blood pressure
Pulse
Temperature

Respiratory rate
Oxygen saturation
CBC
Complete metabolic-chemistry profile
Urinalysis
Stool culture
Xtag GPP stool test
Stool for ova and parasite
Stool leukocytes
Stool Gram stain
Stool for C. Difficile A and B toxin
Blood culture
Polymerase chain reaction (PCR) for individual viruses
Chest x-ray
Abdominal ultrasound
Abdominal CT Scan may or may not be necessary

Treatments of viral gastroenteritis/stomach flu include:

Intravenous fluid with normal saline and glucose plus 20 MEQ of potassium at 150cc per hours

or

Half normal saline and glucose plus 20 MEQ of potassium at 150cc per hour

or

Ringer's lactate at 150cc per hour
Zofran 8mg IV every 8 hours for nausea and vomiting

or

Compozine 5 or 10 mg IM every 6 hours
Pepto-Bismol 1 tablespoon every 6 hours as needed for abdominal cramps

Complications of viral diarrheal disease/gastroenteritis include:

Dehydration
Electrolytes imbalance
Hypotension (low blood pressure)
Cardiac arrhythmias
Kidney failure
Disseminated intravascular coagulopathy
Deaths.

CHAPTER 37

CHOLERA GASTROENTERITIS IN AFRICAN AMERICAN MEN

Cholera associated diarrheal disease/gastroenteritis affects 3-5 million people in the world every year and kills 100-120,000 every year. In the U.S. about 10 cases of cholera are reported every year, half of these cases are acquired outside of the U.S. Deaths are rare from cholera in the U.S. Source: WHO

More recently, 485,000 cases of cholera have been reported in Haiti and 6,700 deaths have been reported because of cholera. According to the U.N. the cholera in Haiti was brought to Haiti from peacekeepers from Nepal.

Cholera Vibrio is a gram-negative bacterium that causes infection of the small bowel trough fecal contamination of foods and water. "The Cholera bacterium releases a potent toxin (CTX) which binds to the intestinal wall, where it interferes with the normal flow of sodium and chloride. This causes the body to secrete enormous amounts of water, leading to diarrhea and rapid loss of fluids and salts. "Two 2 subgroups of Vibrio cholera cause dirrheal disease and there are V. cholera O1 and O139. Vibrio cholera O1 causes the majority of cholera outbreaks in the world.

The majority of people infected with Vibrio Cholera don't get sick even tough, they can transmit the infection to other people. About 10-20 percent of those who become infected develop full blown cholera diarrheal disease/gastroenteritis.

Risks of Cholera diarrheal disease/gastroenteritis include:

Living slums where there are many people with no running water, no bathroom facilities and poor sanitary conditions
Living in overcrowded camps
Consumption of fecal contaminated foods and water
Eating raw and uncooked shellfish
Raw fruits and vegetables
Surface water/well water
Contaminated grains
Travel to developing countries where Cholera epidemic is common
Reduced acid in the stomach (hypochlorhydria), The Cholera organism cannot survive

in an acidic environment)
Type O blood type

Evaluations of Cholera diarrheal disease/gastroenteritis include:

History and physical examination
Temperature
Blood pressure
Pulse
Respiratory rate
Oxygen Saturation
Stool culture
Stool Gram stain
Stool leukocytes
Stool ova and parasites
Stool toxin
Blood culture
CBC
Complete metabolic Chemistry profile
Urinalysis
T4 and TSH
HIV blood test
PT and INR
PTT
Chest X-ray
Abdominal CT scan
Abdominal ultrasound
EKG
Internal medicine consultation
Infectious disease consultation
Gastroenterology consultation
Cardiology consultation
Nephrology consultation

The symptoms of Cholera diarrheal disease/gastroenteritis include:

Watery diarrhea
Nausea
Vomiting
Dehydration
Fever
Seizures
Muscle cramps
Lethargy
Extreme thirst

Sunken eyes
Low blood pressure
Low urine output
Electrolytes imbalance
Cardiac arrhythmia
Sock
Disseminated intravascular coagulopathy (DIC)

Complications of Cholera diarrheal disease/gastroenteritis include:

Hypoglycemia (low blood sugar)
Hypocalcaemia (low serum potassium)
Kidney failure etc
Treatments of Cholera diarrheal disease/gastroenteritis include:
Salty water solution by mouth
Intravenous fluid with Normal Saline plus 20 MEQ of potassium chloride in each liter at 200cc per hour   or
Intravenous fluid with Normal saline and glucose plus 20 MEQ of potassium in each liter at 200cc per hour   or
Intravenous Ringer Lactate at 200cc per hour

Antibiotics in use to treat cholera include:

Doxycycline 300mg single dose adults
Tetracycline 500mg three times per day for 3 days for adults
Trimethoprim/sulfamethoxazole 160 mg for adult
Azithromax 500mg adults
Tetracycline 12.5mg/kg three times per day children
Trimethoprim/sulfamethoxazole 5mg/gk children
Zithromax 250 mg children

Anti-emetics:

Zofran 4mg every 8 hours IV or by mouth as needed for nausea and vomiting
Compozine 10mg by mouth every 6 hours as needed for nausea and vomiting

Anti-pyretic s (anti- fever)

Tylenol 325mg 2 tablets every 4 hours for fever
Aspirin 325mg 2 tablets every 4 hours as needed for fever
Advil 1 tablet every 8 hours as needed
Motrin 400-600mg every 6-8 hours as needed
Don't use Motrin, Advil or Aspirin if the kidney has failed or if there is bleeding.
Prevention of Cholera diarrheal disease/Gastroenteritis includes:
Wash hands thoroughly with water and soap after using the bathroom

Drink only bottled water

Don't drink water unless you boiled it yourself

Don't eat uncooked fish of any kind

Don't eat shellfish

Eat foods that are completely cooked

Don't eat foods from street vendors.

Make sure your physician gives you prescriptions for Tetracycline, Doxycycline, Bactrim or Zithromax and Zofran to carry with you when you travel to developing countries where the incidence Cholera is high.

When there, follow all the suggestions above

When you return, even if you don't feel sick, see a physician to have your stool cultured for Cholera.

CHAPTER 38

CROHN'S DISEASE IN AFRICAN AMERICAN MEN

Cronh's disease is a chronic inflammatory immune disease of the gastrointestinal tract. 700,000 people in the U.S. have Crohn's disease and worldwide and more than five million people have Crohn's and crohn is very common in Men.

Crohn's disease can affect all parts of GI tract and many other parts of the can be affected by Crohn's disease.

The signs and symptoms of Crohn's disease include:

Diarrhea
Bloody diarrhea
Abdominal pain
Abdominal cramps
Bloating
Nausea
Vomiting
Intestinal obstruction
Poor appetite
Fatigue
Weight loss
Fever
Iron deficiency anemia
Malabsorption
Vitamin B12 deficiency
Folic acid deficiency

Extra GI conditions that can be seen in Crohn's disease include:

Osteoporosis
Arthritis
Skin rashes
Pyoderma Gangrenosum
Erythema nodosum
Liver diseases

Inflammation of the eye
DVT
Pulmonary embolism
Kidney stones etc;
Examples of Pyoderma Gangrnosum skin lesions in a person with Crohn's disease

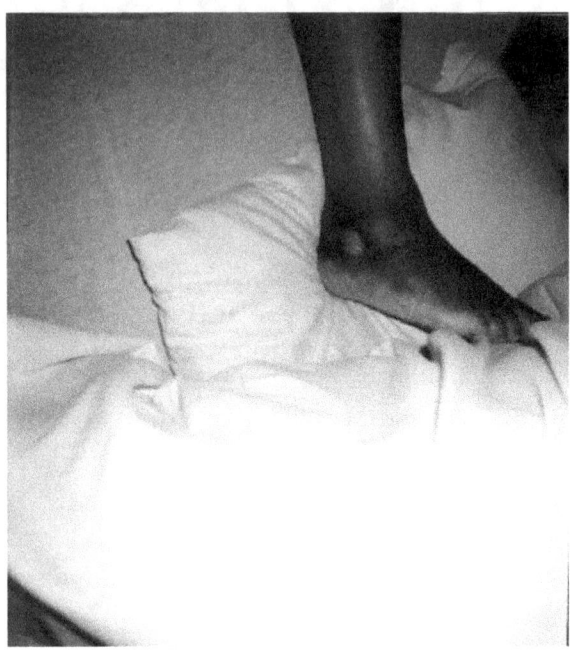

Figure 38:1

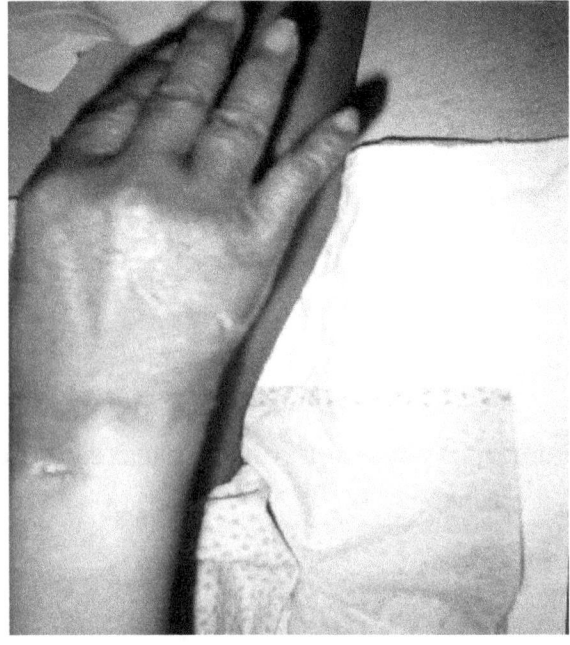

Figure 38:2

Risk factors for Crohn's disease include:

Being of European ancestry
Being of Jewish ancestry (Jews are 3-6 times more likely to have Crohn's disease as compared to other racial groups.)
People who have family history of Crohn's disease
Tobacco smoking
Living in industrialized countries
Being obese
Eating diets rich in saturated fat, sugar
Eating a diets low in fruits and vegetables etc;

Evaluations of Crohn's disease include:

History and physical examination
CBC
Complete chemistry profile
Urinalysis
Serum ferritin
Serum B12
Serum folate level
Vitamin D3 level
Lipid profile
ANA
ESR
Chest-ray
EKG
Abdominal ultrasound
Abdominal CAT Scan
Sigmoidoscopy
Colonoscopy
Barium enema
UGI series
Endoscopy
Capsule endoscopy

Complications of Crohn's disease include:

Intestinal obstruction
Narrowing of the intestine
Abscesses of the colon
Fistula of the colon
Colon cancer
Toxic megacolon
Sepsis

Iron deficiency anemia
Anemia of chronic diseases
Malabsorption
B12 deficiency
Folic acid deficiency
Malnutrition
Poor appetite
Weight loss
Arthritis
Liver diseases
Vitamin D deficiency
Osteoporosis
Gallstones
Infection of the eyes
Ulcers in the mouth
Dental cavities
DVT
Pulmonary embolism
Pyoderma Gangrenosum
Erythema nodosum
Depression
Erectal dysfunction
Menstrual irregularities
Hematuria from kidney stones
Spntaneous abortion etc;

Treatments of Crohn's disease include:

Asacol
Azaulfidine
Steroid
Imuran
Humira
Methotrexate
Remicade
Mesalamine
Cimzia
Cyclosporine
Diphenoxylate
Loperramide
Psyllium
The FDA has just approved Entyvio (vedolizumad) to treat Crohn's disease
When there is infection of the bowel

Appropriate history and physical examination ought to be done including:

CBC
Blood culture
Stool culture
Stool for C. Difficile toxin A and B
Stool for Ova and parasites
Complete chemistry profile
Serum amylase
Serum lipase
Urinalysis
Abdominal CAT Scan
Intravenous Fluid with Normal saline and D5 W with potassium
Cipro IV or by mouth
Flagyl IV or by mouth
Levaquin IV or by mouth
Bactrim IV or by mouth
Ceftriaxone IV
B12 IV or sublingual
Folic acid 1 mg by mouth daily
B-complex vitamin 1 tablet daily
Vitamin D 2000 Units daily
Surgical Consultation when necessary
Psychiatric consult.

CHAPTER 39

ULCERATIVE COLITIS IN AFRICAN AMERICAN MEN

Ulcerative colitis is an immune inflammatory chronic disease of the large bowel.

Worldwide 5 million people have ulcerative colitis and 620,000 people in the U.S. have ulcerative colitis.

It affects men very commonlly and tends to run in families. Ulcerative colitis affects people of all ethnicity, but the disease tends to be more prevalent in people of Jewish descent.

Ulcerative colitis causes inflammation and ulcers in the lining of the colon and rectum.

Symptoms of ulcerative colitis include:

Abdominal pain
Abdominal cramps
Abdominal bloating
Bloody diarrhea
Pain during bowel movements
Weight loss
Fatigue
Loss appetite
Rectal bleeding
Iron deficiency anemia
Weakness
Depression etc;

Extra GI signs and symptoms of ulcerative colitis include:

Arthritis
Ankolyising spondylitis
Sacroilitis
Arthritis of the spine
Uveitis
Iritis

Aphthous ulcer of the mouth
Pyoderma gangrenosum
Erythema nodosum
Autoimmune hemolytic anemia
Deep vein thrombophlebitis
Pulmonary embolism
Clubbing of the fingers
Primary sclerosing cholangitis
Skin rashes
Kidney stones
Osteoporosis
Liver diseases etc;

Evaluations of ulcerative colitis include:

History and physical examination
CBC
Complete chemistry profile
ESR
Urinalysis
Stool culture
Stool for ova and parasites
Stool for C. Difficile toxin A and B
Chest x-ray
Abdominal ultrasound
Colonoscopy
Anoscopy
Barium enema
CT of the abdomen
MRI of the abdomen
Gastroenteroly consult
Colorectal surgical consult
Psychriatric consult etc

Complications of ulcerative colitis include:

Rectal bleeding
Diarrhea
Intestinal obstruction
Abdominal pain
Abdominal pain
Fistula
Intra abdominal abscess
Fever
Chills
Sepsis

Infertility
Ileostomy
Ilioanal Anastomosis
Malabsoprtion
Electrolytes imbalance
Anemia
Weight loss
Loss of appetite
Gall bladder stones
Acute Cholecystitis
Blind loop syndrome
B12 deficiency
Osteoporosis
Kidney stones
Bone fractures
Depression etc;

Treatments of ulcerative colitis include:

Steroid
Entocort (enema)
Remicade
Humira
Imuran
Mercaptopurine
Cyclosporine A
Prograf
Methotrexate
Azathioprine
Azulfidine
Asacol
Rowasa
Canasa
The FDA has just approved Entyvio (veddolizumad) to treat ulcerative colitis.
Antibiotics are used when needed

The antibiotics in use to treat infections in ulcerative colitis include:

Cipro
Levaquin
Flagyl
Ceftriaxone
Fortaz etc;

Multiple different surgical procedures are done to treat ulcerative colitis in different individual cases.

CHAPTER 40

DIVERTICULOSIS IN AFRICAN AMERICAN MEN

Diverticulosis is a condition in which small pouches/sacs arise from the wall of the large intestine. These pouches/sacs develop more frequently in lower left part of the colon called the sigmoid. Each individual pouch/sac is called a diverticulum.

People who suffer from this condition is said to have diverticular disease.

Every now and again fecal materials cause erosion in the walls of diverticuli resulting in bleeding. Once an individual bleeds from diverticuli, he or she tends to have recurrent bouts of diverticular bleeding on and off.

Diverticular disease is more common in developed countries compared to underdeveloped countries. Diverticular disease begins to develop at age 40 and 50% of

People residing in industrial countries have diverticulosis after age 60.

"Diverticular disease of the colon is a common condition, and the prevelance increases with age, affecting up to 60% of persons older than 60 years. Approximately 4% of patients with diverticulosis will develop acute diverticulitis." Source JAMA July 18, 2017 Volume 318, Number 3

A diet poor in high fiber foods plays a major role in development of diverticulosis, hence the reason why diverticulosis is less common in the developing world where people eat a fiber rich diet and the reverse is true in the developed world where people eat a fiber poor diet.

Symptoms of diverticulosis include:

Painless rectal bleeding
Low red blood cells count (Anemia)
Low blood pressure
Shock
Rapid heart rate etc;

Evaluations of diverticular bleed include:

History
Physical examination
Rectal examination
Temperature
Blood pressure
Pulse
Respiratory rate
Oxygen saturation
CBC
Complete metabolic profile
PT/INR, PTT
Serum B12
Serum Folic acid
Chest x-ray
EKG
Bleeding scan
Colonoscopy
ABO blood typing and indirect coomb's screening

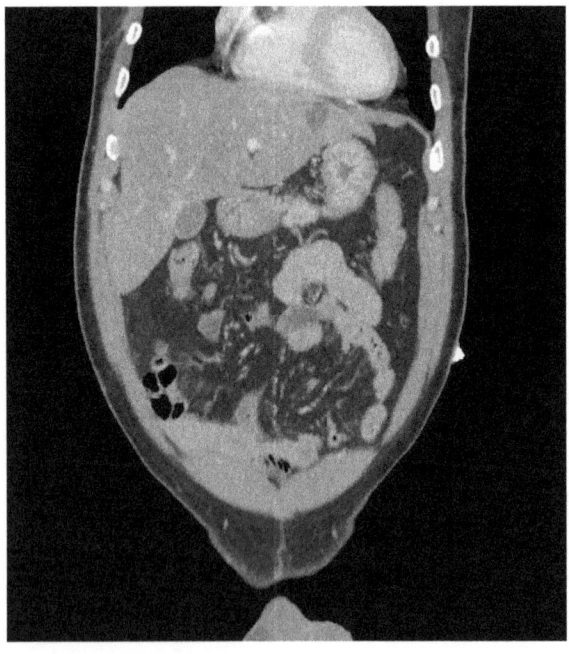

Figure 40:1 CT Scan of the abdomen in a person with diverticulosis

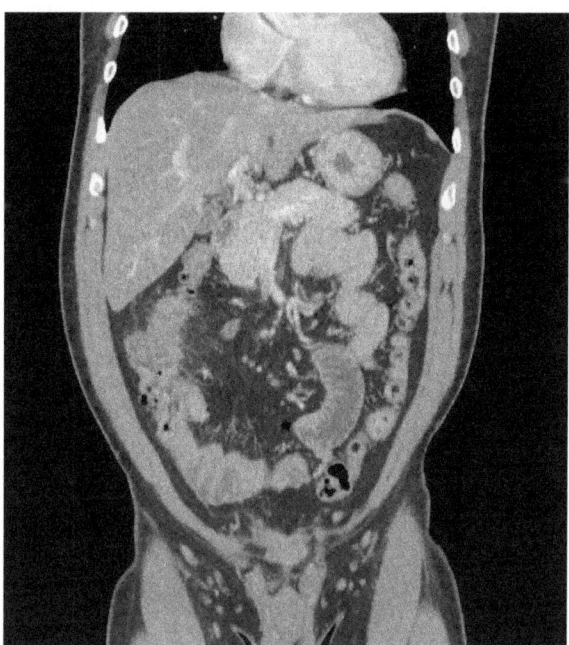

Figure 40:2 *CT Scan of the abdomen in a person with diverticulosis*

Treatments of diverticular bleed include:

Intravenous fluid with D5/normal saline at 150cc per hour
Nasal Oxygen at 2 liter per minute nasal cannula
Transfuse with packed red blood cells if indicated for severe blood loss anemia.
Iron replacement medications

Prevention of diverticulosis/diverticular bleed includes:

Red meat free diet
Low far diet
High fiber diet
Diet full of poultry, fish, vegetables, fruits and grain
Diet free of seeds containing foods
Diet free of hot and spicy foods etc

Complications of diverticulosis include:

Lower GI bleeding
Acute blood loss anemia

Blind loop/bacterial overgrowth syndrome (anytime one sees a very high serum folic acid in an individual who had colon resection surgery, one must think of blind loop/ bacterial overgrowth syndrome, whereby bacteria eat too much B12 that get caught inside the blind loop resulting in very low serum B12 and very high serum folic acid.

If the man never had colon resection surgery and his serum folic acid is very high, then diverticular disease is most like present and is causing blind loop/bacterial overgrowth syndrome, because stools are accumulating inside diverticuli in the wall of the colon resulting in very low serum B12 and very high serum folic acid.)

Low B12 level
Very high folic acid level
Low blood pressure
Rapid heart rate
Rapid respiration
Shock
Acute kidney failure
Death

CHAPTER 41

DIVERTICULITIS IN AFRICAN AMERICAN MEN

Diverticulitis develops when diverticular pouches/sacks become infected because of stools entered inside them or otherwise cause them to become inflamed. 25% of people with diverticular disease develop diverticulitis.

Symptoms and signs of diverticulitis include:

Abdominal pain
Abdominal cramps
Fever
Chills
Nausea
Vomiting
Constipation
Rapid heart rate
Rapid pulse rate
Elevated white blood cells (WBC)
Elevated ESR

Complications of diverticulitis include:

Diverticular abscess
Intestinal perforation
Peritonitis
Sepsis
Death

Evaluations of diverticulitis include:

History
Physical examination
Rectal examination
Stool hemoccult
Temperature

Pulse
Respiratory rate
Oxygen saturation
CBC with differential
Complete metabolic chemistry profile
Serum amylase
Serum lipase
Urinalysis
Urine culture
Blood culture
Chest X-ray
Abdominal sonogram
Abdominal / pelvis CT scan with contrast by mouth and IV
EKG
Surgical consultation
Gastrointestinal consultation
ABO blood typing
Type and screen

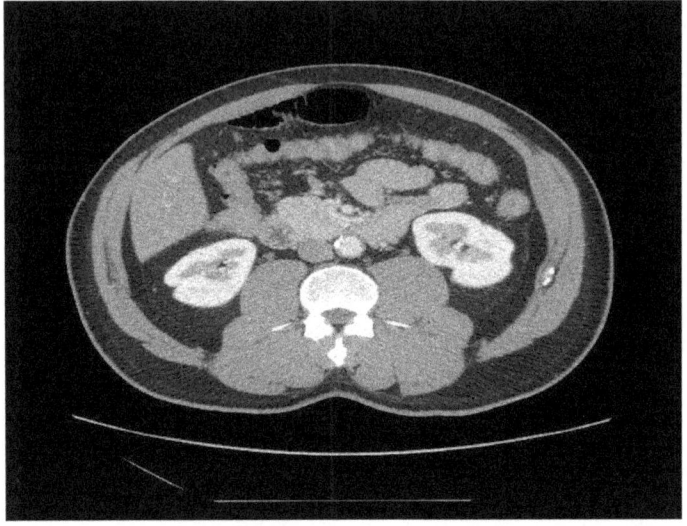

Figure 41:1 CT of the abdomen in a person with acute diverticulitis

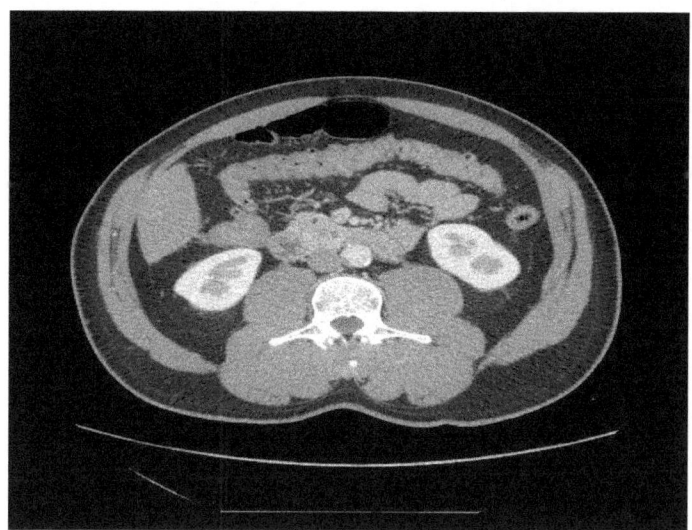

Figure 41:2 *CT Scan of the abdomen in a person with acute diverticulitis*

Treatments of diverticulitis include:

Intravenous fluid with D5/normal saline at 150cc per hour
               or
Normal saline IV at 150cc per hour
Nasal oxygen at 2 liter per minute nasal cannula
Transfuse with blood as needed for anemia
Ceftriaxone 1 gram IV every 12 hours, plus Flagyl 500mg IV every 6 hours
               or
Cipro 500mg IV every 12 hours, plus Flagyl 500mg IV every 6 hours
               or
Levaquin 500mg IV every 24 hours, plus Flagyl 500mg IV every 6 hours
               or
Zosyn 3.375 Gm IV every 6 hours

Prevention of diverticulitis includes:

Avoid eating popcorn
Avoid eating nuts
Avoid eating pumpkin
Avoid eating sunflower
Avoid eating Hot peppers
Avoid eating spicy foods
Avoid eating tomatoes
Avoid eating Zucchini
Avoid eating strawberries
Avoid eating raspberries

Avoid eating poppy seeds
Avoid eating cucumbers
Avoid eating red meat

When a person has diverticulosis/diverticulitis it is ok to eat
Bread
Beans
Whole grain
Cereal
Oatmeal
Poultry
Fish
Shrimps
Eggs
Seedless fruits
Seedless vegetables
Milk
Cheese

People who suffer from diverticulosis/diverticulitis ought to follow the advice of their physicians.

Complications of diverticulitis include:

Diverticular abscess
Sepsis
Shock
Kidney failure
Death

CHAPTER 42

ACUTE APPENDICITIS IN AFRICAN AMERICAN MEN

In the U.S. 680,000 people develop acute appendicitis every year and 1 in 500 people in the world develop appendicitis every year. Appendicitis occurs when inflammation develops in the vermiform appendix.

Signs and symptoms of acute appendicitis include:

Abdominal pain (RLQ) with rebound tenderness
Nausea
Vomiting
Fever
Constipation
Diarrhea

Evaluations of appendicitis include:

CBC
Complete metabolic chemistry profile
ESR
Serum amylase
Serum lipase
Urinalysis
Blood culture
Urine culture
Abdominal CT with contrast by mouth or IV
Chest x-ray
EKG
Surgical consult etc;

Treatments of acute appendicitis include:

Appendectomy
IV antibiotics (According to recent literature antibiotic treatment is just as effective as surgery to treat appendicitis)

IV Fluid with Ringers lactate
                    or
D5 W with normal saline
The best antibiotics to treat acute appendicitis are:
Ceftriaxone 2 grams IV every 24 hours and Flagyl 500mg IV every 6 hours
                    or
Zosyn 3.375 grams IV Q6h

    Complications of appendicitis include:

Ruptured appendix
Peritonitis
Appendiceal abscess
Sepsis
Septic shock
Kidney failure
Death.

CHAPTER 43

GALLBLADDER DISEASES IN AFRICAN AMERICAN MEN

Gallstones (or Cholelithiasis) are very common, about 25 million people in the U.S. have gallstones and several hundred million people worldwide have gallstones. There are three main types of gallbladder stones, and there are

Cholesterol stones -70%
Pigment (bilirubin) stones -20%
Mixed stones-10%
Roughly three fourths of all gallstones in the U.S. are cholesterol stones.

Gallstones are more common in African American men

About 800,000 cholecystectomies are done every year in the U.S. and worldwide several million cholecystectomies are done yearly. The death rates from gallbladder diseases in the U.S. are 0.20% and the worldwide death rates for gallbladder disease are very low as well. It is estimated that gallstone operations cost about $5 billions dollars every year in the U.S.

Risk factors for gallstones include:

Obesity
Fatty diets
Native Americans (most Native American men have gall stones by age 60)
Pima Indian women (80% of them have gallstones by age 30)
Being Hispanics
Being Northern Europeans
Genetics (the ABCG8/ABCG5 gene is highly associated with gallstones development)
Diabetes
Metabolic syndrome
Bariatric surgery
Chronic hemolytic anemia
Sickle cell disease
Beta thalassemia
Alpha thalassemia
Crohn's disease

Cirrhosis of the liver
Lipid lowering medications
Hormones replacement medications
Organ transplants
Acute changes in weights
Extended treatment with IV fluid
Use of cholesterol lowering medications etc;

Signs and symptoms of gallstones disease include:

Ninety percent of gallstones cause no signs and symptoms
Nausea
Bloating
Belching
Heartburn
Regurgitation
Dyspepsia
Right upper quadrant gnawing pain
Vomiting
Loss of appetite
Upper abdominal pain after eating fatty foods
Jaundice etc.

Evaluations of gallstones (cholelithiasis) include:

History and physical examination
Abdominal ultrasound
CBC
Complete chemistry profile
Urinalysis
Abdominal CT
Abdominal MRI
Surgical consultation etc;

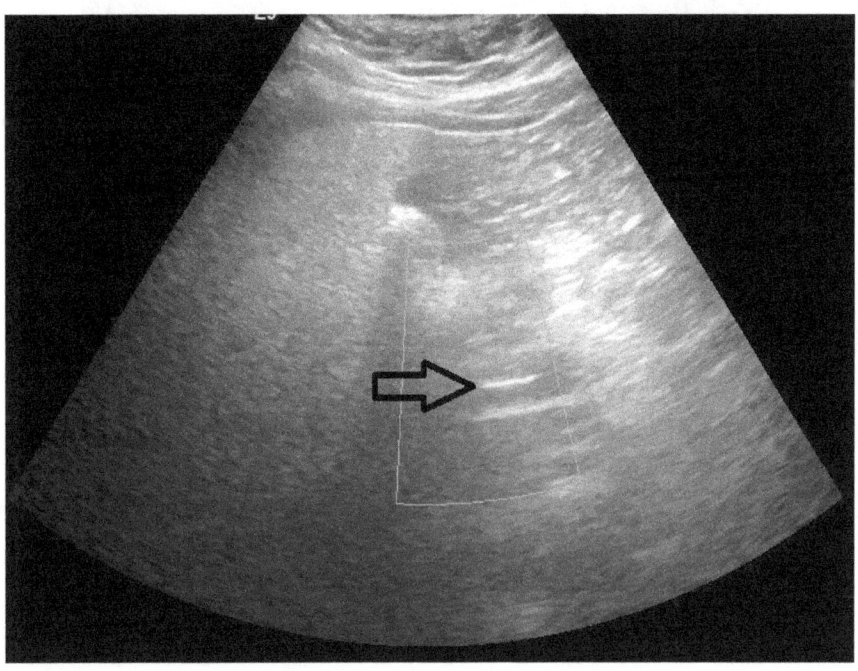

Figure **43:1** *Abdominal sonogram showing stones in the gall bladder*

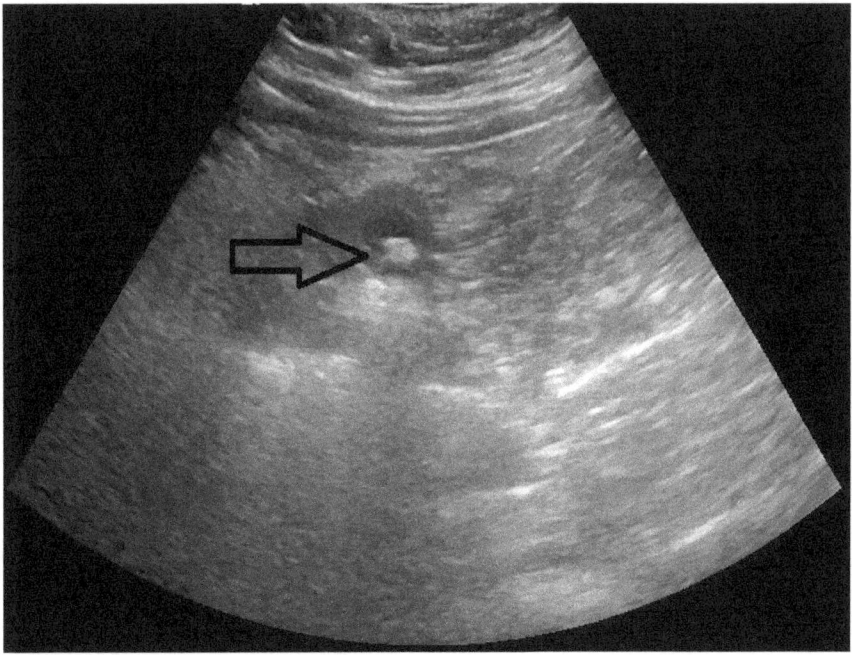

Figure **43:2** *Abdominal sonogram showing stones in the gall bladder*

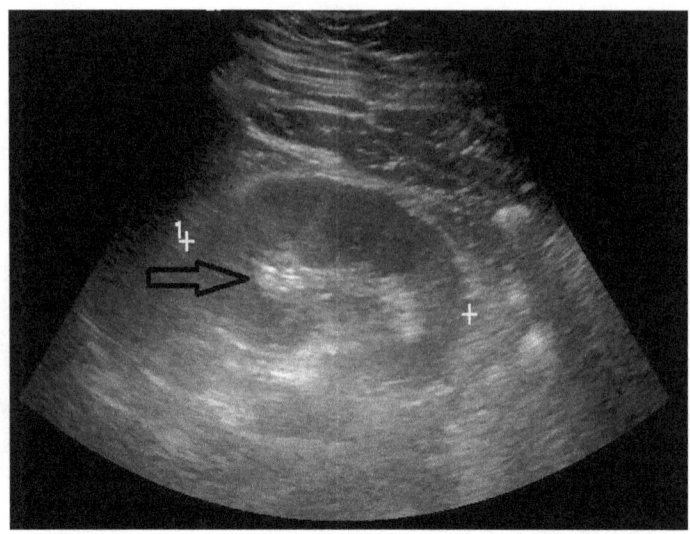

Figure 43:3 *Abdominal sonogram showing stones in the gall bladder*

Treatments of Cholelithiasis include:

Low fat diet
PPI or H2 blockers
Low alcohol intake
Cholecystectomy

Complications of gallstones include:

Acute cholecystitis
Common bile duct obstruction
Jaundice
Itchings
Clay colored stools
Acute gallbladder colic
Chronic cholecystitis
Acute pancreatitis
Chronic pancreatitis
Sepsis etc;

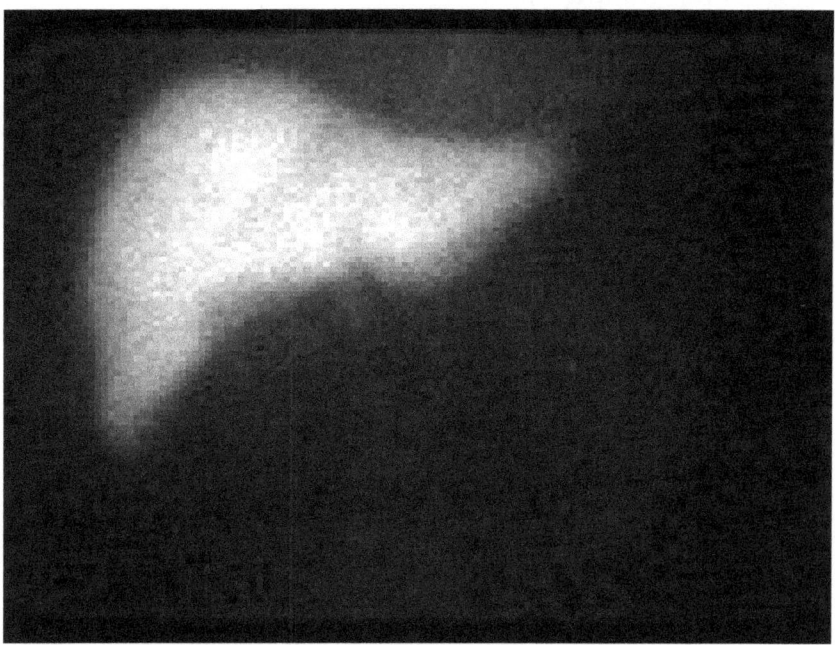

Figure **43:4** *Normally visualized gall bladder in a patient with gallstones Indicating that the gall bladder is not inflammed nor infected Ruling out cholecystitis.*

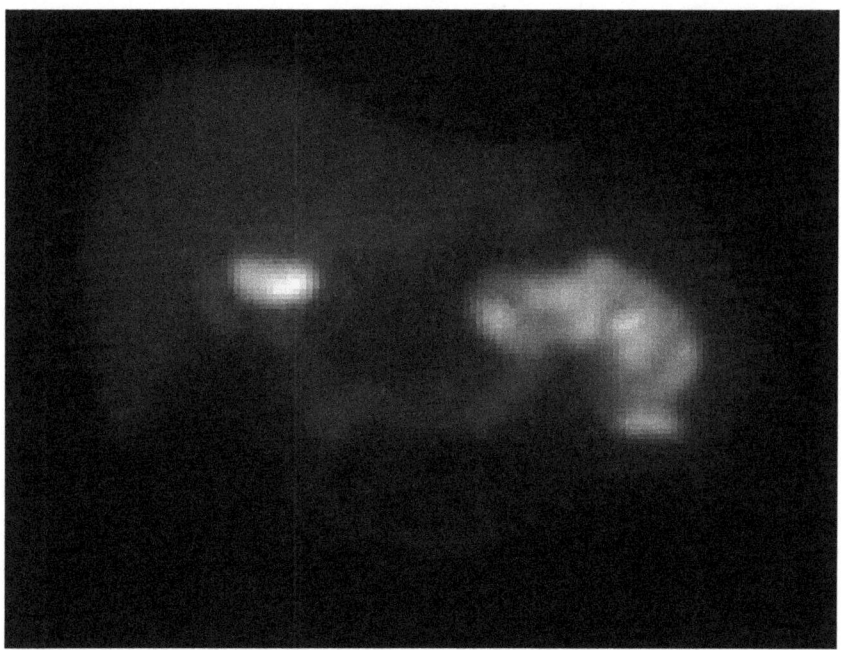

Figure **43:5** *Normally visualized gall bladder in a patient with gallstones Indicating that the gall bladder is not inflamed nor infected Ruling out cholecystitis.*

Prevention of gallstones includes:

Low fat diet
High fiber diet
Eating plenty of fruits and vegetables
Eating plenty of nuts
Decrease sugar intake
Decrease alcohol intaket
Increase coffee intake
Maintaining a good body weight
Weight loss
Xenical (use for weight loss)
Actigall.

CHAPTER 44

ACUTE CHOLECYSTITIS IN AFRICAN AMERICAN MEN

About ninety percent of acute cholecystitis is due to gallstones, and the prevalence of cholecystitis is same in the U.S. as it is in the rest of the world.

Signs and symptoms of acute cholecystitis include:

Right upper quadrant abdominal pain
Tenderness of RUQ on physical examination with rebound
Nausea
Vomiting
Fever
Chills
Jaundice
Itching
Clay colored stools
High white blood cells
High serum amylase
High serum lipase
High direct serum bilirubin
Swollen gallbladder with gallstones on abdominal ultrasound
Abnormal Hida scan

Evaluations of acute cholecystitis include:

History and physical examination
CBC with differential
Complete blood chemistry profile
Serum amylase
Serum lipase
Blood culture
Abdominal ultrasound
Abdominal CT
Hida Scan
Chest x-ray

EKG
Surgical consult

Treatments of acute cholecystitis include:

Broadspectrum IV antibiotics such as
Ceftriaxone 1 gram IV q12 hours
Plus
Flagyl 500mg IV q6h
or
Levaquin 500mg IV q 24 hours
Plus
Flagyl 500mg IV q 6 hours
or
Zosyn 3.375 grams Q6h IV
There are many more combinations of IV antibiotics available to treat acute cholecystitis in use.
Cholecystectomy
When the gallbladder is very infected and swollen, it is best to treat it with IV antibiotics for several days before surgery is performed.
IV fluid with D5 normal or ½ normal saline at 150cc per hour
or
Lacted Ringer at 150cc per hour etc.
Dilaudid 1mg IV q 4 hours for pain
Zofran 4mg or 8mg IV q 4 hours four nausea and vomiting

Complications of acute cholecystitis include:

Gangrene of the gallbladder (more frequently seen in diabetics)
Sepsis
Acute pancreatitis
Chronic cholecystitis
Chronic pancreatitis
Malabsorption
Low vitamin B12
High blood glucose
Death

CHAPTER 45

ACUTE PANCREATITIS IN AFRICAN AMERICAN MEN

Over 300,000 individuals develop acute pancreatic every year in the U.S. and worldwide several million individuals develop acute pancreatitis every year or 73.4 cases per 100,000 of acute pancreatitis occur yearly worldwide.

In the U.S. there are 275,000 hospital admissions for acute pancreatitis annually, costing 2.6 billion dollars every year.

Pancreatitis occurs when the tissues of the pancreas become inflamed.

The most common causes of acute pancreatitis include:

Alcohol abuse
Gallstones
Hypercalcemia
Hyperparathyroidism
Hyperlipidemia
Malnutrition
Hereditary pancreatitis
Abdominal trauma
Post ERCP
Penetrating stomach ulcers
Cancer of the head of the pancreas
Lasix
Thiazides
Vildagliptin
Gliptins
Saxagliptin
Sitagliptin
Linagliptin
Sulfonamides
Tetracycline
Estrogens
Salicylates

Mercaptopurine
Pentamidine
Azathioprine
Trimethoprim-sulfamethoxazole
Valproic acid
Viral hepatitis
Herpes zoster infection
Mumps
Cytomegaly virus
Coxsackievirus
Ascaris infestation
Chinese fluke infestation
Mycoplasma pneumoniae
Pancreas divism
Choledochocele
Fatty liver
Ischemia from bypass surgery
Pregnancy
Cystic fibrosis
Scorpion venom
Eating raw ackee etc;

Signs and symptoms acute pancreatitis include:

Left sided upper abdominal pain
Nausea
Vomiting
Diarrhea
Fever
Chills
Hiccup
Loss of appetite
Dehydration
Hypotension
Shock
Tachycardia
Respiratory distress
Elevated WBC
Elevated liver function tests
Elevated serum amylase
Elevated serum lipase
Elevated ESR
Elevated urine amylase
Electrolytes imbalance
Peritonitis

Sepsis
Pleural effusion
Respiratory distress
ARDS
Respiratory failure
Acute renal failure
Disseminated intravascular coagulopathy etc;

Evaluations of acute pancreatitis include:

History and physical examination
CBC with differential
Complete blood chemistry profile
Serum amylase
Serum lipase
Blood culture
ABG
Urinalysis
PT/INR
PTT
Chest x-ray
EKG
Abdominal sonogram
Abdominal CT
Abdominal MRI
Abdominal MRCP

Ranson Score was introduced in 1974 to evaluate the severity of acute pancreatitis.

At admission
"age in years > 55 years
white blood cell count >16000 cells/mm3
blood glucose > 10 mmol/L (>200 mg/dL)
serum AST >250 IU/L
serum LDH >350 IU/L"

At 48 hours

"Calcium (serum calcium <2.0mmo/L (<8.0 mg/dL)
Hematocrit fall >10 mmol/l
Oxygen (hypoxemia PO2 < 60 mmHg)
BUN increases by 1.8 or more mmol/L (5 or more mg/dL) after IV fluid hydration
Base deficit (negative base excess) > 4 mEq/L
Sequestration of fluids > 6 L "

The APACHE, Balthazar scorings and the Glasgow criteria are also very useful and helpful in helping physicians in the managements of patients with acute pancreatitis.
Fluid loss is a major problem in acute pancreatitis, not only from vomiting, but also from fluid accumulation in the retroperitoneal area of the abdomen.

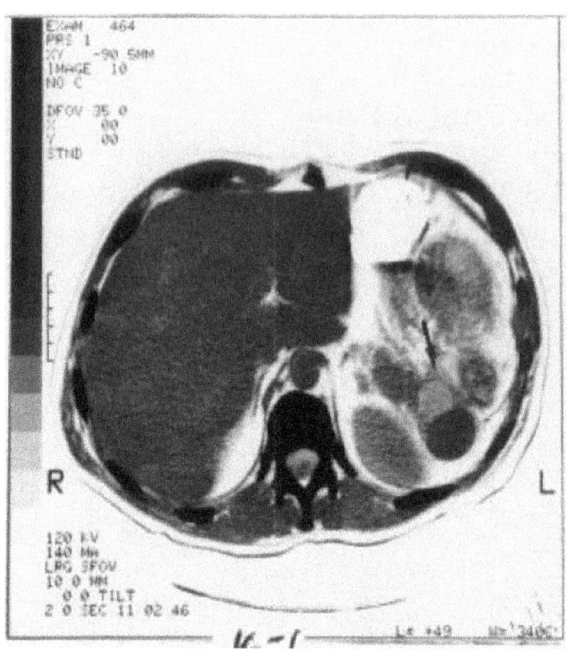

Figure 45:1–CT of acute pancreatitis. *CT of the abdomen showing acute pancreatitis with a pseudocyst of the pancreas (arrow showing swollen pancreas with pseudocyst).*

Treatments of acute pancreatitis include:

No foods by mouth
IV fluid that contains glucose and saline with electrolytes
Dilaudid or Morphine IV for pain (No Demerol)
TPN (total parenteral nutrition)
Nasal oxygen 2 liters per minutes if the PO2 is below 70%
Antibiotics that can be used include:
Levaquin IV 500mg every 24 hours
Cipro 400 mg IV every 12 hours
Ceftriaxone 2 grams IV every 24 hours
Meropenem 2 grams IV every 8 hours
Rocephin 2 grams IV every 24 hours
Zosyn 3.375 gram IV every 6 hours etc;

Complications of acute pancreatitis include:

ARDS
Multiple organs dysfunction syndrome
Hypoglycemia
Pseudo cyst of the pancreas
Pancreatic abscess
Splenic artery pseudo aneurysms
Splenic vein thrombosis
Superior mesenteric vein thrombosis
Portal vein thrombosis
Common bile duct obstruction
Hypovolemic shock
Kidney failure
DIC
Death

CHAPTER 46

CHRONIC PANCREATITIS IN AFRICAN AMERICAN MEN

Chronic pancreatitis occurs because of recurrent inflammation of the pancreas over several years.

Risks of chronic pancreatitis include:

Recurrent attacks of acute pancreatitis
Alcoholism
Gallstones
Malnutrition
Smoking
Cystic fibrosis
Hypocalcaemia
Hereditary etc;

Symptoms of chronic pancreatitis include:

Persistent upper abdominal pain
Nausea
Vomiting
Steatorea
Malabsorption
Diabetes mellitus
B12 deficiency
Weight loss etc.

Evaluations of chronic pancreatitis include:

History and physical examination
CBC
Complete blood chemistry profile
Serum amylase
Serum lipase
Serum B12 level

Serum folate level
Serum vitamin D
Serum ferritin
ESR
CRP
24 hours stools for fat
Abdominal ultrasound
Abdominal CT
Abdominal MRI
EUS
ERCP
MRCP
Chest-x-ray

Treatments of chronic pancreatitis include:

Cessation of alcohol intake
Low fat diet
Insulin treatment for high blood sugar
Analgesics for pain
Replacement of pancreatic enzymes
B12 injection
Surgical drainage of pancreatic abscesses
IV antibiotics to treat pancreatic abscesses

Complications of chronic pancreatitis include:

Abdominal pain
Malnutrition
Weight loss
Malabsoprtion
Steatorea
B12 deficiency
Folic acid deficiency
Macrocytic anemia
Vitamin D deficiency
Iron deficiency anemia
DVT
Pulmonary embolism
Diabetes mellitus
Stroke
Heart attack
Secondary hyperparathyroidism
Kidney stone
Oteoporosis

Pseudo cyst of the pancreas
Cancer of the pancreas
Diabetes mellitus
Pancreatic abscesses
Fever
Chills
Leukocytosis
Peritonitis
Sepsis
Shock
Kidney failure
DIC
Death

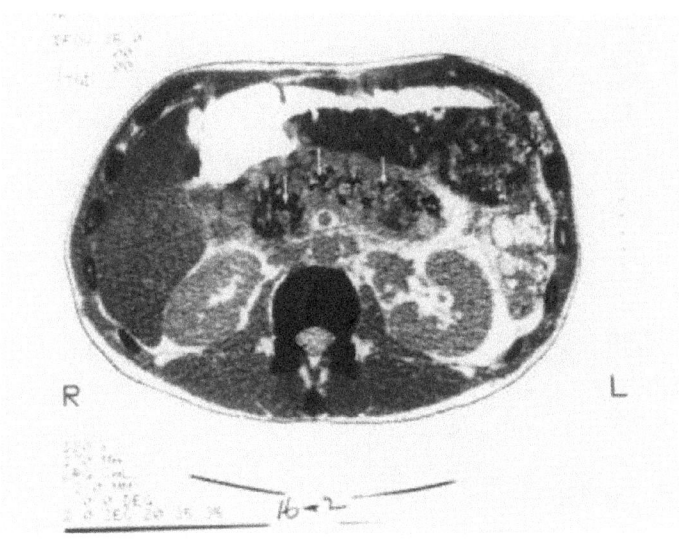

Figure 46:1–CT of chronic pancreatitis.

CT of the abdomen showing chronic pancreatitis with calcifications. Arrows showing swollen pancreas in a patient who abuses alcohol.

CHAPTER 47

HELICOBACTER PYLORI GASTRITIS IN AFRICAN AMERICAN MEN

H Pylori is gram-negative bacterium that infects the human stomach. H pylori gastritis is the number one nosocomial infection in the world. Fifty percent of the world seven plus billion people are infected with H Pylori. Thirty percent of the U.S. population is infected with H Pylori and seventy percent of New York City's population is infected with H Pylori.

H Pylori is brought into the GI tract via the fecal oral route through poor sanitation and eating or drinking contaminated foods and water and other liquids.

Risks of H Pylori infection include:

Living in developing countries
Visiting developing countries
Living in crowded houses
Sleeping on the same bed with a person infected with H pylori
Using the same bathroom with some one infected with H pylori
Husbands, wives, boyfriends and girlfriends infected with H pylori can transfer the infection to each other by sleeping on the same beds and using the same bathrooms.
Using the bathroom without using soap and water to wash one's hands.

Signs and symptoms of H pylori include:

Abdominal pain
Abdominal cramps
Nausea
Bloating
Belching
Gastritis
Peptic ulcer
Upper GI bleeding
Low-grade lymphoma
Iron deficiency anemia
Poor appetite
Chronic fatigue syndrome
Weight loss

Diffuse joints pain
Tiredness
Headache
Insomnia
Depression
Thrombocytopenia (low platelets)
ITP etc;

Evaluations for H. Pylori infection include:

History
Physical examination
CBC
Complete blood chemistry profile
LDH
Blood for H. pylori antibody
Stools for H. pylori antibody
Breathe test for H. pylori
Gastroenterology consultation
Endoscopic examination
Endoscopic biopsy of the stomach
Gram stain of stomach biopsy
Clo test (the gastric juice when tested goes from yellow to red, indication positive clo test for H. pylori)
When antibody is positive in the blood it can be either IGM, IGG or IGA
Complications of H. Pylori include:
Peptic ulcer (H. pylori is the #1 cause of stomach ulcer in the world)
Bleeding from the stomach
Iron deficiency Anemia
Weight loss
Poor appetite
Thrombrotic thrombocytopenic purpura (ITP)
Low platelets count
Lymphoma etc;

Treatments of H. pylori include:

Prev Pac (Lansopazole, Amoxicillin and Clarithromycin) for 14 days

Precautions to prevent H. Pylori infection include:

Avoid traveling to developing countries
Avoid eating fecal contaminated foods, vegetables and liquids
Wash hands with soap and water after using the bathroom
If one member of the household is infected with H. pylori, other members of that household should be tested for H. pylori.

CHAPTER 48

UPPER GASTROINTESTINAL BLEEDING IN AFRICAN AMERICAN MEN

—◦◦◦◦◦—

Upper GI bleeding is a common medical problem. Upper GI bleeding occurs in about 50 to 150 per 100,000 adults per year

The most common causes of upper GI bleeding include:

Peptic ulcer
Gastritis (due to alcohol abuse, Aspirin or NSAIDs ingestion
Chinese fluke infestation (the most common cause of hematemesis in the world)
Cirrhosis of the liver with portal hypertension
Esophageal varices
Cancer of the esophagus
Cancer of the stomach
Lymphoma of the stomach
AV malformation
H. Pylori infection (The number one cause of peptic ulcer disease in the world
Mallory Weiss tear
Meckle diverticulum
Bleeding disorders etc.

Signs and symptoms of upper GI bleeding include:

Dizziness
Shortness of breath
Rapid pulse rate
Upper abdominal pain
Nausea
Vomiting of blood
Black tarry stools (melena due acid mixture with blood down to the small bowel)
Pure blood in the stools (due to fast transit)
Anemia
Hypotension (low blood pressure)
Sock
Possible cardiac arrest and death

Evaluations of upper GI bleed include:

History
Physical examination, including blood pressure and pulse rate
Rectal examination
Occult blood testing of stools
CBC
SMA 20
Serum amylase
Serum lipase
H. Pylori antibody/antigen in the blood
PT/INR
PTT
Serum ferritin
Folic /B12 levels in alcoholic and cirrhotic patients
ABO type and screen
ABO type cross match
EKG
Chest x-ray
Endoscopic examination by a Gastroenterologist

Treatments of upper GI bleeding include:

1. Immediate IV access
2. D5 normal saline at 150cc per hour to maintain a good blood pressure
3. Blood transfusion
4. Nasal oxygen at 2 liter per minutes
5. Transfer patient to ICU
6. Cardiac monitoring
7. Monitor HCT several times per day
8. If patient was taking aspirin or NSAID, give DDAVP 20mcg in 50cc of normal saline over ½ hour to reverse the effect of the drugs on the pastient's platlets
9. Transfuse with platelets if the platelet count is low, as might happens in cirrhotic patients.
10. Treat patient with IV PPI or H2 blocker right away and continue this treatment daily
11. Treat with IV folic acid, magnesium, phosphorous, Thiamine, B complex vitamin, 1 Amp of 50cc glucose and 1 mg of Ativan. (This is the so -called alcoholic cocktail that must be given to all alcoholics who present to the ER. Do remember to always give the IV Thiamine before given the IV glucose to prevent acute Wernicke's encephalopathy.
12. Failure to do so will cause acute agitation, confusion, hallucination and combativeness in alcoholics. (Read chapter on alcoholism for more details.)

If the upper GI bleed is due to portal hypertension resulting from cirrhosis of the liver, then a beta-block ought to be given IV to decrease the portal pressure.

Frrous sultate treatment when the patient is stable.
Chronic treatment with PPI
Rarely is it necessary to treat peptic ulcer with hemegastrectomy in the developed world these days.
Other causes of upper GI bleeding are treated based on the underline causes.

CHAPTER 49

LOWER GASTOINTESTINAL BLEEDING IN AFRICAN AMERICAN MEN

Lower GI bleeding occurs in about 20 to 30 per 100,000 per year and the U.S. lower GI bleeding causes about 300, 000 hospitalizations per year.

The most common causes of lower GI bleeding include:

Hemorrhoids
Ana fisure
Crohn's disease
Ulcerative colitis
Angiodysplasia
Aortoenteric fistula
Diverticular disease
Diverticular bleed
Polyps
Cancer
Ischemic colitis
Cancer of the colon usually develops from polyps.
Cancer of the small bowel

The different types of polyps are:

Inflammatory polyps
Hyperplastic polyps
Adenomatous polyps (adenomatous polyps are usually pre-cancerous)

There are several hereditary polyps and the most common are:

Familial adenomatous polyps
Gardner's syndrome
MYH-associated polyps
Peutz-jeghers syndrome
Serrated polyps syndrome
Lynch syndrome

The risk Factors for colon cancer include:

Family history of colon cancer
Colon polyps
High red meat diet
Crohn's disease
Ulcerative colitis
Obesity
Smoking
Alcoholism
Type 2 Diabetes

Signs and symptoms of colon cancer include:

Occult blood in the stools
Rectal bleeding
Change in bowel habits
Constipation
Diarrhea
Abdominal pain
Bloating
Nausea
Vomiting
High RDW
Low serum ferritin
Iron deficiency
Iron deficiency anemia
Weight loss etc.

Evaluations of lower GI bleeding include:

History
Physical examination
Digital rectal examination
Hemoccult testing of the stools
Colonoscopy
Barium enema (if colonoscopy is not available)
Sigmoidoscopy
Abdominal CT
MRI of the abdomen
Angiography
Scoping of the small bowel
Capsule study of the small bowel
CBC
Serum ferritin

RDW
Complete chemistry profile
PT/INR
PTT
CEA
GI consultation
Colorectal surgery consultation
Capsule study of the small bowel etc;

Treatments of lower bleeding include:

Colonoscopy with removal of polyps
Cauterizing of bleeding site
Clipping of bleeding site
Sclerotherapy of bleeding site
Angiography with embolization of bleeding site
Surgery to excise the part of the colon that is bleeding
Surgery to excise cancer from the colon
Blood transfusion
Iron replacement treatment

CHAPTER 50

SMALL BOWEL BLEEDING IN AFRICAN AMERICAN MEN

Five per cent of GI bleed is due to small bowel bleeding.

The causes of bleeding from the small bowel include:

Angiodysplasia
Crohn's disease
Lymphoma of the small bowel
Adenocarcinoma of the small bowel
Aspirin ingestion
NSAIDs ingestion by mouth
Torodol IM
Meckle diverticulum
Cancer

Signs and symptoms of small bowel bleeding include:

Rectal bleeding
Melena (black stools)
Anemia
Midabdominal pain
Weakness
Dizziness
Low blood pressure
Rapid heart rate
Headache
Low red blood cell count (HCT/Hgb)
High RDW
Low serum ferritin
Low platelets count

Evaluations of small bleeding include:

History and physical examination
Rectal examination
Stools occult blood testing
CBC
Ferritin
RDW
Complete chemistry profile
Endoscopy of the small bowel
Small bowel series
Capsule endoscopy
Gastroenterologist consultation

Treatments of small bleeding include:

Blood transfusion
Ferrous sulfate replacement
Treatment with PPI
Treatment with H2 blocker
Surgery

CHAPTER 51

HIATAL HERNIA IN
AFRICAN AMERICAN MEN

Hiatal hernia is the result of a weakness/herniation that occurs where the esophagus enters into the stomach.

There are 2 types of hiatal hernias, the sliding hiatal hernia and the Para esophageal hernia. Roughly 60% of people 50 years and older suffers from hiatal hernia.

The most common causes of hiatal hernias are:

Obesity
Heavy lifting
Hard and frequent coughing
Violent vomiting
Hard sneezing
Stress
Straining etc.

Signs and symptoms of hiatal hernias include:

Heartburn
Gastroesophageal reflux disease (GERD)
GI bleeding (Para esophageal hiatal hernia) causes more bleeding than sliding hiatal hernia because in Para esophageal hiatal hernia the part of the esophagus involved remains fixed in one place to bath by gastric juice causing irritation and erosion of the gastric mucosa. On the other hand in sliding esophageal hiatal, the part of the esophagus involved slides up and down exposing it less to irritation and erosion by gastric juice resulting in less bleeding.
Iron deficiency anemia
Chest pain
Nausea
Vomiting
Abdominal pain
Dizziness
Headache

Evaluations of Hiatal hernias include:

History and physical examination
CBC
Complete chemistry profile
Serum ferritin
Endoscopy
Upper GI series
Abdominal CT
Abdominal Sonogram etc.

Treatments of hiatal hernias include:

Low fat diet
Decrease alcohol consumption
Sleeping upright with several pillows under upper chest
H2 blockers such as Zantax, Tagamet, Axid and Pedcid
PPI such as Prilosec, Protonix, Aciphex, Nexium, and Prevacid
Mylanta and Maalox are also effective to relieve the dyspepcia that hiatal hernia causes.

CHAPTER 52

GASTEOESOPHAGEAL REFLUX IN AFRICAN AMERICAN MEN

Gastroesophageal disease (GERD) is a very common medical condition. It occurs mostly in adults in their 60 to 70 years of age. Roughly 20% of people in the western world suffer from GERD. GERD develops when there is an abnormal relaxation of the lower esophageal sphincter resulting in gastric acid backing up into the lower esophagus.

The sings and symptoms of GERD include:

Heartburn
Regurgitation
Sore throat
Pain on swallowing
Chest pain
Nausea
Vomiting
Chronic cough
Laryngitis
Laryngopharyngeal reflux
Pulmonary fibrosis
Asthma
Hoarness
Wheezing
Reflux esophagitis
Upper GI bleeding
Low serum ferritin
Iron deficiency anemia
Esophageal stricture
Barrett's esophagus
Adenocarcinoma of the esophagus etc

Causes of GERD include:

Obesity
Hiatal hernia
Zollinger-Ellison syndrome
Scleroderma
Elevated serum calcium
Chronic use of steroid
Chronic use of NSAIDs etc;

Evaluations of GERD include:

History and physical examination
Endoscopic examination
Upper GI series
Barium swallow
CBC
Serum ferritin

Treatments for GERD include:

Zantax 150mg twice per day by mouth
Axid 150mg twice per day by mouth
Pepcid 40mg daily by mouth
Tagamet 300mg twice per day by mouth

or
Prilosec 40mg daily by mouth
Nerxium 40mg daily by mouth
Prevacid 30mg daily by mouth
Protonix 4omg daily by mouth
Aciphex 20mg daily by mouth
Dexilant 60mg daily by mouth
Maalox 1table spoon 4 times per day as needed
Mylanta 1 tablespoon 4 times per day as needed
Low fat diet
Decrease alcohol consumption
Sleeping upright with several pillows under the upper chest
Vitamin B12 1000mcg sublingually daily or 1cc of B12 every 2-3 months IM
All individuals who are on chronic H2 blockers or PPI will require IM B12 or sublingual B12 on regular basis

Surgical treatments for GERD include:

Nissen fundoplication
FDA recently approved Laparoscopic magnetic sphincter augmentation with LINX device achieved GERD symptom control.

CHAPTER 53

ANEMIA IN AFRICAN AMERICAN MEN

The different types and causes of anemia in African Americam men include:

1. Sickle cell disease
2. Beta- thalassemia
3. Alpha-thalassemia
4. Sickle cell C disease
5. Sickle-Beta thalassemia
6. Hemoglobin CC diseases
7. Hemoglobin AC diseases
8. Chronic diseases anemia
9. Mixed collagen vascular diseases
10. Poverty
11. Malnutrition
12. Parasitic infestation
13. Iron deficiency
14. Cirrhosis of the liver
15. Lead poisoning
16. Iron deficiency
17. Vitamin B12 deficiency
18. Folic acid deficiency
19. Scleroderma
20. Kidney failure
21. Alcoholism
22. Intravenous Drug abuse
23. Hepatitis C
24. Hepatitis B
25. Cirrhosis of the liver
26. AIDS
27. Hemochromatosis
28. Lupus
29. Arthritis
30. Cancer
31. Sarcoidosis
32. Endocarditis

33. Diverticulosis
34. Gastrointestinal bleeding
35. Auto immune hemolytic anemia etc;

Five percent of the world population carries the genes for sickle disease and thalassemia. Each year 300,000 babies are born with sickle cell disease in the world.

Two million five hundred thousands black Americans carry the gene for sickle cell anemia and have sickle trait and about 100.000 black Americans have sickle disease.

Anemia is more common in certain racial groups than others because of the fact that some racial groups suffer more from conditions such as abnormal hemoglobin, poverty, and parasitic infestation, AIDS etc;

The racial groups that more affected by anemia include:

Blacks
Greeks
Italians
Asians
South East Asians
Indians
Middle Easterns

What is anemia?

Anemia is a condition in which the human body has low concentration of red blood cells.

Why is too little blood bad for the body?

Low concentration of red blood cells is bad for the body because red blood cells are needed to carry oxygen to all the organs in the body for proper body functioning.

When an individual is anemic, the different organs in the body are deprived of the proper amount of oxygen, resulting in the condition referred to as anoxia. An anoxic organ can become sick because of oxygen deficiency. Red blood cells contain a substance called hemoglobin and hemoblobin is needed to carry oxygen.

Hemoglobin has as its function to bind with oxygen in order to carry it to the different places in the human body where it is needed.

There exists an invisible man-conceived curve in the human body called the Oxygen Dissociation Curve. When the right amount of oxygen is present in the blood, this curve is well balanced in the middle and is shifted to the right to deliver oxygen to the tissues. When something happens that causes anemia to develop, the end result is that the red blood cells hold onto oxygen, and the curve is shifted to the left, resulting in the inability of the red cells to discharge their content of oxygen to the different tissues of the body, resulting in improper perfusion of the tissues with oxygen.

The Oxygen Dissociation Curve is influenced by the pH of the blood and the concentration 2,3-DPG(2,3-Diphosphoglycerate).

What are some of the symptoms of anemia?

To answer this question one must know how long the person has been anemic and how severe the anemia is. Normal hemoglobin in man is 14.0-16.0 grams and normal hematocrit in a man is 45% 50%.

The more acute the blood loss, hemolysis or inability to produce red blood cells the lower red blood cell count, which results in anemia and the less able an individual is to tolerate it. The younger the man who is losing blood is, the better he is able to tolerate the anemia. The older the person is who is acutely losing blood due to bleeding or hemolysis, the less well he is able to tolerate the anemia. Older people are more likely to have underlying medical problems, such as heart disease, kidney disease, hardening of the arteries in the brain, etc., making it easier for the anemia to complicate these already precarious conditions.

People who have had anemia for a long time are better able to tolerate their anemias because they have had enough time for their bodies to adjust to the effects of the anemia. In time, many of these chronically anemic people's vital organs, such as the heart, the brain, the kidneys and many other organs would be affected by the anemic state, but it would happen gradually.

The most common symptoms of anemia are weakness, malaise, headaches, shortness of breath, tiredness, irritability, depression, chest pain, menstrual irregularity, infertility, insomnia.

What conditions must exist in the human body before anemia can occur?

1. A person must be bleeding or must have bled.
2. A person must be hemolyzing red blood cells (that is, breaking up red blood cells in the body).
3. A person's bone marrow must have stopped producing red blood cells because of bone marrow failure, or
4. The bone marrow cavity is replaced by other cells, such as cancer cells etc., leaving little or no room for red blood cells to be made, or
5. The bone marrow may also be replaced by fibrous tissues such as occur in a condition known as myelofibrosis.
    Any combination of the aforementioned conditions interplaying at the same time can result in anemia.

There are three categories of anemia:

Normoproliforative anemia
Hyperproliforative anemia
Hypoproliforative anemia
Normoproliforative anemia occurs when a person is bleeding actively
Hyperproliforative anemia occurs when a person is hemolyzing
Hypoproliforative anemia occurs when a person's bone marrow is not making enough red blood cells.

What are the physical signs of anemia?

The signs of anemia are many and frequently coincide with the type of anemia the person is suffering from.

If a man presents to the emergency room or to the doctor's office and is acutely bleeding, from the rectum, or vomiting blood from an upper gastrointestinal tract or from the urinary tract, his pulse rate will be fast, his blood pressure might be low and he may shortness of breath, he be having chest pain and he may looks pale.

Severe and acute bleeding from any of these sites resulting in about 1800 cc of blood loss or more will likely cause a drop in the blood pressure.

The reason for the rapid heart rate/pulse rate is because the heart is trying to make up the difference by increasing the cardiac output in an attempt to help deliver enough oxygen for proper body functions. If the anemia persists for many years, the heart may fail because of what is called high output heart failure.

Other physical signs of anemia include:

1. Paleness of the skin
2. Pale nail beds
3. Pale conjunctivae in the entire human body the only place where naked vessels can be seen is in the eyes. By looking at the conjunctivae (the white of the eye) the examining physician can see blood vessels with the naked eyes and can tell if these vessels are pale, indicating chronic blood loss.
4. In addition, if the patient is hemolyzing different degrees of icterus in the eyes (yellowishness) can be observed by the examining physician. There are many other conditions having nothing to do with hemolytic anemia that can cause scleral icterus.
5. Rapid breathing
6. Flow heart murmurs, which is a function of the thinness of the blood as it passes through the heart valves.

Evaluations of anemia include:

History and physical examination
Complete blood count with differential
Complete blood chemistry profile
T4 and TSH
Serum ferritin
Serum B12
Serum Folic acid
Hemoglobin electrophoresis
Direct comb's test
Reticulocyte count
Bone marrow aspiration
Bone marrow biopsy

The reticulocyte count categorizes the type of anemia a person has and also directs how the anemia ought to be evaluated.

If the reticulocyte count is normal, it means that the person has a normoproliforative anemia or has anemia of chronic diseases If the reticulocyte count is high, it means that the person is hemolyzing If the reticulocyte count is low, it means that the person is not making enough red blood cells. The normal reticulocyte count is 0.5%-1.5%

Reticulocytes are young red blood cells that are one step to mature red blood cells they still have RNA in their cytoplasm. When peripheral blood smears are stained with Gram Giemsa stain, the RNA in the cytoplasm of youg red blood cells stain blue.

Laboratory technicians count 100 red blood cells on the peripheral blood smear and the number of stained reticulocytes counted among the 100 red blood cells is the percent of reticulocytes. About one percent of circulating blood are reticulocytes.

CHAPTER 54

IRON DEFICIENCY ANEMIA IN AFRICAN AMERICAN MEN

Men have iron deficiency anemia because gastrointestinal bleeding from ulcer, cancer of the esophagus, esophageal varices, cancer of the small bowel, meckel diverticulum of the small bowel, colon cancer, hemorrhoids etc;

As of 2017, the world had over 7.4 billion people. Thirty percent of the world population suffers from hunger. Hunger and malnutrition play a major role in high incidence of anemia. More than 2 billion people in world have iron deficiency anemia. WHO

Eight hundred and sixty eight million people in the world suffer from hunger and malnutrition in 2012 and Fifteen million children die every year because of hunger in the world. WHO

Fifty million people in the U.S. suffer from hunger including 1 in 6 adults and 1 in 5 children and fifty million Americans are getting food stamps. Source: USDA

People who migrated to the United States from regions of the world, such as South America, Latin America, Central America, the Caribbean, Africa and other tropical countries where the incidence of parasitic infestation is high are more likely to be infested with parasites.

Iron deficiency anemia occurs because blood is lost due to worms sucking blood from people's intestines. Parasitic infestation is a serious problem for black people, many of whom are surviving on a meager diet to begin with, while at the same time they are losing a significant percentage of their intake of nutrients to parasites that afford them no symbiosis in return. That is clearly an unfair deal.

Parasitic infestation occurs significantly in the rural South of the U.S. and people most affected are Black people working in the farms.

Many people abuse alcohol to a significant degree and alcohol abuse is associated with many conditions that can cause iron deficiency anemia. For instance, alcohol abuse frequently causes gastritis. The blood that is lost because of gastritis can lead to iron deficiency anemia when the gastritis occurs recurrently, as is often the case.

Alcohol abuse frequency causes esophageal varices with recurrent bleeding, and this too can cause iron deficiency anemia. Alcohol abuse frequently causes damage to the liver resulting in alcoholic liver disease (cirrhosis of the liver), which can cause stomach ulcer, resulting in iron deficiency anemia. The incidence of colon cancer is quite high in blacks in the U.S. and in the world, and one of the most common signs of colon cancer is iron deficiency anemia.

Drinking tea with food in the stomach can cause a person not to be able to absorb iron that is contained in the food, making iron deficiency anemia worse. The reason why drinking too much tea can contribute to low iron level in the blood is because tea contains tannic acid, and tannic acid binds the iron that is in the food, preventing its absorption from the stomach. So people ought to be aware that drinking tea is okay, but it is best to drink tea on an empty stomach.

Evaluate iron deficiency anemia include:

History and Physical examination
CBC
Reticulocyte count
Serum ferritin
Serum for H Pylori antibody
Stools hemoccult
Stools for Ova and parasites
Colonoscopy
Endoscopy
Small bowel capsule study (if colonoscopy & endoscopy are negative)

Iron deficiency as a disease has several stages:

Stage 1 is called prelatent iron deficiency
Stage 2 is called latent iron deficiency state or iron deficient erythropoiesis
Stage 3 is frank iron deficiency anemia. Each millimeter of blood contains 0.5 mg of iron

BLOOD SMEAR IN IRON DEFICIENCY ANEMIA

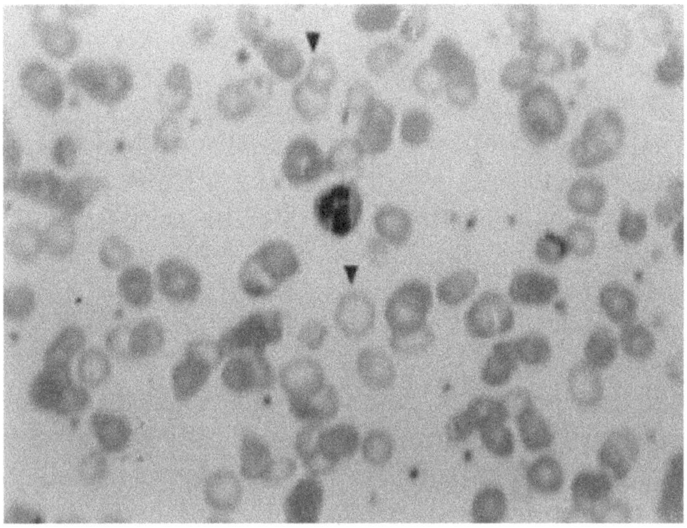

Figure 54:1–Peripheral blood smear showing hypochromic

It is said, according to the World Health Organization, that more than 2 billion people of the 7.4 billion people in the world suffer from iron deficiency anemia.

Iron deficiency is most probably much more common than the 2 billion reported by the World Health Organization for several reasons. Iron deficiency state is one of the leading diseases in the world in blacks. Iron deficiency state is defined as total body iron store depletion that leads ultimately to iron deficiency anemia.

Long before iron deficiency anemia comes about, the loss of blood, and the iron it contains, had already begun.

The first iron a man loses when he is bleeding slowly is the iron from the store, as reflected by the serum ferritin. Iron is stored as ferritin in the bone marrow, the muscles, the spleen, the liver, and other tissues of the body, including the iron that is located in the cytochrome system of the brain, which is needed for proper uses of oxygen by the brain to make the brain function well to carry the daily activities.

When *the iron stored is depleted, even before evidence* of anemia appears, people whose iron store is absent feel tired all the time, can't concentrate well, yawning a lot, become irritable easily, and feel overall unwell. An average size adult man has 2 grams of iron in his circulating red blood cells and 1.5 grams of iron his iron store as strage iron, for a total body iron of 3.5 grams.

The storage iron is manifeated as ferritin. 1 gram of iron is the equivalent of 4 units of blood, because each unit of blood contains 250 mg of iron. Once a man loses the entire iron store, as reflected by a serum ferritin of less than 10 to 15, and then he begins to use up the circulating iron for the production of red cells. As the level of the circulating iron decreases, iron deficiency anemia starts to set in, which gets worse and worse over time, resulting in low hematocrit, low MCV and low red cells per million and high RDW. At this juncture, he looks pale and feels very tired.

It is important for a treating physician to understand iron kinetics because it enables him or her to determine very early whether a person is slowly bleeding and losing iron. When an individual is bleeding slowly and occultly, the very first blood test to become abnormal is the RDW (red cells distribution width). The RDW becomes elevated when an individual begins to lose blood slowly. *The RDW is elevated in all diseases that cause microcytosis, such as thalassemias, iron deficiency anemia, and macrocytic anemias such as B12 deficiency, folate deficiency, and hemolytic anemias.*

The next blood test that becomes abnormal when a person is bleeding slowly and chronically is the serum ferritin. Ferritin is a phase 2 reacting protein and therefore can be falsely high in inflammation and infection. It is therefore prudent to always interpret the serum ferritin with this fact in mind.

Serum ferritin ought to be looked at as a scale, in that if the level of ferritin is going down, that represents blood and iron loss and the patient must be evaluated accordingly.

In the case of cancer of the GI tract, the decreased level of serum ferritin can be detected very early, sometimes as much as four years prior to the person becoming anemic or prior to the person having any symptoms that might make him or her suspect that he or she may have colon cancer. It is, therefore, important to test the stool for occult blood, which is mixed with the rest of the stool, making it difficult for the eye to see. It takes 25 cc of blood in the gut to cause the stool hemoccult to become positive.

The RDW comes with the CBC and, as just mentioned, is elevated in slow chronic bleeding. The serum ferritin test costs only about $44.00 in most clinical laboratories.

The normal ferritin level is from 10-320 ng/ml in men in most laborsatories.

When it is interpreted properly, the serum ferritin can help to save thousands of black men from dying as a result of GI cancer, because, by evaluating black man early, the doctor can remove the precancerous or cancerous lesion either endoscopically via biopsy or via colonoscopic biopsy or surgically.

Polyps do bleed and they bleed intermitantly and they bleed, the serum ferritin level begins to drop. Once it is noticed that the serum ferritin begins to go down from the normal rsange, it is time to investigate the reason why, waiting till anemia appears may be too late.

It takes about 3-5 years for a polyp to become cancerous. So, knowing iron kenatic and using this knowledge on a routine basis will help prevent patients from developing and dying from many types of GI cancers by diagnosing early.

A new test that is now clinically available called the soluble serum transferrin receptor level, which is much more sensitive to diagnosed iron deficiency anemia. This test is not affected by either infection or by inflammation. An elevated soluble serum ferritin level is firm evidence of iron deficiency anemia, even if the serum ferritin is normal or high. Iron is attached to the receptors in the transferrin protein to be carried to the early red blood cells in the bone marrow to produce new red blood cells. When there is no iron, these receptor sites remain unoccupied and, as such, their level is elevated, hence the value of this test.

Starting at age 40, Blacks and Hispanics ought to have a colonoscopy, because the incidence of colon cancer begins to develop at around that age in these groups. Blacks also have larger polyps and seem to have more right-sided colon cancer than do whites. Right-sided colon cancers are missed more often during colonoscopy than left sided cancers.

Other conditions that can cause iron deficiency Black men include:

1. Gastro esophageal reflux disease
2. Peptic ulcer
3. Chronic gastritis associated with ingestion of aspirin or nonsteroidal anti-inflammatory drugs or alcohol abuse
4. Diverticulosis
5. Inflammatory bowel diseases, such as ulcerative colitis, Crohn's disease
6. Bleeding esophageal varices
7. Chronic bleeding from the prostate
8. Chronic bleeding from the urinary bladder
9. Chronic Bleeding from hemophilia
10. Chronic bleeding from Von Willebrand's disease
11. Chronic bleeding from ITP
12. Chronic bleeding H Pylori gastritis
13. AV malformation etc;

What can people do to prevent iron deficiency anemia and what are the best ways to treat it?

1. A simple bleeding test from the tip of a finger done of aspirin for two weeks and of NSAIDS for 12 hours can help to determine if a man has Von Willebrand's disease or not. The normal bleeding time is up to 7 minutes. Von Willebrand's disease consists of qualitative platelet abnormalities which prevent platelets from aggregating properly, resulting in prolonged bleeding. A special Von Willebrand' disease complete profile test is available and very accurate to establish the diagnosis of Von Wllibebran's disease.
2. Von Willebrand's disease is the most common bleeding abnormality in the world, affecting several million individuals to one degree or another. Making the diagnosis can in most instances be quite complicated, so when this diagnosis is being considered, it is a good idea to refer the black men to a hematologist for both evaluation and treatment. Excessive vaginal bleeding, nose bleed, bleeding from the GI tract and

urological tract and, penis etc. due to Von Willebrand's disease is treated with 20 micrograms of Desmopressin (DDAVP) in 50 cc of normal saline IV over half an hour.

3. Blacks and other people from third world countries and African-Americans who reside in the rural South of the U.S. must have their stool tested for parasites, which, if found, can be in part responsible for chronic blood loss due to parasites attaching themselves to the wall of the bowel, sucking up blood, resulting in iron deficiency. Black men, who because of their living condition which place them at high risk for parasitic infestation. Those either lived in the third world before at one point in the past or in the rural South of the U.S. or who visited countries where they could have been infested with parasites, to have their stool checked by the parasitology laboratory for the possibility that parasitism may be partly responsible for their iron deficiency.

4. Still another contributing factor to iron deficiency anemia is drinking tea with one's meal. It is a small contributing factor to iron deficiency, but it is one, nevertheless. Tea contains tannic acid, which binds iron in the stomach, preventing its absorption. The best way for a person to drink tea is on an empty stomach or three or four hours after eating iron-containing foods to allow the stomach a chance to absorb the iron.

If the iron deficiency anemia is severe, sometimes, blood transfusion is necessary. Otherwise, iron deficiency is best treated with iron tablets by mouth. There are several iron preparations on the market such as Ferrous Sulfate, Ferrous Gluconate, Ferrous Fumarate, and Slow Fe, Corvite Fe 150 1 tablet per day, Multigen plus Caplets 1 tablet per day, Multigen Caplets 1 tablet per day and Ferrex Forte 150 1 tab daily.

For people who cannot tolerate iron because of nausea, diarrhea, and constipation or so severely iron deficient, Vonofer IV 100mg per day can be used.

In order to treat iron deficiency properly, patients must take one 325 mg tablet daily for one week with foods, then one tablet twice per day for one week, then one tablet three times per day. 180 mg of iron must be taken daily in order for 60 mg per day can be absorbed. Taking less iron than that, will not correct the anemia properly.

CHAPTER 55

HEMOGLOBINNOPATHIES IN AFRICAN AMERICAN MEN

―⊸⊸⊸⊸⊸―

Hemoglobinopathies are:

1. Sickle cell disease
2. Beta-Thalassemia
3. Alpha-Thalassemia
4. Hemoglobin C C
5. Hemoglobin AC
6. Hemoglobin SC
7. Hemoglobin sickle thalassemia
8. Hemoglobin persistent of hemoglobin F
9. Hemoglobin D
10. Hemoglobin E
11. Hemoglobin Lepore

Hemolytic anemias:

1. Autoimmune hemolytic anemia (warm types)
2. Cold agglutinin hemolytic anemia
3. Paroxysmal cold hemoglobinuria
4. Hereditary spherocytosis hemolytic anemia
5. Paroxysmal Nocturnal hemoglobinuria (PNH)
6. Drug-induced hemolytic anemia
7. G6PD associated hemolytic anemia
8. Cirrhosis of the liver (Hyperslpenism associated hemolytic anemia)
9. Thrombotic Thrombocytopenic Purpura (TTP) associated anemia
10. Disseminated intravascular coagulopathy (DIC) associated anemia
11. Blood transfusion reaction associated anemia etc;

HEMOGLOBIN F

Elevated Hemoglobin F can be seen in different abnormal hemoglobinopathies.

Sickle cell anemia
Beta-thalassemia
Hereditary persistence of fetal hemoglobin (HPFH)
Delta-beta-thalassemia etc.

In sickle cell anemia the level of hemoglobin F level varies.
In hereditary persistence of fetal hemoglobin is moderately elevated, but the hemoglobin A2 is normal and the MCV is also normal. The heterozygous and homozygous carriers are asymptomatic.

In Beta-thalassemia, there is a decrease in the synthesis of chain, resulting in a normal hemoglobin F level and elevated A2 level and low MCV.

In Delta-beta thalassemia there is a reduction in the synthesis of both and chainsynthesis with elevated hemoglobin F, normal A2 and low MCV.

HEMOGLOBIN C DISEASE

There exist a serious misconception in the literature regarding hemoglobin CC and hemoglobin AC. Nowhere in the text books of hematology and text books on hemoglobin is it mentioned that hemoglobin CC and hemoglobin AC cause anemia and SC disease.

The truth it both these conditions cause a microcrystal anemia with erythrocytosis.
I have large number of black patients in my practice with hemoglobin AC with microcytic anemia with erythrocytosis. To resolve this falsehood once and for all, here are the CBC, serum ferritin and quantitative hemoglobin electrophoresis of a 63 year black female patient in my practice with classic hemoglobin AC.

WBC 8.000
HGB 11.0 grams
RBC 3.990.000
HCT 31.4%
MCV 76.7
Serum Ferritin 78
Quantitative hemoglobin electrophoresis hemoglobin A 55.4% hemoglobin C 44.6%.

HEMOGLOBIN D

Hemoglobin D is an autosomal recessive variation of hemoglobin A that develops in the beta-globin chain of hemoglobin A. Hemoglobin D develops because of a substitution of glutamic acid for glutamine at codon 121 of the Bchain.

There are several variants of Hemoglobin D and they are:

Hb D Punjab (hemoglobin Los –Angelese, a substitution of glycine for glutamic acid at codon 121) Hb Ibadan (a substitution of lysine for threonine at codon 7)

Hemoglobin D is seen most commonly in people from:

India
Pakistan
Ireland
England
Australia
Holland
Iran
Turkey
China

Homozygous hemoglobin DD is rare and causes only mild symptoms with an enlarged spleen and a mild hemolytic anemia. Hemoglobin Beta thalassemia is a more severe form of hemoglobin D disease and causes moderate hemolytic anemia.

HEMOGLOBIN E

Hemoglobin E is a hereditary abnormality that occurs as result of a substitution of lysine for glutamic acid at position 26 of the B globin chain. This abnormality causes thalassemia to develop because of decrease in B chain.

Hemoglobin E thalassemia is seen most frequently in people from:

Vietnam
Cambodia
Laos
Thailand
Filipino
China
India
Turkey

Homozygous hemoglobin E causes slpeenomegaly and hemolytic anemia. Other hemoglobin E diseases include hemoglobin sickle/ E disease and hemoglobin E/B. Both these two types of hemoglobin E disease cause hemolytic anemia.

HEMOGLOBIN LEPORE

Hemoglobin Lepore occurs because of a cross over "between the delta and beta globin loci." Hemoglobin Lepore has 2 normal alpha chains and 2 delta fusion chains.

Hemoglobin Lepore is commonly found in people from:

Greek
Italy
Yugoslavia
Rumania
Turkey
Africa
Papua
India

Individuals who suffer with hemoglobin lepore have the same problems as those who have Beta-thalassemia and all its associated complications.

CHAPTER 56

SICKLE CELL DISEASE IN AFRICAN AMERICAN MEN

The genetic abnormalities that cause these different anemias are quite different and, as a result, the severity varies. The severest of these anemias is sickle cell anemia. About 8.0% of the Black-American population carries the sickle cell gene (sickle cell trait). This number is the same for Caribbean Negroes as well as Latinos and 300 million people worldwide have sickle cell trait.

Sickle disease affects million of people mostly in Africa, the Mediterranean and North America. Nigeria alone has about 4 million people with sickle cell disease.

A cardiologist from Chicago Dr. James Bryan Herrick and his intern Dr Ernest E. Irons first discovered sickle cell disease, the clinical entity, in the U.S. in 1910. They made the discovery in a 20-year-old black dental student named Walter Clement Noel studying dentistry in Chicago from the island of Grenada in the Caribbean. This biomolecular abnormality causes the red blood cell of the sickle cell patient to become sticky and deformed and develop into a half-moon or banana-shaped cell. The normal red cell is disc-shaped.

Only about 100, 000 Negroes/Black-Americans actually have sickle cell anemia, the homozygous type (full-blown sickle cell disease) and 3,600,000 have sickle cell trait. At birth, 1:625 Black-American babies born are expected to develop sickle cell disease. Sickle cell disease has an important historical background. This research done in sickle cell anemia gave birth to the entire field of molecular biology and to a great extent modern science and modern medicine. Dr. Linus Pauling made the discovery that the substitution of valine for glutamic acid in position 6 of the beta globulin chain is responsible for the basic abnormality that causes red blood cells to sickle in people who carry the sickle cell gene.

These abnormalities in the red cell membranes cause the red cells to develop a great deal of difficulty passing through small vessels to deliver oxygen to tissues of the heart, the brain, the kidneys, the liver, the bone, the eyes, the spleen, the skin, the muscle and the rest of the tissues of the body. The lack of oxygen delivery to these different organs is responsible for many of the problems associated with sickle cell disease.

Historically, the sickle cell gene can be traced to three main areas of Africa. The most prevalent sickle cell gene came from Benin near Nigeria in Central Africa. Another gene came from Senegal on the West Coast of Africa. The third gene came from the Bantu-speaking area of Central Africa. There are 4 million people with sickle cell disease in Nigeria.

These genes are also known as 1. **BEN** for Benin 2. **CAR** for Central African Republic and **SEN** for Senegal.

The same three genes can be found within North American Blacks and in the Caribbean. The African slaves who were brought here against their will to work the fields and to do forced labor brought these sickle cell genes to the North American continent during the slave trade. Over the close to 500 years since slavery started, the sickle cell gene has had ample time to penetrate the North American Black race, causing much devastation and leaving a lot of pain, suffering, despair and death in its wake. As early as 1670, there is evidence that clinical sickle cell disease existed in a Ghanaian family. Sickle cell disease does not only affect Blacks. Sickle cell disease affects some Indians, Italians, and Arabs, and the same percentage of Hispanics throughout the Americas are affected by sickle cell disease, as are Blacks, which is 8.5%.

Sickle cell disease is a preventable disease, if individuals who carry the gene for this deadly disease would learn the pros and cons of how the disease is inherited. If a black man who is not carrying the sickle cell trait gene marries with a man who is carrying the gene for sickle cell trait and they decide to have children, 50% of the children will be born without the sickle cell gene and 50% will carry it. If both individuals are carrying the sickle cell trait, 25% of their children will be born normal, 25% will be born with the full-blown sickle cell disease, and 50% will be born carrying the sickle cell trait.

If one of them has the full-blown sickle cell disease and the other is normal, 100% of the children will be born carrying the sickle cell trait. If one of these two individuals is carrying the sickle cell trait (AS) and one has the full-blown sickle cell disease (SS), 50% of the children will be born with the sickle cell trait (AS) and 50% will be born with the full-blown sickle cell disease (SS).

If both of these individuals have full-blown sickle cell disease (SS), 100% of their children will be born with full-blown sickle cell disease (SS). Once a person is carrying either the sickle cell trait (AS) or sickle cell disease (SS), many factors interplay to make that person sick and suffer from sickle cell disease.

What makes sickle cell as deadly as a disease is the inability of the hemoglobin S to carry oxygen to the different tissues and organs of the body for proper body functions. The basic effect of the hemoglobin molecule is the substitution of valine for glutamic acid in the beta globulin chain at position 6, as mentioned earlier, which causes sickle cell hemoglobin to gel where there is lack of oxygen.

This process is called polymerization. This basic abnormality is responsible for most of what is wrong in sickle cell disease. Because of polymerization, the red cells become stiff and sticky and therefore are unable to pass freely through small vessels such as venules, arterioles, capillaries and other medium-sized vessels, resulting in vascular occlusion.

Vascular occlusion, which occurs because of these sticky, misshaped, half-moon or banana-shaped red cells prevents red cells from delivering oxygen normally to tissues in the body of people who are affected by sickle cell disease.

White blood cells also contribute to the occlusive processes that occur in sickle cell disease. White cells secrete a series of adhesive proteins that result in an inflammatory reaction within the vessels of the sicklers. This inflammatory reaction participates in the vascular occlusion that occurs in painful sickle cell crisis. Platelets may also contribute to the vascular occlusion processes by secreting abnormal proteins within the vessels of the sicklers.

Sickle cell disease is a multi-system disease and, as such, affects every major and minor organ in the human body, starting with the skin, which is the largest organ in the human body. The lower extremities can develop ulcers due to skin breakdown. The brain of a sickle cell patient is damaged early and severely, resulting frequently in stroke at an early age, from 4 to 6 years old.

All together, there are four types of sickle disease syndrome:

Sickle trait AS
Sickle cell SS
Sickle cell SC
Sickle cell Sickle Thalassemia
Each one of these sickle disease syndromes affects people differently.

Blacks with sickle cell disease frequently present acutely with one or several of the following crises:

1. Painful sickle cell crisis
2. Hemolytic crisis
3. Hypoplastic crisis
4. Acute chest syndrome
5. A combination of all the aforementioned crises occurring in tandem
6. Splenic sequestration in sickle thalassemia or sickle cell C disease

Painful sickle cell crisis

Painful sickle cell crisis occurs because of occlusion of the small vessels in the body due to the misshaped, sticky red cells making it difficult for them to pass through these vessels to carry oxygen for proper perfusion of tissues. The lack of oxygen delivery to these tissues results in tissue anoxia. The anoxic tissues secrete kinins, mentioned earlier, which cause the burning pain in different parts of the body. This pain can at times be quite severe.

The basis of the painful sickle cell crisis is when the body of the sickle cell patient is under stress, such as infection, which raises the pulse rate, causing the need for more oxygen delivery to tissues to be more severe.

When that need cannot be met, that further aggravates the anoxia, causing a painful crisis to be triggered and made worse.

Another frequent predisposing factor in the development of painful crises is cold weather, which causes vasoconstriction, preventing oxygen delivery to tissues in sufficient amounts, causing ischemia to occur in these tissues, and the result is pain.

Most recently, new information has come out in the literature outlining some of the mechanisms responsible for the occlusive nature of sickle cell disease. The sickled red cells cause damage to the inner lining of blood vessels. The damaged inner lining of blood vessels produces a series of adhesion proteins. These adhesion proteins are said to play a major role in causing occlusion of red blood cells, resulting in painful sickle cell crises. It is believed that both white blood cells and platelets produce proteins that play a role in the vascular occlusive nature of sickle cell disease. (Ref.: *American Society of Hematology Education Program Book, 1998*).

Treatment of painful sickle cell crisis

The painful sickle cell crisis is best treated with pain medication such as Dilaudid IM or by mouth, morphine sulfate IM, IV or by mouth, Percocet, by mouth, Toradol by mouth or IM, and IV fluids. Some blacks with sickle cell disease, by virtue of the fact that they have an enlarged heart due to repeated assault to the heart by the sickle cell disease over a long period of time, may be in heart failure chronically, so giving them IV fluids may be detrimental.

It is important that people with sickle cell disease that come to the emergency room with painful crisis be evaluated thoroughly by physical examination and by chest x-ray to be certain that they do not have congestive heart failure before being given large amounts of fluid. Giving too much fluid to a sickler can throw the patient into pulmonary edema, which, if not understood quickly, can result in the death of the patient. Pain medication, oxygen, and transfusion of fresh blood are indicated in the treatment of patients with sickle cell disease who are in pain.

It must be clearly understood that the vast majority of patients with sickle cell disease who suffer with recurrent painful crises are, by necessity, addicted to the pain medications that they have been receiving over the years. In spite of this fact, however, these patients must be given ample amount of pain medication when they are in pain, for this is the only way to help them ease their suffering. If it can be determined that an infection triggers the painful crisis, then that infection must be treated with appropriate antibiotics to help alleviate the crisis.

Tests, such as chest x-ray, blood culture, urine cultures, etc. and CBC with reticulocytes count must be done before starting antibiotic treatment. Trying to treat a patient with painful sickle cell crisis with an underlying infection, without treating the infection, is just not going to work.

The infection must be treated simultaneously, while the pain is being treated in order to handle the situation in its totality.

The most effective pain medication to treat sickle cell painful crisis is morphine sulfate. Demerol (meperidine) is frequently used to treat patients with painful sickle cell crisis, but it is a bad medication for this purpose. The reason that Meperidine (Demerol) is a bad pain medication to use in the treatment of painful sickle cell crisis is because Meperidine breaks down in the body into Normeperidine, which accumulates in the body because of its very long half-life.

Normeperidine has no significant pain-relieving effect. Normeperidine, however, causes insomnia, anxiety, agitation and seizure, all of which are very bad for people suffering with pain due to sickle cell disease. Morphine sulfate therefore is the recommended pain medication to treat sickle cell patients suffering with pain.

Hydroxyurea is effective in treating sickle cell disease painful crisis by increasing the level of hemoglobin F

Crizanlizumab is extremely effective in treating sckle cell disease painful crisis. "Crizanlizumab is a monoclonal antibody, which is a selectin inhibitor, which targets anti –P-selectin, reduces the frequency of pain crisis by nearly half." Source: ASH Clinical News Volume 03 number 07 June 2017 (FDA approval is yet to be given)

The FDA has just approved "Endari (L-glutamic oral powder) to treat patients sickle cell disease 5 years old and older." Endari is effective in treating painful sickle cell crisis.

Hemolytic crisis

People with sickle cell disease hemolyze a certain percentage of their red blood cells at all times, and that is the nature of their disease. It is, however, not clear as to the reason or reasons why suddenly patients with this disease begin to hemolyze grossly. When individuals with sickle cell disease develop the hemolytic crisis, they drop their hematocrit abruptly, resulting in shortness of breath, joint pains, general weakness, and sometimes acute congestive heart failure.

The hemolysis can be so brisk, causing the patients to suddenly develop dark looking urine, then their eyes become as yellow as an orange, when, the day before, the situation was not like that at all, and they need to be quickly brought into the hospital and treated appropriately. Other evidence of the hemolytic crisis is a markedly elevated LDH, total and indirect bilirubin and elevated reticulocyte count.

Treatments of the hemolytic crisis

Once it is recognized that a patient is in acute hemolytic crisis, the patient must be admitted to the hospital and oxygen, nasally or by mask, administered along with fresh packed red blood cells. If the patient shows signs of congestive heart failure, Lasix IV must be given to prevent worsening of the CHF.

Folic acid, either by mouth or by IV, must also be given to the patient.

Treatments of acute hemolytic crisis

People with sickle cell disease hemolyze their red blood cells all the time, which is part of the disease process. The half-life of their red blood cells is extremely short, maybe 10 to 20 days, as compared to 120 days in a normal person. However, under the stress of an infection or some other circumstances, some of them known, some of them unknown, these individuals can acutely begin to hemolyze, resulting in a rapid drop in their hematocrit.

When this happens, a number of things can develop such as acute shortness of breath, chest pain, drop in blood pressure with shock, and an acute heart attack can occur because of this severe drop in hematocrit. This occurs because of the inability of the heart to pump sufficient blood to carry oxygen to the myocardium.

Acute hemolytic crises must be discovered quickly and treated carefully with fresh packed red cells under the cover of IV Lasix or other loop diuretics to prevent acute pulmonary edema from occurring. In addition to a very low hematocrit, high bilirubin, high LDH, and high reticulocyte count also occur in acute hemolytic crisis.

In addition to replacing blood with fresh packed cells, a high dose of folic acid must also be given when the patient is acutely hemolyzing. The recommended dose of folic acid in patients with chronic hemolytic disease such as sickle cell is as much as 25 mg of folic acid per day and not the usual 1 mg per day of folic acid, which is given for nutritional deficiency. One milligram of folic acid is inadequate in people who are chronically hemolyzing.

Failure to understand this fact can result in the inability of the patient who is chronically hemolyzing to make sufficient red cells. As an individual hemolyzes, the body attempts to make new red cells to meet the demand created by the hemolytic state and uses all available folic acid to make new red cells. Everybody who is hemolyzing chronically is, by definition, folate deficient.

The need to give fresh packed red cells to chronically anemic patients has been mentioned earlier. This is a very important concept to understand because when a severely anemic patient needs a blood transfusion, the anemia can be made worse if she is transfused with old packed red cells that have been sitting in the blood bank for a long time. As blood sits in the blood bank, the level of 2–3 Diphosphoglycerate (2–3 DPG) constantly decreases.

Blood that is depleted in 2–3 DPG, when infused in an already anemic person, shifts the oxygen dissociation curve further to the left, making it much more difficult for that person to deliver oxygen to the tissues. What needs to be done do is to give fresh packed cells, less than a week old, so that a sufficient amount of 2–3 DPG can be delivered into the blood stream to shift the oxygen dissociation curve to the right, allowing for better delivery of oxygen to the tissues.

If a person has underlying ischemic myocardial disease, as is frequently the case in people with sickle cell disease, then the ischemic myocardial disease can be made acutely worse, resulting in either worsening of underlying congestive heart failure. This can even lead to an acute heart attack or can cause serious cardiac arrhythmias to occur because of the worsening myocardial ischemia.

Hypoplastic crisis

The hypoplastic crisis usually occurs because of an infection that suppresses the bone marrow or because of folic acid deficiency or some other insult to the bone marrow that causes it to fail. Evidence that a patient has developed hypoplastic crisis is an acute drop in the hematocrit and a low reticulocyte count. Treatment of hypoplastic crisis includes oxygen, blood transfusion, folic acid administration, and treatment of any underling infection if any exists

Acute chest syndrome

Acute chest syndrome is the most serious and potentially lethal of all the sickle cell crises. Next to painful crisis, acute chest syndrome is the second most common reason patients with sickle cell disease get admitted to hospitals, and acute chest syndrome is the cause of death in 25% of all deaths of sickle cell disease patients. Surgery is a major risk factor for the development of acute chest syndrome. Some 25% of patients with sickle cell disease who undergo elective surgery develop acute chest syndrome.

In acute chest syndrome the sickle cell patient usually presents with chest pain, tachycardia, fever, cough, shortness of breath, low oxygen saturation, high white blood cell count, low baseline hemoglobin, low platelet count, together with infiltrates on the chest x-ray.

The nature of the acute chest syndrome appears to be multifactorial and is associated with inflammatory cytokines causing vascular endothelium damage with fat embolism and pulmonary infarction. Secretory phospholipase A2 is an inflammatory substance that is produced in the lungs in ACS and liberates free fatty acids, which in turn cause acute pulmonary fat embolism to occur.

The level of secretory phospholipase A2 is quite high in the blood of patients with ACS and is elevated before the onset of ACS and when detected confirms the diagnosis of ACS. Infection plays a major role in ACS. In patients with ACS, when bronchoscoped, several different microorganisms were found. Included in the list of microorganisms were different bacteria and viruses. The most common bacteria found were Chlamydia pnuemoniae, Mycoplasma pneumoniae, respiratory syncytial virus, Parvovirus, Rhinovirus, etc.

Treatments of acute chest syndrome

1. Patients who are having pain should be given pain medication such as morphine sulfate to relieve their pain.
2. Oxygen must be given.
3. Incentive spirometry every 3–4 hours while awake is crucial to prevent atelectasis and eventual pneumonia.
4. Transfusion of fresh packed red blood cells must be given and if necessary exchange transfusion ought to be given.
5. Broad-spectrum IV antibiotics must be given because they are felt to play a major role both in genesis of ACS and in its complications.
6. Blood for secretory phospholipase A2 should be obtained and the level ought to be used to monitor the activity of the syndrome.
7. Daily chest X-ray is necessary to monitor lung infiltrates if there are any.
8. Frequent arterial blood gas is needed to monitor the lung functions of these patients.
9. It is very important to avoid giving too much IV fluid to patients with ACS so as to prevent the development of pulmonary edema and other complications such as adult respiratory distress syndrome (ARDS), etc.
10. The FDA has just approved Endari (L-glutamine oral powder) Endari is effective in treating acute chest syndrome.

Splenic sequestration

Splenic sequestration as a sickle crisis is seen most frequently in infants, but can also be seen in adults who have either sickle C disease or sickle thalassemia.

The reason why patients with SC or sickle thalassemia can have this form of sickle crisis is because frequently they have spleens and these spleens are enlarged.

Therefore, when patients in this category present with acute left-sided mid-abdominal pain, splenic sequestration with impending rupture of the spleen must be considered and an abdominal CT scan and a surgical consult must be obtained immediately. Oftentimes, people who carry the sickle cell trait (AS) do not realize that the AS state carries its own list of medical problems. These problems include prominently:

1. Hematuria with occasional severe gross bleeding from the kidney because of papillary necrosis of the left kidney more often than the right kidney, as mentioned earlier.
2. Arthritis of the hips, knees, and spine.
3. Inability to concentrate the urine properly, although general kidney function is normal.
4. Infraction of the spleen can occur in situations where ambient oxygen pressure is too low in people with sickle cell trait, but people with sickle cell trait are able to tolerate simulated high altitude with no problem. People with the sickle cell trait have been engaging in strenuous physical activities, including professional sports, with no difficulty. Usual medical management with analgesics, iron by mouth, with IV fluids,

blood transfusions, when necessary, and high-dose folic acid, up to 25 mg per day, are the mainstay in the everyday treatment of patients with sickle cell disease. The usual 1 mg dose of folic acid given daily is grossly inadequate as outlined earlier.

5. Recently, several reports have appeared in the medical literature outlining evidence of sudden cardiac arrest and deaths in young athletes with sickle cell trait during strenuous athletic activities.

Other acute complications of sickle cell disease include:

1. Gross hematuria due to papillary necrosis of the kidney
2. Acute chest syndrome
3. Pulmonary Embolism
4. Acute myocardial infarction (heart attack)
5. Congestive heart failure, which is due to the cardiomyopathy associated with the secondary hemochromatosis.
6. Acute gouty arthritis, due to the rapid red cell turnover associated with the chronic hemolytic state
7. Stroke
8. Acute multi-organ damaged syndrome
9. Sickle cell disease hemolytic transfusion reaction syndrome.

There are several more recently described complications of sickle cell disease, such as the effect of increased viscosity due to high hematocrit in a person with sickle cell anemia. A hematocrit of 30%–35% or higher interferes with oxygen delivery to the tissues, resulting in hypoxia and can be associated with thrombosis (clot formation). As part of this increased viscosity scenario another syndrome, called acute multi-organs damage syndrome, can occur. Because of the hypoxia associated with increased hematocrit, several organs can become damaged at the same time, resulting in an acute medical emergency. These are the most frequently damaged organs during this syndrome:

1. The kidneys causing hematuria (blood) in the urine, or the kidneys can fail (acute renal failure)
2. Necrosis of the liver can occur
3. The bone marrow may become necrotic, resulting in the propagation of fat emboli
4. Acute pancreatitis can occur
5. Acute stroke as well as acute myocardial infarction can occur.

To prevent the acute multi-organs damaged syndrome, the hematocrit of the sickle cell patients ought to be kept between 27%–29% (Ref: *American Society of Hematology Education Program Book,* Dec. 2000).

Still another serious complication of sickle cell disease is a hemolytic transfusion reaction that can occur in patients being transfused with red blood cells to treat anemia associated with sickle cell disease.

This problem is called sickle cell transfusion reaction syndrome. Some of the indications that a patient with sickle cell may be experiencing sickle cell transfusion reaction syndrome include:

1. Worsening of the painful crisis while receiving blood transfusion
2. A marked drop in the patient's hematocrit and acute inability to make new red blood cells, as manifested with a low reticulocytes count
3. A rapid drop in the hematocrit after receiving blood transfusion (the hematocrit drops to a lower percentage than before the transfusion of red cells were given)
4. Subsequent transfusions of red blood cells may make the anemia worse and, at times, this situation can be severe enough to cost the affected black man his life.

This problem must be recognized quickly and when and if it occurs, to avoid transfusing a patient who is suffering from this problem.

BLOOD SMEAR SHOWING SICKLE CELLS

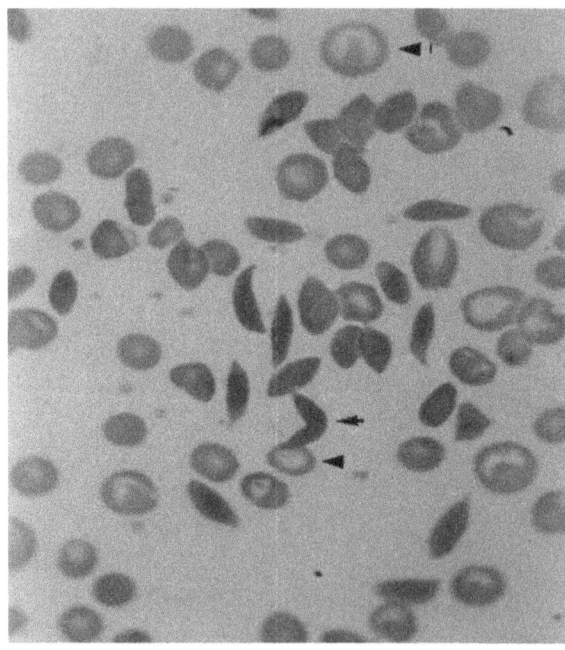

Figure 56:1–*Arrow showing sickle cell (banana-shaped cell). Arrowhead showing a target cell in a Negroe/black person with sickle cell anemia, with thalassemia combined (sickle thalassemia).*

Other types of anemias seen in Negroes/blacks are folic acid deficiency, B-12 deficiency and autoimmune hemolytic anemia. Sickle cell disease frequently affects the bone and brain of individuals suffering from it.

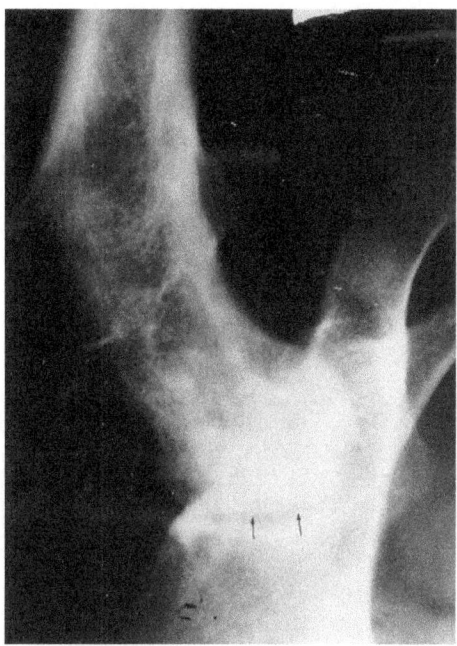

Figure 56:2– *Arrows showing avascular necrosis (lack of blood flow to bone) of femoral head with flattening necrosis of head bone in a Negroe/black person with sickle cell disease.*

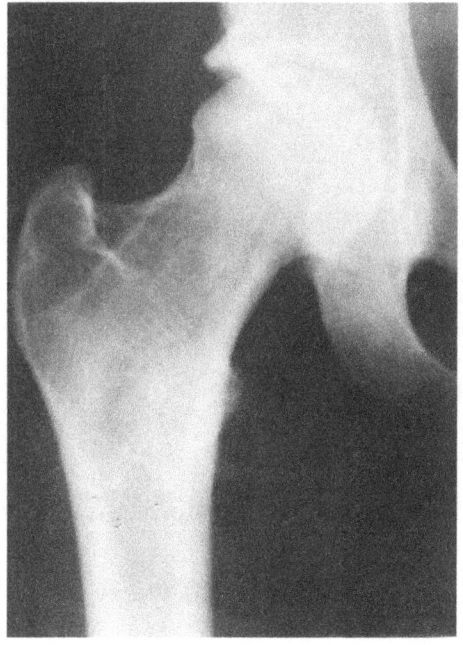

Figure 56:3– X-ray of a normal hip

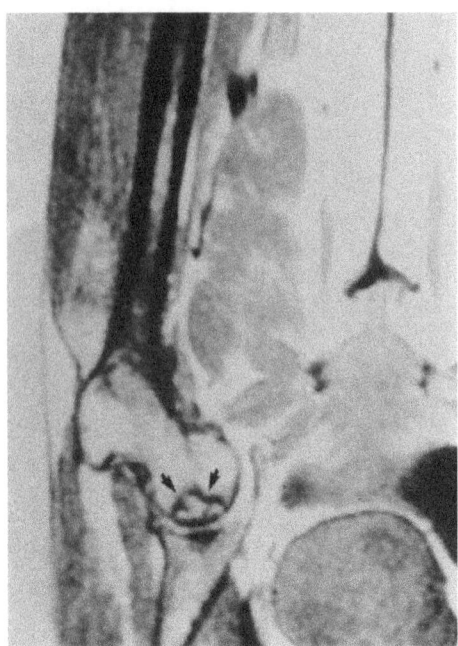

Figure 56:4–MRI *of femoral head of hip of a black person with sickle cell disease. Arrows showing avascular necrosis.*

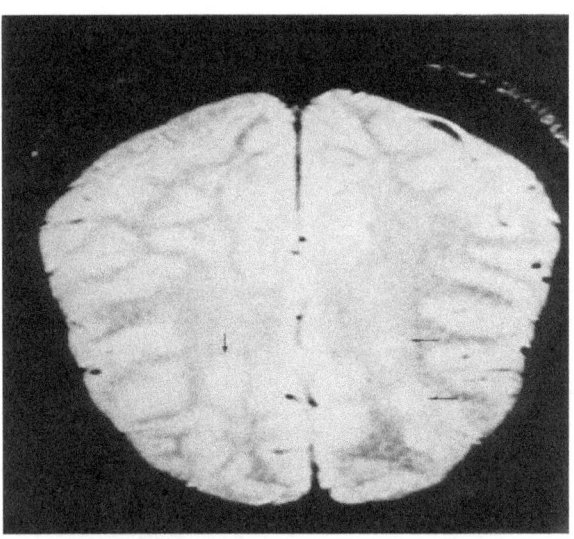

Figure 56:5– *Arrows showing multiple infarcts (stroke) in the brain of a Negroe/black person with sickle cell disease as documented by brain MRI.*

The treatment of sickle cell hemolytic transfusion reaction is administration of corticosteroid intravenously. A rising reticulocytes count and hematocrit is an indication that the patient is getting better (Ref: *American Society of Hematology Education Program Book,* 2000**).**

The heart is always affected in a rather severe way in patients with sickle cell disease. The mechanism through which the heart gets affected in sickle cell disease is similar to all the other affected organs, through a vascular occlusive mechanism. The vessels carrying blood to the heart to deliver oxygen are of all different sizes.

The smaller they are, the easier it is for them to get occluded by the very nature of the sickle red cells. Sickled red cells just cannot pass through these small vessels easily, and there lies the basis of the ischemia that occurs in the muscle of the heart in black men suffering with sickle cell disease. The ischemia causes the release of substances called kinins, which are chemicals that tissues of all types release once they become ischemic (starved for oxygen).

Once the kinins are released they cause a burning pain, and this burning pain is responsible not only for chest pain, but also is, in fact, the basis of the painful sickle cell crisis, which is most common of the sickle cell crises. The myocardial ischemia that occurs in patients with sickle cell disease is just as detrimental as any other ischemia that affects the heart. It leads to muscle scarring and if one or more of the coronary arteries were to become occluded then acute myocardial infarction can occur.

Nevertheless, more commonly, what happens is that the small vessels that carry blood to the heart muscle is occluded, causing myocardial ischemic disease to occur. Along with the ischemia of the myocardial muscle that occurs in black men with sickle cell disease, the red blood cells of these people constantly hemolyze. The homolysis causes lots of iron to be deposited in the bloodstream, resulting in a serious condition called hemochromatosis. This secondary hemochromatosis results in elevated serum ferritin.

This storage iron gets deposited in many organs in the body, in particular the heart muscles, the liver, the pancreas, the joints, the testicles, etc. The iron, once it accumulates in the heart muscles, causes the heart to become enlarged (a condition called cardiomyopathy). When the iron breaks down, it releases free radicals, which damage myocardial tissues, as well as many other tissues.

The enlargement of the heart in turn makes blood pumping very difficult, resulting in congestive heart failure. Cardiac arrhythmias of different types can also occur in this situation. The pumping of the heart becomes so sluggish at times that blood within its chambers becomes stagnated, which can cause a clot to form, and this clot can be carried to different organs as emboli. An organ that is particularly vulnerable to this situation is the brain. If a clot gets loose and becomes lodged in the brain, then an acute stroke can occur. To prevent such a problem from arising, these patients with cardiomyopathy are frequently treated with Heparin or Coumadin (blood thinners) to thin the blood to prevent the development of emboli.

As just mentioned, these individuals frequently develop different rhythm irregularities of the heart and one of the most common rhythm disturbances seen in this situation is a condition known as atrial fibrillation.

The reason why this particular rhythm abnormality is so serious is that in the acute setting it can make the affected black man quite sick. Atrial fibrillation can cause the heart to decompensate, but it can also cause a stroke to develop. Digitalis is used to control the rate of the heart and Coumadin is used to prevent a clot from forming.

Hemochromatosis (too much iron in the body) in people with sickle cell disease is quite serious because of what it can do to the liver, pancreas, heart, and the joints, etc.

The two most effective treatments are phlebotomy (removing one unit of blood 500 cc from the body at a time) and Desferal (a chelating agent). Desferal, when used in the proper fashion, chelates the iron, removing it from the body and passing the iron out in the urine, thereby decreasing the level of iron in the body. Also available to remove excess iron from the body is a new drug called Exjade (deferasirox). It is used by mouth at 20-30 mg/kg/day on an empty stomach.

In addition to the problems just outlined, people who suffer from sickle cell disease (SS), sickle thalassemia, or sickle cell C disease, commonly have a spectrum of clinical manifestations of disease that causes them to be frequently quite sick.

What is the mechanism through which sickle cell disease causes stroke to occur?

Stroke occurs in sickle cell disease patients because the misshaped and sticky red cells clog the small vessels within the brain preventing oxygen from getting to vital parts of the brain. This lack of oxygen results in ischemia, which in turn causes ischemic stroke to occur, and depending on the extent and location of the stroke paralysis may result.

Other major problems that arise as a result of stroke induced by sickle cell disease, even in a child, are inability to control bowel and urinary functions, and aphasia may occur (the inability to speak), sometimes permanently. The stroke frequently causes difficulty in swallowing, which is quite common, and this can sometimes result in recurrent aspiration pneumonia, which may lead to lung abscesses, bronchiectasis, and, sometimes, pulmonary death is the result.

Other frequent complications are seizures. These seizures can be quite troublesome even when anti-seizure medications are used. Pulmonary problems are also quite common in sickle cell patients such as pneumonia, pulmonary embolism, congestive heart failure, causing marked difficulty in breathing with severe hypoxia (lack of oxygen).

Along with these new concepts and mechanisms in sickle cell disease are the proposed newer treatments of sickle cell disease. Hydroxyurea works in sickle cell disease by raising hemoglobin F. In addition, it decreases the level of white blood cells and platelets and helps to improve the symptoms of sickle cell disease.

So, sickle cell patients on hydroxyurea, even if their hemoglobin F level does not go up, benefit because of the lowering of white cells and platelets (Ref: *American Society of Hematology Education Program Book,* 1998).

Other proposed treatment modalities include inhalation of nitric oxide gas to dilate blood vessels, allowing for better tissue perfusion. Another proposed new modality of treatment for sickle cell disease is low-dose aspirin, which works as an anti-inflammatory medication against the effects of the adhesion proteins. Aspirin also works to prevent platelet aggregation, resulting in better blood flow through blood vessels and decreasing the incidence of sickle cell painful crises (Ref:. *American Society of Hematology Education Program Book,* 1998).

Another common problem that frequently occurs in blacks people suffer from sickle cell disease is gall bladder disease. If gall bladder disease is allowed to go undiagnosed it can cause severe problems for the patient. It usually presents with acute abdominal pain, nausea, and vomiting. This constellation of symptoms is usually due to acute cholecystitis. Because blacks with sickle disease and other chronic hemolytic diseases hemolyze constantly, they dump large amounts of bilirubin pigments into their bloodstream. These bilirubin pigments in turn form bilirubin-containing gall bladder stones.

Over time, these gall bladder stones cause the gall bladder to become inflamed and sometimes infected, resulting in a spectrum of acute and chronic gallbladder diseases. The diagnosis and treatment of gallbladder disease is described elsewhere in this book.

Other frequent problems that people with sickle cell disease have to cope with are things such as:

1. Sickle cell retinopathy (bleeding into the eyes) is seen more frequently in SC disease than in SS disease.
2. Leg ulcers are seen more frequently in SS didease
3. Aseptic necrosis of different bones, such as the shoulder joints, the elbow joints, the hip joints, and the knee joints.
4. Microscopic or gross hematuria due to papillary necrosis is quite common.
5. It is seen more often from the left kidney than the right kidney. The reason why papillary necrosis is seen more frequently from the left kidney is that the anatomical position of the two kidneys is different. The left kidney is located higher than the right kidney.

The position of the left kidney places it in a situation where it is less able to receive appropriate amount of oxygen as compared to the right kidney. In normal people that doesn't matter, but in people who have sickle cell disease, that becomes a major problem and in the left kidney where that situation occurs, papillary necrosis occurs frequently, resulting in gross hematuria.

People with sickle cell disease have the propensity of getting infected with capsular bacterial organisms such as pneumococci and Haemophilus influenza.

It has been said that patients with sickle cell disease get infected in the bone frequently with salmonella bacteria, resulting in osteomyelitis.

The spleens of people with sickle cell anemia (SS) variety get destroyed by the time these people become teenagers, due to the recurrent insults of the sickling phenomena to the splenic circulation. The hypo -splenic state that results causes people with SS disease to become immunoincompetent, thus causing them to get infected much more easily.

It is therefore recommended that these individuals get vaccinated with pneumococcal vaccine about every three years or so. It is also recommended that these people get treated with penicillin 250 mg daily as a prophylaxis against pneumococcal organisms.

These organisms are exquisitely sensitive to penicillin. If the patient is allergic to penicillin, Erythromycin 250 mg daily or twice a day can be used as a substitute. People with sickle thalassemia or sickle C disease tend to have large spleens.

People with sickle cell disease are prone to develop sickle hepatopathy (sickle cell liver disease), with large engorgement of the liver, which frequently causes right upper abdominal pain.

Another common problem that individuals with sickle cell disease suffer from is disease of the kidneys. At first the manifestation of the kidney disease appears as different degrees of renal insufficiency in the blood chemistry tests that evaluate kidney function. As the sickle cell disease progresses, chronic renal failure develop, forcing these individuals to be placed frequently on chronic hemodialysis.

Before the kidneys fail completely, hypertension frequently develops, complicating the picture even more because the hypertension can cause strokes or congestive heart failure. As outlined earlier in this chapter, people with sickle cell disease have the propensity to develop strokes and cardiomyopathy. When the blood pressure becomes elevated, it is superimposed on an already sick heart and sick brain, risking decompensation of these and other organs that are frequently affected by elevated blood pressure.

There are several medications and methods available to treat the disease. Hydroxyurea is being used to treat patients with sickle disease to improve the symptoms of the disease.

Hydroxyurea works to improve the symptoms of sickle cell disease in some patients by raising the level of hemoglobin F. Hemoglobin F is an excellent carrier of oxygen and by increasing hemoglobin it enables oxygen to be carried to tissues much more easily, thereby preventing ischemia from occurring.

The result is less pain and improvement in the overall symptoms of the affected patients.

Sodium butyrate has been shown in a recent setting to be able to increase hemoglobin F level as well. Recombinant human erythropoietin (Epogen or Procrit) is being used in combination with hydroxyurea to increase hemoglobin F and red blood cells levels.

Another common complication of sickle anemia is chronic sickle cell lung disease.

Bone marrow transplantation is the only curative treatment available to treat sickle cell disease. Bone marrow transplantation to treat sickle disease was first used in 1984 successfully for the first time. Since that time, a total of 1,200 bone marrow transplants have done successfully using compatible siblings throughout the world.

Genetic counseling remains a very worthwhile approach for those who are affected with sickle cell disease.

Pulmonary hypertension is a major complication of sickle disease.

The best tests to diagnose pulmonary hypertension in people with sickle cell anemis are echocardiogram, pulmonary function test, EKG and chest x-ray and cardiac catherization. Pulmonary hypertension exists when a person mPAP >25 mmHg is present on the echocardiogram. Right heart catheterization is often done to confirm the diagnosis of pulmonary hypertension.

Treatments of pulmonary hypertension include:

Oxygen
Calcium channel blocker
Viagra (it works in PH because it dilates blood vessels)
Cialis (it works in PH because it dilates blood vessels)
Levitra (it works in PH because it dilates blood vessels)
Anticoagulation Source: American Society of Hematology Education Program Book December 10-13, 2011
The annual cost for treating sickle cell disease in the U.S. is over 1.1 billion dollars.

CHAPTER 57

ALPHA THALASSEMIA IN AFRICAN AMERICAN MEN

Alpha thalassemia

Alpha thalassemia affects several hundred million people in the world. The areas of the world most affected by alpha thalassemia are Africa, North Africa, Mediterranean, Asia, South East Asia, India, Middle East and North America, and The Americas.

In alpha thalassemia, the silent carrier is missing one alpha globin chain, and the alpha thalassemia trait missing two alpha globin chains taken together is among the most common genetic disorder in the world. About 32% of Negores/black Americans carry the alpha thalassemia genetic abnormality. Of that figure, 30% are missing one alpha globin chain and 2% are missing two alpha globin chains.

Blacks don't have any symptoms from this abnormality. Those who are missing two alpha globin chains from opposite sides of the alpha globin chain may have a mild microcytic anemia and are said to have alpha thalassemia trait or alpha thalassemia minor. People with immediate African ancestral genes always miss the two alpha globin chains from opposite sides of the alpha globin chain. On the other hand, Asian people and others, when they are missing two alpha globin chains, always miss the chains from the same side of the alpha globin chain, creating an unbalanced alpha globin chain situation.

This is what happens in hemoglobin constant spring, which causes anemia and symptoms in individuals who are afflicted with it. Individuals who are missing three alpha globin haplotypes have hemoglobin H and severely anemic. Hine's bodies are seen in the red blood cells of these individuals on blood smears. When four alpha globin chains are missing, that is Hemoglobin Bart's (hydrops fetalis) and the fetuses that these women carry die in utero, resulting usually in spontaneous abortion.

How to diagnose alpha thalassemia

The best way to diagnose alpha thalassemia is to do a CBC and a quantitative hemoglobin electrophoresis. In alpha thalassemia, the CBC shows microcytosis, low MCV, erythrocytosis, and high RDW. The erythrocytosis (elevated red blood cell count) differentiates thalassemia from iron deficiency. For every 10% of the hematocrit there are 1 million of red blood cells and where there is a discordance of about 400,000 or greater, there exists a thalassemia syndrome in the patient.

If all the aforementioned conditions exist and hemoglobin A2 and hemoglobin F are normal on the quantitative hemoglobin electrophoresis, then the patient has alpha thalassemia of one degree or another.

The treatments for alpha thalassemia are folic acid, blood transfusion, and Procrit/ Epogen when necesary.

CHAPTER 58

BETA THALASSEMIA IN AFRICAN AMERICAN MEN

Beta thalassemia/Cooley's anemia

Beta thalassemia affects about 3% or 201 million of the world population and its distribution are worldwide. The people who are most affected by Beta thalassemia are some Greeks, Italians, Turkish, Iranians, Syrians, Arabics, Pakistanis, Indians, Asians, Northern China, Southeast Asians; Kurdish Jews; and, in North America, Blacks and Hispanics. Beta thalassemia has also been reported in some Northern European people as well.

The cause of beta thalassemia is the deficiency in the beta globin chains of the hemoglobin molecule. Normal hemoglonin has 2 globin beta chains and 4 alpha globin chains.

In beta thalassemia the quantity of the beta chain is deficient and the degree of this deficiency determines the degree and severity of the disease.

Beta thalassemia has three clinical categories: beta thalassemia minor, beta thalassemia intermedia and beta thalassemia major.

Beta thalassemia minor causes no clinical manifestation or disease. Beta thalassemia intermedia cause a hypochromic microcytic anemia with moderate degree of iron overload, but growth is normal and life span is also not affected.

Beta thalassemia major causes a severe anemia, serious symptoms, and high iron overload, endocrine abnormalities with growth retardation, large spleen, large liver, large heart, and congestive heart failure along with cardiac arrhythmias etc. Without early, effective, and aggressive treatment, many individuals with thalassemia major die before reaching adulthood.

How to diagnose beta thalassemia

The CBC in beta thalassemia major shows low hemoglobin and hematocrit, low MCV, high red blood cell count, high RDW and the blood shows many target cells. The quantitative hemoglobin electrophoresis shows elevated hemoglobin A2 or F or both.

An example of what a CBC, serum ferritin and Hemoglobin electrophoresis of a person with beta thalassemia trait looks like. This person has the increased HGB A2 variant of beta thalassemia with normal HGB F level.

WBC	8.6	(4.0 – 10.5)	TH/MM3
RBC	6.37	(4.2 – 5.8)	MIL/MM3
HGB	13.4	(13.0 – 17.0)	G/DL
HCT	42.1	(38.0 – 50.0)	%
MCV	66.1	(80 – 96)	FL
MCH	21.0	(27 – 32)	UUG
MCHC	31.8	(33 – 35.5)	%
RDW	15.4	(11.0 – 14.5)	%
PLT	21.9	(130 – 400)	TH/MM3
MPV	9.0	(6.8 – 11.0)	FL
NEU	69.6	(43 – 75)	%
LYMPH	21.4	(15 – 45)	%
MONO	7.5	(3 – 12)	%
EOS	1.0	(0 – 5.5)	%
BASO	0.5	(0 – 2.0)	%
NEU#	6.0	(1.7 – 7.9)	TH/MM3
FERRITIN	673	(12 – 282)	NG/ML
hemoglobin A	93.4	(94.7 – 98.2)	%
hemoglobin a2	5.80	(1.8 – 3.3)	%
hemoglobin f	0.80	(0.0 – 2.0)	%

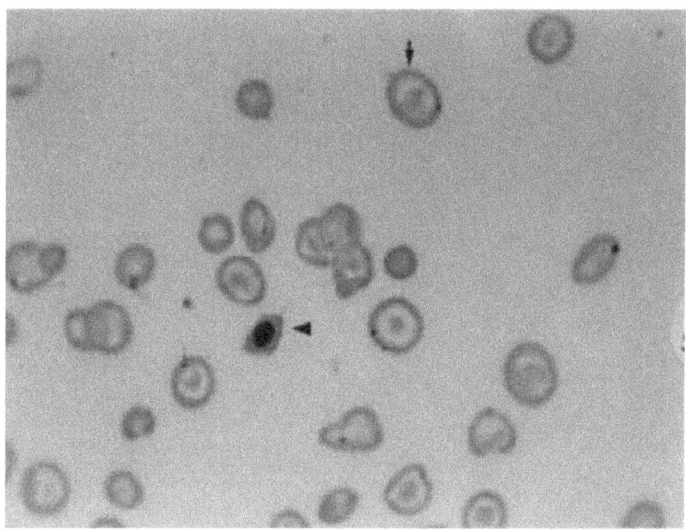

***Figure* 58:1–** *Thalassemia (arrow head) showing nucleated red cell, small arrow showing howel jolly body. Big arrow shows target cell.*

How to treat beta thalassemia major

The most effective treatments for beta thalassemia major consist of:

1. Blood transfusion
2. Chelation therapy using Desferal, Deferiprone, or Exjade
3. Folic acid
4. Bone marrow transplantation
5. Prenatal diagnosis during the first 9–10 gestation can be done, using chorionic villus sampling for DNA fetal analysis. This procedure allows the parents of the unborn fetus to know whether the fetus is homozygous or heterozygous for beta thalassemia major.
6. Preimplantation genetic diagnosis (PGD) is also available for couples who carry the beta thalassemia genes and wish to use this modality to secure the birth of a child free of the beta thalassemia that can be used as a bone marrow donor for a sibling who is sick with beta thalassemia major.

The thalassemias as well as the major sickling diseases are in great measure responsible for the preservation of the new world from the old world because these diseases allowed some people who lived in the old world to survive the ravages of malaria, mainly because the malarial organism could not flourish inside these abnormal red blood cells.

CHAPTER 59

AUTOIMMUNE HEMOLYTIC ANEMIA IN AFRICAN AMERICAN MEN

Autoimmune hemolytic anemia affects hundred of millions people in the world. Autoimmune hemolytic anemia develops when the body develops antibodies against its red blood cells. There are warm and cold autoantibodies. Fifty percent of warm antibodies are idiopathic and fifty percent are secondary.

In idiopathic autoimmune hemolytic anemia, immunoglobulin G (IgG) bins to red blood cells at 37-degree temperature (body temperature) and causes red blood cells hemolyse (burst).

The diseases that are associated with autoimmune hemolytic include:

Chronic Lymphocytic leukemia
Non-Hodgkin's lymphoma
Ovarian cancer
Systemic Lupus Erythematosus (SLE)
Multiple myeloma
AIDS
Hepatitis
Rheumatoid arthritis
Mixed collagen vascular diseases etc.

Drugs that are associated with autoimmune hemolytic anemia include:

Quinidine
Methyldopa
Hydralazine
Tylenol
Ibuprofen
Alfa interferon
Cephalothin
Insulin
Sulfa drugs like Bactrim
Hydrochlorothiazide
Rifampin
Streptomycin
Penicillin etc.

Secondary warm autoimmune hemolytic is associated with diseases like

Lymphoproliferative disorders such as lymphoma and chronic lymphocytic leukemia
SLE
Rheumatoid arthritis
Mixed collagen vascular diseases
Ulcerative colitis
ITP/Evan's syndrome
Myasthenia gravis etc;

Cold autoimmune hemolytic anemia occurs because of autoantibodies of immunoglobulin M (IgM). The IgM antibodies bind o red blood cells causing the red blood cells to hemolyze (burst) when the body temperature drops to 32˚C.

The diseases that are associated with cold autoimmune hemolytic anemia include:

Infectious mononucleosis
Mycoplasma pneumonia
Lymphoma
Paroxysmal cold hemoglobinuria
Syphilis
Mumps
Measles etc.

Symptoms of autoimmune hemolytic anemia include:

Fatigue
Weakness
Fever
Pale skin
Dizziness
Tiredness
Headache
Low blood pressure
Enlarged liver
Enlarged spleen
Rapid heart rate
Flow heart murmur
Chest pain
Jaundice
Dark urine
Anemia
High reticulocyte count
Low platelets in Evan's syndrome etc;

Evaluations of autoimmune hemolytic anemia include:

History
Physical examination
Blood pressure
Pulse
Temperature
Respiratory rate
Oxygen saturation
CBC
Peripheral blood smear (shows rouleaux formation, spherocytes, macrocytes, polychromasia)
Direct coombs test
Serum complement level
IgG/C3 test
In warm autoimmune hemolytic anemia the IgG/C3 test is positive
In cold autoimmune hemolytic anemia C3 is positive
Lactic dehydrogenase
Indirect bilirubin
Haptoglobin
Urinalysis
Cold agglutinin titer (positive when >1:64)
Bone marrow aspiration and biopsy
Donath-Landsteiner test (to be done only when paroxysmal cold hemoglobinuria is suspected)
EKG
Chest x-y
Abdominal CT scan with contrast both IV and by mouth

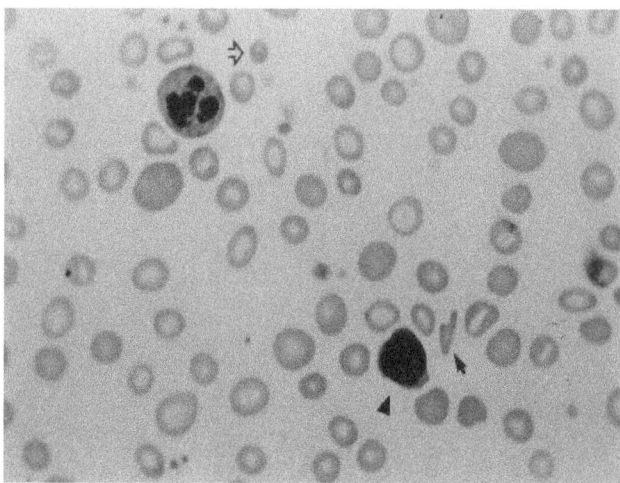

Figure 59:1–Hemolytic anemia (arrow head) showing nucleated red cell in a person. Arrow showing schistocyte (fragment of red blood cell). Open arrow showing spherocytes (very small red cell full with hemoglobin).

Treatments of autoimmune hemolytic anemia include:

Steroid
Folic acid
Intravenous Immunoglobulin
Blood transfusion (a person is having chest pain due to low blood count)
Slpenectomy (when all other treatments have failed)

CHAPTER 60

B12 DEDIFIENCY IN AFRICAN AMERICAN MEN

B12 deficiency is a very common disease B12 is necessary in the myelination of nerve cells in the brain, and is also necessary in the maintenance of the myelination of these nerve cells for normal brain functions.

In addition, B12 is needed to mediation of nerve cells in the cervical, thoracic dorsal, lateral columns of the spinal cord, cranial and peripheral nerves. When B12 level is low in the body, degeneration of myelin sheets occurs. B12 deficiency also causes demyelination of the white matter of the brain. Myelin is lipid like substance that forms a sheet around the axons of nerve. All cells that grow in the body require B12 to grow, including red blood cells, white blood cells and platelets.

The different things that cause B12 deficiency are:

1. Nutritional deficiency (diet deficient of B12)
2. Parasitic infestation (Diphyllobothrium latum, a Fish tape worm)
3. Blind loop syndrome
4. Atrophic gastritis (being elderly)
5. Gastrectomy
6. Malabsorption
7. Pernicious anemia
8. Inhalation of nitrous oxide
9. Xerostomia
10. Inflammatory bowel disease
11. Divirticulosis (diffuse)
12. Sprue
13. Tropical sprue
14. B12 deficiency itself can cause malabsoprtion because low B12 causes the cells in the GI tract to become macrocytic resulting in malabsorption of B12.
15. Gastric bypass
16. Chronic use of H2 blockers, such as Zantac, Tagamet, Pepcid and Axid.
17. Chronic use of PPI such as Prilosic, Prevacid, Nexium, Aciphex and Protonix
    Both H2 blockers and PPI interfere with B12 absorption by decreasing acid production in the stomach. For B12 to be decomplexed properly to allow for its absorption with

the help of intrinsic factor, an acidic milieu is necessary to facilitate this process. Since PPI and H2 cause a decrease in acid production they prevent proper B12 absorption leading to B12 deficiency.

18. Chronic pancreatitis causes malabsoroption resulting in B12 deficiency

How do these different things cause B12 deficiency?

The total store in the body is about 5000 micrograms. The body loses about 1–4 micrograms of B12 per day and the daily requirement for B12 is in the range of 2 micrograms per day. B12 is found in liver, milk, eggs, cheese, and meats.

Nutritional B12 deficiency is usually found in strict vegetarians and in people who don't have access to the food products just mentioned.

Diphyllobothrium latum is the fish tapeworm most commonly associated with B12 deficiency. This worm causes malabsorption of B12 to occur.

The tapeworm takes up the B12; thereby preventing its absorption from the ileum, and the result is B12 deficiency.

Small bowel blinds loops/bacterial overgrowth, small bowel diverticulosis, and other pouches and fistulae cause B12 deficiency because the bacteria eat the B12, making it unavailable for absorption. In this condition, the level of folate is quite high.

Atrophic gastritis causes B12 deficiency because as an individual age the stomach is less able to produce acid and an acidic milieu is necessary in order for intrinsic factor to properly work to allow B12 to be absorbed. Along the same line, the elderly are prone to develop B12 deficiency because of a deficiency that occurs in the mouth due to a lack of certain salivary enzymes that are necessary to begin the process of B12 digestion.

Millions of elderly individuals, who have macrocytic anemia, have B12 deficiency that can cause severe medical problems, including dementia. B12 deficiency state does not always mean B12 deficiency anemia. It takes years before B12 deficiency state becomes B12 deficiency anemia. Anemia is the last stage of the multiple stages of B12 deficiency disease. A person can be very sick from B12 deficiency and not yet develop macrocytic anemia. A good example of that is dementia.

Gastrectomy can cause B12 deficiency 5–10 years post gastrectomy because the bulk of the intrinsic factor-producing surface was removed during the gastrectomy, leaving very little or no intrinsic factor behind, so B12 cannot be absorbed, resulting in B12 deficiency. It would take that long to deplete the B12 store of about 5000 micrograms. Therefore patients who have undergone hemigastrectomy ought to receive B12 injection monthly for life about 5 years after the procedure.

Malabsorption of B12 occurs in chronic pancreatitis because of exocrine enzyme insufficiency. It also occurs in Zollinger-Ellison syndrome because of low pH in the ileum; it occurs as well in regional enteritis involving the terminal ileum in Crohn's disease. Chronic hemodialysis can also cause malabsorption of B12. Therefore, individuals who are affected by these conditions ought to receive B12 injection on a regular basis.

Pernicious anemia is an autoimmune condition involving an interaction between the stomach and intrinsic factor. This antigen-antibody reaction prevents intrinsic factor from attaching itself to B12 to allow it to be absorbed from the terminal ileum into the bloodstream, where it is taken to the bone marrow and incorporated in the early red cells for the production of red blood cells.

Pernicious anemia can be seen in association with hyperthyroidism, hypothyroidism, vitiligo, diabetes mellitus, Addison's disease, and sometimes cancer of the colon.

The previous standard way of making the diagnosis of pernicious anemia was by doing the Schilling test is no longer practical because the radioactive B12 that is used to be employed to carry out this test is no longer routinely available in this country.

Using the patient's symptoms, the low serum B12, the high MCV, the megaloblastic features on the bone marrow smear and the positive intrinsic factor antibody, will suffice to establish the diagnosis of pernicious anemia.

If the diagnosis of pernicious anemia is established, then ANA, T4, TSH, fasting blood sugar, serum electrolytes, and colonoscopic evaluation of the patient in question ought to be done, for the reasons previously described.
Nitrous oxide interferes in the biochemical pathway of B12 in a way that leads to B12 deficiency and megaloblastic anemia. People who chronically inhaled nitrous oxide are likely to develop this form of anemia and all its medical complications if left untreated.

How to diagnose B12 deficiency

The first thing to do is to take good history and do a good physical examination. The next thing to do is to order CBC, serum B12, serum homocysteine, and if the serum B12 is borderline or normal and the diagnosis is still suspected, then serum methylmalonic acid ought to be done.
The serum methylmalonic acid is much more accurate in making the diagnosis of B12 deficiency than the serum B12. Methylmalonic acid is elevated in true B12 deficiency. In B12 deficiency both the methylmalonic acid and the homocysteine are elevated, but in folate deficiency, only the homocysteine is elevated.

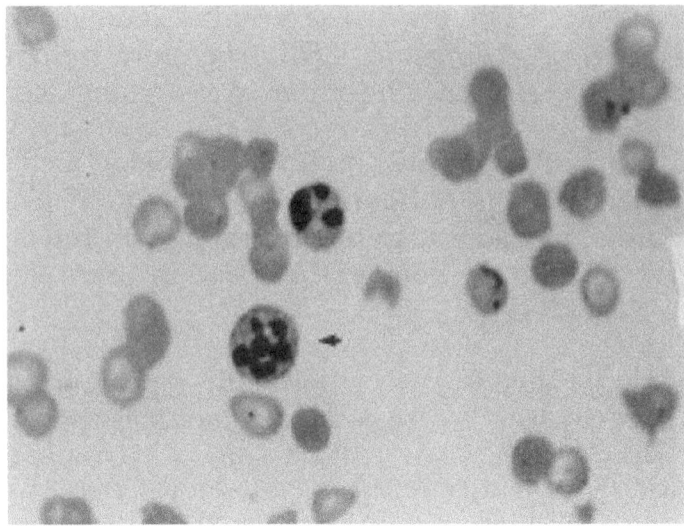

***Figure* 60:-1** *B12 deficiency on a person (big arrow showing segmented polynucleated white cell with 7 lobes, typical of macrocytic anemia). Small arrow showing macrocytic (large immature red blood cells).*

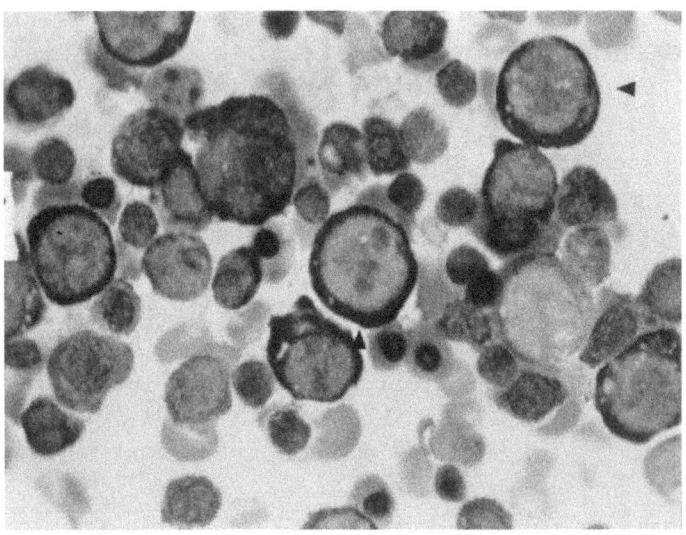

***Figure* 60:2**–*Bone marrow aspiration smear in a person (arrow heads) showing megaloblastic red cells (very large immature red cell and pernicious anemia due to B-12 deficiency).*

Complications B12 deficiency include:

The brain:
Memory loss
Dementia
Depression
Mania (psychosis)

Paranoia
Irrititabilty
Delusison
Lability
Insomnia etc.

Spinal cord:
Myelopathy
Parasthesia
Numbness and tingling in feet and toes
Numbness in hands and fingers
Ataxia of gait
Weakness of legs
Incontinence
Hypotension when standing
Sexual impotence (ED)
Glossitis (redness of tongue)
Loss of taste
Optic atrophy
Infertility
Low WBC
Low Red cells count
Low platelets count
Hypersegmented polys
Low reticulocytes count
High indirect bilirubin
High LDH
Decreased Haptoglobin
Elevated methylmalonic acid
Elevated homocysteine
High MCV
Megaloblastic anemia
High megaloblasts in the bone marrow etc;

How to treat B12 deficiency

The first thing to do to treat is the underlying problem or problems responsible for the B12 deficiency:

1. In the case of nutritional deficiency, B12 can be given IM at first then added to the diet.
2. In the case of fish tapeworm infestation, treat with anti-tapeworm medication and replace B12 by injection at first, then by mouth until the macrocytic anemia is corrected and the store of B12 is replenished.

3. In the case of blind loops, treat the problem surgically if possible, give B12 by injection, give tetracycline, physical examination and history that the malabsorption has resolved and add B12 by mouth till the store has been replenished.

As for atrophic gastritis, give injection of B12 monthly for life.
For post-gastrectomy, give injection of B12 monthly for life.
For malabsorption, treat the same as for blind loops.
For pernicious anemia, give 1 mg of B12 IM daily for 7 days, and then give 1 mg of B12 IM three times per week for three weeks and then gives 1 mg of B12 IM monthly thereafter for life.

It is prudent when treating truly B12-deficient patients with B12 injection to do the followings in the beginning of the treatment.

1. Take the patient's baseline weight.
2. Weigh the patient weekly.
3. Listen to the patient's lungs carefully for evidence of heart failure (rales).
4. Listen to patient's heart for evidence of heart failure (S3 gallop).
5. Check the patient's serum potassium weekly for the first 4 weeks.

Patients with true B12 deficiency who receive B12 injection are likely to respond quickly by increasing their blood volume markedly, as though they have just been given 2–3 units of blood, which can throw them into acute congestive heart failure and death. Acute weight gain would be an indication of water retention and congestive heart failure.

In order to make new red blood cells potassium is needed to be incorporated into RNA; this process can cause an acute depletion of body potassium, resulting in chest muscle weakness with inability to breathe, as well as acute cardiac arrhythmia and death. Therefore, treating a person for true B12 deficiency is serious business and to be carried out by physicians experienced in dealing with this disease.

As for nitrous oxide, those who are exposed to it ought to find ways to decrease their exposure and those who use it, as an addicting drug ought to seek help to resolve their addiction and stop using it. B12 injection at first, followed by B12 by mouth, is the treatment of this form of B12 deficiency.

If an individual who is B12 deficient remains untreated, he or she can develop severe megaloblastic anemia, combined system disease with severe neurological problems, dementia and psychosis. The neurological problems associated with B12 deficiency are not reversible if remained for 5 years or more.

CHAPTER 61

FOLIC ACID DEFICIENCY IN AFRICAN AMERICAN MEN

The other common cause of macrocytic/megaloblastic anemia is folic acid deficiency.

Folic acid deficiency occurs in:

1. Nutritional deficiency
2. Alcoholism
3. Hemolytic anemia
4. Drug-associated folic acid deficiency
5. Tropical sprue etc
6. Non-tropical sprue
7. Cirrhosis of the liver
8. Gastric bypass
9. Chronic pancreatitis
10. Malabsoption
11. Chemotherapy treatments etc.

How folic acid deficiency occurs

Nutritional deficiency causes folic acid deficiency because of poor intake of folic acid. The total body folic acid store is about 5000 micrograms and in 2–4 months the body can become depleted of folic acid. The daily requirement for folic acid in an adult is about 400 micrograms. In fact the body is incapable in a normal individual to absorb more than 400 mcg of folic acid per day. The foods that are richest in folic acid are vegetables. Poor nutrition causes folate deficiency if a person stays on a folate-free diet for about 2–4 months.

Alcoholism causes folic acid deficiency via three main mechanisms:

1. Alcoholics as a rule eat a diet that is poor in folate.
2. Alcohol as a substance, when consumed in excess, poisons the folate biochemical pathway.
3. When the alcoholic develops cirrhosis of the liver, portal hypertension develops, which in turn causes hypersplenism with secondary hemolysis, making folic acid deficiency worst.

Medications such as Dilantin, Phenobarbital, Mysoline, and Methotrexate, to name a few, are known to cause folic acid deficiency. Both tropical and non – tropical sprue is known to cause folic acid deficiency because of the malabsorption that they cause.

How to diagnose folic acid deficiency

To diagnose folic acid deficiency, do a serum folate, CBC and a reticulocyte count. In folic acid deficiency, the serum folate is low, the hematocrit is low, the MCV is high and the reticulocyte count is low. Sometime the folate level may be in the range even though the patient is folate deficient. That may happen because the folate level reflects the last folate-containing meal that the patient ate before the blood was drawn.

The most accurate test to do to measure folate level is red blood cells folate level, but this test is not routinely available and is therefore not practical. The bone marrow aspirate in folate deficiency shows megaloblastic changes in the red blood cells and a left shift in the early white blood cells. (See 60:1 & 60:2 above because bone marrow aspiration in people with folte deficiency looks the same way.)

How to treat folate deficiency

The best treatment for folate deficiency is folic acid by mouth or IV/IM. If the patient is very anemic, then blood transfusion can be given. To treat tropical sprue and non-tropical sprue folic acid 1 mg per day, tetracycline 250 mg 4 times per day ought to be given. Chronic hemolytic anemia is treated with high doses of folic acid, up to 25 mg per day in order to keep up with constant destruction of red blood cells that is taking place.

CHAPTER 62

ANEMIA OF CHRONIC DISERASES / INFLAMMATORY DISEASES IN AFRICAN AMERICAN MEN

Anemia of chronic disease is mediated by cytokines IL1 and TNFα (Interleukin 1 and Tumor Necrosis Factor alpha), these substances cause an inflammatory reaction to occur, which then result in the production of nitric oxide, which in turn suppresses the ability of erythroid blood progenitors (early red blood cells) from being able to make red cells. In this setting iron moves from the blood into to the tissues where it is stored and not made available for red blood cell production.

In addition, it is believed that "during inflammation, inflammatory cytokines stimulate the production of hepcidin by the liver. Hepcidin leads to the internalization and degradation of the cellular iron exporter ferroportin, which is expressed on liver cells and reticuloendothelial cells that store iron and on duodenal cells that absorb dietary iron.

When ferroportin is reduced in the cell membrane of those cells, less iron is released into the blood stream and circulating iron levels decrease-meaning that less iron is available for erythropoeisis in the bone marrow. Inflammation-induced production of hepcidin ultimately leads to iron restriction of the bone marrow, contributing to the development of anemia." Source: ASH Clinical News, October 2014

Apparently, this is the body's way of protecting itself from invading microorganisms, such as bacteria, viruses, and fungi, by depriving them of iron for their growth. In addition, the body seeks to protect itself from cancer by depriving the cancer cells of iron, which is necessary for their growth.

The second apparent advantage of anemia of chronic disease is to deprive cancer cells and microorganisms of sufficient oxygen needed for their growth and their proliferation by not making enough red cells to carry oxygen to them.

The third proposed advantage of anemia chronic disease is that the lack of circulating iron strengthens the cell-mediated immune system. The third advantage mentioned seems to make sense, since having cancer in the human body, by itself, creates an immune deficiency-type state (Source: *American Society of Hematology Education Program Book,* pages 42–45, 2000).

Evaluations of anemia of chronic diseases/inflammatory diseases include:

History
Physical examination
CBC with differential
Reticulocytes count
Serum ferritin
Soluble serum transferrin receptor level
Complete metabolic chemistry profile
Urinalysis
T4/TSH
Serum B12
Serum folate
PSA
Hemoglobin electrophoresis
Chest x-ray
Abdominal ultrasound
Abdominal CT scan
Chest CT Scan when indicated
PPD TB skin test
QuantiFeron TB Gold blood test
HIV/AIDS test
Hepatitis B screen blood test
Hepatitis C screen blood test
VDRL
ANA
ENA
Rheumatoid factor
ESR etc.

The different chronic diseases that are treated with Procrit/Epogen and Aranesp are:

1. Hemochromatosis/Iron overloads both primary and secondary, when the
2. Patient is anemic
3. Rheumatoid arthritis
4. End stage renal failure
5. Sickle cell anemia
6. Beta thalassemia
7. Alpha thalassemia
8. AIDS
9. Chronic hepatitis B with iron over overload and anemia
10. Chronic hepatitis C with iron overload and anemia

11. Chronic auto immune hemolytic anemia
12. Other chronic hemolytic anemia
13. Chemotherapy/radiotherapy associated anemia
14. Chronic osteomyelitis with anemia
15. Myelodisplastic syndrome
16. Sideroblastic anemia
17. All other diseases that cause anemia and iron overloads
18. Cirrhosis of the liver with iron overload
19. Mixed connective tissue diseases with anemia and iron overload

Treatments of anemia of chronic diseases/anemia of inflammatory diseases:

Treat the chronic diseases with medications or surgical means etc. as appropriate for each disease.

Use Procrit or Epogen 10,000 units SC to over the inflammatory block and to mobilize the iron from the reticuloendothelial cells into the pro-erythroblasts in the bone marrow to produce red blood cells to raise the hematocrit and improve the anemia. Tow things are being achieved with this treatment. 1. The iron is being removed from tissues and 2. The anemia is being treated.

Depending on the severity of the anemia, sometime Venofer IV can be used to help correct the anemia faster.

In reality, anemia of chronic disease/inflammatory diseases is iron deficiency anemia eventough the ferritin is high.

CHAPTER 63

HEMOCHROMATOSIS/IRON OVERLOAD IN AFRICAN AMERICAN MEN

A very serious complication of chronic hemolytic diseases is iron overload, known as hemochromatosis, which was discussed earlier in the section on sickle cell disease.

Primary hemochromatosis is a very common hereditary disease in the U.S. and around the world. It affects 1 million white Americans, which is about 1 in 300 white

Americans. Several million Black, Latino and Asian Americans are also affected by hemochromatosis. The total number of hemochromatosis in these other racial groups is not known because most physicians are not testing nonwhites for hemochromatosis.

This is wrong because there are 3 more genes plus hepcidin deficiency that cause hemochromatosis other than the C282Y gene. The non -hematology literature seems only interested in talking about the C282Y gene seen in whites, if as tough whites are the only people in existence in America. Of course they did not say that, they just get their facts wrong.

Some articles the literature say "1 million Americans or 1 in 300 have hemochromatosis" and hemochromatosis is the most common hereditary disease in America". This is blatantly false.

The truth is that, while primary hemochromatosis is most common in white Americans, it is not the most common hereditary disease in the U.S.

For instance, there are about 52 million Latinos in America and 8.5% of them have sickle trait (representing 4.4 million) and there are about 44 million Blacks in America and 8.5% of them have sickle trait (representing 3.7 million). In addition, 32% of Blacks in America have Alpha thalassemia either as silent carrier or as alpha thalassemia minor (representing 14 million). These diseases are hereditary and can be transmitted from parents to their children. All together, there are 3,600,000 people in this country with sickle cell trait.

Now you can clearly see how blatantly false the assertion that "hemochromatosis is the most common hereditary disease in the U.S." is. Worldwide hemochromatosis affects 1 in 400 people or 28 million people.

A serum ferritin of 500 or greater at some point during a person lifetime represents hemochromatosis. Hemochromatosis/iron overload must be treated with a low iron diet or phlebotomy to bring the iron level to below 200 if the person is not anemic. If the person is anemic, Procrit or Epogen 10,000 units SC must given either every week or 2 x per weeks for 4-8 weeks to bring the serum ferritin down.

Genetic testing is positive for the C282Y gene (HFE) in less than 50% in Caucasians with hemochromatosis/iron overload. Genetic testing for the C282Y gene is hardly ever positive for hemochromatosis/ iron overload in known Caucasians.

There is only one reported case in the literature of the C282Y gene (HFE) having found in a black person and this author made such a discovery and published it. (See below)

The basis for the other cases primary hemochromatosis/iron overload has recently been published The Journal The hematologist ASH NEWS AND REPORTS August/September 2005 volume 2 issue 4. According to this article, it is a deficiency of hepcidin, which causes the level of ferroportin to remain unchecked resulting in both over absorption of iron from the small bowel and over production of iron from dying red blood cells under the influence of ferroportin.

Other genetic reasons to explain hemochromatosis/iron over load are:

1. Type 2 Hemochromatosis 2nd to G320V mutations
2. Type 3 Hemochromatosis 2nd to TFR2 receptor mutations
3. Type 4 hemochromatosis 2nd to 977 GYC mutations

The hemochromatosis seen in the individual who suffers from hemoglobinopathies is the secondary type as compared to the idiopathic type or primary hemochromatosis. About 10% of the U.S. population carries the gene for primary hemochromatosis, and in certain sub groups, as much as 1:200 or 1:2000 have hemochromatosis.

Primary hemochromatosis-affected people over-absorb iron because of a genetic defect that forces them to absorb too much iron. In secondary hemochromatosis, which is the result of hemoglobinopathies, the iron gets dumped into the bloodstream because of shortened red cell survivals, resulting in hemolysis. In the full-blown thalassemia, these children classically have bronze skins due to iron deposits under the skin.

The iron gets deposited in different tissues and organs in the body of these children who are suffering from thalassemia and sickle cell disease or any other chronic hemolytic anemia. The organs that are most affected by iron deposits are the heart, the liver, the endocrine organs such as the adrenal glands, the pituitary, the gonads and the pancreas. Iron deposits also affect the joints. Iron deposits cause damage to tissues and organs because as iron particles lie in the tissues they break down, releasing free radicals.

These free radicals are extremely toxic to human tissues, damaging the tissues, resulting in diseases such as cardiomyopathy with resulting heart failure. As the free radicals are released they damage the liver, resulting in cirrhosis, which results in scarring of the liver, which can result in hepatocellular carcinoma of the liver. One of the most sensitive ways to diagnose iron deposits in the liver is by doing an MRI of the liver, which, if positive with iron deposits, shows a starry sky-type picture.

Damage caused by iron deposits in the gonads can result in sexual dysfunction and sexual underdevelopment. Damage of iron deposits into the pancreas often result in diabetes mellitus Type II, because the beta cells within the pancreas get damaged and destroyed. These beta cells that are responsible for the production of insulin, and without insulin, sugar cannot be broken down to be used as fuel for proper body functions.

Osteoarthritis is a common disease in people who are affected by hemochromatosis, and black men are particularly afflicted by this because black men, as a result of their lower economic status, are forced to do heavier work to earn a living, which places their bone structure at most stress and also their musculoskeletal structures at most stress, causing osteoarthritis. When iron deposits are superimposed on this condition, osteoarthritis is made worse.

The free radicals that are released from the breakdown products of iron deposits in the joint spaces cause an inflammatory reaction to occur, which results ultimately in destruction of the joints, causing severe arthritis in these joints and chronic pain. Many blacks do not know that they have hemochromatosis and that is really a major issue.

The worst-case scenario is that oftentimes they are carrying abnormal hemoglobin, which predisposes them constantly to smoldering hemolysis with secondary iron being dumped in their body. At the same time, they may be carrying the gene for hemochromatosis, which is also causing them to over-absorb iron, having, therefore, two problems affecting them simultaneously, resulting in more frequent problems associated with iron overload.

Primary hemochromatosis is believed by some to be a disease that is found usually in Caucasians of Scandinavian and European descent. This in fact turns out not to be so. While the disease is more common in whites, it does occur with significant frequency in blacks and other races. The gene that is responsible for primary hemochromatosis is located in the short arm of chromosome 6 and is on the HLA locus.

Many people with no abnormal hemoglobin frequently have high serum ferritin consistent with hemochromatosis/iron overload state with clinical features of primary hemochromatosis. **The author was the first physician in the world to discover the C282Y gene in a black man, in the year 2000, documenting that this gene, which is responsible for primary hemochromatosis, is also found in Blacks in very rare instances. The so-called African Iron Overload Syndrome probably does not exist at all and never existed, but rather those who described it were in fact describing hepcidin deficiency with ferroportin excess.**

There are in fact many whites who have primary hemochromatosis/iron over load and are treated for it and yet the C282Y (HFE) gene is absent in them and they are said to have primary hemochromatosis/iron over load.

However, when Blacks have clear and unquestionable primary hemochromatosis/iron over load, many physicians would say that they have "African Iron Overload Syndrome".

This is nothing more than an attempt to say that Blacks cannot possibly have the same disease that Whites have. Which is total racial nonsense because the human race began in Africa and all human beings are the same from a DNA standpoint, except for a few minor differences, and since skin color happens to be one of these minor differences, some choose to make a big deal of it for their own psychosocial and economic advantages.

"Prevalence of Iron Overload in African-Americans- A Primary Care Experience —
Revised" *Prestige Medical News*, February 2003, Vol. 5 No. 3 pp 1–22
By Valiere Alcena, M.D., FACP.
Le Negre Publishing
37 Davis Avenue
White Plains, NY 10605

Evaluations of hemochromatosis/iron overload include:

History and physical examination
CBC
Complete blood chemistry profile
Serum ferritin
ESR
Rheumatoid factor
ANA
Hemoglobin electrophoresis
C282Y blood test
Serum hepcidin
Serum ferroportein level
Soluble serum transferrin receptor level

The C282Y (HFE) test to diagnose primary hemochromatosis of different degrees is available in several commercial clinical laboratories. The best way to determine if someone has hemochromatosis is to do a serum ferritin. A serum ferritin costs about $44.00 to do and it is immensely important. The serum ferritin gives an evaluation of the total body iron. A serum ferritin of 500 or greater establishes a possible diagnosis of hemochromatosis.

The organs most affected by hemochromatosis include:

The hematopoietic (blood system)
The liver
The skin

The reproductive organs of men
The bones
The adrenal glands
The kidneys etc;

The best treatments for hemochromatosis/iron overload include:

Phlebathomy
Chealating medications
Vitamin C by mouth
Procrit
Epogen

During that procedure 500 ml of blood is removed. Each time 500 ml of blood is removed, 250 mg of iron is removed with it. Each 1 cc of blood contains 0.5 mg of iron. It is important that the person whose blood is being removed is examined by a physician, to be certain that she is not anemic or has no active cardiac disease that can contraindicate the removal of that much blood from him or her.

The only other treatment available to remove iron from the body is a chelating agent called Desferal, which works to remove iron from the body by chelating the iron from the body and excreting it through the kidneys, into the urine. Desferal is given subcutaneously as a continuous infusion over 12 hours together with 100 to 200 mg of Vitamin C. The Vitamin C helps to mobilize iron in the tissues, making it easier for the chelating agent to remove it from the body into the urine and out.

This is a unique property that Vitamin C has. Because Vitamin C is able to mobilize iron from the body, it is dangerous for someone to take Vitamin C, unless a physician prescribes it.

If an individual has hemochromatosis and does know it, and is taking Vitamin C, the Vitamin C would help to enhance the absorption of iron from the stomach. The vitamin C will help to mobilize a lot of iron into vital organs such as the heart, liver, pancreas the joints etc., resulting, in a multitude of diseases, such as diabetes mellitus, cirrhosis of the liver, cancer of the liver and cardiomyopathy etc.

Vitamin C is plentiful in fruits, juices, bananas, and vegetables and, when consumed as food products, is both nutritious and helpful to keep the body in good Vitamin C balance.

People who have secondary hemochromatosis due to hemolytic diseases, such as sickle cell disease, thalassemia, or other diseases such as, rheumatoid arthritis, chronic renal failure with high body iron store. And blacks who have secondary hemochromatosis and are anemic at the same time, can be given injection of Procrit, 10,000 units SQ twice per week or Epogen, 10,000 units SQ, twice per week, to use the iron in their bodies to make red cells, thereby decreasing the iron level while at the same time treating their anemias.

Deferosirox (Exjade) is available to treat secondary hemochromatosis-iron overload.

The daily dose of Exjade is 17.3 mg /kg/day by mouth. This medication is very effective in iron overload due to multiple blood transfusions.

Deferipone (Ferripox) is another medication in used to treat iron overload in thalassemia. The usual dose is 75-100 mg /Kg/day 3 times per day by mouth.

Complications of hemochromatosis/iron overload include:

Anemia
Arthritis
Cardiomyopathy/enlarged heart
Congestive heart failure
Cardiac arrhythmias
Cirrhosis of the liver
Hypogonadism
Erectal dysfunction
Infertility etc;

CHAPTER 64

OSTEOPOROSIS IN AFRICAN AMERICAN MEN

⟞⟞⟨⟍⟋⟩⟝⟝

OSTEOPOROSIS causes softening of bones that causes pain, arthritis, and fractures. The bones become soft due to decrease in bone mass. When looking under the microscope at a bone in a person suffering from osteoporosis, what is seen is a decrease in what is called cortical thickness of the bones. Osteopenia is the beginning of the softening process that leads ultimately to osteoporosis.

Osteoporosis / osteopenia affect about 44 million Americans and 55 percent of the U.S. population 50 years or older have osteopenia. Worldwide 200 million people have osteoporosis.

The percentage of whites and Asians affected by osteoporosis is greater than the percentage of blacks that are affected by this disease. Blackmen have higher bone density than white men do and as such, blackmen have stronger bones.

However, blackmen suffer significantly from osteopenia/osteoporosis because 90% of blackmen and other people with dark have vitamin D insufficiency and about 70% of them have vitamin D deficiency risking them to the development of osteoporosis/ osteoporosis. 90% of Hispanics have low vitamin D, 75% of Whites and 75% of Asians have low vitamin D.

The fact blacks and other people with dark skin make it harder for them to produce vitamin when they are exposed to the sun's rays. The sun's rays activate Ergosterol under the skin to produce vitamin D. Other sources of vitamin D include egg yolk, milk, cheese, butter, salmon, and cod liver oil.

In addition, 75% of blackmen have lactose intolerance and this further adds to their propensity to developing osteopenia/osteoporosis.

The fragile bone fractures associated with osteoporosis amount to about 1.5 million per year in the USA. Between the ages of 40 and 50 years, cortical bone loss is somewhere in the range of 0.2% to 0.5% per year. Loss of bone mass per year ranges anywhere from about 40% to 50% in some individuals.

Women tend to lose bone mass much earlier than men do, and this loss of bone mass seems to progress more rapidly after menopause.

The difference in the incidence of osteoporosis in blacks versus whites and other racial groups seems to be due to the fact that blacks have higher bone minerals than other racial groups, hence the lesser incidence of osteoporosis seen in blacks.

Risks of osteoporosis include in African American men:

1. Smoking
2. Alcohol abuse
3. Low dietary calcium
4. Vitamin D
5. Lack of exercise
6. Malabsorption
7. Malnutrition
8. Low serum magnesium
9. Heparin use chronically
10. Primary hyperparathyroidism
11. Secondary hyperparathyroidism
12. Chronic use of steroid
13. Kidney failure
14. Cushing syndrome
15. Thyrotoxicosis
16. Calcium deficiency
17. Systemic mastocytosis
18. Rheumatoid arthritis
19. Scurvy
20. Rickets
21. Homozygous osteogenesis imperfecta
22. Heterogygous osteogenesis imperfecta
23. Hemochromatosis
24. Marfan's syndrome
25. Gigantism
26. Multiple myeloma etc;

There is a form of osteoporosis called idiopathic, which occurs in children and adolescents of both sexes. The two most common forms of osteoporosis are Type I osteoporosis, which occurs in postmenopausal women between the ages of 51 and 75. It causes loss of trabecular bones, and fractures of vertebral body and distal forearm are quite common. Type II osteoporosis is seen in people over the age of 70 and these people suffer frequently from fractures of the femoral neck, proximal humeral, proximal tibia and pelvis. Collapse of vertebral bodies frequently occurs, resulting in kyphosis, scoliosis and other deformities as these people get older, and fractures of the hips are quite common, as well.

Among the cancers that may be associated with osteoporosis causing bone pain, and vertebrae fractures.

1. Multiple myeloma
2. Leukemia
3. Lymphoma
4. Metastatic cancer to bones

Multiple myeloma is the most common cancer that is associated with osteopenia/osteoporosis. To diagnose multiple myeloma using x-rays, skeletal survey is the most accurate. Bone scan is the most sensitive test to diagnose metastatic cancer to the bones. Plain x-ray study is the best test to diagnose multiple myeloma, because multiple myeloma causes an osteolytic process.

Bone scan is the best test for metastatic cancer to the bones because metastatic cancer to bone is an osteoblastic process. MRI of bones will show cancer in bones, in both osteolytic and osteoblastic processes. However, MRI is an expensive test and is not routinely done to diagnose cancer to the bones, but is done when either the bone scan or the plain x-rays are not definitive. Still a better test to diagnose bone cancer is PET scan.

Another common disease that causes osteoporosis is primary hyperparathyroidism. The reason why primary hyperparathyroidism is associated with osteoporosis is because of bone resorption.

The bleaching of calcium from the bone causes the bone to become soft and painful, and because the bones are soft, they break easily, resulting in even more pain.

Still, another more common cause of osteoporosis is steroid treatment Steroid treatment has many major and minor side effects, and prominent among these side effects is osteoporosis. Among the reasons why steroid treatment causes osteoporosis is the fact that it reduces calcium absorption from gastrointestinal tract and increases calcium loss in the urine. As calcium is lost in the urine, the bones become calcium deficient, which ultimately causes soft bones (osteoporosis).

Non-black people weighing in the 127-pound range are roughly two times more likely to have fractures of the hip, pelvis, and ribs, as compared to non-black whose weight is in the 161-pound range. Blacks with small frame are not at higher risk for fractures of the arm, elbow, wrist, ankle, and foot.

Bone density measurement is the best test to diagnose osteoporosis. This is a painless test, which is quite accurate in diagnosing bone loss of different degrees. In addition to the bone density study, regular bone x-ray is capable of showing osteopenia/osteoporosis and different degrees of fractures that occur because of osteoporosis.

The following are two examples of osteoporosis as seen on x-rays and MRI done on individuals suffering from osteoporosis:

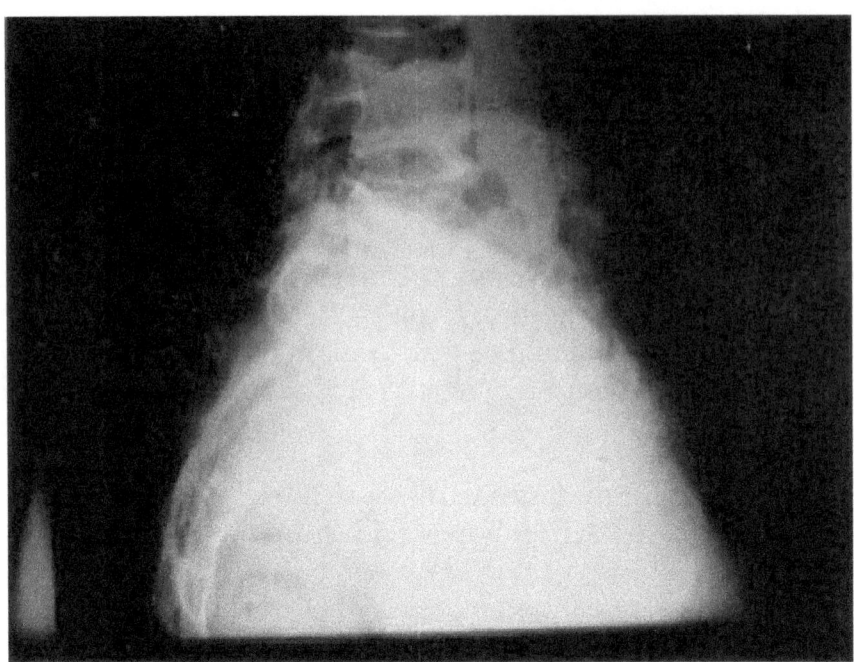

Figure 64:1–Plain x-ray of the lumbar spine of a person with osteoporosis; multiple wedge compression on osteoporosis with mark osteopenia at L1, L2, L3 and L4.

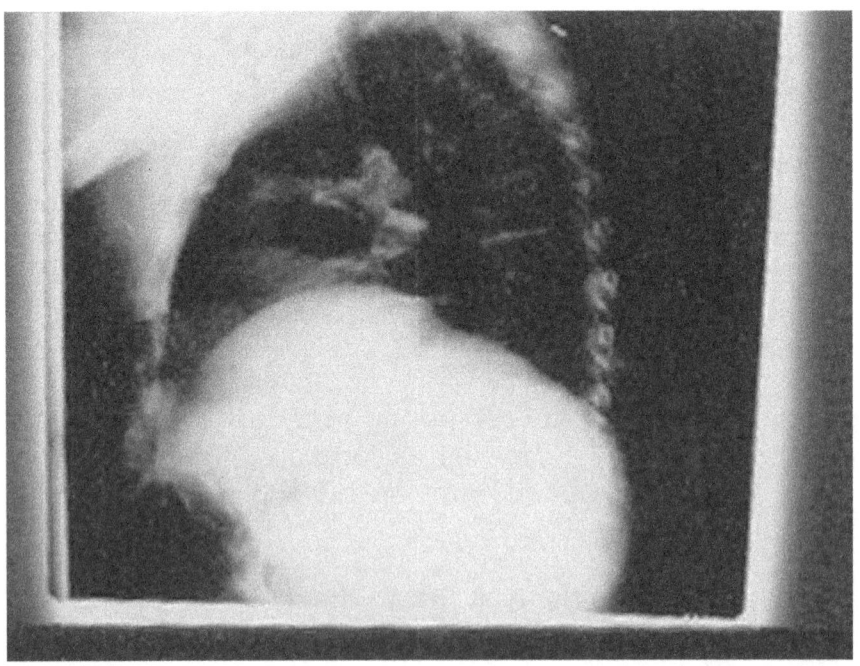

Figure 64:2–Plain x-ray of the thoracic spine of a person with osteoporosis; multiple wedge compression on osteoporosis with mark osteopenia at T9, T10, T11, and T12.

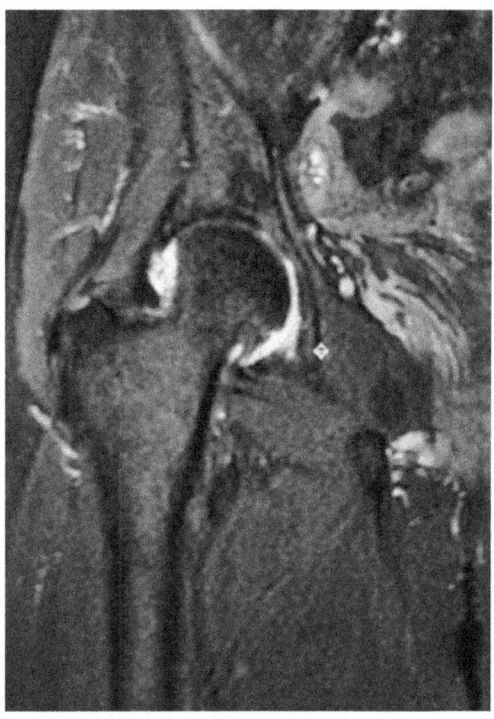

Figure 64:3 Osteoporosis and inflammation of the hip bone of a person with adult Ricket's/Oeteomalacia

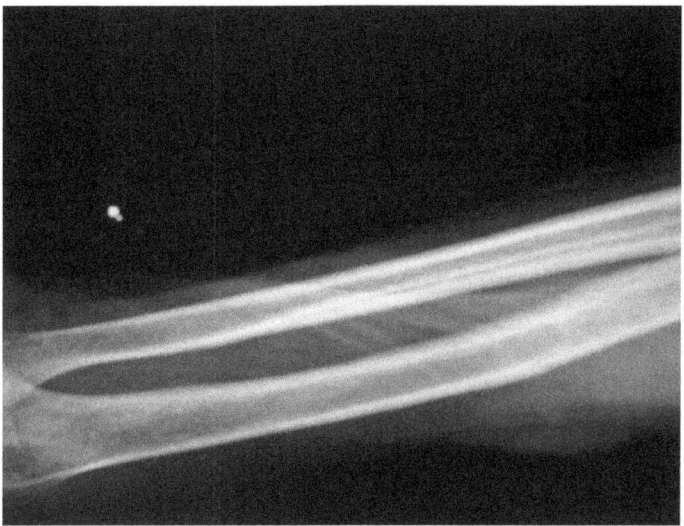

Figure 64:4 Osteoporosis and inflammation of the forearm of a person with adult Ricket's/Osteomalacia

An adult needs to take in 0.8 grams of calcium daily in a diet, in order to be in calcium balance. The body of an adult male contains 800 grams of calcium.

Prevention of osteoporosis is extremely important to avoid the complications of osteoporosis and their associated morbidities and mortality.

Diet plays a major role both the cause and in the prevention of osteoporosis. Other Foods that are rich in vitamin D and calcium include:

Cheese
Yogurt
Beans
Eggs
Kale
Cauliflower
Chard
Molasses
Rhubarb
Beets
Almonds
Cabbage,
Bran
Carrots
Celery
Dates
Chocolate
Figs
Lettuce
Lemons
Oranges
Oysters
Pineapples
Raspberries
Shellfish
Spinach
Walnuts
Watercress
Parsnip etc.

While several of the aforementioned do have good calcium source, it must be kept in mind that because some of them are very rich in cholesterol, they must be consumed in moderation. Some of these cholesterol-rich foods are milk, cheese, egg yolk, oysters, shellfish, etc. It is a good idea to consume skim milk, as well as cheese made with skim milk, to decrease the amount of cholesterol intake.

The human skin contains a substance called ergosterol, and sunlight, as well as ultraviolet radiation from the sun, activates this substance, which leads to the production of Vitamin D, hence, the importance of sunlight exposure.

Many people are not exposed to sunlight on a regular basis because they work in offices. In addition, elderly people are confined to their places of residence and have no sun exposure. In addition, people who cannot tolerate dairy products because of lactose intolerance, depriving them of an importance of source of vitamin D and calcium.

Another important reason why blacks and others with dark skins have such high rate of vitamin D insufficiency/deficiency is because their skins have high concentration of melanin making it very difficult for the sun rays to penetrate their skins to stimulate vitamin D production.

As mentioned above ninety percent of blacks, ninety percent of Hispanics, South Asians, Arabs, other people with dark skins, and seventy-five percent of whites have vitamin D insufficiency in the U.S. According to a published report by the CDC on March 30th 2011, "one third of Americans are not getting enough vitamin D".

Vitamin D deficiency can cause osteoporosis, rickets, caries, secondary hyperparathyroidism, low magnesium, low phosphorous, renal tubular acidosis, congestive heart failure, uncontrolled essential hypertension (low vitamin D causes over activation of the rinin-angiotensin-aldosterone system which can lead to elevated blood pressure), increase infection by suppression of the immune system, and a multitude of possible other skeletal malformations. Increase exercise plays a major role in the prevention of osteoporosis.

The normal vitamin D-25 OH level in the blood is between 30-100 NG/ML. Vitamin D is insufficient when the level of D-25 OH in the blood is between 10-29 NG/ML and vitamin D-25 OH is deficient when the level in the blood is between 1-9 NG/ML.

When the vitamin D OH is deficient in the blood, it is necessary to check the levels of magnesium, phosphorous and parathyroid hormone in the blood to rule out Adult Rickets /Osteomalacia. In Rickets/Osteomalacia, the serum magnesium and phosphorous will be low and the parathyroid hormone level will be elevated. It is always necessary to do a bone density test in people 50 years and older.

The effects of low level of vitamin to the kidney are significant. Low vitamin can cause the kidney to excrete magnesium and phosphorous in the urine and elevated parathyroid hormone in the blood, which in turn can lead to renal tubular acidosis. Renal tubular acidosis is a serious kidney disease.

This combination of medical problems affecting the kidney prevent the kidney from properly metabolize vitamin D 25 OH which takes place in the kidney. The form of vitamin D in the liver is vitamin D 125 OH. Vitamin D 125 OH must go the kidney to be activated to vitamin D 25 OH to be used in the body for normal functions.

Therefore, a disease kidney cannot do this, hence the reason kidney failure causes low vitamin D, and low vitamin can cause kidney insufficiency/failure. Both conditions lead to osteoporosis.

Treatments of osteoporosis

Medications that are available to treat osteoporosis include:

1. Fosamax
2. Actonel
3. Evista
4. Miacalcin
5. Calcium supplements, and
6. Vitamin D in age-appropriate dosages.
7. Zoledronic injection once per year
8. Boniva

The National Academy of Sciences, in 2002, recommended the daily intake of Vitamin D to be:

0–50 years 200 IU/day (International Unit)
51–70 years 400–600 IU /day
71 years and older 600–800 IU /day

The National Academy of Sciences in 2002 also recommended the following daily intake of calcium:

0–6months	200 mg/day
7–12 months	270 mg/day
1–3years	500 mg/day
4–8 years	800 mg/day
9–18 years	1,300 mg/day
19–50 years	1000 mg/day
51 years and older	1,200 mg/day until menopause
51 years and older	1,500mg/day after menopause

In people whose vitamin D level is abnormally low, it is necessary to treat them with 50,000 units of vitamin D 2 tablets per week for either for 4 weeks, 8 weeks or 12 weeks depending on how low the vitamin D level is. Once vitamin D level is corrected to normal, the person can be placed maintenance dose of vitamin D of either 1000 units per day or 2000 units per day for life.

Understanding the different causes of osteoporosis and knowing the different subgroups of individuals in society who have a predisposition to developing it, will help to prevent it by providing the right diet and treatments for these people.

CHAPTER 65

OSTEOARTHRITIS IN AFRICAN AMERICAN MEN

WHAT IS ARTHRITIS?

Arthritis is an autoimmune/inflammatory condition that affects mainly joints resulting in swelling, pain, restriction of movement and, ultimately, deformity of the joints and bones, as a result. In addition, chronic bony destruction and edematous destruction also occur. However, certain types of arthritis, at times, can be multi-system, affecting a multitude of organs such as the heart, the lungs, the kidneys and the blood system, etc.

The most common forms of arthritides are:

1. Osteoarthritis
2. Rheumatoid arthritis
3. Gouty arthritis
4. Ankylosing spondylitis
5. Psoriatic arthritis
6. Reiter's dyndrome with arthritis
7. Systemic lupus erythematosus associated with arthritis
8. Polymyalgia rheumatica
9. Infectious arthritis
10. Lyme disease associated with arthritis
11. Sickle cell disease-associated arthritis etc.

Different types of arthritis affect 50 million Americans, but osteoarthritis is the most common form of all the arthritides. Twenty seven million Americans suffer from osteoarthritis and six hundred millions people in the world have osteoarthritis. The process that ultimately leads to osteoarthritis begins in the cartilage.

The cartilage apparently releases a certain enzyme, which causes its destruction and in time causes breakdown of the joints to occur. Cartilage is a gelatinous substance whose function is to provide cushion in between joints. Once the cartilage dries out, overtime; the areas in between the joints rub against each other, resulting in bone destruction and deformities.

Worldwide, about 60% of the population ages 60–70 have osteoarthritis of one joint or another. Certain ethnic groups seem to be affected with arthritis of some part of their body structure to a lesser degree than others do. For example, Africans and southern Chinese's have less arthritis in their hip joints. The knees seem to be the joint most frequently affected by osteoarthritis in all ethnic groups. Hundreds of million of people in the world are affected by osteoarthritis.

A study published in 2008 showed that 33.8 percent of blacks have osteoarthritis compared to 26.6 percent whites. The aging process plays a major role in the development of osteoarthritis. In most cases, people over age 40 will develop osteoarthritis by virtue of getting older.

Obesity plays a major role in causing osteoarthritis of the knees in older individuals leading to morbidity and mortality.

The joints, most frequently affected by osteoarthritis are:

Knees
Hips
Hands
Fingers
Spine
Feet
Ankles
Shoulders
Neck
Wrists
Jaws
Ribs
Toes
Osteoarthritis is classified as primary or secondary.

TABLE 1:

Classification of Osteoarthritis

I. Primary-Idiopathic

A. Localized
1. Hip, superolateral, superomedial, medial, inferoposterior
2. Knee, medial, lateral patellofemoral
3. Spinal apophyseal
4. Hand, interphalangeal, base of thumb
5. Foot, first metatarsophalangeal joint, midfoot, hindfoot
6. Other, shoulders, elbows, wrists, ankles

B. Generalized
1. Hands, Heberden's nodes
2. Hands and knees; spinal apophyseal generalized osteoarthritis

II. Secondary

A. Dysplastic
1. Chondrodysplasia
2. Epiphyseal dysplasias
3. Congenital joint displacement
4. Developmental disorders, Perthes' disease, epiphysiolysis

B. Post-traumatic
1. Acute
2. Repetitive
3. Postoperative

C. Structural failure
1. Osteonecrosis
2. Osteochondritis

D. Post-inflammatory
1. Infection
2. Inflammatory arthropathies

E. Endocrine and metabolic
1. Acromegaly
2. Ochronosis
3. Hemochromatosis
4. Crystal deposition disorders

F. Connective tissue
1. Hypermobility syndromes
2. Mucopolysaccharidoses

G. Etiology obscure
1. Kashin-Beck disease"

Primary osteoarthritis occurs as part of the aging process; secondary arthritis occurs because of some form of abnormality that occurs in the joint causing it to be misaligned, resulting in the abnormalities that ultimately result in the formation of arthritic changes. Sometimes these changes are the result of injuries to the joints or the result of a person's occupation, which exposes the joints to repeated stress, resulting in the development of arthritis.

If a joint becomes infected and the infection is not treated quickly, then that joint can develop post-inflammatory changes, which could develop arthritic changes ultimately.

Both primary and secondary hemochromatosis are conditions that cause iron to be deposited in joints and breaks down within the joints into free radicals that can cause breakdown of the tissues and the bones in the joints. The result is the development of arthritis. Blackmen and Hispanic men have a high percentage of secondary hemochromatosis, because of such diseases as sickle cell anemia and thalassemia that cause a large amount of iron to be deposited in their bloodstream from hemolyzed red blood cells. Many Italians, Greeks, Arabics, Indians, Whites and Asians men, and men also suffer from primary and secondary hemochromatosis with resulting high incidence of osteoarthritis.

People who suffer from sickle cell disease can develop aseptic necrosis of joints such as the hips, shoulders, elbows, etc. This occurs because the sickling phenomenon impedes the ready flow of blood with oxygen to these joints, resulting in ischemic changes in the bony parts of these joints, which can lead to the development of aseptic necrosis and different stages of arthritis. People who use steroid chronically frequently develop aseptic necrosis of the hip and other joints.

There are many other people of different ethnic background who, because they suffer from thalassemia, either beta or alpha, have secondary hemochromatosis, which can cause them to develop osteoarthritis due to the deposition of iron in their joints.

Obesity is a major predisposing factor in the development of osteoarthritis. The knees are most prone to the development of arthritis because of the stress placed on them by the excess weight. About 76% of black Americans are overweight/obese and 2/3 of Americans adults are obese/overweight. Worldwide there are 502 million obese adults. As a result, osteoarthritis is quite common in these groups

The chances of a person developing osteoarthritis of the knees can be determined by the body mass index of that person. The greater the body mass index of a person, the greater his or her chances of developing osteoarthritis changes in her knees, hip, ankles, and feet.

TABLE 2:

Determining Body Mass Index (BMI) from Height and Weight Body Mass Index* (kg/m2)

Body Mass Index* (kg/m2)													
	19	20	21	22	23	24	25	26	27	28	29	30	35
Height (in) Body weight (lb)													
58	91	96	100	105	110	115	119	124	129	134	138	143	167
59	94	99	104	109	114	119	124	128	133	138	143	148	173
60	97	102	107	112	118	123	128	133	138	143	148	153	179
61	100	106	111	116	122	127	132	137	143	148	153	158	185
62	104	109	115	120	126	131	136	142	147	153	158	164	191
63	107	113	118	124	130	135	141	146	152	158	163	169	197
64	110	116	122	128	134	140	145	151	157	163	169	174	204
65	114	120	126	132	138	144	150	156	162	168	171	180	210
66	118	124	130	136	142	148	155	161	167	173	179	186	215
67	121	127	134	140	146	153	159	166	172	178	185	191	223
68	125	131	138	144	151	158	164	171	177	184	190	197	230
69	128	135	142	149	155	162	169	176	182	189	196	203	236
70	132	138	146	153	160	167	174	181	188	195	202	207	243
71	136	143	150	157	165	172	179	186	193	200	208	215	250
72	140	147	154	162	169	177	184	191	199	206	213	221	258
73	144	151	159	166	174	182	189	197	204	212	219	227	265
74	148	155	163	171	179	186	194	202	210	218	225	233	272
75	152	160	168	176	184	192	200	208	216	224	232	240	279
76	156	164	172	180	189	197	205	213	221	230	238	246	287

Body mass index, or BMI, is the measurement of choice to determine obesity. BMI is a formula that takes into account both a person's height and weight. BMI is a person's weight in kilograms divided by height in meters squared (BMI=kg/m2). The table printed above has already done the conversions. To use the table, find the appropriate height in the left-hand column. Move across the row to the given weight. The number at the top of the column is the BMI for that height and weight.

In general, a person age 35 or older is obese if he or she has a BMI of >27. For people age 34 or younger, a BMI of >25 indicates obesity. Obesity is an indication for further clinical evaluation.

The BMI measurement poses some of the same problems as weight-for-height tables. BMI does not provide information on a person's age or body fat or take into consideration the person's body fat distribution.

As published by the American Diabetes Association

To evaluate pain in a particular joint or joints, a history and physical examination must be carried out. Once that is done, then, certain blood tests ought to be done.

Included among these blood tests are:

CBC
Complete blood chemistry profile
Serum uric acid
Urinalysis
Erythrocyte sedimentation rate (ESR)
Rheumatoid factor
Anti-nuclear antibody (ANA)

In addition, radiological evaluation of the joint or joints in question must be done. These tests include:

Plain x-ray
Ultrasound
CT Scan
MRI

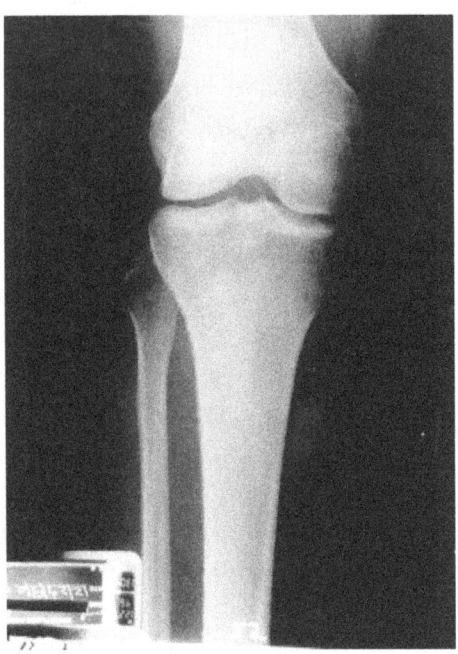

Figure 65:1– X-ray of a normal knee

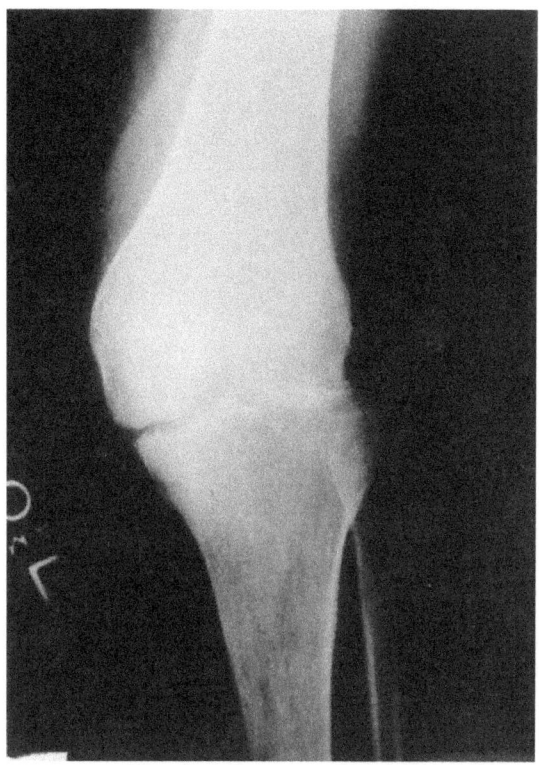

Figure 65:2–X-ray of a knee affected with osteoarthritis

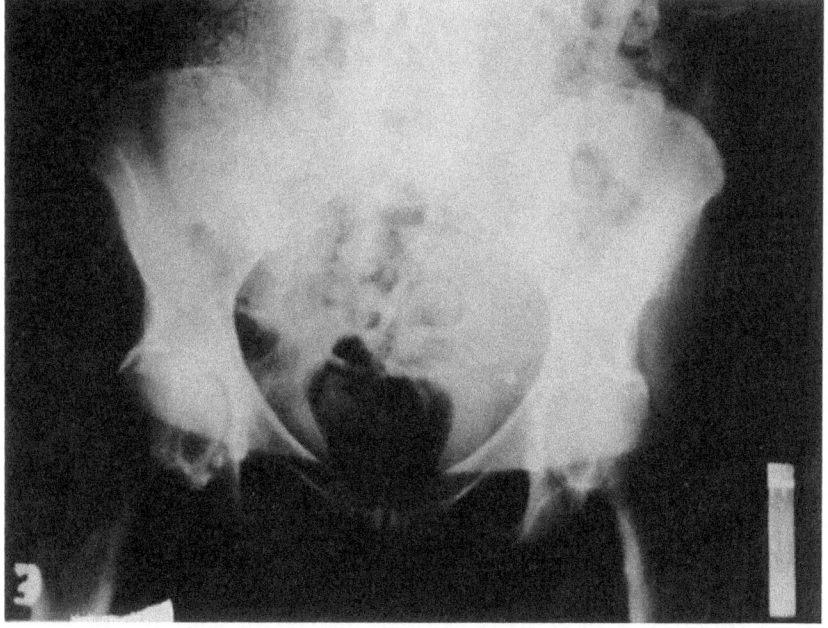

Figure 65:3- X-ray of hip joint affected with osteoarthritis

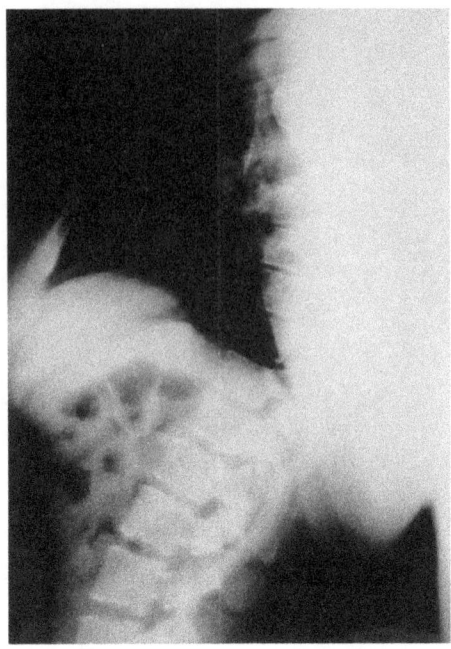

Figure 65:4- X-ray of lumbar spine affected with osteoarthritis

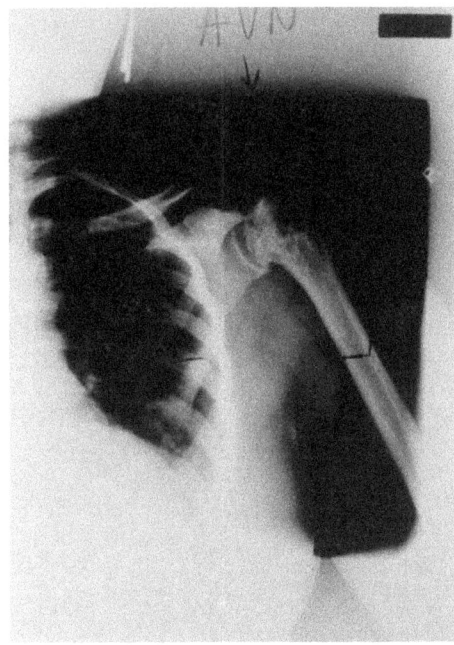

Figure 65:5- X-ray of shoulder joint showing aseptic necrosis in a
patient with sickle cell anemia

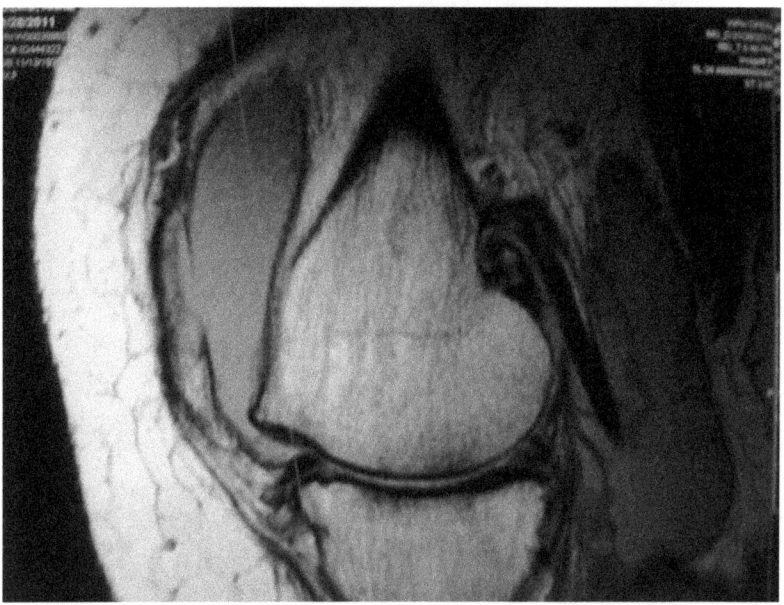

Figure 65:6- MRI of right of a patient with severe osteoarthritis showing a large Joint effusion, a large Baker's cyst measuring 4.5 x 2.0 x 7.2 cm and a high grade tear of the anterior cruciate ligament, and partial tears of the posterior cruciate ligament and collateral ligament.

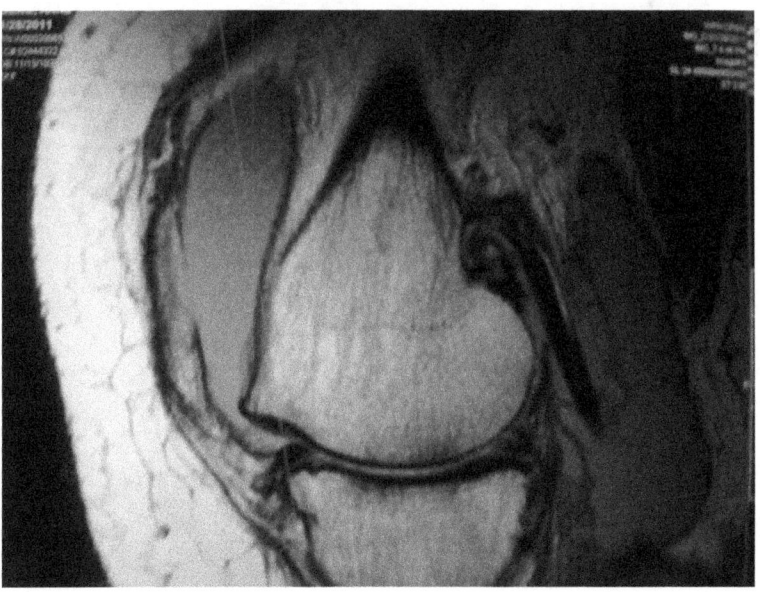

Figure 65:7 Another view of the MRI of the same knee showing a complex tear of the posterior horn of the meniscus and many degenerative arthritic changes.

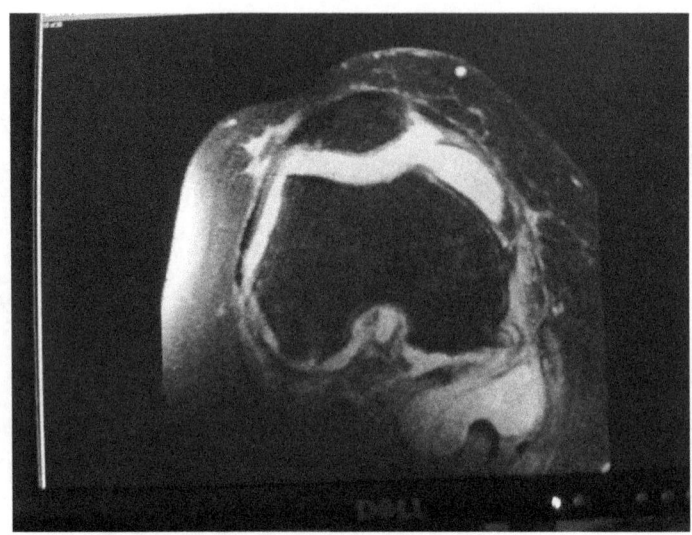

Figure 65:8 MRI of hip in a patient with adult Rickets showing osteoporosis, inflammation and arthritic changes

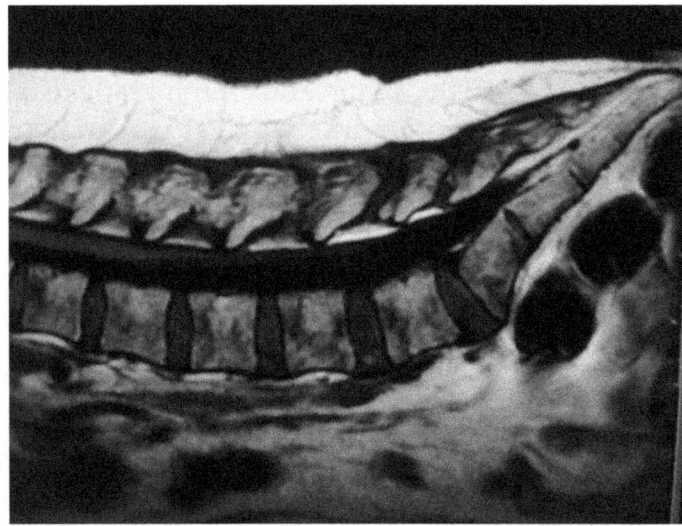

Figure 65:9 MRI of lumbar spine in a patient with adult Rickets / osteomalacia showing degenerative changes.

Osteoarthritis is a painful condition, and it can be very disabling disease.

The medications in use in the U.S. to treat osteoarthritis are:

Motrin
Advil
Aleve
Naprosyn
Anaprox

Daypro
Relefan
Indocin
Celebrex (COX2)
Aspirin
Athrotec
Voltaren
Flector
Toradol
Mobic
Tylenol
Steroid
Ultram etc;

Other modalities of treatments include:

1. Surgical repair of joints
2. Surgical replacements of Knees, hips etc.
3. Physical therapy
4. Heat treatments
5. Application of different cream/ointments to affected bony parts
6. Acupuncture

These medications work by interfering with the inflammation that occurs locally in the affected joints, thereby easing the pain. Physical therapy works by relieving the stiffness and by strengthening the affected joint or joints.

When these treatments are no longer effective and the pain and discomfort persist, then surgical intervention is often considered as an option to treat the arthritic joint.

Surgical replacement of hips, knees and other joints, etc., has become common practice these days, provided the affected individual is not too obese to allow for the operation to have a chance of success, or provided there are no other contraindications, such as associated major medical problems etc.

Osteoarthritis is both more common and more severe in minorities than whites are. Many minorities work as factory workers, housekeepers, construction workers, sanitation workers, farmers etc; and these types of work require a lot of physical activity, which places a lot of stress on the joints of the fingers, shoulders, elbows, knees, lumbar spine, cervical spine and the hip joints. Low back pain is one of the most common causes of work related disability in the world causing hundred of billions of dollars in lost income worldwide.

Osteoarthritis, as a disease, is also common in athletes, no matter what form of athletic activities they are engaged in. Preventive measures such as eating a proper diet to maintain an ideal weight and wearing proper sports equipment during athletic activities would help to decrease the incidence of osteoarthritis.

Paget's disease of the bone is another type of arthritis that is frequently seen in some people with osteoarthritis.

CHAPTER 66

RHEUMATOID ARTHRITIS IN AFRICAN MEN

Rheumatoid is an autoimmune/inflammatory disease that affects close to 2.1 million Americans. Rheumatoid arthritis is 2-3 more common in women than in men. People who smoke seem to have a higher incidence of rheumatoid arthritis. Black men with RA develop serious complications. RA affects people of all ethnic backgrounds.

Worldwide 140 million people are afflicted with Rheumatoid Arthritis and 1.3 million people in the U.S. have rheumatoid arthritis.

When left untreated, or when treatment fails, causes chronic deformity of the bones with destruction of the affected joints. In point of fact, even when appropriate and effective treatments are provided to a person suffering with rheumatoid arthritis, joint deformities ultimately develop in the majority of patients with rheumatoid arthritis.

The joints frequently affected by rheumatoid arthritis are:

Feet
Ankles
Hands
Fingers
Elbows
Wrists
Shoulders
Hips
Neck
Lumbar spine
Thoracic spine

The cause of rheumatoid arthritis is unknown. Although many theories have been proposed, none has so far been proven.

Rheumatoid arthritis is a multi-system disease, but the joints, bones, muscles, skin, and blood system are affected most frequently.

Other organs that can be affected by RA include:

Heart
Lung
Brain
Blood system
Kidney
Skin
Neurological system,

In the beginning, the symptoms of rheumatoid arthritis can be insidious and difficult to discern. At times, a person may present with vague symptoms such as:

General malaise
Fatigue
Weakness weight loss
Aches and pains
Headache
Fever

Morning stiffness in different joints that improves as she starts to move around, doing daily chores.

As the disease progresses, then the signs of synovitis with swelling of the joints with pain and warmth become evident.

The disease affects black men between the ages of 20 and 50 years, although some black men are afflicted earlier and some are afflicted at a later age. Women are affected three times more often than men with R A also affect children, resulting in juvenile arthritis,

TABLE 1: Classification of Rheumatoid Arthritis

Revised, as Published by the American College of Rheumatology

1. *Guidelines for classification*
   Four of seven criteria are required to classify a patient as having rheumatoid arthritis
   Patients with two or more clinical diagnoses are not excluded
2. *Criteria*
   a. Morning stiffness: Stiffness in and around the joints lasting 1 hr before maximal improvement.
   b. Arthritis of three of more joint areas: At least three joint areas, observed by a physician simultaneously, have soft tissue swelling or joint effusions, not just bony overgrowth. The 14 possible joint areas involved are right or left proximal interphalangeal, metacarpophalangeal, wrist, elbow, knee, and ankle and metatarsophalangeal joints.

c. Arthritis of hand joints: Arthritis of wrist, metacarpophalangeal joint, or proximal interphalangeal joint.
d. Symmetric arthritis: Simultaneous involvement of the same joint areas on both sides of the body.
e. Rheumatoid nodules: Subcutaneous nodules over bony prominences, extensor surfaces, or juxtaarticular regions observed by a physician.
f. Serum rheumatoid factor: Demonstration of abnormal amounts of serum rheumatoid factor by any method for which the result has been positive in less than 5% of control subjects.
g. Radiographic changes: Typical changes of RA on postero-anterior hand and wrist radiographs, which must include erosions or unequivocal bony decalcification localized in or most marked adjacent to the involved joints.

Criteria a-d must be present for at least 6 weeks. A physician must observe criteria b-e.

Taking a thorough and detailed history is crucial in a person in whom the physician suspects rheumatoid arthritis. Equally important is a thorough physical examination. Eliciting the fact that other immediate members of the family have rheumatoid arthritis or symptoms suggesting rheumatoid arthritis is quite important, because there is clear evidence that rheumatoid arthritis can run in the family.

No one test is diagnostic of rheumatoid arthritis, but a series of blood tests together with x-ray examination of certain joints, such as the hands and the fingers, may add up to confirming the diagnosis of rheumatoid arthritis. X-rays of the proximal interphalangeal, metacarpal phalangeal, metatarsal phalangeal, have distinct characteristics that are seen mainly in rheumatoid. Chronic changes of the hands and wrists resulting in swan neck deformity is classic for rheumatoid arthritis, but these are late bony changes.

X-ray of the wrist and hand joints showing arthritic changes in a patient with rheumatoid arthritis

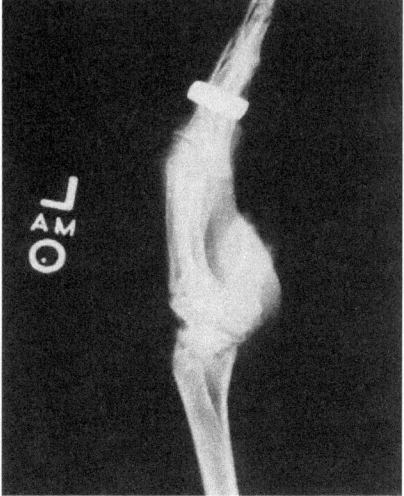

Figure 66:1

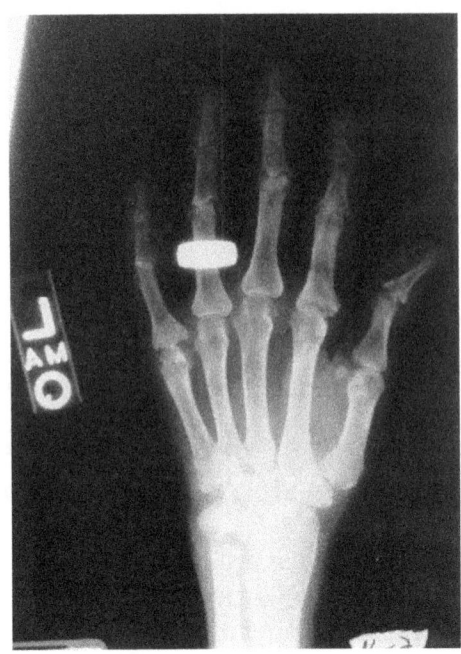

Figure 66/:2 Deformed finger's joints in person with rheumatoid arthritis

Other systemic involvements of rheumatoid arthritis include:

1. Vasculitis involving medium-sized vessels.
2. The lungs may become involved because of pleural effusion, resulting in shortness of breath, and diffuse interstitial fibrosis may develop, resulting in chronic lung disease.
3. The eyes may become involved with a condition called keratoconjunctivitis sicca (also known as Sjoren's Syndrome) causing dry eyes.
4. In about 10% of individuals with rheumatoid arthritis, the spleen is enlarged. Frequently, when the spleen is enlarged in rheumatoid arthritis, the white blood cell count is also low. (This is called Felty's Syndrome.)
5. Some adults with rheumatoid arthritis develop a clinical picture similar to children with rheumatoid arthritis called Still's disease, with fever spike, polyarthralgia, myalgia, a maculopapular rash, pericarditis, pneumonitis, sore throat, large spleen, lymphadenopathy and pain in the abdomen.
6. The heart can, at times, be involved and pericarditis can occur. Aortic regurgitation and conduction abnormalities of the rhythm of the heart can also occur.

People with rheumatoid arthritis may develop peripheral neuropathy because of vasculitis of the vasa nervorum. Further, neurological problems may result when, because of tenosynovitis of the wrists, compression of the median nerve occurs, resulting in carpal tunnel syndrome.

The hematopoietic system (blood system) is markedly affected by rheumatoid arthritis. Anemia is the most serious and most common blood abnormality seen in rheumatoid arthritis. A characteristic of the anemia seen in rheumatoid arthritis is normochromic, normocytic (meaning the sizes and the hemoglobin contents of the red cells are normal, but there are not enough red cells produced, resulting in anemia). The serum iron is low, the TIBC (total iron binding capacity) is normal, but the serum ferritin is high.

Although there is plenty of iron in the body, as reflected by the high serum ferritin, anemia exists because there is an abnormality involving the release mechanism of the iron from the transferrin to the early erythroblasts (early red blood cell precursors). The iron accumulates in the reticulo-endothelial cells. This failure to release iron to the erythroblasts is what is responsible for the hypoproliferative anemia that is seen in rheumatoid arthritis (anemia of chronic disease/anemia of chronic inflammatory diseases).

In effect, the rheumatoid person suffers from iron deficiency anemia because she has an inability to use the iron in the body (iron-deficient dyserythropoiesis).

Recent evidence in the literature suggests that some cytokines play a major role in this process of anemia of chronic disease (now also referred to as anemia of inflammatory diseases).

Leukopenia (low white blood cell) is frequently seen in rheumatoid arthritis and in particular when there is splenomegaly (known as Felty's Syndrome as mentioned earlier).

Evaluations of RA include:

History and physical examination
CBC
Complete blood chemistry profile
Urinalysis
ESR
Rheumatoid factor
ANA
Anti-cyclic citrullinated peptide
Chest x-ray
Joints xray
CT of joints
MRI of joints etc;

Indicators of the presence of RA include:

1. Elevated ESR (erythrocyte sedimentation rate)
2. Elevated rheumatoid factor (latex fixation)
3. Positive ANA (antinuclear antibodies) is elevated in up to 60% of patients with rheumatoid arthritis.
4. Positive Anti-cyclic citrullinated peptide (anti-CCP)

An ESR of 100 mg/hr or greater, together with a high latex fixation and rheumatoid nodules as seen in some joints represents not only severe rheumatoid arthritis, but also a very poor prognosis.

The symptoms of rheumatoid arthritis and the overall clinical course of rheumatoid arthritis is worse in blacks than in whites because most blacks are engaged in heavier physical work than their white counterparts. Poverty and heavier physical work and poor working conditions in the factories, housekeeping and domestic work are more closely associated with black men.

Therefore, people whose life circumstances place them in these poor working conditions, while at the same time being afflicted with rheumatoid arthritis, have a harder task to cope with it. Trying to work to earn a living using stiff, painful, and swollen joints of the hands, elbows, shoulders, knees, feet and lower back is a very difficult task, to say the least.

There are several modalities available to treat rheumatoid arthritis although there is no cure for this disease. Rheumatoid arthritis is primarily treated with medications such as:

Aspirin
Indocin
Motrin
Naprosyn
Clinoril
Feldane
Daypro
Relafen
Anaprox
Celebrex
Methotrxate
Arava
Minocin
Steroid
Imuran
Cytoxan
Orencia
Kineret etc.

Treatments for RA include:

Physical therapy as a modality plays a major role in the treatment of rheumatoid arthritis to prevent weakness, contractures, atrophy, and other assorted problems affecting the joints of people suffering with rheumatoid arthritis.

At times, surgical intervention must be carried out to help alleviate some of the deformities that rheumatoid arthritis causes in the joints of its victims. Anti-inflammatory medications, such as aspirin, Indocin, Excedrin, and all the NSAIDS, can cause gastrointestinal bleeding in up to 10% of individuals taking them with major medical complications. A higher number, up to 30%, of individuals taking these medications chronically develop a multitude of stomach symptoms, such as heartburn, etc.

People with kidney disease, such as renal insufficiency, ought to be very careful with NSAIDS because not only can these medications themselves cause kidney disease, *de novo*, they can make kidney disease worse. When taking these medications, these individuals ought to be supervised closely by a physician, in order that their blood counts, their liver function tests, and their kidney functions test can be closely monitored.

The most effective and the only medication approved by the FDA to prevent bleeding from the stomach (gastric ulcer) caused by aspirin and NSAIDS is misoprostol (Cytotec). Cytotec is used as 100 mcg three times per day with food. Cytotec is a prostaglandin analog.

1. Increase the pH of the gastric juice;
2. Increase mucous production by the stomach; and
3. Increase blood flow to the lining of the stomach, thereby preventing erosions and ulcerations of the stomach wall. .

Methotrexate has major side effects to the liver and bone marrow, so physicians must observe individuals taking Methotrexate closely with blood count and liver function tests, etc;

The Author was the very first person in the world to have shown that Methotrexate prevented the production of antibobies when injected into mice while working as medical a technologist as a supervisor of an immuno-heamotoplogy laboratory at a Hospital in Brooklyn New York in 1966-68.

The Physician in whose laboratory I was working published my research work without given any credit to me when he published the article containing my research. I gave him all my research data as I was leaving to go to medical school and fully explained to him how I did the experiment.

I am therefore entitled to the legitimate credit every time Methotrexate is used to treat any rheumatological diseases any where in the world.

> Of all the original ideas and major contributions I made in the field medicine, this one was the first one I made. I must in fairness say that the physician in whose laboratory I worked at a Hospital in Brooklyn NY did help me to get into medical school by given me an outstanding letter of Recommendation. I hold no grudges against him he treated me very well while working for him and without the chance he gave me to work in his laboratory, I probably would not have gotten into medical school.

All the new biologic medications in use on the market presently to treat RA and other diseases were made in the laboratory using DNA recombinant technic based on my original research experiment using methotrxate in mice, which was duplicated in humans. This was most likely done in part to bypass the toxicity of methotrxate in the treatment of RA, and other rheumatological diseases, such as mixed connect tissue diseases, psoriasis, psoriatic arthritic, ulcerative colitis, crhon's disease etc. The biologics are superb medications and credit goes to those who developed them.

To this day, methotrexate is being used all over the world to treat RA and other rheumatological diseases.

CHAPTER 67

GOUT IN AFRICAN AMERICAN MEN

Gout is a very common disease that affects 8.3 millions people in the U.S. and many more millions people in the world are affected by gout.

Three are other forms of arthritis are interconnected in that their symptoms are similar, and must be differentiated one from the other all the time.

They are as follows:

1. Acute gouty arthritis
2. Acute pseudo-gout
3. Septic arthritis

High serum uric acid affects 43.3 million American adults, representing 21 per cent of the U.S population. Diseases such as obesity and hypertension are associated with increased incidence of gout.

Acute gouty arthritis is one of the most painful conditions known in the field of medicine and to mankind. It usually occurs in a single joint such as the big toe, the ankle, the knee, the foot, or the wrist etc.

The affected joint is usually markedly swollen, painful, and tender. Gouty arthritis occurs because of either too much production of uric acid or a decreased excretion of uric acid. Thirty two million people in the U.S. have elevated uric acid. Source: International Medical news December 2010. In addition, 8 million Americans suffer from Gout and many of them are black men.

Primary overproduction of uric acid occurs because of deficiency of hypoxanthine-guanine-phosphoribosyltransferase.

This enzyme deficiency causes an increased level of 5-phosphoribosyl-1-pyrophosphate (PRPP), which accelerates purine biosynthesis and results in an increased production of uric acid.

The reduced excretion of uric acid leads to uric acid accumulation. Reduced filtrations, enhanced resorption, and decreased excretion are three other processes that lead to accumulation of uric acid in the blood.

Several other conditions can cause elevated uric acid and they include:

Diuretic treatment
Lymphoma
Leukemia

Rapid cells turn over ca.n cause acute and massive release of purines into the bloodstream as a result of chemotherapy-induced cells breakdown, resulting in marked increase of serum uric acid.

This is a crucial point to remember when treating patients who present with this form of cancer requiring acute chemotherapeutic treatment, so that IV fluid must be provided together with Allopurinol to prevent acute renal failure because of purine accumulation in the blood from clogging up the kidney tubules, causing them to fail.

Gout, which is the disease responsible for gouty arthritis, is an interesting disease, but it is not under discussion here, but one of the many problems that it can cause, namely arthritis, is under discussion.

Gout causes the production of monosodium crystals, which accumulate in joints. These crystals cause an acute inflammation leading to swelling, warmth, and severe pain of the affected joints. When this attack occurs in the big toe, it is called podagra.

Acute gouty arthritis is one of the most painful conditions known to humanity. Another gouty condition that causes acute and chronic pain in joints is pseudo-gout. Pseudo-gout occurs most frequently in older men.

The inflammatory reaction that occurs in pseudo-gout is due to calcium pyrophosphate dehydrate crystals. These crystals are seen under the microscope as weakly positive birefringent using polarized light. Similarly, the monosodium urate crystals are seen in synovial fluid taken from the joint and examined under the microscope.

The blood test that is elevated in gout is uric acid. The uric acid can be tested in the blood as part of the blood chemistry profile. The normal uric acid in the blood is 2.8 to 6.0 mg/dl. The higher the level of uric acid in the blood the more likely that it will accumulate in joints, causing inflammation to occur. The repeated inflammatory reactions that occur in the joints can result in chronic destruction of these joints to different degrees.

It is important to realize that in an acute gouty arthritic attack the uric acid level may be normal to low. The reason is that the uric acid is moving from the blood to the joints, thereby reducing its level in the blood. When someone presents with an acute, swollen, hot, and painful joint, there are really three major considerations:

1. Gout
2. Pseudo-gout
3. Septic arthritis or
4. Trauma

Septic arthritis can occur because of bacteria in the blood settling into a joint, causing inflammation to occur.

Many clinical conditions can be associated with septic arthritis:

1. Gonorrheal infection is probably the most common in sexually active individuals;
2. Pneumonia with bacteremia;
3. Sub-acute bacterial endocarditis (SBE) as seen frequently in IV drug-abusing individuals or any non-IV drug addict with SBE;
4. Penetrating trauma in a joint, etc.

To differentiate gouty arthritis in the joint from septic arthritis, one must tap synovial fluid off the joint and send it to the laboratory for evaluation. In thelaboratory, the fluid will be evaluated for:

1. Turbidity or cloudiness
2. The total number of white blood cells
3. The level of protein
4. The bacterial content of the fluid by gram stain
5. Bacterial growth on bacterial cultures
6. The presence or absence of crystals in the fluid etc.

Further evaluations include history and physical examinations and x-ray studies of the affected joint.

To treat gouty arthritis the physician has to determine the extent and severity of the symptoms.

The most effective treatment to treat acute gouty arthritis includes:

Colchicine
Colcrys
Indocin
Motrin
Naprosyn
Anaprox
Steroid

Allopurinol during an acute attack of gout might lead to an idiosyncratic reaction, worsening the condition.

Once the acute attack has been brought under control, Allopurinol 300 mg per day is given to lower the level of uric acid in the blood and colchicine 0.6 mg two times per day is given along with it.

NSAIDS or Indocin may be given clinically to prevent acute attacks from occurring. For reasons that are not quite clear, acute gouty arthritic attacks seem to occur in spite of the fact that the patient is on a good dose of prophylactic medications.

Both gout and pseudo-gout can lead to markedly deformed joints with chronic arthritic pain.

It is said that a diet that contains sweetbread, shellfish, too much red meat and red wine can all contribute to bring about acute attacks of gout. Therefore, dietary management with a decreased intake of this type of foods is a reasonable approach in the management of patients with gout and frequent gouty arthritic attacks.

As for septic arthritis, this diagnosis must be made without failure, or the affected joint will be destroyed. The treatment of choice for septic arthritis is antibiotics given intravenously. Once the suspicion is strong that septic arthritis may exist, the joint must be tapped and fluid sent to the lab for studies and IV antibiotics must be given to the affected individual immediately. The type of antibiotics given depends on the clinical profile of the patient involved. Physicians are trained to know precisely what to do, and how to do it in these circumstances.

CHAPTER 68

MIXED CONNECTIVE TISSUE DISEASES/ OVERLAP SYNDROME IN AFRICAN AMERICAN MEN

Another series of rheumatological diseases that are very common are mixed collagen vascular diseases MCTD also called overlap syndrome. About 5 million people in the U.S. have MCTD and 1 in 100,000 people in the world have MCTD. Frequently these diseases are seen in conjunction with SLE, scleroderma, polymyositis, dermatomyosis, rheumatoid arthritis, polymyositis, sjogren' syndrome and psoriatic arthritis

MCTD is an autoimmune disease of unknown cause. MCTD affects people of all ethnicity, but is more common in women than men and is more common in Blacks, Chinese, and Japanese than Caucasians. MCTD affects 1 in 100,000 or 70,000 people in the world.

The symptoms of MCTD include:

Malaise
Fatigue
Fever
Joints pain
Pain in muscles
Swelling of hands, fingers, wrists ankles, feet, and elbows
Raynaud's disease

MCTD can affect several organs including lungs, heart, joints, bones, skin, eyes, mouth, esophagus, stomach, small bowel, large bowel, blood system etc.

Evaluations of MCTD include:

History
Physical examination
CBC
Complete metabolic profile (SMA20)
Urinalysis
ESR

Rheumatoid factor
ANA
Anti-dsDNA
ENA
Anti-RNP
Anti- Ro/SSA antibody
La/SSB antibody
Anti-Jo 1 antibody
Anti-Smith antibodies
Anti-Scl 70 antibodies

Other tests to do in evaluating a person for MCTD include:

Chest x-ray
CT of the chest
MRI of the chest
Esophogram
Endoscopy
Esophogram motility study
Colonoscopy
Abdominal CT etc.

Treatments of MCTD include:

Motrin
Advil
Aleve
Naproxen
Anaprox
Celebrex
Steroid etc;
Because MCTD is often an overlap syndrome with other diseases
Such as SLE, RA, Scleroderma, Dermatomyositis, Polymyositis, Sojgreen syndrome,
treatments are usually prescribed based on associated diseases and symptoms.

CHAPTER 69

SCLERODERMA / SYSTEMIC SCLEROSIS IN AFRICAN AMERICAN MEN

Scleroderma is an autoimmune disease of unknown that causes an over growth of collagen to develop. Three hundred thousand people in the U.S. have scleroderma. More women than men have scleroderma. According to the literature, "the risk systemic sclerosis is 4-9 times higher in women than in men" Two third of people with scleroderma have the limited form of the disease and one third have the systemic form. Systemic sclerosis is 10 times higher in blacks and other minorities than as compared to whites.

Scleroderma/systemic sclerosis affects the skin, muscles, blood vessels, lungs, esophapus, stomach, small bowel, large bowel, heart, hands, fingers, kidneys, genitourinary, endocrine system, neurological system etc.

Some of these different symptoms can lead to a condition called CREST syndrome.

CREST syndrome stands for:

Calcinosis
Raynaud's phenomenon
Esophageal dysfunction
Sclerodactyly
Telangiectasias
However, CREST usually occurs in the systemic part of scleroderma.
Scleroderma usually develops in people who are between ages of 30-50.

Symptoms of scleroderma include:

Hardness of skin
Hair loss
Thickening of skin
Shiness of the with no hair
Stiffness of fingers, hands, arms
Sores and ulcers of fingers and toes
Expression less of face
Waxy looking face
Blueness, redness, blanching of fingers, toes to heat, and cold

Weight loss
Fatigue
Weakness
Shortness of breath
Joints pain
Chest pain
Numbness of hands and feet
Swelling of joints, hands, arms, wrists and feet
Cough
Wheezing
Difficulty swallowing
Bloating
Heartburn (GERD)
Vomiting
Diarrhea
Constipation
Dizziness
Malabsorption
Hypertension
Congestive heart failure
Pulmonary hypertension
Pulmonary fibrosis
Kidney failure
Cardiac arrhythmias (heart block etc.)
Erectile dysfunction
Hypothyroidism
Anemia of Chronic diseases
Menstrual irregularity
Vaginal dryness
Fibrosis of the urinary bladder etc;

Evaluations of scleroderma/systemic sclerosis include:

History and physical examination
CBC
Complete metabolic profile
ESR
Urinalysis
Antinuclear antibody
Rheumatoid factor
Anticentromere antibody
Anti-SCL-70 antibody
Endoscopy
Colonoscopy
Muscle biopsy
Skin biopsy
Small bowel scoping and biopsy

Radiological examinations to in evaluating scleroderma/systemic sclerosis include:

Chest x-ray
Chest CT
EKG
Echocardiogram
Pulmonary function test

Treatments of scleroderma/systemic sclerosis include:

Steroid
Imurin
Cytoxan
Methotrexate
NSAID

In addition, people with scleroderma/systemic sclerosis are treated for different medical complications that individual patients may suffer from.

Sometimes, individuals with scleroderma/systemic sclerosis have no external signs of the disease. Therefore, it is important to always be vigilant to look for internal symptoms like heart, lungs, kidneys, esophagus, small bowel, large bowel etc.

Several years ago, I received a long distant phone call on a late Friday afternoon from lady. A patient of mine referred her to me. Her complaint was many years of diarrhea, with 20-30 bowel movements per day and marked weight loss. Her weight was down to 65 ponds. She was had been admitted to hospitals in her hometown, Washington DC and Atlanta Georgia and no one could tell her what was wrong with her.

I admitted her to a Hospital in White Plains N.Y. on a Monday and began to evaluate her. I ordered CBC, SMA20 chemistry profile, urinalysis, ESR, ANA, ENA, RNP, anti-dada, anti-Centro mere antibody, EGK, Chest X-ray, stools culture, stools ova and parasites, stools for clostridium difficult and skin biopsy. In addition, I started her on IV fluid with glucose/normal saline with added potassium chloride.

Two days later, the results came back with positive ANA, positive RNP and positive anti- centromere antibody, establishing the diagnosis of systemic sclerosis of the small bowel causing malabsorption and diarrhea.

Subsequently, the skin biopsy, which was sent to a special laboratory confirmed scleroderma/systemic sclerosis as the diagnosis.

I treated her with IV solu-Medrol and 2 days later, her bowel movements decreased to 6 bowel movements per day. She responded well to treatments and discharged home on tapering dose of prednisone and 50mg of cytoxan. To this day, she remains on daily cytoxan, off prednisone. Her normal weight has returned and she has returned to work having been on disability for several years.

CHAPTER 70

PSORIATRIC ARTHRITIS IN AFRICAN AMERICAN MEN

The cause of psoriatic arthritis is not known and psoriatic arthritis is a chronic inflammatory disease of the skin that affects both skin and joints. There is a genetic component to psoriatic arthritis.

In addition, psoriatic arthritis can be systemic and affects the eyes, lungs, heart, and kidney. Psoriasis affects about 2 % of whites in the U.S. It affects about 8% of people with psoriasis and is less common in blacks as compared to whites.

It usually found in people between the ages of 40-50 years. Most of the time, psoriasis precedes psoriatic arthritis by 15-20 years. However, sometime arthritis precedes psoriasis by as much as 20 years. 7.5 million People in the U.S. have psoriasis and 30% of people with psoriasis develop psoriatic arthritis.

About 5 million people in the U.S. have psoriatic arthritis and 125 million people in the world have psoriasis and about 30% of them have psoriatic arthritis. People of all racial backgrounds have psoriatic arthritis.

Symptoms psoriatic arthritis includes:

Swollen and pain in knees
Swollen and pain in ankles
Swollen and pain wrists
Swollen, stiffness and pain hands
Pain and stiffness in shoulders
Pain and stiffness in neck
Pain and stiffness in lower back
Pain and stiffness in upper back
Pain and stiffness in buttocks
Pain and stiffness in the elbows
Shortness of breath
Chest pain
Blurry vision etc
The diagnosis of psoriatic arthritis is made clinically.

Evaluations of psoriatic include:

History
Physical examination
CBC
Chemistry profile
ANA
ESR
RF
CRP
T4 and TSH
B12 level
Vitamin D level
Serum Ferritin
HIV blood test (some patients with AIDS do develop a psoriatic rash)
RPR
Serum uric acid
Blood test for HAL-B27 gene (50% of people with psoriatic arthritis are positive for this gene)
Skin biopsy
Chest x-ray
EKG
Echocardiogram
Eye examination by an Ophthalmologist (some people with psoriatic arthritis develop iristi and become blind)

Medications available to treat psoriatic arthritis include:

NSAIDs
Steroid
Methotrexate
Plaquenil
Celebrex
Endrel
Exercise etc;

CHAPTER 71

PSORIASIS IN AFRICAN AMERICAN MEN

Psoriasis is very common skin condition. Worldwide 125 million people have psoriasis. In the U.S. 7.5 million people have psoriasis.

Psoriasis is the most common autoimmune disease in the U.S., about 10-30% of people with psoriasis develops psoriatic arthritis. Psoriasis is prevalent in 1.3% African Americans and 2.5% in whites.

Risk factors for psoriasis include:

Bacterial infection
Viral infection
Insect bites
Cuts on the skin
Skin burn
Medications
Too much sunlight
Not enough sunlight
Stress
HIV/AIDS
Non -HIV autoimmune disease
Chemotherapy

Symptoms of psoriasis include:

Dry skin
Flaky skin
Pink/red color skin
Thick and raised skin Lesions in the male genital area of men
Scaly/reddish lesions over elbows
Scaly/reddish lesions over knees
Scaly/reddish lesions over abdomen and chest wall
Severe dandruff on the scalp
Thick plaques and red patches over multiple parts of the body
Joints pain

Evaluations of psoriasis include:

History and physical examination
CBC
ESR
ANA
HIV 1 and 2 bloods test
Complete chemistry profile
VDRL test for syphilis
Rheumatoid factor
Lactic dehydrogenase (LDH)
Skin biopsy
Chest x-ray
Abdominal CT
Chest CT etc;

Treatments /medications to treat psoriasis include:

Steroid ointments
Steroid Creams
Steroid lotions
Prednisone
Tramcinolone
Kenalog-40
Ointments that have Vitamin D and vitamin A
Shampoos
Enbrel
Humira
Amevive
Remicade
Stelara
Clobex
Tazorac
Dovonex
Soriatane
Temovate
Methotrexate
Saltz
Phototherapy etc;

CHAPTER 72

EYE DISEASES IN
AFRICAN AMERICAN MEN

The incidence of eye diseases and blindness are more common in blacks and other minorities than in their white counterparts. Many of the diseases that predispose the development of diseases in the eye are much more common blacks and other minorities.

For example, diseases such as hypertension, diabetes mellitus, and glaucoma are much more common in blacks than in whites and other racial groups.

"285 million people are visually impaired worldwide, 39 million are blind and 246 million have low vision. About 90% of the world visually impaired lives in developing countries. "Source: WHO

The incidence of glaucoma is five times higher in blacks and other minorities than in whites. 60.5 million People in the world are diagnosed with glaucoma yearly.

Diabetes is among the most common causes of blindness. Twenty six million Americans have diabetes. According to the American College of Ophthalmology, about 5 million Americans have glaucoma. Both hypertension and diabetes mellitus predispose a person to the development of glaucoma. Of the 5 million or so Americans who have glaucoma, a very large percentage of them are blacks. For reasons that are not yet clear, blacks have a higher propensity to develop glaucoma than whites do.

Glaucoma runs in families. About 80,000 individuals go blind in the U.S. because of glaucoma yearly. What makes glaucoma so dangerous is the fact that it causes no pain. So, a person whose intraocular pressure is high, which is the first step to the development of glaucoma, will not know that the pressure inside the eye is high unless she goes to the ophthalmologist to have her eye pressure tested.

As is the case for many other diseases, blacks and other minorities often present for medical evaluations when the disease they are suffering from have already gone too far. Sometimes, these conditions are too fargone to be helped, even with the best medications or the best of medical procedures.

There are four different types of glaucoma:

1. Primary open angle glaucoma
2. Secondary glaucoma
3. Angle closure glaucoma
4. Congenital glaucoma

One-fourth of all cases of glaucoma presents at birth and are due to congenital reasons. According to the Center for Health Statistics, in Bethesda, Maryland, 1.2 out of every 100 individuals have some form of eye disease. Though this is a high percentage, the incidence is much higher among the blacks and other minorities than in whites.

The reasons are:

The higher incidence of hypertension, leading to hypertensive retinopathy with hemorrhage inside the eyes, which, if left untreated, will cause permanent blindness,

The higher incidence of diabetes in blacks and other minorities and in particular obese Blacks, Hispanics, American Indians, and Alaskan Natives who have the propensity to develop diabetes mellitus because of obesity, which then leads to diabetic retinopathy with different degrees of bleeding inside the eyes that can lead to blindness if left untreated.

The high incidence of trauma to the eye which occurs much more frequently in blacks and other minorities as compared to whites because blacks and other minorities are more likely to get exposed to riskier jobs that predispose them to a higher likelihood of being injured in their eyes on the job.

Besides glaucoma, diabetes mellitus, and hypertension, other diseases that affect the eyes include cataracts, syphilis, sarcoidosis, sickle cell disease, AIDS, temporal arteritis, vitamin deficiency, and malignant tumor etc.

In adults there are three different types of glaucoma:

1. Primary open angle glaucoma
2. Angle closure glaucoma
3. Low tension glaucoma

There are about 5 million reported cases of glaucoma in the United States. Glaucoma is the third leading cause of eye problems leading to blindness in blacks and other minorities in the United States and around the world. It is the number one cause of blindness in the world.

The incidence of blindness because of Glaucoma is 7 to 8 times higher in blacks and other minorities than in whites. Blacks and other minorities between the ages of 44 and 65, and in particular, those who are hypertensive and have a family history of glaucoma have a 15 to 17 times greater possibility of developing glaucoma than whites.

According to published reports, 30% of glaucoma patients have family history of glaucoma.

Open-angle glaucoma

The cause of open angle glaucoma is an inherited defect in the function of the endothelial cells of the cellular meshwork inside the eyes. The result is increased production of aqueous humor fluid inside the eyes on the one hand, and on the other hand, failure of drainage of the aqueous humor fluid, resulting in increased pressure inside the eyes.

The normal intraocular pressure is 13 to 20 mm/Hg. While an intraocular pressure of 13–20 mm/Hg is normal for whites, it is not necessarily normal for blacks and other minorities. This fact must be kept in mind because blacks and other minorities have a higher incidence of glaucoma; it is also true that glaucoma is much more aggressive in its progression in blacks and other minorities than it is in whites. Therefore, an intraocular pressure above 14 in a minority person must be watched closely and evaluated more frequently.

When the pressure inside the eyes is elevated, it damages the optic nerve. The optic nerve is the nerve that allows the eyes to see. Once the optic nerve is damaged, vision becomes impaired. Though the intraocular pressure is elevated, it causes no pain, and therefore, a person suffering from elevated intraocular pressure has no way to know about it until an ophthalmologist examines him or her.

The test done to evaluate the pressure inside the eye is called tonometry. The test used to evaluate the optic nerve is called a visual field. Elevated intraocular pressure does not mean glaucoma. If the intraocular pressure is allowed to remain high for an extended period of time months to years the optic nerve will become damaged. Once the optic nerve is damaged, then glaucoma ensues.

Open-angle glaucoma is responsible for more than 90% of all cases of blindness. The first sign that a person has glaucoma is when the person loses his or her peripheral vision. About 5% of first-degree relatives of people with open angle glaucoma 50 years or older develop open angle glaucoma, as compared to 1% of people in the general population.

Three things happen clinically in open angle glaucoma:

1. Intraocular pressure of 24 mm/Hg or greater
2. Cupping of the optic disc
3. Visual field loss

Typically, the first modality of treatment in someone with open angle glaucoma is eye drop medication to either reduce the production of aqueous humor fluid and/or increase the drainage, thereby lowering the intraocular pressure.

Some frequently used eye drops include:

1. Pilocarpine
2. Timoptic
3. Ocupress
4. Trusopt
5. Carbachol
6. Phystignine salicylate
7. Desmocranium bromide (Humorsol)
8. Acetazolamide (Diamox)
9. Isofurophate (Floropryl)
10. Btaxololhydrochloride (Betoptic)
11. Optipranolol
12. Propine
13. Latanoprox solution (Xalatan)
14. Betagan,
15. Cosopt
16. Alphagan P
17. Travatan etc.

If maximum eye drop treatment fails to bring the intraocular pressure down and visual field abnormality starts to develop, then laser treatment is carried out to facilitate drainage of aqueous humor fluid from the eye, thereby reducing the intraocular pressure.

As stated before, the peripheral vision is the first vision to go when increased intraocular pressure damages the optic nerve.

Angle-closure glaucoma

It is reported that angle closure glaucoma occurs mostly in individuals who are farsighted and are above age 55. About 5% of first-degree relatives of people with angle closure glaucoma are affected with the same condition in their later years.

There are three different stages of angle closure glaucoma:

1. Sub-acute angle closure glaucoma
2. Acute angle closure glaucoma
3. Chronic angle closure glaucoma

As just outlined, angle closure glaucoma occurs principally because of blockage to the proper drainage of the aqueous humor fluid that is produced inside the eyes.

In sub-acute angle closure glaucoma, the drainage is occurring in an insidious way so that the patient's eyes find ways to compensate, keeping the intraocular pressure intermittently normal.

In acute angle closure glaucoma, the intraocular pressure rises suddenly, resulting in a painful red eye, with reduced ability to see in that eye. When the examining physician places his or her finger on the affected eyeball, it is rock-hard and quite painful. On tonometric examination, the intraocular pressure may be as high as 50 mm/Hg. The affected patient feels very sick, with pain and nausea, and may even vomit.

Next to trauma to the eye, acute angle closure glaucoma is the severest emergency seen in the field of ophthalmology.

The first step in the treatment of acute angle glaucoma is to try to bring the intraocular pressure down as quickly as possible. To do that, a doctor is likely to treat the eye with Pilocarpine eye drops 2% to 4% for five minutes. Later 0.5% Timolol solution is placed in the affected eye. If this does not work then 500 mg of Diamox IV is given to bring the pressure down.

If the intraoc ular pressure fails to come down in spite of these treatments, then IV Mannitol can be given to reduce the intraocular pressure, while the eye doctor is getting the patient ready for surgery to open the eye to allow the aqueous humor fluid to drain, bringing the intraocular pressure down to save the eye. Frequently after surgery, eye drops are used to maintain a normal pressure in the eye.

As angle closure glaucoma affects both eyes, in treating acute angle closure glaucoma, the non-affected eye must also receive immediate treatment with 0.5%–1% Pilocarpine, followed by Timolol or other beta-blocker like eye drops.

The Pilocarpine is used every four hours and the beta blocker twice a day until prophylactic laser surgery can be done to that eye to prevent a similar event from occurring as that which has occurred in the acutely affected eye.

Other forms of glaucoma include:

1. Low-tension glaucoma
2. Congenital glaucoma
3. Secondary glaucoma, which can result from using iridocyclites, steroid treatment, either directly into the eye or when taken by mouth for long periods of time.

Low-tension glaucoma is seen most often in elderly individuals who suffer from severe circulatory diseases impeding blood flow. Glaucoma occurs more frequently in blacks and other minorities than in whites. The ratio is about 5-6:1 black versus white.

Glaucoma also occurs in blacks and other minorities at a younger age than in whites and it is more aggressive in blacks and other minorities and leads to blindness more rapidly than in whites. The most important thing to do is to get the eyes examined in order that if the pressure inside the eye is found to be elevated then appropriate treatments and other measures can be instituted to prevent progression to blindness.

Cataract

Another common disease of the eye is cataract. The most common form of cataract is age-related cataract or senile cataract. Cataract is an opacification of the lens of the eyes. 24.4 million Americans have cataracts and 50 million people worldwide are diagnosed with cataracts yearly.

The second form of cataract is a congenital cataract, which is usually the result of maternal rubella or cytomegalovirus infection during the first trimester of pregnancy.

Other causes of cataract include diabetes mellitus, systemic use of steroids, myotonic dystrophy, uveitis, cigarette smoking, heavy alcohol consumption, etc.

Trauma to the eye is also a common cause of cataract. Traumatic cataract is more common in blacks and other minorities than in whites because the economic circumstances of blacks and other minorities is worse, as compared to that of whites, exposing blacks and other minorities to more work-related trauma to the eyes.

The first sign of cataract is blurry vision, which progresses over months to years, with no pain, or redness to the eye and obvious clouding of the lens of the eyes when examined with the ophthalmoscope.

There are three types of cataract:

1. Posterior subcapsular cataract
2. Cortical cataract
3. Mixed cataract

Treatment of cataract

Once the diagnosis of cataract is established, the first mode of treatment is glasses to improve vision. This is the conservative management. When this treatment fails, then surgical removal of the cataract is recommended to the patient. There are two types of surgical cataract removal procedures:

1. Extracapsular cataract removal with implantation of an intraocular lens.
2. Intracapsular cataract removal

The second type of surgical procedure is much less popular because of the advent of microsurgery, which facilitates the first procedure. Cataract removal surgery is carried out in the operating room with the patient being able to go home in a few hours after the operation has been completed with a patch on the operated eye, to be followed by the surgeon in his or her office. The patient is fully awake during the time of the surgery. Only the eye being operated on is anesthetized.

Hypertensive retinopathy:

Hypertension has many complications associated with it and if left untreated will cause serious damage to occur in many organs. Prominent among these organs are the eyes. The increase in pressure within the vessels of the eye causes different degrees of damage to occur within the lumen of these vessels. The damaged vessels then trap platelets and other materials from the blood on the inner surface of these vessels, starting a nidus, which leads to plaque formation.

Leakage of fatty material occurs out of these damaged vessels, making the situation more complicated. This process perpetuates itself over time, causing different vascular abnormalities to occur inside the eyes, resulting in hypertensive retinopathy.

Hypertensive retinopathy is graded as 1, 2, 3, and 4, depending on the severity of the vascular abnormalities.

Grade 1 shows arteriolar narrowing.
Grade 2 shows arterio-venous nicking, some exudates, and hemorrhages.
Grade 3 shows retinal edema, hemorrhage, and cotton wool spots. Grade 4 shows a combination of Grade 3 plus papilledema.

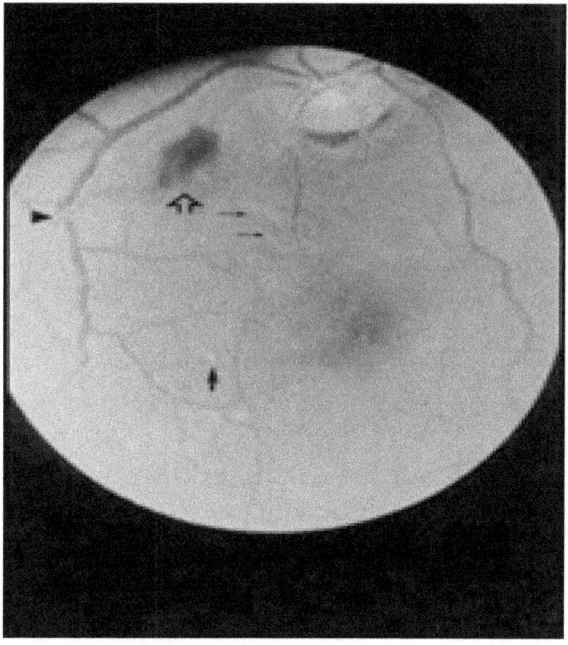

Figure 72:1 Showing different types of abnormalities in the eye of a hypertensive patient (hypertensive retinopathy). Small arrow showing silver wiring. Big arrow showing hand yellow exudates. Open arrowhead showing blot hemorrhage. Arrowhead showing A-V nicking.

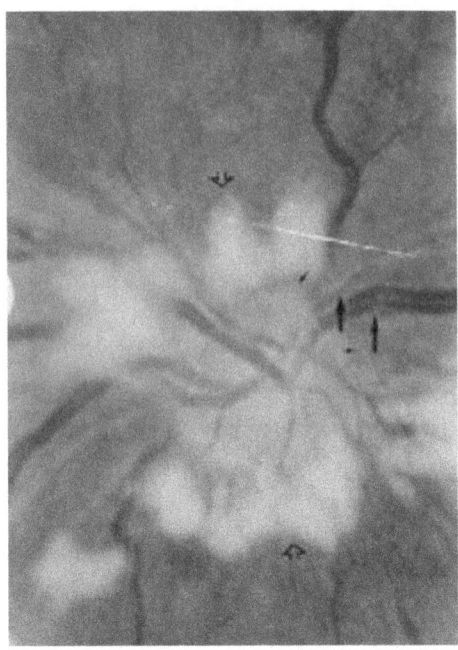

Figure 72:2: *Showing different types of abnormalities in the eye of a hypertensive patient (hypertensive retinopathy). Small arrows showing early papilledema. One big arrow pointing to vein engorgement (larger vessel). The other big arrow pointing to arterial attenuation (smaller vessel); open arrow showing cotton wool exudates.*

If proper treatment is not provided for these abnormalities, the patient often develops blindness. Hypertension is a very common disease, according to the latest estimates, occurring in about 73 million individuals in the United States. About 42% of these individuals go untreated for hypertension. Hypertension is the number-one disease among blacks in the United States.

The percentage of hypertension is higher among blacks and other minorities than whites are because there are many more obese blacks. In fact, 76% of black Americans are overweight/obese, and obesity has a major impact in both the causation of hypertension and in making it worse.

It is common knowledge that many blacks and other minorities with hypertension are being treated inappropriately because many of them are receiving the wrong medications, namely they are not being treated with water pills. Thiazide water pill (diuretic) is the most appropriate and the most effective medication to treat blacks with hypertension the world over.

According to a recent report that appears in the literature, it costs about 7–10 cents per day to treat patients with diuretic, as compared to an ACE inhibitor and calcium channel blocker that costs about $1000 per year each. This amount of money represents about 8% of the Social Security income of many people who are on Social Security.

This report confirms the inappropriateness of the treatment that some people are receiving for their hypertension. The result is that they are getting treatments for their blood pressures that cause their blood pressure to go without proper control, resulting in end organs damage. The eyes are one of the end organs. The medication prescribed is often too expensive to buy, so the condition goes untreated, resulting in progression of their hypertension.

Therefore, the percentage of people with untreated hypertension is much higher in blacks and other minorities than it is in whites, as most blacks and other minorities often are forced to do without adequate health care. It is, therefore, not difficult to see why there is such a high incidence of glaucoma and other hypertension-associated lesions in the eyes of many people, leading to their very high incidence of blindness.

Diabetes mellitus and its effects on the eyes

Type II diabetes mellitus is very common among blacks and other minorities and this is in part due to the fact that the incidence of overweight/obese among blacks and other minorities is very high and obesity is highly associated with diabetes. According to the American Diabetic Association, there are roughly 24 million individuals diagnosed with diabetes mellitus in the United States.

Worldwide, there are 1.9 billion people who are overweight and 2.1 billion people who are obese.

All diabetics are at risk of developing diseases of the eyes, such as cataracts, glaucoma and diabetic retinopathy with hemorrhage inside the eyes. One out of every 14 African-Americans is likely to develop diabetes. This rate is 30% to 40% higher in blacks and other minorities than that seen in whites. Therefore, blacks and other minorities are 30% to 40% more likely to have diabetes eye diseases compared to whites.

Diabetic retinopathy

Diabetic retinopathy is a very serious disease, which causes blindness in a significant number of blacks and other minorities who are diabetics. The same is true for any individuals who suffer from diabetes mellitus. Some of the lesions that can be seen in patients who are suffering from diabetes mellitus are as follows:

1. Micro-aneurysm
2. Arteriolar narrowing
3. Retinal edema
4. Hard exudates
5. Venous abnormalities
6. Soft exudates
7. Vitreus hemorrhages
8. Retinal hemorrhages
9. Retinal detachment etc;

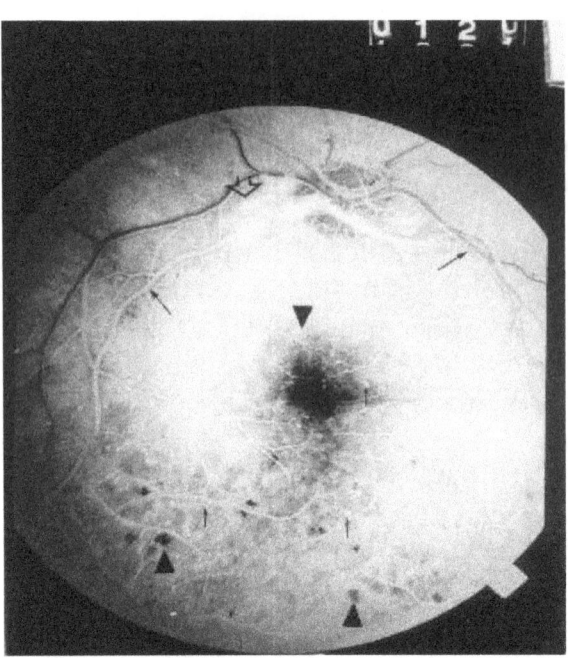

Figure 72:3–Showing different degrees of abnormalities in the eye of a patient with diabetes mellitus (diabetic retinopathy). Fluorescein angiogram shortly after injection of dye in patient's eye. Dye in arteries (white) and just starting to enter veins (large arrow). White area off NH is neovascular tuff (open arrow). White spots are hemorrhages (arrow heads). Tiny white spots are micro-aneurysms (small arrow).

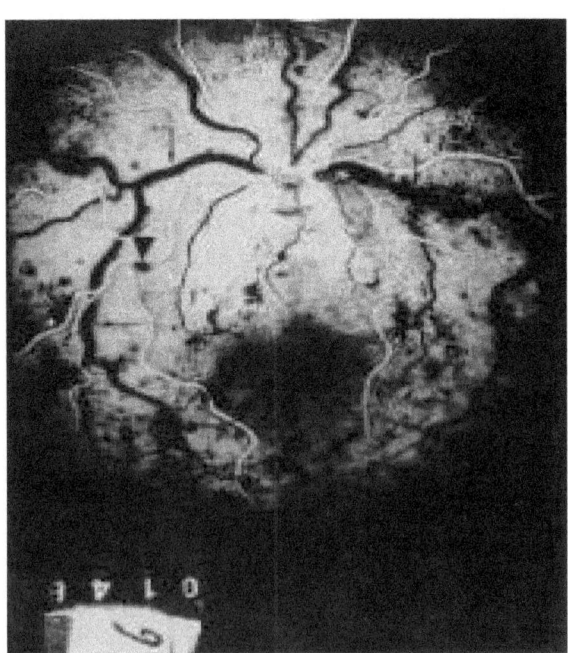

Figure 72:4–Showing different degrees of abnormalities in the eye of a patient with diabetes mellitus (diabetic retinopathy). Large arrows showing dilated veins. Arrow heads showing hemorrhages inside the eye.

It should be noted that eye symptoms and abnormalities may be the first signs that a person is suffering from diabetes mellitus. Very often, the patient presents to the ophthalmologist complaining of blurry vision, and the examining ophthalmologist, if he or she suspects diabetes mellitus as a cause of the blurriness of the eyes, can then order the blood sugar to confirm whether it is elevated blood sugar that is causing the blurry vision.

As just stated, if the diabetic retinopathy is not very advanced, the fact that the blood sugar is elevated is enough to cause eye symptoms like blurry vision. Once the patient presents with symptoms of diabetes and is diagnosed with diabetes, the treating physician should refer the patient to an eye doctor for an appropriate eye evaluation to prevent unnecessary blindness due to diabetes mellitus. Because the incidence of diabetes mellitus is on the rise, diabetes-associated blindness is also on the rise among all people.

It is very important that individuals with diabetes mellitus understand that if they present themselves to the eye doctor early enough and keep their blood sugar under tight control, and remains under constant care of a qualified ophthalmologist; they can prevent eventual blindness secondary to the effects of diabetes mellitus to the eyes.

Diabetes and ischemic diseases of the eyes

Diabetes mellitus causes ischemia because it causes plaque depositions to occur, the same way it causes plaque depositions to occur within vessels of the legs. The same process also causes deposition of plaque in the vessels of the eyes. When these very delicate vessels within the eyes have plaque within their lumens, and lipid material leaks out of these vessels, platelet deposition and plaque deposition take place, resulting, gradually, in the occlusion of these vessels to different degrees.

The occlusion causes rupture of these vessels and hemorrhage to occur, leading to different types and degrees of diabetic retinopathy. That is the underlying pathophysiology as to why, how these conditions occur, and why they lead to blindness if left untreated.

The eye is the only organ in the human body where an examining physician can actually see a vessel with the naked eye and the use of an instrument called the ophthalmoscope. It is very important that all referrals are made to an ophthalmologist, who is a physician trained and experienced to both evaluates and treats diseases of the eyes.

Hemoglobinopathies and eye disease

Sickle cell disease is the number-one abnormal hemoglobin disease that causes eye disease in those affected. Many three different types of sickle cell diseases that can cause retinopathy:

1. Sickle cell disease retinopathy (SS)
2. Sickle cell-C retinopathy (SC)
3. Sickle thalassemia retinopathy

The most severe retinopathy among these three conditions is seen in sickle cell-C disease. There are two types of retinopathies seen in sickle disease: the proliferative type and the non-proliferative type. The proliferative type is more common in SC disease and sickle thalassemia than in SS disease.

The problems occur because of sludging of red blood cells inside the small vessels of the eyes. The red cells in sickle cell disease are mal-shaped and sticky, making it difficult for them to pass through these vessels. The result is occlusion of these vessels, resulting in a multitude of vascular abnormalities within the eyes.

The types of vascular abnormalities range from arteriovenous anastomosis and neovascularization that result in leakage of blood through these newly formed vessels and cause different degrees of hemorrhages.

Retinal tear and detachment commonly occur as well. Flurocescin angiography is used to demonstrate these abnormalities. Photo-coagulation can be used as a treatment modality and laser is used to treat these conditions in the eyes of sicklers with retinopathy.

Sarcoidosis and its effects on the eyes

Sarcoidosis is quite common in blacks and the eyes are frequently affected in this condition. In fact, eye symptoms are often the presenting symptoms of sarcoidosis. Redness and swelling of the eyes with blurry vision are often seen. The eye doctor usually looks for anterior uveitis, which is often present when sarcoidosis involves the eyes.

Slit-lamp examination is usually carried out to evaluate the eyes when sarcoidosis is suspected. If sarcoidosis is not recognized and treated early with Prednisone, the end result often means total blindness in the affected eye. Glaucoma is also seen in chronic untreated sarcoidosis of the eye. The angiotensin-1-converting enzyme blood test is often elevated in individuals affected with sarcoidosis, and the serum calcium may be elevated as well.

AIDS and eye disease

AIDS, as a viral illness, frequently affects the eyes. The most common infection that is seen in the eyes of AIDS patients is cytomegalovirus (CMV). CMV causes an infection of the eyes called retinitis. Blacks are affected more than whites with AIDS-associated CMV retinitis are because the percentage of blacks with AIDS is much higher than that of whites.

CMV retinitis in AIDS is quite difficult to treat and eradicate. The most effective medication is Ganciclovir. This medication has serious side effects and must be given IV in the hospital setting.

Temporal arteritis and eye disease:

Temporal arteritis (giant cell arteritis) is a condition seen in middle-aged to elderly individuals The diagnosis of temporal arteritis cannot be missed, and, in fact, must not be missed, for if it is missed, the end result is permanent blindness in the affected eye.

Usually, the patient comes to see the physician with headache, general malaise, and visual abnormality, and may report having a low-grade fever. Following a physical examination, a diagnosis can quickly be established by doing an erythrocyte sedimentation rate (ESR). If the ESR is very high (normal ESR is from 10– 30 ml/hr) then the diagnosis of temporal arteritis is very likely.

The next step is to admit the patient to the hospital for treatment with high-dose IV steroids. The ophthalmologist always must always be involved in the care of the patient, to carry out a thorough eye examination of the patient.

The next step is to call a surgeon in to do a temporal artery biopsy. It is not necessary to wait for the biopsy before starting steroid treatment. If the physician waits for the results of the biopsy, it may be too late to save the eyes. A negative temporal artery biopsy does not rule out the diagnosis of temporal arthritis (giant cell arthritis) because this disease is often a segmental disease and a normal segment of artery could easily have been biopsies, leaving behind the abnormal segment.

Vitamin deficiency and eye disease

As alcoholism is quite common among all people, and certain vitamin deficiencies are likely to occur. One of the frequent vitamin deficiencies that occur in this setting is Vitamin B6 (thiamine). Thiamine deficiency can cause ocular motor palsy. It can also lead to Wernicke's disease, which is associated with nystagmus, ptosis, retinal hemorrhage, diplopia, and internal strabismus.

Treatment consists of injection of thiamine to replete the store, followed by B-complex vitamins by mouth, which contains all the B vitamins, and abstinence from alcohol is the key. Thiamine by mouth can also be given following the acute repletion of the stores.

Malignant tumor and eye symptoms

Malignant tumors, such as primary melanoma, tumor of the lid of the eye (associated with xeroderma pigmentosum), can affect the eye. The eye can also be affected by sarcoma.

Malignant melanoma is a particularly troublesome disease that can lead to the demise of the patient if not diagnosed quickly and treatment started right away.

Metastatic cancer may first show signs of its presence in the eye. This is believed to be due to an autoimmune phenomenon (the body reacting to the cancer as a foreign agent), thereby producing an antibody against it, causing an inflammatory reaction to occur in the eye, resulting in eye symptoms.

Sexually transmitted diseases and eye diseases include:

AIDS (see CMV retinitis above)
Syphilis
Herpes simplex infection

Syphilis and eye problems

In the latter stage of syphilis, a variety of different eye problems can occur. One problem may be small, irregular pupils that sometimes react to accommodation, but does not react to light. Another problem might be the Argyle-Robertson pupils (the result of atrophy of the iris), which is seen in neurosyphilis. Neurosyphilis is common in people suffering from AIDS.

Other problems that can occur in neurosyphilis include iritis and photophobia. Adhesion of the iris to the lens of the eye can also occur, which can cause a fixed pupil. These problems can all be picked up through a good eye examination by an internist who can then refer the affected person to an ophthalmologist for further evaluation and treatments.

According to The Center for Disease Control and Prevention (CDC) guidelines, treatment for neurosyphilis must include blood VDRL and FTA-ABS. A lumbar puncture ought to be done to obtain cerebrospinal fluid (CSF). The CSF fluid must be sent for VDRL and FTA-ABS. If it is positive, then treatment for neurosyphilis must be started by giving 10 to 20 million units of aqueous penicillin daily IV for ten days.

In addition, a three-week course of 2.4 million units of Bicillin for 7.2 million units must be given. If the patient has HIV infection (AIDS) and a positive VDRL, FTA-ABS in the blood, even if the CSF is negative or if the patient refuses a lumbar puncture, the same protocol as just outlined ought to be employed to treat the patient.

This ought to be done because neurosyphilis is quite prevalent in individuals with AIDS. If a person is allergic to penicillin, then Erythromycin 2 grams by mouth daily for 30 days or Tetracycline 2 grams daily for 30 days should be prescribed to treat the syphilis. Keep in mind that if a person is pregnant she ought not to be treated with Tetracycline.

In summary, eye diseases are very common in blacks, for the reasons outlined in this chapter. Diseases such as diabetes mellitus, hypertension, trauma in the workplace to the eyes, sickle cell disease, sarcoidosis, AIDS, Syphilis, all of which participate in the rising incidence of glaucoma that is five times higher in blacks than whites. (See the section on sarcoidosis in the previous chapter above)

The overall economic and educational situations of the majority of blacks will have to be improved drastically if it is expected that a real impact can be made to decrease the accelerated rate of blindness from which some blacks are suffering.

CHAPTER 73

DEPRESSION IN AFRICAN AMERICAN MEN

Mental illness is one of the most common illnesses in the world. One in every four individuals or 25% of people in the world suffers from some types of mental illnesses.

The world population in 2013 is 7,103,804 people and 25% or 1,775,951,000 of them suffer from mental illnesses. 350, 000,000 in the world suffer from depression, in the world 25, 000, 000 suffer from schizophrenia, 2.4 % people in the world suffer from bipolar disorder, 5.7 000,000 American adults suffer from bipolar disorder, 24, 000,000 suffer from schizophrenia, 20,000,000 Americans suffer from depression and

Worldwide 140, 000,000 million suffer from alcoholism. Source: WHO According to the Surgeon General, there are 44 million Americans with mental illness one in 4 Americans suffers with a diagnosable mental illness. Every year 19 million Americans suffer from some form of mental illnesses.

"22.5% of US Adults Had At Least One Mental Disorder in 2013"
"According to a report by the Substance Abuse and Mental Health Services Administration in conjunction with the National Institute of Mental Health, nearly a quarter of American adults experienced at least one mental health disorder in the past year." The report found that 22.5% of American adults (51.2 million people) had at least one mental in the past year." Some 17 million Americans (7.4% of the adult population) suffered mood disorders, including major depression and bipolar disorders."

"About one in six American adults reported at least one psychiatric medications, usually an antidepressant or an anti-anxiety medication and most had been doing so for a year or more". JAMA Internal Medicine December 12, 2016

"More than 20 %of white Americans reported reported being prescribed psychiatric medications, compared to about 9% Hispanic adults, nearly10% of black adults and close to 5% Asian."

Mental illness affects all racial groups, both sexes and all social strata. However, Black Americans, Hispanic Americans other American minorities and other minorities in the world are affected by depression more than whites are. Mental is the number one cause of suicide. Every day 3000 people in the world commit suicide because of depression and 90% of suicide is due to mental illness.

"Death by suicide occurs every 40 seconds."
"Around the world an estimated 804,000 people killed themselves in 2012, a rate of about 11.4 per 100,000 populations. "Men were almost twice as likely as females to kill themselves. "In the U.S. of the 43,361 Americans, who killed themselves in 2012, 34,055 were males and 9,306 were females." Source: WHO

Depression is more common than cancer, heart disease and HIV/AIDS combined.

There are different types of depression:

1. Transient situational depression
2. Permanent or chronic situational depression
3. Depression associated with taking medications for a medical condition
4. Depression associated with alcohol abuse or drug abuse
5. Minor classical depression
6. Major classical depression
7. Depression associated with anxiety reaction and panic attacks
8. Manic depression,
9. Smoking associated depression etc.

According a report published on 7/18/14, smoking increases the rate of suicide by a factor of 4. Suicide is 4 times higher in smokers than in non-smokers.

(The concept of permanent or chronic situational depression is the author's own developed concept.)

Incidence of depression

Depression is 3 to 4 times more common in black men and other minority. In the U.S. more than 17 million individuals (about 1 in 10 adults) suffer from a depressive episode at least once per year and more than 80% of the time these episodes go untreated.

According to some study, blacks and other minorities suffer more from mental illnesses than do whites.

Black men, Hispanicmen and other minority men experience more depression, anxiety and panic attacks than whites do. Being poor is a depressive state of being and, therefore, 100% of poor people suffer from one form of depression or another, at one time or another worldwide. The difference is in the cultural expression of these symptoms and the cultural conditioning and reluctance to express the symptoms of these illnesses for fear of being ostracized by their communities. Being poor, it is a miserable state, however, is not a shame and many people have worked themselves out of poverty.

In any African ancestral society, mental illness is taboo because it is seen as a sign of weakness. A failure to be able to endure whatever it is that the majority of society can dish out and not only surviving it, enduring it and to be able to live long enough to tell one's children and grandchildren about it, is an essential part of the indigenous black culture.

Black men and Hispanic men and other minority men see mental illness as a label that can be used to discriminate against them by the medical community, the job market, and the legal community and, by the law enforcement community to prevent them from getting ahead. Because these people do not want any mention of mental illness on their records if they can help it, they hide their symptoms of depression and suffer in silence.

When an interviewer tries to elicit mental illness from them, they would not tell him or her about it. They frequently do not tell a physician/therapist about their mental illness either, unless they absolutely have to.

TABLE 1

Some of the symptoms of major depression:

Five (or more) of the following symptoms have been present during the same 2-week period and represent a change from previous functioning: at least one of the symptoms is either depressed mood or loss of interest in pleasure, excluding symptoms that are due to medical illnesses.

(1) Depressed mood most of the day, nearly every day as indicated by either subjective report (e.g., feels sad or empty) or observation made by others (e.g., appears tearful). **Note:** In children and adolescents, can be irritable mood.
(2) Markedly diminished interest or pleasure in all, or almost all activities most of the day, nearly every day (as indicated by either subjective account or observation made by others.)
(3) Significant weight loss when not dieting or weight gain (e.g., a change of more than 5% of body weight in a month), or decrease or increase in appetite nearly every day. **Note:** In children, consider failure to make expected weight gains.
(4) Insomnia or hypersomnia every day
(5) Psychomotor agitation or retardation nearly every day (observable by others, not merely subjective feelings of restlessness or being slowed down)
(6) Fatigue or loss of energy every day
(7) Feelings of worthlessness or excessive or inappropriate guilt (which may be delusional) nearly every day (not merely self-reproach or guilt about being sick)
(8) Diminished ability to think or concentrate, or indecisiveness, nearly every day (either by subjective account or as observed by others).
(9) Recurrent thoughts of death (not just fear of dying), recurrent suicidal ideation without a specific plan, or a suicide attempt or a specific plan for committing suicide.
A. These symptoms do not meet criteria for a mixed episode.
B. The symptoms cause clinically significant distress or impairment in social, occupational, or other important areas of functioning.

C. The symptoms are not due to the direct physiological effects of a substance (e.g., a drug of abuse, a medication) or a general medical condition (e.g., hypothyroidism).
D. The symptoms are not better accounted for by bereavement, i.e., after the loss of a loved one, the symptoms persist for longer than 2 months or are characterized by marked functional impairment, morbid occupation with worthlessness, suicidal ideation, psychotic symptoms, or psychomotor retardation.

As modified from DSM IV

Depression as seen in blacks is a very complex disease with many associated components. Classical minor depression is defined as 3 or 4 depressive symptoms for 2 weeks or longer. Major depression is defined as 5 or more depressive symptoms for 2 weeks or longer.

TABLE 2

Some symptoms of minor depression:

A. A distinct period of abnormally and persistently elevated, expansive, or irritable mood, lasting at least 1 week (or any duration if hospitalization is necessary).
B. During the period of mood disturbance, three (or more) of the following symptoms have persisted (four if the mood is only irritable) and have been present to a significant degree.
(1) Inflated self-esteem or grandiosity
(2) Decreased need for sleep (e.g., feels rested after only 3 hours of sleep)
(3) More talkative than usual or pressure to keep talking
(4) Flight of ideas or subjective experience that thoughts are racing
(5) Distractibility (i.e., attention too easily drawn to unimportant or irrelevant external stimuli)
(6) Increase in goal-directed activity (either socially, at work or school, or sexually) or psychomotor agitation
(7) Excessive involvement in pleasurable activities that have a high potential for painful consequences (e.g., engaged in unrestrained buying sprees, sexual indiscretions, or foolish business investments)
C. These symptoms do not meet criteria for a mixed episode.
D. The mood disturbance is sufficiently severe to cause marked impairment in occupational functioning or in usual social activities or relationships with others, or to necessitate hospitalization to prevent harm to self or others, or there are psychotic features.
E. The symptoms are not due to the direct physiological effects of a substance (e.g., a drug of abuse, a medication, or other treatment) or a general medical condition (e.g., hyperthyroidism).

Blacks, Hispanics and other minorities worldwide can suffer from the classic forms of depression such as:

1. Minor depression.
2. Major depression.
3. Manic depression.

1. A mixed form of depression associated with anxiety and panic attacks.
2. Transient and permanent situational depression.
3. Depression associated with alcohol abuse and drug abuse.

Criteria used to make the diagnosis of major depression:

Blacks, as well as Hispanic, are extremely reluctant to go to the psychiatrist because of the fear of being labeled "crazy" in the case Hispanics "loco". Both these groups culturally deal with mental illness the way in which mental illness is dealt with in the African culture.

In the African culture, when a person of African ancestry is troubled with a mood disorder, he or she goes to an elder or group of family members within that family for advice in order to deal with the problem. Sometimes this group is organized as a committee, as is done frequently in the third world. Never in this setting is the word mental illness used. In fact, in the third world it is unlikely that a man would marry into a family that has an immediate member with a history of being mentally ill.

Because of racism, different degrees and different types of racial insensitivity and the suspicion and distrust that it causes, Blacks and Hispanics in the U.S. and in the world are almost exclusively reluctant to seek help for mental illness, and in particular depression, because most of the psychiatrists-therapists are Caucasians.

The reasons Blacks, Hispanics and other minorities give for refusing to see Caucasian or non-minority psychiatrists-therapists are as follows:

"Why should I go to the white and non-Hispanic, non-black psychiatrist-therapist to open up my innermost secrets to them, when they are partly responsible for my problems to begin with?"

Q. *"You mean the psychiatrist-therapist is the source of your problem?"*
A. **"No, not him or her in particular, but he or she belongs to the group of people that is the underlying cause of my depression in the first place."**
Q. **"How so, could you elaborate?"**
A. **"Well, you know, racial insensitivity and bigotry are so pervasive and widespread you don't know who to trust and who not to trust."**
Q. **"Is it that you have a problem trusting anyone?"**
A *"No, I just have difficulty opening up my inner soul to the people who I know don't like me in the first place." And have a predetermined negative notion about me.*

It is a known fact that when Blacks, Hispanics and other minorities are evaluated for mental illness by white psychiatrists-therapists, oftentimes the diagnosis made is wrong. The literature outlines cases of Blacks, Hispanics and other minorities that were diagnosed as schizophrenics, when in fact they were not.

Because of subjectivity that is often involved in the diagnosis of mental illnesses, very frequently psychiatrist-therapists and others involved in dealing with Blacks, Hispanics and other minorities who have mental illness tend to give them a worse diagnosis rather than a better diagnosis, and clearly racism, racial insensitivity, bigotry, racial insensitivity and intellectual condescendence play a major role in that particular situation.

Transient situational depression occurs in all groups regardless of ethnic background. In what normally would have been transient situational depression because of a loss of a job, a boyfriend, a girl friend, a death in the family, or the death of a close friend, etc. can sometime ends up in a severe form of depression.

The depression would seem to last longer because underneath exists a mental fragility born out of constant exposure to racial injustices, making it easier to cross over the line to a more permanent situational depressive state.

Permanent and chronic situational depression in blacks in the U.S. is a condition born out of constant and relentless barrages of daily exposure to racial discrimination and injustices at all levels of American society. Many several sub-cultures in the world communities whose poor people have been conditioned or brainwashed into the belief that their poverty is the result of divine will.

These folks then are coerced through different means to pray to God for easing of their earthly suffering to get to heaven, to get their divine rewards. This concept does not seem to be as prevalent among blacks in the U.S. as elsewhere in the world.

It does not matter if a black person in America works as a sanitation worker or as physician or a judge in a court of law; he or she has to deal with racial discrimination and racial confrontations, be it in different forms and different circumstances.

Granted, the less educated and less financially able a person is, the more he or she feels the stings and often the bites of racism eating away at his or her flesh, heart and soul. Because racism has become an accepted part of the American culture, Blacks and Hispanics and other minorities feel a sense of constant persecution that is "real" and, therefore, they are more prone to become chronically situationally depressed.

Most Caucasians and most non-blacks individuals leaving in America constantly discriminate racially against blacks in America. They do it because they see white Americans doing it, so they do it too. In particular, black men are the most discriminated against human beings in the U.S. by all other racial groups.

Some blacks in America and around the world have developed coping mechanisms to both survive racism and its depressive nature. Some blacks have chosen to excel at whatever it is that they do; they go beyond that which is necessary as a mechanism of coping, not just to be accepted necessarily, but also to be respected.

Professional respect means a lot to any professional person, but more so to blacks and other minorities. Professional blacks and other minorities typically would say, "Though you don't like the color of my skin and many other things about me, but I dare you to doubt my ability to beat you at your own game and do my work with excellence" and more often than not, much better than you.

Some blacks and other minorities have chosen to become activists and community organizers, to wake up other blacks and minorities, to fight for their rights. Still, others have chosen to give up and allow racism to engulf all aspects of their beings by becoming welfare recipients and part of the culture of the have-nots.

Many people are on welfare because of physical or mental disabilities, and this is both acceptable and understandable, but many minorities have become so chronically passive, and dependent, they do not care a damn anymore, so welfare has become a way of life for them.

Still many blacks and other minorities have allowed their anger and despair to cause them to fall into the trap of drug, alcohol and other substance abuse, which have totally taken over their lives to a degree that their very humanity represents nothing to them. Therefore, the lives of other individuals have not much value to them either. It is this state of being, that causes some of them to commit unspeakable crimes against their neighbors, and their communities (see the chapters on drug abuse and alcohol abuse).

Depression, associated with anxiety and panic attacks, is extremely common in minorities. However, this type of depression is much more common in minorities than in whites based on the fact most minorities have more reasons to be anxious, and even more reason to be panicky.

This is so because blacks and other minorities have to face racism, poor education, and lack of jobs, lower economic status, raising children without a father around to help, and many other unspeakable injustices to cope with. All the above problems create a constant state of negative anger, disappointment, uncertainty, and the result is anxiety, panic attacks, and depression.

THE WAY TO SUCCEED AS A BLACK PERSON IN THE U.S. AND THE WORLD IS TO AVOID THE NEGATIVE ANGER SYNDROME; RATHER, IT IS BEST TO BE POSITIVELY ANGRY.

NEGATIVE ANGER IS SELF-DESTRUCTIVE, POSITIVE ANGER IS SEL-MOTIVATING AND CONSTRUCTIVE.

What makes this whole situation even more serious is the fact that more often than not, these Blacks, Hispanics and other minorities go without being diagnosed and without being treated for their mental illnesses. A small sub-group of educated and professional Blacks, Hispanics and other minorities does seek help and are receiving psychological treatment.

How to evaluate Blacks, Hispanics and other minorities when they come in for evaluation of depression to a primary care physician.

In the black community, the primary care physician is likely to be the one who is most likely to see the vast majority of blacks with depression. This is so because these blacks are extremely resistant to the concept that they may have a need for psychological care. This reluctant to admit mental illness is a cultural fact and it must be understood, respected and dealt with, with the greatest of care and ethnic sensitivity.

TABLE 3

Some of the most common symptoms of depression:

Depression
Persistent sad, anxious, or "empty" mood
Loss of interest or pleasure in activities, including sex
Feelings of hopelessness, pessimism
Feelings of guilt, worthlessness, helplessness
Sleeping too much or too little, early-morning awakening
Appetite and/or weight loss or overeating and weight gain
Decreased energy, fatigue, feeling "slowed down"
Thoughts of death or suicide, or suicide attempts
Restlessness, irritability
Difficulty concentrating, remembering, or making decisions
Persistent physical symptoms that do not respond to treatment, such as headaches, digestive disorders, and chronic pain
Mania
Abnormally elevated mood
Irritability
Severe insomnia
Grandiose notions
Increased talking
Racing thoughts
Increased activity, including sexual activity
Markedly increased energy
Poor judgment that leads to risk-taking behavior
Inappropriate social behavior

A thorough diagnostic evaluation is needed if five or more of these symptoms persist for more than two weeks, or if they interfere with work or family life. An evaluation involves a complete physical checkup and information gathering on family health history.

(As published by the National Institute of Mental Health)
Some of the symptoms of panic attack:

1. Palpitations, pounding of heart, or accelerated heart rate
2. Sweating
3. Trembling or shaking
4. Sensation of shortness of breath or smothering
5. Feeling of choking
6. Chest pain or discomfort
7. Nausea or abdominal distress
8. Feeling dizzy, lightheaded, or faint
9. Derealization (feelings of unreality) or depersonalization (being detached from oneself)
10. Fear of losing control or going crazy
11. Fear of dying
12. Paresthesias (numbness or tingling sensation)
13. Chills or hot flashes
14. Abdominal pain
15. Diarrhea
16. White-out spells
17. Urinary frequency
18. Hyperventilation
19. Leg cramps
20. Insomnia

Partially modified from DSM IV

The first step in evaluation someone with depression includes a complete history and physical examination. The next step is a series of specific laboratory tests such as:

1. CBC
2. Chemistry profile (SMA 18)
3. Thyroid profile T4, TSH
4. Urinalysis
5. Serum ferritin
6. Serum B12
7. Chest x-ray
8. EKG
9. Mammogram, if the man is 40 years or older; or younger if a mass is felt in the breast or if there is a family history of breast cancer
10. A CT Scan of the brain or MRI of the brain, if there is headache, dizziness, and forgetfulness, or symptoms of neurological signs are found during the history and physical examination. In fact, it may be important to do a CT scan anyway, even though there may be no obvious neurological signs or symptoms.

Other specific blood tests may become necessary based on the physician's assessment of the case.

Approaching the patient in this way allows the physician to ascertain whether or not the patient's signs and symptoms of depression, anxiety or panic attacks have no organic basis (that is, nothing medical can explain her symptoms).

Diseases such as diabetes mellitus, hyperthyroidism, hypothyroidism, cancer, iron deficiency anemia, kidney failure, heart disease such as mitral valve prolapsed, atherosclerotic heart disease with angina pectoris, congestive heart failure with low cardiac output and poor brain perfusion, B12 deficiency, etc. (if a person remains B12 deficient for 3 to 5 years, he or she may develop permanent neuropsychiatric problems).

It is not unusual to find a patient in a psychiatric hospital who is permanently committed as a result of B12 deficiency that either was not diagnosed at all or was diagnosed too late, resulting in permanent neurological and mental disease.

Brain tumor may first present with symptoms of psychiatric disease. It is, therefore, always necessary for a person who manifests symptoms of depression to undergo a thorough medical evaluation by a primary care physician before any definite statement can be made regarding the proper psychiatric diagnosis of that man.

Both hyperthyroidism and hypothyroidism can manifest symptoms of depression. As part of the evaluation of depression, serum B12, T4, TSH, and brain CT ought to be done.

It is important that prior to starting any psychotropic medications, a CBC, liver function tests and EKG be done, because many of the psychotropic medications have many side effects that can cause the white blood cell count, the platelets, the red blood cell count as well as the EKG and liver function test to be abnormal.

Some of these medications can affect the rhythm of the heart in different ways, so a baseline EKG must be done before starting these medications. In fact, periodically CBC, kidney function tests such as BUN, creatinine, electrolytes, liver function tests, T4, TSH must be done during the course of psychotropic medication therapy.

Treatments of depression

Depression is treated usually with medications, psychotherapy and, at times, with ECT. Some of the medications used to treat depression are the following:

Serotonin-specific reuptake inhibitors such as:

1. Zoloft
2. Paxil
3. Prozac
4. Celexa

5. Lexapro
6. Paxil
7. Celexa
8. Luvox etc;

Serotonin non-selective reuptake inhibitors such as:

1. Effexor
2. Effexor XR
3. Cymbalta etc.

Other anti-depression medications:

1. Wellbutrin
2. Wellbutrin SR
3. Remeron
4. Ludiomil, which is basically a dopamine-active medication
5. Norpramin.
6. Serzone
7. Symbyax
8. Desyrel
9. Pristiq etc;

Anti-Anxiety medications include:

1. BuSpar
2. Klonopin
3. Xanax
4. Lithium
5. Ativan
6. Valium
7. Serax
8. Valium
9. Klonorpin
10. Centrax
11. Serax
12. Librium
13. Tranxene etc.

Tertiary amines such as:

1. Elavil
2. Tofranil
3. Anafranil
4. Sinequan
5. Pamelor

6. Ascendin
7. Anafranil
8. Surmontil
9. Vivactil etc;

MAOIs or monoamine oxidase inhibitors such as:

1. Parnate
2. Eldepryl
3. Nardil etc.

The usual dosages and side effects of these medications are:

1. **Zoloft–** The initial dose is 50 mg per day; this dose can be increased up to 200 mg per day. There are several tolerable side effects of Zoloft, and liver function tests and EKG must be closely monitored along with blood levels while the patient is on Zoloft.
2. **Paxil–**The usual starting dose of Paxil is 20 mg per day and this dose can be increased up to 50 mg per day for those people who fail to respond to the 20 mg dose. Paxil can cause several tolerable side effects, but liver function tests and EKG must be monitored along with Paxil blood level.
3. **Prozac–**The usual dose of Prozac is 20 mg per day. If a patient fails to respond to 20 mg per day, the dose can be increased up to 80 mg per day. Prozac has several side effects, and liver function tests and EKG ought to be monitored along with blood level of Prozac.
4. **Effexor–**The usual starting dose of Effexor is 25 mg three times per day. The dose may be increased up to 150 mg per day in divided doses, and in rare circumstances, the dose may be raised to as high as 275 mg per day in divided doses. Effexor has many tolerable side effects, but liver function tests and periodic EKG ought to be done along with blood level of the medication.
5. **Wellbutrin SR–**The usual dose of Wellbutrin SR is 150 mg two times per day; at times a dose of 200 mg two times per day can be given. Wellbutrin SR has several tolerable side effects, but is important to monitor liver function tests, EKG and blood level of Wellbutrin SR.
6. **Ludiomil–**The usual dose of Ludiomil is 75 mg per day. In the elderly, as little as 25 mg per day may be effective. Doses as high as 150 mg to 225 mg may be used in hospital patients. Ludiomil has several tolerable side effects, but periodic EKG, liver function tests should be done.
7. **Norpramin–**The usual dose of Norpramin is 100 mg to 200 mg per day. This dose may be increased to as high as 300 mg per day. This medication is not recommended for use in children. Norpramin is not to be used in conjunction with MAO inhibitors. In fact, it cannot be used up to two weeks after stopping MAO inhibitors. Norpramin has several tolerable side effects, but CBC, liver function tests, EKG; and blood thyroid function must be done before starting this medication. These same tests must be done periodically while a patient is on Norpramin.

8. **Pamelor**–The usual dose of Pamelor is 25 mg 3–4 times per day. At times, the dose may be raised up to 150 mg per day. Pamelor has several tolerable side effects. While on this medication, EKG, CBC, liver function tests ought to be done along with blood level of Pamelor.

9. **Lithium**–The usual maintenance dose of Lithium is 450 mg, two times per day, but doses as high as 1,350 mg per day may be given. Lithium has several tolerable side effects. Before starting a patient on Lithium, CBC, liver function tests, kidney function tests, blood thyroid function tests, and EKG must be done. While on Lithium, these same tests must be done and monitored closely. Blood level of Lithium must also be monitored. The kidneys are particularly sensitive to the effects of Lithium, and at the first signs of blood kidney function test abnormalities, the treatment must be stopped. Lithium can cause thyroid function tests to become abnormal. The WBC can sometimes go down as a result of Lithium.

10. **Desyrel**–The usual starting of Desyrel is 150 mg in divided doses, but a dose up to 600 mg per day in divided doses can be used. Desyrel has several tolerable side effects; therefore, an EKG ought to be done before starting this medication and periodically ought to be done while the person is on this drug.

11. **Asendin**–The usual dose of Asendin is 200–300 mg per day in divided doses. Asendin has several tolerable side effects. Blood chemistry tests, CBC and EKG should be done while the patient is on Asendin.

12. **Klonopin**–The initial dose of Klonopin is 1.5 mg per day in divided doses. Sometimes the dose can be raised to as high as 20 mg per day. This medication is quite effective in individuals with anxiety reaction associated with depression. It allows the patient to get a good night's sleep. CBC, liver function tests and EKG ought to be done before starting the medication and the same tests should be monitored while the patient is on the medication.

13. **BuSpar**–The usual dose of BuSpar to treat anxiety is 10 mg two times per day and the dose can be raised up to 30 mg per day in divided doses.

14. **Xanax**–The usual dose of Xanax to treat anxiety is 0.25 mg three times per day. A dose up to 4 mg per day can be used in divided doses, in certain cases. In treating panic disorder, the dose can be as high as 4 mg in divided doses. Xanax has several tolerable side effects, but laboratory tests are not required during the treatment of patient on Xanax.

15. **Elavil**–The usual dose of Elavil is 75 to 300 mg per day in divided doses. Elavil has several tolerable side effects. EKG, CBC, liver function tests, along with Elavil blood level should be done periodically while the patient is on Elavil.

16. **Tofranil**–The usual dose of Tofranil is 75 mg per day. The dose may be increased up to 150 mg per day. Tofranil has several tolerable side effects; EKG, CBC, liver function tests along with Tofranil blood level should be done periodically.

17. **Anafranil**–The usual starting dose of Anafranil is 25 mg per day and the dose may be increased up to 200 mg per day in divided doses. EKG, CBC, liver function tests, along with Anafranil blood levels, should be done periodically while a patient is on Anafranil.

18. **Doxepin**–The usual starting dose of Doxepin is 75 mg per day. The dose may be increased up to 300 mg per day. EKG, CBC, blood chemistry tests should be done periodically while the patient is on Doxepin.

19. **Parnate**–The usual starting dose of Parnate is 30 mg per day in divided doses. The dose may at times be increased to as high as 60 mg per day in divided doses. Frequent monitoring of blood pressure, EKG, CBC, blood chemistry tests ought to be done while the patient is on this medication. Parnate has a long list of medications that it cannot be used with. Further, there are several food products that must be avoided while on Parnate; among those are cheeses, foods high in tyramine, sour cream, Chianti wines, sherry, beer, liquors, caviar, anchovies, pickled herring, canned figs, raisins, bananas, avocados, chocolate, soybean, sauerkraut, yogurt, yeast extracts, etc.

ECT remains an effective modality of treatment for depression. ECT is used under a general anesthesia and muscle relaxants, decreasing convulsions and eliminating the possibility of fractures and other injuries to the patient. ECT is most appropriate for patients who cannot take medications or whose associated illnesses contradict them taking an antidepressant medication. In addition, in certain life-threatening situations, when all other antidepressant medications fail, then ECT is most appropriate and useful.

Psychotherapy

Psychotherapy is a non-medication effective modality of treatment for certain types of depression. Psychotherapy involves counseling. The mental health professionals who provide psychotherapy treatments are psychotherapists, psychiatrists, and certified social workers. Primary care physicians are well equipped to provide psychotherapy counseling, if they have the time to do it. The incidence of depression is 3 to 4 times more common in blacks than in their male counterparts.

Many people fear being stigmatized with mental illness and refrain from seeking psychiatric treatment for depression, until the depression is too far advanced and more difficult to treat.

These people avoid going to the psychiatrist for treatment of depression because of the stigma associated with mental illness. This situation is gravest among working poor and working Blacks, Hispanics and other minorities and poor people the world over. This is true for all minority people no matter their status.

Upper-class Blacks, Hispanics and other minorities are less concerned about going to the psychiatrist because they have money and enjoy a high social standing, and they do not fear the stigma of mental illness, and the economic and social negativities associated with it.

In addition, most of these individuals seem to have high trust in the Caucasian therapists who dominate and control the field of psychiatry, psychology and social work.

It is common for Blacks, Hispanics and other minorities to seek counseling from their priests, pastors and their elders. The primary care physician of color is the first one to diagnose and treat depression in minorities, because these affected minorities feel more comfortable with him or her whom they have known for a long time and trust.

Therefore, primary care physicians of color are providing the bulk of the treatment for depression in minorities because these minorities feel more comfortable with these doctors as just outlined.

Depression is a very common disease and much more so in minorities than in whites. Depression has many bases, many causes, and many manifestations. In minorities, depression can be gravest because of the penetrating and pernicious nature of racism, which fosters so much distrust of those in control of U.S. and the world societies, that it makes it difficult for minorities to seek help for their depressive illnesses.

Minorities have a higher propensity for the development of depression as compared to whites, as already stated, and the fact that they are under more stress and many of the have a lesser level of education, lesser economic status and a lower social standing, creates a situation that makes their depression more grave, more serious, more multifactorial and much more difficult to treat.

What can be done to lessen the propensity of minorities to develop depression?

It is crucial to educate these Blacks, Hispanics and other minorities about the seriousness of mental illnesses. The fact is that 80% or more of individuals who suffer from depression can be successfully treated and the best people to seek treatment from for depression are those who have the professional training and expertise to treat these treatable diseases.

It is also important to sensitize the professionals who are in the position to treat minorities, by considering their cultures, their daily economic and social struggles and other things that trouble them.

Different and more racially sensitive approaches must be undertaken in order to provide appropriate and better treatments for minorities with mental illnesses.

It is foolish and potentially harmful to attempt to impose the majority's views, hypocritical values, and traditional treatment modalities to minorities whose psychiatric problems are unique in many instances.

The bases and factors that are contributing to their state of mind are themselves unique because of their unique societal circumstances. So if the professionals from the majority community do not take it upon themselves to familiarize themselves with the culture, and the circumstances of life and other different dynamics that inter- play leading to these depressive illnesses, they will fail most of the time in their attempt to treat them for these very serious, but treatable, mental diseases.

The training programs whose job it is to train these individuals must include several components of the cultural diversity as it relates to minorities and minority people's issues in general, into their training programs. Future mental health professionals need to acquire special skills and techniques that are necessary to deal with the psychological problems of mionorities and their unique features.

Those in charge of organizing training programs in the field of psychiatry, psychology etc., ought to set up a required sub-specialty in cultural diversity of minority people and in their mental health training programs.

This will prepare their trainees for the real world of the twenty-first century, using a model that mirrors the reality of those individuals and all aspects of their lives.

The number of people of color in the mental health profession needs to be increased significantly to help in correcting the problems just outlined.

In so doing, many of the barriers of mistrust will be lowered to a significant degree, making it easier for Blacks, Hispanics and other people of color in the U.S. and around the world to be more receptive to the care that the mental health professionals are providing for them.

CHAPTER 74

ALCOHOLISM IN
AFRICAN AMERICAN MEN

Alcoholism is a very commonly abused substance in the United States and in the world.18 million people in the U.S. and 140 million people in the world abuse Alcohol. One in twelve adults in the U.S. abuses alcohol. However, more people abuse alcohol than those who are registered. Worldwide 2 billion people drink alcohol. Source: WHO.

Alcohol abuse affects all segments of society. At any one time, there are roughly 18 to 21 million individuals in the United States receiving one treatment or another for alcohol abuse and its multitude of associated medical and psychosocial problems.

" The racial break down of the number people who drank alcohol on a regular basis in the year 2001, were white females 65%, black females 45.9%, white males 74.2% Black males 62.6%, American Indian males 65.48%, American Indians females 51.6% Alaska Natives 38.6%, Asian males 61.5%, Asian females 36.1%, Native Hawaiians and other Pacific Islanders 30.1%, Hispanic males 69.99% and Hispanic females 49.52%. "

(Source: National Institute on Alcohol Abuse and Alcoholism 2001- 2002)

According to a recent report by the CDC 1 in 10 deaths that occur in working American adults is the result of excessive alcohol drinking. This adds up to 88,000 deaths per year and cost $222 billion per year. Source: CDC June 27, 2014

"The ten countries with highest per capita consumption of alcohol are:

1. Luxembourg
2. Ireland
3. France
4. Hungary
5. Denmark
6. Czech Republic
7. Spain
8. Portugal
9. Austria
10. Switzerland "

The annual cost of alcohol abuse and its associated medical complication is 223.5 billion dollars and alcoholism causes 79,000 deaths annually in the U.S.: N Engl j MED 368; 4 January 24, 2013. Worldwide 2.5 million people die from alcohol abuse yearly Source: WHO

Alcohol abuse is one of the most serious medical problems known to humankind. What makes alcohol use so easy and so widespread is that a person does not need a prescription to buy it. Alcohol is sold in liquor stores, bars, restaurants, airport shops, supermarkets, etc. Some people start drinking alcohol in their teens, as a recreational habit or because of peer pressure.

Frequently, teenagers see their parents abusing alcohol at home and getting drunk in front of them and they think it is OK for them to do the same thing (obviously it is not).

It is not too difficult to see how some teenagers can drink alcohol, are not reprimanded by their drinking parents, because the parents do it in front of them, so they think it is all right, and "cool" to do the same thing.

It is said, according to the literature, that some form of alcoholism is hereditary. Parents, it is said, transfer an alcoholism gene to their offspring, resulting in them becoming alcoholics as well. The evidence is quite compelling that this may indeed so.

On average, it would appear that whites start drinking at an earlier age than Blacks, Hispanics and other minorities do. Whites on the aggregate have a high incidence of alcohol abuse than do Blacks, Hispanics and other minorities do, but Blacks, Hispanics and other minorities suffer more from the physical effects of alcohol abuse than do whites.

For example, Blacks, Hispanics and other minorities seem to have a greater incidence of cirrhosis of liver due to alcohol abuse than do Whites. In fact, the death rate from cirrhosis of the liver is two times as high for Blacks, Hispanics and other minorities as compared to Whites.

Blacks, Hispanics and other minorities suffer from more health problems because of alcohol abuse, than do Whites. Diseases such as cancer, hypertension, malnutrition, birth defects, and obstructive pulmonary disease are much more prevalent in alcoholic Blacks, Hispanics and other minorities as compared to alcoholic Whites.

The risk of fetal alcohol syndrome (FAS) is seven times higher for Black, Latinos and other minority babies than it is for white babies. In 2013, it was estimated that 17 million Americans have alcohol-related health problems and worldwide 75 million people have alcohol related health problems. In the U.S. every year 85, 000 people die from alcohol related health problems and worldwide 2.5 million people die every year from alcohol health related problems. Alcohol consumption costs 188 billion dollars annually in the U.S.

The estimated annual cost for alcohol health care in the U.S. was 223 billion dollars in 2013.

Alcohol abuse is a multi-system disease. The organs that are most frequently affected by alcohol are the following:

1. The brain
2. The heart
3. The lungs
4. The liver
5. The spleen
6. The pancreas
7. The breasts
8. Female genital organs
9. Male genital organs
10. Male erectal functions
11. Females fertility
12. Males fertility
13. The gastrointestinal system
14. The blood system
15. The endocrine system
16. The mouth, throat, and esophagus
17. The neurological system
18. The psychological system
19. The skin
20. Frequently, many of the organs and systems are affected in combination in the same person.

According to a recent report alcohol abuse increases the risk of stroke.

When a person drinks alcohol, the brain is the first organ to be affected. When a person drinks alcohol, first it is absorbed from the stomach into the bloodstream. Once in the bloodstream, the alcohol goes to the brain. The effect of alcohol on the brain depends on the level of alcohol in the blood of the person drinking alcohol and the length of time that person has been drinking alcohol.

The level of alcohol that causes drunkenness in one person is different in another individual. In other words, different individuals respond differently to the effect of alcohol. The weight of a black man determines how quickly she becomes intoxicated. Blood alcohol concentration (BAC) is measured as milligrams of alcohol per deciliter of blood.

This same number can be converted in percent of alcohol concentration in the blood: 100 mg of alcohol per deciliter in the blood equals 100 mg percent or 0.1 percent of alcohol in the blood. For example, a person weighing 200 lbs., who drinks six drinks of hard liquor in one hour, will likely develop a blood alcohol level of 100 mg per deciliter. A person who weighs 150 lbs. will reach a blood alcohol concentration of 100 mg per deciliter by drinking four drinks of hard liquor in one hour.

Alcohol is both a stimulant and a neuro-suppressor (brain suppressor). The first thing that happens when alcohol reaches the brain is to calm the person who drinks it. It relaxes the person at first. Then as more alcohol is consumed, a feeling of elation or euphoria ensues. Associated with this level of drinking is a mild form of excitement, and the person may become talkative and giddy.

Mild social drinking of 2–3 glasses of wine, or 1–2 drinks of hard liquor, or 2–3 twelve-ounce bottles of beer per day should not be harmful to the human body. Further consumption of alcohol can create a state of drunkenness associated with excitation, rude behavior, and physical dis-coordination. Another way of saying the same thing is that a standard drink of alcohol is usually expressed as a can of twelve ounces of beer, 1½ ounces of liquor/whiskey, vodka, etc., or 5 ounces of wine.

Different individuals metabolize alcohol differently, and when taken with food in the stomach, alcohol absorption is slowed. If alcohol is consumed on an empty stomach, its full effects are felt quicker.

Impairment due to the effects of alcohol occurs in a person when the alcohol concentration reaches 50 mg per deciliter. Blacks and elderly individuals show impairment from drinking alcohol at lower concentration, probably 25–30 mg per deciliter.

The risks of causing an automobile crash starts to occur when the blood alcohol concentration reaches 40 mg per deciliter. This risk rises when the blood alcohol concentration reaches 100 mg per deciliter. When the blood alcohol concentration reaches between 50– 70 mg per deciliter, most drivers are alcohol impaired and are unsuitable to drive.

At this blood alcohol concentration, a person loses coordination (he or she cannot walk straight). At an alcohol level concentration of 100 mg per deciliter, a person has a more pronounced inability to walk, and would be stumbling around, and if that person attempts to drive, that person would be driving while drunk.

When the blood alcohol concentration reaches 200 mg per deciliter, the person becomes confused, disoriented and may actually lose consciousness (alcohol blackout). When the blood alcohol concentration reaches 400 mg per deciliter, coma may ensue and death may occur.

Blood alcohol levels that are deem unsafe for driving a car is different in different states in the USA. Examples of different blood alcohol levels from different states in the in the U.S. that are considered safe or unsafe to drive a motor vehicle:

TABLE 1

Alaska	0.10/0.00	90 days	after 30 days	Yes
Arizona	0.10/0.00	90 days	after 30 days	No
Arkansas	0.10/0.02	120 days	Yes	Yes
California	0.08/0.01	4 months	after 30 days	Yes
Colorado	0.10/0.02	3 months	No	Yes
Connecticut	0.10/0.02	90 days	Yes	No
Delaware	0.10/0.02	3 months	No	Yes
District of Columbia	0.10/0.02	90 days	Yes	No
Florida	0.08/0.02	6 month	Yes	No
Georgia	0.10/0.02	1 year	Yes	Yes
Hawaii	0.08/0.02	3 months	after 30 days	Yes
Idaho	0.08/0.02	90 days	after 30 days	Yes
Illinois	0.06/0.00	3 months	after 30 days	Yes
Indiana	0.10/0.02	180 day	after 30 days	Yes
Iowa	0.10/0.02	180 days	Yes	Yes
Kansas	0.08/0.02	30 days	No	Yes
Kentucky	0.10/0.02	—	—	No
Louisiana	0.10/0.02	90 days	after 30 days	Yes
Maine	0.08/0.00	90 days	Yes	Yes
Maryland	0.10/0.02	45 days	Yes	Yes
Massachusetts	None/0.02	90 days	No	No
Michigan	0.10./0.02	—	—	Yes
Minnesota	0.10/0.00	90 days	after 15 days—	No
Mississippi	0.10/0.08	90 days	No	No
Missouri	0.10/0.02	30 days	No	Yes
Montana	0.10/0.02	—	—	Yes
Nebraska	0.10/0.02	90 days	after 30 days	Yes
Nevada	0.10/0.02	90 days	after 45 days	Yes
New Hampshire	0.08/0.02	6 months	No	No
New Jersey	0.10/0.10	—	—	No
New Mexico	0.08/0.02	90 days	after 30 days	No
New York	0.10/0.02	variable	Yes	Yes

North Carolina	0.08/0.00	10 days	No	Yes
North Dakota	0.10/0.02	91 days	after 30 days	Yes
Ohio	0.10/0.02	90 days	after 15 days	Yes
Oklahoma	0.10/0.00	180 days	Yes	Yes
Oregon	0.08/0.00	90 days	after 30 days	Yes
Pennsylvania	0.10/0.02	–	–	No
Rhode Island	0.10/0.02	–	–	Yes
South Carolina	None/–	–	–	No
South Dakota	0.10/–	–	–	No
Tennessee	0.10/0.02	–	–	Yes
Texas	0.10/0.00	60 days	Yes	Yes
Utah	0.08/0.00	90 days	No	Yes
Vermont	0.08/0.02	90 days	No	No
Virginia	0.08/0.02	7 days	No	Yes
Washington	0.10/0.02	–	–	Yes
West Virginia	0.10/0.02	6 months	Yes	Yes
Wisconsin	0.10/0.02	6 months	Yes	Yes
Wyoming	0./10/–	90 days	Yes	No

(Insurance Institute for Highway Safety)

Alcohol abuse is a worldwide serious medical problem and the list of countries below highlight the extent of this problem.

"List of countries by alcohol consumption per capita

This is a list of countries by alcohol consumption measured in equivalent litres of pure ethanol consumed per capita per year.

Contents

1. OECD statistics
2. WHO statistics

OECD statistics

The table below lists OECD countries by the annual consumption of pure alcohol in liters, per person, aged 15 years old and over, as published in the 2013 OECD Health Data. Note that the methodology to convert alcoholic drinks to pure alcohol may differ across countries. Typically beer is weighted as 4–5%, wine as 11–16% and spirits as 40% of pure alcohol equivalent.

This table is an accurate reflection of the annual consumption of pure alcohol in litres by OECD countries.

Rank	Country	Litres per capita [1]	Relative size	Year
1	Estonia	12.3		2011
2	Austria	12.2		2011
3	France	12		2011
4	Ireland	11.7		2011
5	Czech Republic	11.5		2011
6	Hungary	11.4		2011
6	Portugal	11.4		2007
6	Spain	11.4		2009
9	Germany	11		2011
10	Belgium	10.8		2008
11	Denmark	10.6		2011
11	Slovenia	10.6		2011
13	Poland	10.4		2011
14	Finland	10.1		2011
15	Australia	10.0		2010
15	Switzerland	10.0		2011
15	United Kingdom	10.0		2011
18	Slovakia	9.9		2011
19	Netherlands	9.4		2009
20	New Zealand	9.3		2012
21	South Korea	8.9		2011
22	Chile	8.6		2009
22	United States	8.6		2010
24	Greece	8.2		2009
25	Canada	8.0		2011
26	Sweden	7.4		2011
27	Iceland	7.3		2008
27	Japan	7.3		2011
29	Italy	6.9		2009
30	Norway	6.6		2011
31	Mexico	5.1		2011
32	Israel	2.4		2007
"33	Turkey	1.6		2012

"WHO statistics

The table below uses 2010 data from the WHO report published in 2014. The methodology used by the WHO calculated use by persons 15 years of age or older. All data in columns refer to year 2010. The column "recorded" refers to the average recorded consumption for the period 2010. Unrecorded consumption was calculated using empirical investigations and expert judgments. Total is the sum of the recorded and unrecorded consumption. The next four columns are a breakdown of the recorded alcohol consumption by type. Beer refers to malt beer, <u>wine</u> refers to grape wine, <u>spirits</u> refers to all distilled beverages, and the column "other" refers to all other alcoholic beverages, such as <u>rice wine</u>, <u>sake</u>, <u>kumi kumi</u>, <u>kwete</u>, <u>mead</u> and <u>cider</u>.

Pure alcohol consumption among adults (age 15+) in litres per capita per year, 2010[2]

Country	Total	Recorded consumption	Unrecorded consumption	Beer (%)	Wine (%)	Spirits (%)	Other (%)	2015 projection
Belarus	17.5	14.4	3.2	17.3	5.2	46.6	30.9	17.1
Moldova	16.8	6.3	10.5	30.4	5.1	64.5	0	17.4
Lithuania	15.4	12.9	2.5	46.5	7.8	34.1	11.6	16.2
Russia	15.1	11.5	3.6	37.6	11.4	51	0	14.5
Romania	14.4	10.4	4	50	28.9	21.1	0	12.9
Ukraine	13.9	8.9	5	40.5	9	48	2.6	11.8
Andorra	13.8	12.4	1.4	34.6	45.3	20.1	0	9.1
Hungary	13.3	11.3	2	36.3	29.4	34.3	0	12.4
Czech Republic	13	11.8	1.2	53.5	20.5	26	0	14.1
Slovakia	13	11.4	1.7	30.1	18.3	46.2	5.5	12.5
Portugal	12.9	11	1.9	30.8	55.5	10.9	2.8	12.5
Serbia	12.6	9.6	2.9	51.5	23.9	24.6	0	12.9
Grenada	12.5	11.9	0.7	29.3	4.3	66.2	0.2	10.4
Poland	12.5	10.9	1.6	55.1	9.3	35.5	0	11.5
Latvia	12.3	10.5	1.8	46.9	10.7	37	5.4	10.6
Finland	12.3	10	2.3	46	17.5	24	12.6	11.9
South Korea	12.3	9.8	2.5	25	1.6	2.9	70.5	10.9
France	12.2	11.8	0.4	18.8	56.4	23.1	1.7	11.6
Australia	12.2	10.4	1.8	44	36.7	12.5	6.8	12.6
Croatia	12.2	10.2	2	39.5	44.8	15.4	0.2	11.7
Ireland	11.9	11.4	0.5	48.1	26.1	18.7	7.7	10.9
Luxembourg	11.9	11.4	0.5	36.2	42.8	21	0	11.2
Germany	11.8	11.3	0.5	53.6	27.8	18.6	0	10.6
Slovenia	11.6	10.6	1	44.5	46.9	8.6	0	10.9
United Kingdom	11.6	10.4	1.2	36.9	33.8	21.8	7.5	12
Denmark	11.4	10.4	1	37.7	48.2	14.1	0	10.2
Bulgaria	11.4	10.3	1.1	39.3	16.5	44.1	0.1	11.3
Spain	11.2	10	1.2	49.7	20.1	28.2	1.8	10.6
Belgium	11	10.5	0.5	49.2	36.3	14.4	0.1	10.8
South Africa	11	8.2	2.9	48.1	17.8	16.7	17.4	11.5
New Zealand	10.9	9.3	1.6	38.2	33.9	15.2	12.5	11.2
Gabon	10.9	8.9	2	68.3	11.9	19.8	0.1	11.8
Namibia	10.8	6.8	4	96.7	0.3	0.9	2.1	11.8
Switzerland	10.7	10.2	0.5	31.8	49.4	17.6	1.2	10.4
Saint Lucia	10.4	10.1	0.2	29.7	12.6	56.1	1.5	10.4
Austria	10.3	9.7	0.6	50.4	35.5	14	0	8.5
Estonia	10.3	9.5	0.8	41.2	11.1	36.8	10.9	9.4
Greece	10.3	8.3	2	28.1	47.3	24.2	0.4	9.3
Kazakhstan	10.3	6.8	3.5	31.8	3.1	65.1	0	8.2
Canada	10.2	8.2	2	51.2	22	26.8	0	10.3
Nigeria	10.1	9.1	1	8	0.4	0.9	90.7	11.3

Netherlands	9.9	9.4	0.5	46.8	36.4	16.9	0	9.6
Uganda	9.8	8.3	1.5	9.4	0.1	1.9	88.6	10.5
Rwanda	9.8	6.8	3	11.1	0	0.4	88.4	10
Chile	9.6	7.6	2	29.9	40.7	29.4	0	9.3
Argentina	9.3	8.3	1	40.7	48	5.5	5.8	7.6
Burundi	9.3	6.3	3	24.5	0	0.1	75.4	9.8
United States	9.2	8.7	0.5	50	17.3	32.7	0	9
Cyprus	9.2	8.2	1	40.9	24.7	33.7	0.7	9.1
Sweden	9.2	7.2	2	37	46.6	15.1	1.4	8.7
Venezuela	8.9	7.7	1.3	75.6	0.8	23.4	0.2	8.3
Paraguay	8.8	7.3	1.5	51.1	18.2	28.8	2	9.6
Brazil	8.7	7.2	1.5	59.6	4	36.3	0.1	9.1
Sierra Leone	8.7	6.7	2	6.4	0.5	0.7	92.3	8.2
Montenegro	8.7	4.9	3.9	10.9	47	41.7	0.4	13.3
Belize	8.5	6.8	1.7	67.6	2	30.3	0.1	8.3
Cameroon	8.4	5.8	2.6	63.9	22.1	13.8	0.2	7.7
Botswana	8.4	5.4	3	56	11.8	11.5	20.7	7.7
Saint Kitts and Nevis	8.2	7.7	0.5	44	7.4	48	0.6	7
Guyana	8.1	7.1	1	23	0.3	76.6	0.1	8.6
Peru	8.1	6.1	2	46.8	6.1	47.1	0	5.2
Panama	8	7.2	0.8	69.2	4.6	26	0.2	7.7
Niue	8	7	1	47	1.7	51.3	0	7.7
Palau	7.9	6.9	1	77.7	5.9	16.4	0	
Norway	7.7	6.7	1	44.2	34.7	19	2.1	7
Tanzania	7.7	5.7	2	11	0.2	1.8	87	8.1
Georgia	7.7	5.4	2.3	17	49.8	33.2	0.1	6.7
Uruguay	7.6	6.6	1	30.6	59.9	9.5	0	7
Angola	7.5	5.9	1.6	64.3	13.7	17.4	4.7	7.6
Laos	7.3	6.2	1.1	35.6	0	64.4	0	7.5
Japan	7.2	7	0.2	19.2	4.1	52	24.7	7.5
Mexico	7.2	5.5	1.8	75.7	1.5	22.2	0.5	6.8
Ecuador	7.2	4.2	3	67.3	1.2	31.5	0	6.1
Dominica	7.1	6.6	0.5	13.7	7.1	77.9	1.2	6.6
Iceland	7.1	6.6	0.5	61.8	21.2	16.5	0.5	6.9
Thailand	7.1	6.4	0.7	27	0.4	72.6	0	8.3
Bosnia and Herzegovina	7.1	4.6	2.5	73.3	9.7	17	0	7.5
São Tomé and Príncipe	7.1	4.2	2.9	23.5	60.2	16.3	0	6.8
Malta	7	6.6	0.4	39.4	32.7	27.2	0.7	7.2
Albania	7	4.9	2.1	31.8	19.8	48.4	0	6.6
Bahamas	6.9	6.3	0.5	34	14.6	50.4	1	4.2
Dominican Republic	6.9	6.2	0.7	54.5	2.7	42.7	0.1	7.6
Mongolia	6.9	4.9	2	27.6	2.8	69.6	0	7.8
Cape Verde	6.9	4	2.9	44.4	1.2	0.2	54.2	7.2
Barbados	6.8	6.3	0.5	39.7	10.2	49.3	0.8	6.5
Burkina Faso	6.8	4.3	2.5	10	3	3.1	83.8	7.4
Italy	6.7	6.5	0.2	23	65.6	11.5	0	6.1

Trinidad and Tobago	6.7	6.4	0.3	54	2	43.8	0.3	6.6
China	6.7	5	1.7	27.8	3	69.2	0	7.6
Macedonia	6.7	3.9	2.8	47.4	39.9	12.6	0	5.7
Saint Vincent and the Grenadines	6.6	6.3	0.3	33.4	3	63.1	0.5	7.2
Equatorial Guinea	6.6	5.8	0.8	27.8	72.2	0	0	8.1
Suriname	6.6	5.6	1	40	2.3	57.2	0.5	6.5
Vietnam	6.6	2	4.6	97.3	0.6	2.1	0	8.7
Lesotho	6.5	2.8	3.7	51.3	0.2	18.9	29.6	6.4
Haiti	6.4	5.9	0.6	0.2	0.2	99.6	0	5.9
Cook Islands	6.4	5.9	0.5	0	22.6	77.4	0	4.8
Colombia	6.2	4.2	2	66.1	1.1	32.5	0.3	6.6
Ivory Coast	6	4	2	16.1	3	0.4	80.5	6.5
Bolivia	5.9	3.8	2.1	76.8	3.8	19.3	0.1	5.8
Swaziland	5.7	4.7	1	33.6	0.8	0.7	65	6.4
Zimbabwe	5.7	4.7	1	23.7	1.7	6.8	67.7	4.8
Seychelles	5.6	4.1	1.5	67	22.2	10.8	0	6.7
Cambodia	5.5	2.2	3.3	45.7	0.8	53.5	0	6.1
Puerto Rico	5.4	4.9	0.5	66.6	6.7	26.4	0.3	-
Netherlands Antilles	5.4	4.9	0.4	36.4	16.4	47	0.3	3.2
Philippines	5.4	4.6	0.9	26.9	0.3	72.7	0	5.6
Costa Rica	5.4	4.4	1	59.3	4.7	35.5	0.5	5.1
Armenia	5.3	3.8	1.5	9.7	5.3	84.9	0	5.5
Cuba	5.2	4.2	1	38.8	2.2	58.9	0	5.5
Nicaragua	5	3.5	1.5	38.8	0.5	60.6	0	4.6
Jamaica	4.9	3.4	1.5	42	4.9	51.4	1.6	5.1
Ghana	4.8	1.8	3	30	9.7	2.9	57.3	5.4
Liberia	4.7	3.1	1.6	10.8	1	88.1	0	5.2
Uzbekistan	4.6	2.4	2.1	18.3	6.3	75.4	0	4.8
Chad	4.4	0.4	4	66.3	3.4	3.8	26.5	4.4
United Arab Emirates	4.3	2.8	1.5	10.3	2.9	86.7	0	4.3
Kyrgyzstan	4.3	2.4	1.9	22.6	4.2	72.9	0.3	3.9
India	4.3	2.2	2.2	6.8	0.1	93.1	0	4.6
Turkmenistan	4.3	2.2	2.2	15.4	26.1	58.4	0	5
Kenya	4.3	1.8	2.5	56.1	1.8	21.6	20.4	4
Ethiopia	4.2	0.7	3.5	49.7	0.6	8.2	41.4	4.3
Honduras	4	3	1	40.1	1.1	58.7	0	4
Guinea-Bissau	4	2.5	1.5	19.6	14.9	22.4	43	4.3
Zambia	4	2.5	1.5	22.7	2.9	13.6	60.7	4
Republic of the Congo	3.9	1.7	2.2	78.4	9.8	10.9	0.8	3.9
Guatemala	3.8	2.2	1.6	41.9	1.6	56.3	0.2	3.9
Central African Republic	3.8	1.8	2	16.2	0.6	2.1	81.1	3.8
North Korea	3.7	3.2	0.5	5.1	0	94.9	0	4.4
Sri Lanka	3.7	2.2	1.5	13	0.1	85.2	1.7	4.5
Mauritius	3.6	2.6	1	66.2	12.3	21.3	0.2	4
Samoa	3.6	2.6	1	70.9	16.6	12.5	0	

Democratic Republic of the Congo	3.6	2.3	1.3	24	0.7	2	73.3	3.4
Nauru	3.5	1	2.5	85.4	14.6	0	0	3
Gambia	3.4	2.4	1	5.6	0.7	0.3	93.5	3.2
Federated States of Micronesia	3.3	2.3	1	47	14.1	38.9	0	3.5
El Salvador	3.2	2.2	1	41.7	1.7	56.6	0	3.5
Fiji	3	2	1	67.7	0.9	31.1	0.2	3.2
Papua New Guinea	3	1.5	1.5	51.3	0.9	47.7	0	3.1
Kiribati	3	1	2	36.9	2.2	60.9	0	2.9
Tajikistan	2.8	0.3	2.5	10.2	1.1	88.7	0	2.4
Israel	2.8	0.3	2.5	44	6.2	49.5	0.3	3.1
Sudan	2.7	1.7	1	8	0	13.5	78.5	2.7
Malawi	2.5	1.5	1	9.1	1.2	13.4	76.2	2.5
Lebanon	2.4	1.9	0.5	18.2	29.1	52.4	0.3	2.2
Azerbaijan	2.3	1.3	1	28.7	7.6	63.3	0	2.1
Mozambique	2.3	1.3	1	63	7.3	25.4	4.3	2
Togo	2.3	1.3	1	48.9	26.9	2.4	21.8	1.9
Nepal	2.2	0.2	2	47.7	0.9	51.4	0	2.1
Brunei	2.1	2	0.1	36.6	6.3	57	0.1	2.4
Benin	2.1	1.1	1	54.6	21.7	7.2	16.5	2.2
Singapore	2	1.5	0.5	70.1	13.5	14.7	1.7	2.9
Turkey	2	1.4	0.6	63.6	8.6	27.9	0	2.4
Madagascar	1.8	0.8	1	56	9.5	34.5	0	1.9
Solomon Islands	1.7	1.2	0.5	81.1	2.1	16.7	0	1.6
Tonga	1.6	1.1	0.5	57.9	7.6	34.3	0.1	2.1
Tunisia	1.5	1.3	0.2	68.6	27.7	3.7	0	1.2
Tuvalu	1.5	1	0.5	10	15.5	74.5	0	1.3
Qatar	1.5	0.9	0.6	1.2	13.9	84.6	0.3	1.3
Vanuatu	1.4	0.9	0.5	40.5	22.8	36.7	0	1.2
Djibouti	1.3	1.1	0.2	23.2	5.3	71.5	0	0.9
Malaysia	1.3	0.3	1	76.2	2	21.8	0.1	1.7
Syria	1.2	1	0.3	8.5	27.9	63.5	0	1.4
Maldives	1.2	0.7	0.5	29.1	29.4	41.2	0	1
Mali	1.1	0.6	0.5	13.3	1.5	2.1	83.1	1
Eritrea	1.1	0.5	0.6	63.6	0	0.1	36.3	1.4
Algeria	1	0.7	0.3	62.6	35.5	0	2	0.6
Iran	1	0	1	24.8	52.1	1	1	
Oman	0.9	0.7	0.2	54.6	3.3	42.2	0	0.9
Brunei	0.9	0.6	0.3	89.8	2.3	7.2	0.7	0.8
Morocco	0.9	0.5	0.5	43.5	36.5	19.9	0	0.7
Jordan	0.7	0.5	0.2	22.4	2.1	75.4	0.1	0.7
Bhutan	0.7	0.4	0.3	100	0	0	0	1.1
Guinea	0.7	0.2	0.5	78.9	16.3	3.7	1.1	0.7
Myanmar	0.7	0.1	0.6	82.6	5.7	11.8	0	0.7
Afghanistan	0.7	0	0.7	18.9	38.3	1	1.2	
Senegal	0.6	0.3	0.3	55.1	41.3	3.6	0	0.5
Indonesia	0.6	0.1	0.5	84.5	0.1	15.3	0	0.6

Timor-Leste	0.6	0.1	0.5	9.3	75.9	14.8	0	1.2
Iraq	0.5	0.2	0.3	76.1	1	22.9	0	0.5
Somalia	0.5	0	0.5	9.2	19.2	0.5	0.5	
Egypt	0.4	0.2	0.2	53.8	5.4	40.3	0.5	0.3
Niger	0.3	0.1	0.2	46	13.2	40.7	0	0.3
Yemen	0.3	0.1	0.2	100	0	0	0	0.2
Comoros	0.2	0.1	0.1	23.3	22.2	54.6	0	0.2
Saudi Arabia	0.2	0.1	0.1	0	1.9	97.9	0.2	0.2
Bangladesh	0.2	0	0.2	9	17.6	0.2	0.2	
Kuwait	0.1	0	0.1	58.1	10.8	30.7	0.4	0.1
Libya	0.1	0	0.1	2.5	5	0	0	
Mauritania	0.1	0	0.1					0.1
Pakistan	0.1	0	0	1.2	3	0.1	0.1	

" Source WHO and OECD

What is alcoholism?

Alcoholism is a disease. It is a disease that affects the human mind and the human body. Alcoholism is a serious disease causing both psychological and medical complications of all sorts to the human body. The psychological dependence on alcohol is real and has devastating consequences on the affected individual and his or her family and society.

People who suffer from alcohol dependency have great difficulty stopping being dependent on alcohol. These people are addicted to alcohol and crave it when they stop drinking. There are different patterns of alcohol dependency.

Some people drink alcohol in excess every day and feel the need to drink every day.

A significant percentage of these blacks are able to go to work and function reasonably well on the job. They usually start drinking at lunchtime.

They often consume 2–3 drinks with lunch, after work they will drink 3–4 more drinks, in a bar on their way home or at job-related functions, and when they get home they will again have 2–3 more drinks with dinner. This is about 10 drinks of hard liquor per day. On weekends, that number quadruples. These people are what are called functioning alcoholics. They work, they make money, and they support their families. These people are found at all levels of society from the very rich to the poor, and to the middle class.

They are referred to as people who can handle their alcohol.

There is another group of people who are working alcoholics, who must drink as soon as they get up in the morning to get going and they drink hard liquor at different times throughout the working day. Very often, people know that these people are alcoholics, but tolerate them or cover up for them because they are oftentimes polite, very nice, and jovial, and when sober, they are productive at their work. Frequently, these people miss work because of heavy alcohol drinking and very often come up with very creative excuses as to why they were absent from work.

There is still a larger group of people who drink alcohol in large quantities and on such a regular basis that they become sick so frequently that they are unable to maintain a job. These are the hardcore, non-functioning alcoholics, who are entirely preoccupied with alcohol drinking on a daily basis. People in this group are found also in all segments of society, in all professions and most religious groups.

Alcohol abuse and peer pressure

Peer pressure plays a significant role in alcohol abuse in teenagers, as there is peer pressure to get them involved in illicit drugs. There is also peer pressure to force other young teenagers to drink alcohol. Peer pressure also exists among adults to get together in a bar after work for a drink or two. The incidence of alcohol abuse is quite high among blacks of all ethnic backgrounds.

Alcohol abuse among people starts at an early age (from adolescence to teenage years). Poor people drink alcohol for the same reasons that other rich people drink alcohol, to socialize with their friends and to be less inhibited. This use of alcohol frequently increases to drinking alcohol alone at home on a daily basis.

Eventually, these individuals become dependent on the alcohol, and once that happens, they become preoccupied with alcohol drinking, resulting in alcoholism. Frequently, these individuals grow up in homes where there is either a father or mother who abuses alcohol. They have either a husband who drinks alcohol, or a boyfriend who drinks alcohol, and they drink in order to please their husbands or boyfriends.

They drink because they saw their mothers or fathers doing it and they thought it was all right for them to start doing it also.

Some of these people are heads of the household, single parents with children to bring up with no fathers around and all the stress associated with running a house alone.

In addition, all the problems associated with poverty, racism, low level of education, unemployment etc; leads to heavy alcohol use in some people.

The working-class people group also has many alcohol abusers among it. The people in this group have similar problems with alcohol abuse, and the reasons are the same stress, single parenthood, poverty, racism and all its associated perniciousness, and in more instances, domestic violence and all the awful things that are associated with it.

Middle-class people who abuse alcohol do so for similar reasons as just outlined. The main difference is that this group of Blacks, Hispanics, Asians and rich whites with financial means, which help them to be able to cover up their alcoholism.

As for upper-class people, most of them are professionals, businessmen, athletes, entertainers, husbands and children, are in a position that allows them to cover up their alcoholism.

The wealthy and privileged people who abuse alcohol do so for similar reasons, except that they are not poor. Yes, some minority folks do discriminate against other minority folks; especially light skin minority's people frequently discriminate against darker skin minorities in America and elsewhere in the world.

Because of their money, social and professional status, doors are frequently opened for them that allow their alcoholism to appear more acceptable to their friends, colleagues and their associates. The effects of alcohol on their bodies, however, is the same as that of the poorest minority people, because alcohol cares not how much money a person has, or for that matter, how privileged he or she is or how well a person is able to eat.

The best caviars, the best cheeses, or the finest filets mignons in the world cannot protect the human body from the ultimate devastation of alcohol abuse. Alcoholism affects the human body to the same degree, regardless of a person's nutritional state, with a few minor transient circumstances.

For example, if a black man is undernourished and went on an alcohol binge and does not eat, the fact that he has low storage of carbohydrates in his liver from poor eating over an extending period of time, this person may develop hypoglycemia (low blood sugar) quicker than the person who drinks heavy, but eats a better diet. That being said, the long-term toxic effects of alcohol are the same in everyone who drinks alcohol heavily.

Even though black and Hispanic men and other minority men start drinking alcohol at a later age than their white counterparts do, the signs of alcoholism seem to appear earlier in them than in whites. Undoubtedly, poverty and racism play a major role in these differences.

Poor folks do not have as much money as rich folks to go to the doctor for check-ups. White folks have more money than blacks do. (The top 2 per cent of the U.S. population most of whom whites, owns 98 per cent of the wealth in the U.S. totaling 45 trillion dollars).

White men get physical examinations more often than do Black, Latinos and other minority men do.

According to the literature, rich people get better medical care and live longer. Diseases such as cancer of the mouth, throat, esophagus, liver, and pancreas, which are quite common in alcoholics, get picked up earlier in rich white alcoholics than they get picked up in poor black, Hispanic and other minority alcoholics.

Alcohol is one of the most frequently abused drugs because it is legal to buy alcohol without a prescription. Alcohol is readily available and any person over age 21 that whishes to dink it.

Different states set up different age limits at which a young person can legally buy alcohol. On a yearly basis, alcohol abuse and its associated problems lead to more than 100,000 deaths in the United States.

Of this number, close to 40,000 is due to cirrhosis of the liver and other associated medical complications of alcohol on the human body. The rest are due to alcohol-associated accidents on the highway (DWI) and homicides, liver cancer, pancreatic cancer, cancer of mouth, throat esophagus etc.

The amount of alcohol that a person must drink on a long-term basis to cause damage to the liver is 80 grams of alcohol per day over an extended period, anywhere from 7 years to 15 years. Eighty grams of alcohol can almost be found in a six-pack of 12 ounces of beer, because each 12-ounce can of beer has 13.1 grams of alcohol. If one multiplies this, it adds up to 78.6 grams of alcohol, and some blacks drink twice that much beer per day. As stated above, if a person drinks this amount of alcohol on a regular basis, that person will develop liver disease, as time goes on.

If a person drinks wine regularly (3.5 fluid ounces of wine), which is a glass of wine, it has 9.6 grams of alcohol. A bottle of wine usually has about 5–6 glasses of wine in it. People who drink 2–3 glasses of wine with dinner every night do not develop liver disease. It takes a minimum of 80 grams of alcohol per day on a regular basis over several years to develop fatty infiltration of the liver, which leads to metamorphosis of fat, leading to necrosis, resulting in alcoholic liver disease with subsequent development of cirrhosis.

The same thing applies to champagne. One glass of champagne has 11 grams of alcohol in it; some champagne has 13 grams of alcohol per glass, depending on how dry the champagne is. Therefore, it would take a tremendous amount of champagne consumption to add up to 80 grams of alcohol.

About 11-plus glasses of champagne daily over many years can cause a person to develop alcoholic cirrhosis. Most people do not drink that much champagne.

However, if a person drinks martinis, this is a different situation. Each martini has 18.5 grams of alcohol. If a man drinks five martinis per day, he is already drinking what is in fact in excess of the minimum amount of alcohol that is needed to cause liver disease. Five martinis equal to 92 grams of alcohol.

A Manhattan, for instance, has 19.9 grams of alcohol in it. Five Manhattans equal to 99.65 grams of alcohol. A gin Ricky has 21 grams of alcohol. Five gins Ricky equal 105 grams of alcohol. A High Ball has 24 grams of alcohol in it.

Five High Balls equal 120 grams of alcohol. A mint julep has 29.2 grams of alcohol in it. Five mint juleps equal 146 grams of alcohol, etc. Therefore, it does not take very many of these alcoholic drinks on a daily basis for a man to develop alcoholic liver disease. The organs most affected by alcohol abuse are the followings:

1. The brain
2. The liver
3. The pancreas
4. The spleen
5. The GI system
6. The blood system
7. The bones
8. The reproductive organs
9. The coagulation system
10. The skin
11. The behavioral system etc.

As described here, alcohol is very toxic to the brain. Acute alcohol ingestion alters a person's behavior by creating a state of excitation, restlessness, and poor social behavior. The agitated state leads to poor physical coordination, which frequently progresses to a state of drunkenness, leading to stupor and, at times, to coma.

When intoxicated, the alcoholic is a danger to herself or himself, and a danger to others around him or her. The adult brain is affected by alcohol in many ways.

For instance, a person who abuses alcohol risks losing his or her ability to function properly on her job. He or she is likely to develop serious psychological problems, which can cause disruption of his or her family life, which often results in break-ups of personal relationships such as marriages etc;

Serious damage to the brain tissues leading to dementia is quite common in chronic alcoholics. Chronic alcohol abuse can lead to Korsakoff syndrome, because of long-term vitamin B deficiencies. It is also known to be associated with acute episodes of encephalopathy, such as Wernicke's encephalopathy due to thiamine deficiencies.

Chronic alcohol abuse is also associated with other neurological abnormalities, such as ataxia (inability to walk in a straight line), altered mood functions with suicidal ideations, and peripheral neuropathy.

A chronic alcoholic is prone to develop seizures, either because of alcohol withdrawal, or because of recurrent traumas to the brain.

The chronic alcoholic is often deficient in folic acid, all the B vitamins, magnesium, protein, and phosphate.

Alcohol affects the liver, because it is a direct toxin to the liver tissues. In other words, because alcohol is directly toxic to liver tissues, therefore, the amount of alcohol consumed, the frequency of that consumption, and the length of time an individual abuses alcohol determines the extent of the liver damage.

In some individuals, the damage to the liver occurs quicker than in others, but one thing is certain, as long as a person abuses alcohol, his or her liver will be damaged by it. In some instances, the liver becomes acutely swollen, which can in turn lead to acute enlargement of the spleen due to acute elevation of the portal pressure and the consequence can be acute rupture of the spleen, endangering the life of the affected person, if it is not diagnosed properly and treated surgically quickly.

More chronically, however, alcohol causes tissues within the liver to become inflamed and the recurrent inflammatory reaction in time leads to scarring of the liver tissues, resulting in cirrhosis of the liver.

Once the liver becomes cirrhotic, a multitude of clinical problems can occur. The liver is needed to synthesize (produce) different proteins, which are needed for good body functions. The liver is needed to make most of the coagulation factors required to prevent bleeding from occurring. The liver is needed to store carbohydrates and to break down carbohydrates into usable sugars to use as fuel in the body.

The liver is needed to produce bile, which is needed to break down fats that humans eat, plus a multitude of other essential functions. The liver is the largest organ in the body next to the skin and the skeletal system and it contains the largest supply of reticuloendothelial cells that are needed to participate in the immune system etc.

In addition, the liver is needed to help remove a multitude of breakdown products that the human body produces constantly. So when the liver is sick and is unable to produce needed materials for proper body functions, and is too sick to help remove waste materials from the body, the human person becomes very sick.

In other words, when the liver is too sick to function properly and fails, life cannot go on. Another way of putting it is when the liver fails, the person dies, and alcohol abuse can frequently cause the liver to fail.

The pancreas is another organ that is quite sensitive to the toxic effects of alcohol. Pancreatitis is a common complication of heavy and chronic alcohol abuse.

It is not exactly clear as to the number of years a person has to abuse alcohol before her pancreas becomes sick some say, after seven years of alcohol abuse.

However, again, different individuals have different degrees of resistance and tolerance to the effects of alcohol. Alcohol damages the pancreatic tissues, causing at first acute inflammation to occur. The inflammation causes marked swelling of the pancreas, resulting in acute pancreatitis. After repeated attacks of acute pancreatitis, over several years, scarring of the pancreatic tissues occur which in turn results in chronic pancreatitis?

The third scenario is when the chronicity of the pancreatic disease causes destruction of the pancreatic tissue, leaving empty spaces within the pancreas, causing pancreatic pseudocysts to develop. Quite often, these pancreatic pseudocysts become infected, which in turn can lead to abscesses within the pancreas. Still other sequelae of chronic pancreatitis is pancreatic failure, meaning the pancreas is so damaged that it is no longer able to produce the different enzymes that it was able to produce before it became damaged.

These enzymes are necessary to aid in the digestive process of ingested fat that humans eat. Failure of the pancreas to produce these necessary enzymes causes the development of greasy diarrhea to occur. To further cause matters to get worse, if the African American man with pancreatic failure now becomes diabetic, because the pancreas has failed, it is not able to produce insulin for sugar metabolism; not to mention the constant and intense left-sided abdominal pain this person has to endure.

The effects of alcoholism on the spleen

The spleen becomes sick with chronic use of heavy alcohol intake because of cirrhosis of the liver. When alcohol damages the liver, this damage occludes the blood vessels that run through the liver. These damaged vessels cause narrowing and obstruction of the circulation inside the liver to occur.

Because of intra-liver obstruction of these vessels over time, the pressure within the liver and the portal system rises to the spleen, causing portal hypertension to develop. Portal hypertension then leads to enlargement of the spleen, resulting in a condition called hypersplenism. The enlarged spleen can at times become quite bulky, resulting in severe and chronic left-sided abdominal pain.

The upper gastrointestinal system is quite frequently involved in this scenario and becomes quite sick because of the effects of cirrhosis of the liver and portal hypertension. Because of the destruction and obstruction of these intrahepatic and (intra-liver) circulation, the elevation of the portal pressure causes neovascularization (formation of new vessels) to occur (which is the body's way of trying to bypass the obstructed circulation in the intrahepatic system).

The new vessels, however, are superficial, meaning that they grow on the surface of the esophagus, resulting in esophageal varices.

Because these new vessels, called varices, are superficially located on the outer surface of the esophagus, they tend to rupture quite easily and bleed profusely.

Therefore, esophageal bleeding is a major complication of cirrhosis of the liver with portal hypertension.

Another frequent complication of chronic and heavy alcohol abuse is gastritis, resulting in upper gastrointestinal bleeding. Because alcohol is an irritating drug, it damages the superficial lining of the stomach, causing bleeding to occur, which at times can be quite severe and copious.

Still another common problem that at times occurs in the chronic alcoholic is a condition called Mallory-Weiss syndrome. Mallory-Weiss syndrome develops because of a tear that occurs at the junction of the gastroesophageal area. This occurs because of alcohol abuse and severe vomiting and retching. The force of the retching causes the tear to occur, resulting in upper gastrointestinal bleeding. In all these cases, the bleeding can be severe enough to cause the patient to go into shock with all its multitudes of complications.

Another frequently affected system is the hematopoietic system (blood system). The effects of alcohol on the blood system are many and varied. Acutely, alcohol can suppress the bone marrow, resulting in the lowering of white blood cells, red blood cells, and platelets.

Chronic alcoholism can cause anemia because of recurrent upper gastrointestinal bleeding on the one hand, and on the other hand, alcohol abuse always leads to folic acid deficiency, resulting in folic acid deficiency anemia. In other instances, chronic alcohol abuse can result in a condition called hypersplenism, as mentioned earlier, which causes hemolysis of red blood cells, causing anemia.

Hypersplenism can also cause leukopenia (low white blood cells) and Thrombocytopenia (low platelet count). These abnormalities in the blood system are the result of splenic sequestration (because the spleen is enlarged, it soaks up these cells within it and destroys them).

Chronic alcoholism with liver disease (cirrhosis) causes the white blood cells to not function well; as a result, affected blacks are not able to fight infection properly.

Chronic alcoholic abuse also affects the endocrine systems. For instance, the sick alcoholic liver is unable to break down estrogen effectively, which then allows the excess estrogen to remain in the blood, resulting in over stimulation of the uterus, causing breakthrough vaginal bleeding, worsening their iron deficiency state. Through this same mechanism, estrogen, resulting in swelling and pain in their breasts, over stimulates alcoholic's breast tissues.

The most frequent cardiac problem that occurs in alcohol intoxication is abnormal rhythm of the heart, such as "fast heartbeat" (tachycardia):

1. Atrial fibrillation
2. Super-ventricular tachycardia
3. Multifocal ventricular contractions (PVCs)
4. Atrial premature contradictions PACs.
5. Heart blocks, etc.

Chronic effects of alcohol on the heart cause damage to the heart muscles, resulting in enlargement of the heart (alcoholic cardiomyopathy). Alcoholic heart disease frequently results in congestive heart failure

Lung disease in alcoholics

Blacks who abuse alcohol frequently develop aspiration pneumonia. Pneumonia develops because when these people get drunk, they lose control of their gag reflux and the consequence of that is that they aspirate their vomitus into their lungs, causing aspiration pneumonia. The overall poor nutritional and health state of people who abuse alcohol predisposes them to community-acquired pneumonias. Smoking cigarettes or cigars is part of the alcohol abuse subculture.

The result of the tobacco abuse/ alcohol abuse that some blacks are involved with is that, here is a high incidence of lung cancer in alcoholic blacks who smoke. There is also a high incidence of head and neck cancer in this subgroup of blacks as well; there is a high incidence of cancer of the esophagus in this subgroup of blacks because of the adverse effects of alcohol and cigarette on esophageal tissue.

The take-home lesson is not to use tobacco in any form and not to abuse alcohol. Alcohol is a drug and can be quite addicting when used in large quantities over a long period. Alcohol has the potential to be toxic to the entire human body. The literature clearly shows that alcohol in moderate quantities, such as one or two glasses of wine with dinner, is good in the prevention of coronary artery heart disease. Alcohol does so through different mechanisms:

1. It makes platelets less sticky, thereby, preventing them from aggregating and in so doing lowering the possibility of clot formation.
2. It increases the level of high-density lipoprotein, the good cholesterol. However, it is prudent that anyone with a propensity to alcohol abuse refrain from alcohol altogether.
3. Both white wine and red wine help to decrease the incidence of coronary artery heart disease when consumed in moderate quantity.

It is believed that the phenols found in red grapes function as antioxidants and prevent the damage to coronary arteries.

Clinical management of alcohol-induced clinical problems:

Clinically, acute alcohol intoxication causes the intoxicated alcoholic to be agitated, unreasonable, sometimes violent, and frequently confused. This set of symptoms and behavior can cause intoxicated people to get into fights and other altercations that can cause problems for their spouses, their children and other members of society with whom they meet.

Alcoholics frequently are brought to the emergency room after fights during which they were traumatized, or brought to the emergency room due to upper gastrointestinal bleeding or due to fever and abdominal pain and other alcohol-associated problems. Once the intoxicated alcoholic arrives in the emergency room, he or she must be evaluated immediately.

Vital signs, such as blood pressure, pulse, temperature, and respiratory rate must be quickly taken and documented. It is very important to examine the abdomen, the head, the eyes and inside the ears, looking for evidence of blunt trauma.

Then, an intravenous access must be quickly established. Blood must be drawn and sent for CBC, SMA 20, serum magnesium, serum amylase, lipase, B12, folate, blood alcohol concentration, and urine, must be sent for drug screening. The urine also must be sent to the laboratory for urinalysis to make sure that there is no blood in it, which may indicate that the patient has had some trauma to the kidneys during a fight.

The examining physician must pay particular attention to the examination of the head area, looking for signs of trauma.

It is important to examine inside the ears, looking for signs of blood coming out of the inner ears. The examination must be complete and must include a rectal examination, looking for signs of blood grossly, and if none is found, the stool must be tested for blood using the hemoccult test.

The neurological examination is extremely important, looking for signs of agitation, confusion, hallucinations, stupor etc.

It is necessary to do a CT SCAN of the brain on alcoholics who present to emergency room for medical to rule out intracranial bleeding.

As soon as the physical examination is completed, the alcoholic must be started on the so-called alcoholic cocktail. The alcoholic cocktail is composed of:

1. IV glucose (50% in one ampule)
2. Thiamine 100 mg IV or IM
3. Folic acid 1 mg IV, IM, or PO if the patient can take PO
4. Magnesium sulfate 1-gram IV or IM
5. B complex vitamin IM, IV, or PO
6. Ativan IV or IM

It is crucial that thiamine is given before the glucose is infused. If the glucose is infused before the administration of thiamine, this will lead to an acute depletion of whatever trace of thiamine is left in the body.

This acute thiamine depletion will lead to a condition called Wernicke's encephalopathy. Acute Wernicke's encephalopathy causes acute agitation, confusion, hallucination and combativeness. The reason why acute Wernicke's occurs when 50% of glucose is infused in the alcoholic is because the alcoholic is frequently deficient in carbohydrates and all B-complex vitamins such as thiamine and folic acid.

Alcoholics do not eat enough foods that contain these vitamins. Thiamine is a necessary biochemical vitamin in the metabolism of glucose (the Krebs cycle, a biochemical pathway reaction that contains many substances that are necessary to metabolize sugars) to help make this reaction.

Therefore, the acute depletion of thiamine causes Wernicke's encephalopathy to occur. Sugar is needed in the acutely intoxicated alcoholic because she is likely to be starved and therefore has hypoglycemia (low blood sugar).

The acutely sick alcoholic needs folic acid because he or she is always folate deficient, and because he or she does not eat enough foods that contain folic acid. Further, alcohol as a drug poisons the folate biochemical pathway. As a result, all alcoholics by definition are folate deficient.

The acutely sick and intoxicated alcoholic needs magnesium, because all chronic and heavy alcoholic users are magnesium deficient, even though the laboratory may report the blood magnesium level as normal. Alcohol is a form of diuretic and as such, the alcoholic loses large quantities of magnesium in the urine.

Low magnesium can cause low serum calcium. Both low serum calcium and low magnesium in an individual can cause seizures, muscle cramps, and (in some cases) rhythm abnormalities of the heart. Hypoglycemia (low blood sugar) can cause seizures to occur. Another frequent substance that chronic alcoholics are frequently deficient in is phosphate.

Phosphate is a by-product of protein breakdown and since the alcoholics are too preoccupied with alcohol to eat properly, they are frequently deficient in protein and phosphate. Further, the alcoholic urinates frequently because of the diuretic effect of alcohol, and thereby loses large quantities of phosphate in the urine, causing hypophosphatemia (low serum phosphate).

Low serum phosphate can cause acute seizures and chronically can cause hemolytic anemia. This is so because phosphate is needed to provide for a normal level of 2-3 D-PG (2-3 diphosphoglycerate).

In some instances, low serum phosphate can cause severe rhythm disturbances of the heart.

Once the alcoholic passes through this first stage of her stay in the hospital, the next step is to evaluate her for acute or chronic disease in the usual manner. If it is decided that the alcoholic needs to be hospitalized, then all the medications in the alcoholic cocktail must be continued for several days except for the magnesium and the 50% dextrose.

The next step in providing acute care for the alcoholic is to watch for the possible development of delirium tremens (DTs). Both the blood alcohol concentration level and how the patient looks clinically are important in deciding when to start anti-DT treatment. Equally important is to try to ascertain when the patient last drank alcohol.

Most alcoholics will start showing signs of DTs 36–48 hours after they had their last drink of alcohol. It is important to keep in mind the fact that chronic alcoholics can have a blood alcohol concentration of 100–200 mg per deciliter in the blood and do not appear drunk. Because of this fact, the chronic alcoholic can go into DTs with an alcohol level concentration that is this high because their bodies are accustomed to having a higher concentration of alcohol in it.

Delirium tremens is a clinical syndrome that results from the craving for alcohol that occurs when an alcohol abuser has been kept away from alcohol for several days. The part of the brain that controls addiction misses the alcohol and the alcoholic goes into withdrawal, due to the loss of alcohol in her bloodstream to satisfy the brain's need for the alcohol.

DTs have several stages: Stage I, Stage II, Stage III, Stage IV and Stage V.

Stage I: The first stage of DTs manifested with tremors (the shakes), restlessness, increased heart rate, insomnia, diarrhea, and irritability.

Stage II: The second stage is all of the Stage I signs, plus sweaty palms and confusion.

Stage III: All the symptoms of I and II plus sweating, rise in blood pressure, rise in pulse, palpitations and hallucinations.

Stage IV: All the preceding signs, plus seizures.

Stage V: All of those in the preceding stages, plus coma.

To prevent DTs from developing, it is recommended that the patient be given Ativan 1–2 mg four times per day, prophylactically by mouth as soon as the patient gets to the emergency room and consciousness level has been evaluated to be clinically satisfactory. If the patient cannot take medication by mouth, Ativan can be given IM or IV.

Alternatively, the patient can be treated with Librium 10 mg PO, four times per day IM or PO. Librium is not absorbed well IM and is not a medication to be used if the patient has severe liver disease, because the liver metabolizes Librium.

The liver metabolizes Ativan differently and, therefore, it can be used even if the liver is severely sick.

Other things that are essential in the treatment of DTs are fluid and electrolyte replacement intravenously. It is very important to keep the sick alcoholic in an anabolic state, by making sure there is always sugar in the IV fluid being given to him or her. D5 ½ normal saline or D5 normal saline is preferred. If the patient is hypertensive, the IV can be D5 ¼ normal saline, along with specific medications to treat the hypertension. If seizure develops, then the patient must be treated first with IV Valium then with Dilantin. A brain CT scan without contrast, followed by an EEG at the appropriate time, must always be done.

Two medications in use to help alcoholics stop drinking are Antabuse (Disulfiram) and Naltrexone. Naltrexone is available to be used intramuscularly as well. Both of these medications have side effects and a person who is drinking alcohol must not take them. If a person drinks alcohol and takes Antabuse, he or she can become acutely ill and in fact can die as a result. Naltrexone works apparently on the brain to decrease the desire of the alcoholic to drink alcohol. Antabuse (Disulfiram) works by converting acetaldehyde, which is a breakdown product of alcohol to acetic acid in the liver that causes an increase in serum acetaldehyde anywhere from five to ten times the normal level.

Because of that, the black man can hyperventilate and can develop flushing of the skin, nausea, vomiting, headache, and respiratory distress along with anxiety, palpitations, and sometimes hypertension.

That is why it is important that people do not drink alcohol and take Disulfiram at the same time.

The usual dose of Disulfiram is 250 mg. A 500 mg dose is also available, but frequently the 250 mg dose is sufficient to prevent someone from craving alcohol. The usual dose for Naltrexone (ReVia) is 50 mg daily for about 12 weeks as a prophylactic treatment against alcohol abuse.

Driving while intoxicated remains a major safety problem in the United States, and every year many thousands of people die because of accidents resulting from DWI. Drunken drivers remain a menace to society, and different states have different laws defining what DWI is.

The following is a complete list of the different listings of the blood alcohol concentrations that are considered legal for any person to drive a car, as published by the Insurance Institute for Highway Safety.

Alcohol affects two parts of the fetal brain more severely, the hippocampus and the cerebellum. A breakdown product of alcohol called acetaldehyde causes the bulk of the problem.

Many individuals who abuse alcohol also abuse cocaine, heroin, and prescription drugs, such as Valium, Librium, Ativan, Xanax, etc. Drinking alcohol and taking these drugs is quite dangerous and can cause a person to die. Alcohol is a neurological, cardiac and pulmonary suppressant, so when a person has too much alcohol in his or her bloodstream, and adds illicit or prescription drugs on top of the alcohol, he or she increases the possibility of cardiac arrhythmia, respiratory failure, coma, and death. Drinking alcohol and then taking drugs is to be avoided, because it can be lethal.

Alcohol abuse is quite prevalent among African Americans, but alcohol abuse is much more prevelent among whites compared to whites. 58% of white Americans abuse alcohol and 36% black Americans abuse alcohol.

It is variably reported that there is 18 million registered alcoholics in the USA, plus anywhere from eight to ten million other individuals who abuse alcohol to different degrees. Alcohol abuse contributes to about 100,000 deaths per year in the United States, making it the third leading cause of preventable death in the United States, after tobacco and obesity and its associated health risks. Based on statistics provided by the National Institute of

Alcohol Abuse and Alcoholism (NIAAA), the cost of caring for alcohol and substance abuse problems in the United States is 166 billion dollars in 2010.

Presently in the USA, this great, powerful, and wealthy country with 10 million millionaires, every night about 17 million children go to bed hungry, and altogether 50 million Americans live in poverty and over all11 million children have no health insurance coverage, and overall about 52 million Americans have no health insurance.

While according to a recent report, the U.S. has 10 million millionaires, 50% of the U.S. population is reported to be poor and 45 trillion dollars of the U.S. wealth are in the hand of the top 2% of the U.S. population.

How cans this happen in the U.S.? The answers are multifaceted and complex, but lie mostly in the philosophy that the rich are to supposed get richer and the poor are suppose to get poorer.

How sad! And how awful! How a great and generous country like the United States of America can allows such a condition to exist? Poverty in the U.S. and around the world affects all racial groups, although minorities bare the heaviest burden.

Whites abuse alcohol many more times than Blacks, Latinos and other minorities in the U.S. and around the world do, and some of the reasons people think that minorities drink more alcohol than do whites, and that is absolutely no true.

Most minorities abuse alcohol in part because of the stress associated with racial discrimination, broken homes, raising children without a man in the home, loneliness, stress in the workplace, unemployment, and pain associated with chronic diseases such as arthritis, depression, anxiety, panic attacks, other mental illnesses etc.

Many people abuse alcohol as the drug of choice to use while partying because this is socially acceptable. Since white men possess more money than black do, they spend more time partying and drinking more alcohol in the process. Many people also resort to alcohol abuse as a way of coping with their problems.

Alcohol, when used in small quantities, can be helpful in increasing the good cholesterol (HDL) one drink of hard liquor per day, or two glasses of wine with dinner, red or white wine, both of which can increase the HDL.

Furthermore, it is clear that alcohol decreases the stickiness of platelets (a cell in the blood necessary in forming clots); in so doing, there is less probability of clot forming in the coronary arteries, thereby decreasing the incidence of heart attacks.

When alcohol is used in excess, the advantage is nullified, because alcohol abuse can cause disease to develop in the heart muscles (cardiomyopathy). In addition, alcohol abuse can cause elevation in the blood pressure, which over time can cause hypertensive heart disease along with coronary artery heart disease.

Light to moderate alcohol consumption can be helpful, while heavy alcohol consumption is harmful to the human body.

Anyone at risk for alcohol abuse ought not to drink alcohol in any amount, because it might get him or her to start drinking alcohol heavily again.

The vast majority of blacks and other minorities in the world live in poverty of different degrees and also suffer from racial discrimination of different types, along with ethnic and religious bigotry, social depredation, domestic abuse of different types, male chauvinism, second-class citizenship, and yet many of these individuals do not abuse alcohol.

By stopping alcohol abuse, an alcohol-abusing people will have a healthier lives, hearts, brains, nervous systems, endocrine systems, reproductive systems, gastrointestinal systems, pancreases, blood systems, psychological systems, emotional systems and overall a healthier, less painful and longer lives.

CHAPTER 75

DRUG ADDICTION IN AFRICAN AMERICAN MEN

Drug addiction is a common addictive habit in the United States and around the world. According to published reports there are 22 million drug addicts in the United States and 200 million drug addicts worldwide in 2013. About 800,000 addicts are addicted to heroin in the U.S. and 15 million people in the world are addicted to heroin, opium or morphine resulting in annual market of 65 billion dollars and the total illicit drug industry costs 320 billion dollars per year worldwide.

"6/12/2017Washington Post Analysis: Opioid Crisis Increases Death Rates For Most American Racial And Ethnic Groups"

"Since the beginning of this decade, death rates have risen among people between the ages of 25 and 44 in virtually every racial and ethnic group, according to" a front-page analysis by the Washington Post 6/9,2017 which found "the death rate among African Americans is up 4 percent, Hispanics 7 percent, whites 12 percent and Native Americans 18 percent." The Post added "after a century of decreases, the overall death rate for Americans in these prime years rose 8 percent between 2010 and 2015," increased "in large measure by drug overdoses and alcohol abuse, mortality data from the U.S. Centers for Disease Control and Prevention." Robert Anderson, chief of mortality statistics for the CDC, said that based on preliminary 2016 data, "I think we're in for another steep increase in the drug overdose deaths overall." Leandris Liburd, director of the CDC's Office of Minority Health and Health Equity, asserted, "The data [are] very concerning." Source CDC

"Two million Americans addicted to opioids, report says"

NBC NightlyNews 7/31, 2017 story 4, 2:15, that a "startling new report" from federal health officials shows that "in 2015, nearly 92 million American adults used a prescription opioid." More than "11 million reported misusing opioids, and nearly two million said they were addicted." "Almost half of those who misuse opioids get them from family and friends." "Source : CDC

According to some report, the U.S. spends about 1 trillion dollars annually on the war on drug to no avail.

"The vast majority of drug users are whites" Source: Huffington Post January 4, 2011

Many more millions of people in the world use and abuse elicit drugs of different types; they are also considered addicts.

Every year 200,000 people in the world die because of illicit drug use and in 2017 50,000 people have died from opioid overdose in the U.S.

The part of the brain stimulated by drugs that results in pleasurable feelings is the dopamine center, which is located at the base of the brain. Drugs such as heroin, cocaine, marijuana, opiates and amphetamines activate dopamine to release neurotransmitter substances, resulting in a pleasurable feeling called a "high," which drug addicts crave to experience.

The dopamine center also functions to allow for the experience of sexual pleasure, enjoyment of foods, music, art, and beautiful things, and other aesthetic things that are pleasing to the ears and the eyes. Once an individual becomes addicted to any drug such as heroin, cocaine, crack-cocaine, marijuana, etc., he or she craves these drugs when the level of the drug decreases in the bloodstream. The craving for the drug oftentimes is quite painful.

Drug craving can lead to severe withdrawal symptoms such as sweating, headache, runny nose, abdominal cramps, diarrhea, poor appetite, insomnia, nightmares etc.

So, addiction to a drug, in particular cocaine, heroin and crack-cocaine, can drive addicts to do anything to get money to buy the drugs in order to satisfy the drug craving on the one hand, which is the more powerful and intense feeling, and to avoid going into drug withdrawal feelings.

On the other hand, once a person becomes addicted to drugs, it is very difficult to give it up. The addicted person becomes dependent on the drug and spends a great deal of time preoccupying himself with finding money to get the next fix. He will spend rent money, food money, mortgage money, or he will lie, steal, and commit crimes of different types and magnitude in order to get the money to pay for the drug. Frequently, he prostitutes himself to get money to pay for the drug.

Drug addiction is quite common among all racial groups in the U.S. and around the world. Drug addiction is common in all social and economic status. Wherever there is poverty and ghettos, there is a high incidence of illicit drug use.

However, illicit drug use has become prevalent in the suburbs of the United States, around the world and elsewhere, involving middle and upper class people. More than 15 million people in the U.S. abuse prescription drugs and many more million worldwide abuse prescription drugs. Statistically, more whites' abuse prescription drugs than Blacks, Latinos and other minorities in the U.S. and around the world.100, 000 people in the U.S. die every year from prescription drugs.

In 2009, the U.S. population was 307,006,000 and 47.1% of the population-abused drugs and 118,705,000 used illicit drugs.

The most frequently abused illicit drugs in the U.S. are:

Marijuana usage 104,446,000
Cocaine usage 36,599,000
Crack usage 8,359,000
Heroin usage 3,683,000
Methamphetamine usage 12,837,000
Psychotherapeutics usage 51,771,000
Ecstasy usage 14,234,000
Hallucinogens usage 37,256,000
Painkillers usage 35,046,000
Alcohol usage 208,545,000

Heavy alcohol abuse 17,129,000 (In 2010 17.6 million people registered as alcoholic in the U.S.) Source: Substance Abuse and Mental Health Services Administration, (2009).

Illicit drug abuse is common in every community in the United States, around the world and in all communities. The people involved in abusing illicit drugs include the very poor who reside in the inner cities of the United States, and around the world in the working class, to the middle class and all the way up to the upper class.

Illicit drug abuse is common in all professions to one degree or another and all sexes are involved in the illicit drug subculture. Blacks use more heroin and crack-cocaine, and whites use more cocaine, marijuana, and amphetamines.

Cocaine has, however, made an entry into black, Hispanic, Asian, Native American, Pacific Islander and Latino ghettos in recent years, because the price of cocaine has gone down to a point where some poor people can now afford to buy it.

Outside forces from the communities fuel the illicit drug subculture where these drugs are produced. People who do not live in these communities are bringing the drugs into these communities. The big question is who are these people? What are their motives? Is it just for the money, or is it something else?

Some have said that infiltration of illicit drugs into the minority communities is a well-planned conspiracy to destroy generations of young people of color. Whether or not proof exists to substantiate these allegations is not quite clear. One thing is certain are that the illicit drug subculture is highly associated with criminal behavior of different types and different degrees. The result is that communities where illicit drugs are prevalent also are beset with high crime rates.

Per capita, more whites use illicit drugs than blacks, but fewer whites get arrested for using drugs and even fewer of them get sent to jail for using drugs than blacks.

Of all the modern countries in the world, the United States has more people in jail at any one time than any other country. According to U.S. Bureau of Statistics, there are 2.4 million people in jail in the United States as of 2017.

The U.S. represents 4% of the world population and yet 25% of all people in jails around the world are found in the U.S. All together, there are 9 million people in the jail in the world and half of them are found in China, Russia and the U.S.

Though Blacks represent about 15% of the United States population and Hispanics represent 17%, together that represent 32.5%, of the U.S. population. In 2012, 43.91 per cent of those in jail were Blacks, 18.26 per cent of them were Hispanics, and 34.72 per cent were Whites. So, a total of 62.17 % of those in jail in the U.S. were a combination of Blacks and Hispanics, which is an outrageous number, although these two groups Blacks and Hispanics made up 32.5% of the total population of the U.S. of 319 millions 1 out 36 every Hispanics is in jail in the U.S. and 1 out of 15 Blacks is in jail in the US.

Overall 1 out every 100 people in the U.S. is in jail. In the year 2005, 7 per cent of those in jail in the U.S. were females. There were 107,518 Blacks in jail in the U.S. in 2005. A third of blacks that are in jail are there for drug-related offenses.

In 2017, the U.S. population is 326,474,010 and the world population is now 7.5 billion.

The overall rate of illicit drug use reported in United States black population, age 12 and older, was 11.9%. Relative to the total United States blacks population, Native Americans users of illicit drug are 19.8%, Puerto Ricans 13.3%, Mexican-Americans 12.7%, Asian Pacific Islanders 6.5%, Caribbean-Americans 7.6%, Central Americans 5.7% and Cuban-Americans 8.2%.

"The 2009 National Survey of Drug Use and Health reports that 39 percent whites used an illicit drug in the past year. For blacks, the rate was 34 percent."

According to the National Center on Addiction and Substance Abuse at Columbia University, 21.5 million blacks in the United States smoke, 4.5 million are alcoholics; 3.5 million blacks misuse prescription drugs and 3.1 million blacks use illicit drugs.

The psychological and physical manifestations of drug addiction

The mindset that causes people the world over to abuse drugs is no doubt similar to the mindset of people all over the world. However, the circumstances of life that are associated with drug abuse are quite different in some measure different in minorities than they are in whites. Most people that are drug addicts start out using marijuana recreationally.

They then gradually move on to harder drugs, such as amphetamines, LSD, other psychedelic drugs. As the addiction deepens, they move on to using cocaine, heroin and crack-cocaine. These people are financially able to support their addictions, because they have good jobs with good pay, which enables them to pay for these drugs. Some of these people are in the entertainment world (the sports world, the business world and the art world, a world that predisposes some of them to drug addiction). Minorities are in a different set of circumstances as whites, in that they do not have money to support their drug habits.

A significant percentage of people are addicted to prescription drugs and the most frequently abused prescription drugs are the followings:

1. Valium
2. Librium
3. Xanax
4. Ativan
5. Tranxene
6. Klonopin
7. Codeine
8. Vicodin
9. Demerol
10. Morphine
11. Hydrocodone
12. Ambien
13. Restoril
14. Methadone etc.

Some people become addicted to prescription drugs because of chronic pain associated with illness, such as cancer, arthritis, headaches, sickle cell disease, diabetic neuropathy and many other chronic diseases, which require chronic pain medications for relief.

Sometimes these individuals continue to get the prescription for these medications for a long time, but once they are no longer able to obtain these prescriptions, they resort to illicit drugs to ease their pain.

Some of these people become chronic drug addicts in this way. Drug addiction and all other addictions are psychological illnesses. The craving associated with drug addiction is controlled by neurotransmitters within the brain, in particular the dopamine center.

When the urge comes upon an addicted person to get a high, that person will do just about anything to get the money to buy the drug. Drug addiction is a mental illness and ought to be treated as such. Percentage-wise, IV drug addiction is more common among minorities, as compared to whites.

This is so, because this type of drug addiction is more closely associated with the inner cities where most poor people live around the world. Although it is a known fact, the incidence of IV drug use is on the rise in the middle class as well as in the upper class communities of the United States and the world. In other words, illicit drug use is also on Wall Street, Madison Avenue and most definitely in the suburbs and where rich people work and live all over the world.

The brain is affected by illicit drug use in many other ways. For example, heavy marijuana use is known to affect the brain in ways that lead to slow and slurred speech and memory loss. Both cocaine and heroin use are associated with seizures. When heroin and cocaine are used intravenously, sepsis and bacterial endocarditis can occur. Infected emboli can be thrown to the brain from the heart valve, resulting in brain abscesses.

Most importantly, the brain is frequently affected by drug overdose causing coma and sometimes deaths.

Different illicit drugs affect the brain in different ways, examples include:

"Marijuana causes
Relaxation
Distorted sensory perception
Euphoria
Impaired coordination
Increased heart rate
Increased appetite
Impaired learning
Impaired memory
Anxiety
Panic attacks
Psychosis
Frequent respiratory infection
Addiction
Possible brain damage"

Heroin affects the brain and the rest of the body in these ways:

Euphoria
Impaired coordination
Drowsiness
Dizziness
Confusion
Nausea
Vomiting
Sedation
Constipation
Respiratory failure
Hepatitis
Endocarditis
Addiction
Coma
Death"

Cocaine affects the brain and the rest of the body in these ways:

"Increase heart rate
Increase blood pressure
High temperature
Exhilaration
Mental alertness
Tremors
Poor appetite
Anxiety
Panic attacks
Paranoia
Violent behavior
Psychosis
Weight loss
Insomnia
Arrhythmias
Seizure
Stroke
Heart attacks
Addition
Coma
Death"

Other illicit drugs that frequently abused include:

Methamphetamine
Crystal
Speed
PCP
LSD
Dextromethorphan
Anabolic steroid
Nitrous oxide etc;

Source: National Institute on Drug Abuse (National Institutes of Health)

The lungs are affected by drug addiction in many ways as well. Addicts who use cocaine or heroin intravenously frequently develop symptoms of upper airway diseases such as coughing, wheezing, and bronchitis. Acute pulmonary edema (when the lungs become filled with fluid) can occur as an idiosyncratic reaction to heroin use. Another complication involving the lungs in heroin and cocaine use is pulmonary embolism (a clot to the lungs). This happens because the addicts use veins in their legs to infuse the drug and sometimes the vessels in the groin and legs get damaged and infected and become swollen.

These conditions can lead to stasis, which in turn can lead to clot formation, deep vein thrombophlebitis (DVT). The clots can then migrate through the blood vessels into the lung, causing acute pulmonary embolism. Infected emboli can also be thrown to the lungs from infected vegetation from the heart valves (a condition called bacterial endocarditis). Still another frequent pulmonary complication of the IV drug abuser is pneumonia, which occurs often in IV drug abusers because of their overall poor physical condition predisposing them to the development of different types of lung infection.

The incidence of AIDS is the highest among all minority groups in the U.S., and around the world. The incidence of the lung infection called pneumocystis carinii (PCP) is the highest among minority people with AIDS. PCP is a most serious lung infection and frequently is the cause of death of people with AIDS. The incidence of pulmonary tuberculosis has decreased in the general population over the last several years, but it has gone up in people with AIDS.

The effects of illicit drug use on the heart

The heart suffers immensely from illicit drug use, be it use of amphetamines, LSD, marijuana, prescription drugs, cocaine, crack-cocaine, heroin, etc. The heart is likely to become affected by any one of these drugs once in the bloodstream and is more so when used in excess.

Once in the bloodstream, the drugs stimulate the heart, causing it to beat too fast and frequently, irregularly.

Cocaine use can cause sudden death due to acute myocardial infarction (heart attack). Other cocaine-associated complications of the heart include cardiac arrhythmias, which sometimes can be lethal, myocarditis (inflammation of the heart muscle), cardiomyopathy (enlargement of the heart), and coronary spasm (spasm of the vessel that carries blood around the heart). The heart can, at times, become very slow (bradycardia). The heart rate can also be slowed by cocaine.

At times, in the middle of acute cocaine intoxication, it has been reported that the heart can actually rupture abruptly, resulting in sudden death. It is believed that it is a metabolite (breakdown product) of cocaine that causes the toxicity to the heart.

Acute heroin intoxication can cause the heart to slow down (bradycardia) as well as suppression of the respiratory system, which can result in cardiopulmonary failure. Many things can happen to the heart of an intravenous drug abuser, but one of the most serious is a condition called bacterial endocarditis.

There are two forms of endocarditis: 1) acute bacterial endocarditis, 2) sub-acute bacterial endocarditis. Endocarditis occurs when bacterial organisms enter the bloodstream of the individuals, injecting drugs into their veins. Once in the bloodstream, the bacteria multiply, resulting in a condition called sepsis.

Bacteria then settle on the heart valve, damaging it, causing different types of cardiac decompositions. In drug addicts, the valve most frequently affected is the tricuspid valve (54% of the time), followed by the aortic valve (25%), then by the mitral valve (about 20%), and the rest (6%) can be mixed right-sided and left-sided endocarditis. The bacterial organism most frequently found in drug addicts is staphylococcus coagulase positive, followed by streptococci; fungi, such as Candida and aspergillus, can also cause bacterial endocarditis.

Gram-negative organisms of different types can also settle on the heart valves, causing endocarditis. Staph coagulase negative can also settle on the heart valve, causing bacterial endocarditis in the drug addicts. In intravenous drug abusers, when the tricuspid valve is the affected valve, 80% of the time the Staph coagulase positive is the organism isolated.

They can also become infected with Methicillin-Resistant Staph Aureus. (MRSA). In acute bacterial endocarditis, the affected person becomes acutely ill with fever, chills, shortness of breath, chest pain, sometimes, cardiac arrhythmia and the development of an acute heart murmur, which was not there before with congestive heart failure.

Other physical findings may include distended neck veins, decreased blood pressure; fast pulse rate, increased respiratory rate, cardiac rub, and rales in the lungs can be heard. An enlarged and tender liver can occur and a large spleen can be palpated. Acute pain in the lower back is frequently present in an individual who is septic.

Headache with nausea and vomiting can also occur.

Laboratory findings include a high white blood cell count, low red blood cell count, elevated erythrocyte sedimentation rate, low platelet count, positive ANA, and elevated liver function test.

A chest x-ray may show diffuse infiltrates in the lungs. EKG may show fast rate with regular rhythm or fast rate with irregular rhythm, a slow rate with decreased voltage indicating that the heart is being compromised with fluid around the sac, a condition called cardiac tamponade. Arterial blood gases may be grossly abnormal with low O2 SAT. An echocardiogram may show valvular abnormalities such as vegetation, and an enlarged heart may be seen.

A transesophageal echocardiogram may show the presence of vegetation on the heart valves if the regular echocardiogram does not show it. Sometimes, a Tran thoracic Echocardiogram can also be done if the technology is available in that particular institution. It is a much better test to detect heart valve vegetation than the regular echocardiogram.

The urine may show the presence of protein and red blood cells because of emboli to the kidneys. Septic emboli can also affect the skin, causing assorted skin lesions. Acute bacterial endocarditis is a severe medical emergency requiring the help of a cardiologist and cardiac surgeon to quickly take over the management of the patient, in order to try to replace the heart valve and save the individual's life. If any significant delay takes place, the chances of recovery may not be very good in acute bacterial endocarditis.

What happens is that the bacteria sit on the valve and literally eat it away and then blood flows back and forth, resulting in acute cardiac decomposition with impending deaths, because of the valve having been acutely destroyed.

As for management, these individuals frequently have to be incubated if they are in acute congestive heart failure. They cannot breathe.

They need assistance to breathe and 100% oxygen has to be provided for them. Blood cultures ought to be taken and if they are positive, then clinical decisions must be made to provide appropriate antibiotic treatment for these patients. If staph is suspected, which it frequently is, Vancomycin IV is an excellent choice in antibiotic with coverage for gram-negative organisms. Vancomycin also covers MRSA.

Once the organism is identified, and then an appropriate antibiotic should be provided based on the sensitivity. In the case of enterococcus, Gentamicin, along with Ampicillin, will be the drug of choice; if pseudomonas, then Fortaz will be a very good medication and if it is staph and it is sensitive to penicillin, then Oxacillin IV will be switched, as the medication of choice and the Vancomycin will be stopped.

If it is Methicillin-resistant staph, then the medication of choice clearly in this case is Vancomycin as stated above.

The other infection frequently involving the heart is sub-acute bacterial endocarditis. Sub-acute bacterial endocarditis can be more insidious and often is more insidious in its development, causing difficulty, at times, in arriving at a diagnosis. Sub-acute bacterial endocarditis manifests itself as a febrile illness with chills, general malaise, joint pain, low back pain, and headache.

At times, a person with sub-acute bacterial endocarditis might present with general weakness, pallor, intermittent low-grade fever, and a general feeling of unwellness.

In this instance, a high index of suspicion must be brought into play so as not to mistake the diagnosis for something else. The profile of the patient is of major importance, i.e., in an intravenous drug abuser who is prone to sub-acute bacterial endocarditis by virtue of her habit of using drugs and sharing dirty needles with other drug addicts, the index of suspicion is quite high. Sometimes, these individuals use water from the toilet bowl to prepare the drug, in this way injecting themselves with contaminated materials.

The liver is a frequently affected organ in drug addicts. For those who abuse prescription drugs, the liver may get sick from these drugs, in particular when alcohol is combined with these drugs, as is frequently the case. Intravenous drug abusers' livers get sick most frequently because of hepatitis B and hepatitis C. In rare circumstances, they can also be infected with hepatitis A and hepatitis D, but these types of viral hepatitis occur less frequently in intravenous drug users.

Hepatitis A, B and C can be sexually transmitted and many drug addicts, when they are high on drugs, have sexual intercourse with whomever, wherever and whenever. Some drug addicts prostitute themselves either for drugs or for money to buy drugs.

These loose behaviors predispose the drug addicts to contracting sexually transmitted diseases, such as hepatitis A, B and C, syphilis, gonorrhea, Chlamydia, genital herpes, human papilloma virus (HPV), HIV etc;

Several of these sexually transmitted diseases, such as hepatitis A, B and C, syphilis, gonorrhea, and HIV can be spread to different parts of the body, resulting in all sorts of different symptoms and damage to the human body. In particular, hepatitis B and C can cause chronic liver disease such as chronic active hepatitis, chronic persistent hepatitis, and cirrhosis of the liver, with all its associated complications, including liver cancer and death.

Drug addicts can also get infected with hepatic a through needle sharing, Because of that, sub clinical, acute hepatitis A can develop as well as fulminant hepatitis resulting in acute liver failure. It is therefore a very good idea to do a complete hepatitis profile on drug addicts, to include hepatitis, A, B, and C including DNA-PCR for Delta hepatitis. Delta hepatitis virus needs the presence of hepatitis B to support its growth in the body.

An other very important to remember is that drug addicts must be vaccinated against the hepatitis viruses that they are not infected with, so as to prevent them from becoming infected with other hepatitis organisms on top of an already sick liver, which can have lethal clinical consequences.

The gastrointestinal tract is affected in drug addicts in several ways. One of the most common gastrointestinal symptoms that drug addicts suffer from is abdominal pain associated with craving for drugs.

Secondly, drug addicts suffer frequently from diarrhea. The diarrhea has two bases: 1) nervousness and anxiety associated with craving for drugs; 2) parasitic infestation, which they contract during anal intercourse, transmitting organisms such as amoebae and Giardia lamblia. Upper gastrointestinal bleeding can occur as well when these people become cirrhotic because of chronic hepatitis. The bleeding occurs because of esophageal varices.

The kidneys are affected by intravenous drug addiction in several ways. As part of the sepsis and septic shock, the kidneys frequently fail in drug addicts, who present to the hospital with bacterial sepsis. As part of sub-acute bacterial endocarditis, septic emboli because of septic vegetations being thrown from the heart valves to the kidneys can affect the kidneys. Nephrotic syndrome occurs in intravenous drug addicts. This is probably due to antigen-antibody complexes, which form and circulate in the bloodstream either because of low-grade chronic infection or as a result of the different materials that are used to cut and mix either cocaine or heroin that the addicts use.

These complexes settle in the tubules of the kidneys, causing nephrotic syndrome. Kidney abscesses can also occur in some IV drug addicts.

The men's genital organ is also affected by liver disease resulting in cirrhosis causing small and shiny testicles because of the inability of the liver to break down estrogen in cirrhotic men's liver, and erectal dysfunction can also develop.

Intravenous drug addicts, because they having sexual intercourse with multiple sexual partners, have a high incidence of cervical cancer. Sexually transmitted disease is quite common in drug addicts. When these people are under the influence of drugs they have the propensity of engaging in risky sexual intercourse with multiple sexual partners without regard to barrier protection, exposing their genital organs to being infected with gonorrhea, Chlamydia, herpes simplex virus, human papilloma virus, and HIV infection.

The spread of the AIDS virus through the IV drug addicts is the main reason why there is such a high incidence of AIDS in drug addicts in the United States and all over the world. (See chapter on AIDS).

The blood is one of the most commonly abused systems by drug addicts. This is so because the blood is the entry point of most of the drugs that are used and abused by drug addicts. Once the drugs reach the bloodstream, it gets carried to all parts of the body.

Frequently, the blood of drug addicts gets infected with bacterial organisms such as staphylococcus aureus, staphylococcus epidermidis, streptococci pneumonia, pseudomonas, klebsiella pneumonia, E. coli, hemophilus influenza, and pneumococci. Other Methicillin-Resistant Staph Aureus (MRSA) and fungi such as Candida, aspergillus, and viruses such as hepatitis A, B, C, D, E, and G can all enter the bloodstream through injection of drugs into the blood system.

As described earlier, all these different microorganisms have at one point or another caused infection in drug addicts. The blood cells of the body are all affected by drug addiction. Different drugs that are abused by addicts affect the bone marrow by suppressing it. The suppression of the bone marrow that these drugs can cause leads to anemia, leukopenia, or thrombocytopenia to occur acutely.

Leukocytosis can occur, reflecting the presence of the infection. Pancytopenia can also occur because of an acute infection such as sepsis, as well as hepatitis-induced cirrhosis of the liver, with secondary portal hypertension. When an IV drug abuser is infected with the AIDS virus, parvovirus #B-19 can enter the bloodstream, resulting in pure red cell aplasia. Hepatitis can at times cause aplastic anemia. Both hepatitis C and B have been described in aplastic anemia, and in some instances hepatitis A has been described in some part of the world as being responsible for aplastic anemia.

Bacteria also get into the blood through broken and rotten teeth. However, more often, the bacteria get into the blood through skin abscesses that drug addicts develop during skin-popping or infected veins or dirty needles that addicts use to inject drugs. Another disease that can occur in drug addicts in IVDA is bone infection (osteomyelitis), a condition that results when bacteria that are circulating in the bloodstream infect the bone.

Different bones can become infected in drug addicts, but the lumbar spine, the thoracic spine, the hip joints and the knees, etc. can frequently become infected. Often drug addicts present to the hospital with high fever, severe low back pain, or a swollen knee with effusion. When that happens, the back has to be evaluated with a CT scan and/or an MRI looking for the possibility of destruction of bones because of infection. Sometimes a bone scan might add some more information to the clinical presentation.

When the bone is found to be infected an orthopedic surgeon must be brought into the picture to try to surgically remove the infected bone. In addition, the individual requires several weeks of IV antibiotics. That often is a problem because it is difficult to keep an IV drug abuser in the hospital for as long as six weeks; he or she oftentimes elopes so she or he can go back to continue his or her destructive habits of using drugs.

The skin is the most frequently abused organ by the intravenous drug addicts. The heroin or cocaine addicts who inject drugs have to go through the skin to get the veins or arteries to inject themselves. Frequently, the skin is dirty because of lack of proper cleansing. Some addicts, when they run out of veins to inject, inject drugs under their skin, a practice called skin-popping. Some addicts have multiple sores over their legs, abdomen, buttocks, neck, and arms with very little good skin left. These open sores represent a ready entry point for infection to enter into the bloodstream, resulting in blood infections of different types.

The blood is the main vehicle through which drugs are introduced into the bloodstream. Other routes through which illicit drugs are introduced into the body are smoking, snorting, and skin-popping. Once the drugs are in the bloodstream, and if the doses of the drugs are excessive, the result is frequently drug overdose, resulting in different degrees of mental aberration. Frequently, confusion, stupor, seizures and, oftentimes, coma can develop. Once coma develops, if immediate medical attention is not provided, death may result.

Treatment of drug addicts and drug addiction

Drug addiction is a serious mental illness that affects people in all segments of society. Some people are addicted to prescription drugs, some people are addicted to illicit drugs, and some people are addicted to a combination of illicit drugs and prescription drugs. Drug addiction treatment requires a multi-team effort.

The mental aspect of drug addiction requires treatment from mental health professionals and drug counselors and these individuals ought to go to drug treatment clinics and hospitals, both on an outpatient basis and when necessary on an inpatient basis for long-term drug rehabilitation treatments.

The medical treatments of drug addicts must be both organs and systems directed. One of the key components of intravenous drug abuse treatment is Methadone treatment. Methadone is a synthetic drug that is used to relieve the drug craving of heroin addicts. There are roughly 3.8 million chronic and regular drug addicts in the United States. They represent about 20% of the total drug addicts in the United States, which means that there are about 19 million drug addicts in the United States. 25 million individuals are addicted to illicit drugs in the U.S in 2011 and worldwide 200 million people use illicit drugs.

Methadone use contributes greatly in reducing HIV infection in IV drug abusers.

It helps put people to work and to some degree; it helps to decrease the crime rate because these addicts do not have to commit crimes to find money to buy their drugs. According to published report, only 1.7 million drug addicts can get into a Methadone program in the United States. It is said that only 115,000 of the 800,000 chronic users of heroin are getting Methadone. In New York City, about 35,000 of the 200,000 hardcore drug users are able to get into a Methadone Program. Methadone according to some people is encouraging drug addiction.

This is untrue because Methadone is a form of medical treatment for heroin addiction. Drug addicts can abuse Methadone also. Some addicts take the Methadone from the clinic and sell on the street. Some people on purpose lie about the actual dose of Methadone and as a result too much Methadone is given to them and they can overdose on Methadone on that basis. Because of Methadone overdose, they can go into coma. Some addicts abuse the Methadone Program and stay on it permanently as a form of work disability.

These problems with the Methadone Program are not widespread, and overall the Methadone Program is useful and constructive. The hardcore drug users in the ghettos of the United States use a significant percentage of heroin, cocaine and crack-cocaine. However, according to recent reports, Whites and people in the middle class, upper middle class and celebrities in the sports and entertainment world use more cocaine, heroin and crack cocaine than people of color who live in the ghettos of the U.S.

Because Blacks, Hispanics and other minorities both in the U.S. and around the world are arrested, persecuted and put in jail more often than whites for drug offenses, there is a misconception that they use more of these drugs, than whites, that is, in fact, not the case.

As mentioned above, there are 2.2 million people in jail in the U.S. This is the highest rate of incarceration than any industrial country in the world. In 2009, 754 people per 10,000 were in jail in the U.S. One of 32 American adults is in jail, either on probation or on parole.

At anytime, there are 7 million people in the U.S. in jails, either on probation or on parole. "The U.S. has 5% of the world' population and 25% of the world's prison population" Sixty-five million people in the U.S. have a criminal record. Source: U.S Justice Department.

Many of the people in State prisons or Federal prisons are there for drug related offenses." Currently, the United States houses over 500,000 prisoners for drug related offenses. The drug addiction subculture is associated with criminal behavior because it is illegal to distribute and to use illicit drugs; the trafficking of drugs is controlled by the criminal elements of society. Blacks and Hispanics are more frequently sentenced for drug related offenses. 23% of Blacks, 21% Hispanics, and 15% of whites are sentenced for drug related crimes. The three strikes, you are out send more blacks to jail than other racial groups.

"In 2007, 4,618 black males per 100,000, 1,747 Hispanics males per 100,000, and 773 white males per 100,000 were incarcerated in the U.S." As of April 2010, there were 211,455 people in Federal prisons in the U.S.

Poverty, racial discrimination, poor education, poor housing, lack of economic opportunities, and the chronic depressive state of mind associated with being in the underclass of society contribute to the factors that persist for the proliferation of drugs in the ghettos.

The dynamics for the penetration of drugs into the suburbs are altogether different from that which exists for the poor people's communities. Rich folks get into the drug use subculture for recreational purposes, or to be in with a particular crowd or to be "cool." Either way, drug addiction is drug addiction and a drug addict is a drug addict.

Providing treatment for drug addiction and addressing the multiple and different issues that make drug addiction what it is take a back seat to the building of jails, stiff sentences, and the "Three strikes, you are out" policies of the U.S. and different state governments. There are people in jail serving life sentences because they were arrested for possessing marijuana.

It is utterly absurd that an individual can be thrown in jail for life for using crack-cocaine and most frequently, these individuals happen to be people of color. Individuals in the upper echelon of the United States society can be arrested for using cocaine or heroin, and get away at times with just a slap on the back of the hand. It would seem clear that these laws are placed in the books specifically to punish people of color, simply to get them out of society and throw them in jail.

This seems to be grossly unfair, though no one should condone the use of drugs of any kind, because that is illegal. However, putting it in its proper context, clearly there is some inequity in the way the law is being used as it relates to blacks, versus blacks in the majority community.

It is not hard to envision that these problems would be resolved rather promptly if the hardcore drug users in the United States were white middle class and the white community was being devastated by these drugs.

Marijuana, cocaine and heroine use are now very common in the white Community resulting in a lot of damages to that community causing many Deaths. Drug addiction is no longer a minority people problem in the U.S. and in the world. In addition, chronic use of marijuana is known to cause damage to the brain resulting in a multitude behavioral problems including dementia

The following States in the U.S. have legalized marijuana for recreational use:

Colorado
Oregon
Washington State
Alaska

It is fair to say that a Marshall type of plan would have to be put into effect to deal with the drug problems, and as certain as the sun rises in the east and sets in the west, these problems would have been solved, if not completely, but certainly much better than they are being dealt with now. According to the International Centre for Prison Studies At King's College in London England, "more people are behind bars in the United States than in any other country. China ranks second with 1.5 million prisoners, followed by Russia with 870,000."

The brain is frequently evaluated when drug addicts present with headaches, fever and seizures. Evaluation and treatment include brain CT, brain MRI, EEG, echocardiogram, CBC, SMA 18, PT, PTT, chest x-rays, urinalysis, blood cultures and lumbar punctures. Treatments directed towards possible acute brain disease in the IV drug abuser are based on any abnormal results the aforementioned tests may show. If all the tests are normal, or the results are pending, empirical treatments must be started promptly.

For the seizure, Valium IV followed by Dilantin IV or by mouth should be started. For the fever, broad-spectrum antibiotics are given IV. In this setting, Vancomycin IV is given to cover for gram-positive organisms, and Fortaz or other broad-spectrum gram-negative antibiotic is given to cover for gram-negative organisms. There are multitudes of other antibiotic combinations that can be used to cover both for gram-negative and gram-positive organisms in this setting.

Treatments of acute lung disease in IV drug abusers when they present with fever and shortness of breath are tailored to the findings on physical examination and/or chest x-ray. If the patient is afebrile, but shows signs and symptoms of acute pulmonary disease, then arterial blood gas is done and oxygen is quickly started, and if the signs and symptoms are consistent with congestive heart failure, then treatment is given with IV Lasix right away.

If signs and symptoms are consistent with acute pulmonary embolism, then a lung scan must be ordered along with ultrasound of the lower extremities. If the suspicion is strong and these tests are not readily available, then the patient should be given IV Heparin, if there is no contraindication to anticoagulation.

If all signs, symptoms and findings on chest x-ray and CBC are consistent with pneumonia, then broad-spectrum antibiotics with Vancomycin IV and with Fortaz ought to be started immediately. If the patient is able to cough up sputum, then the sputum ought to be sent to the laboratory for gram stain and culture prior to starting the antibiotics.

Infection of the heart is one of the most common infections seen in IV drug abusers. Anytime an IV drug addict presents to the hospital with fever, heart valve infection such, as acute bacterial endocarditis or sub-acute bacterial endocarditis must be suspected. Once the blood cultures have been obtained, broad-spectrum antibiotics with Vancomycin IV and Fortaz IV must be started to cover for the possibility of bacterial endocarditis.

In acute bacterial endocarditis, the patient's cardiopulmonary system can become decompensated quickly, resulting in acute shortness of breath and acute congestive heart failure (pulmonary edema) because of acute destruction of the heart valve. This happens because bacteria settle on the affected heart valve and destroy it.

As stated earlier, the most frequently affected valve in intravenous drug abuser is the tricuspid valve, followed by the aortic valve, followed by the mitral valves.

This is an acute medical emergency necessitating evaluation by a heart surgeon for replacement of the affected valve surgically.

It is important when treating a patient for possible bacterial endocarditis to frequently listen to the patient's heart, looking for the development of a new heart murmur, which would be the first sign of possible cardiac decompensation. Sub-acute bacterial endocarditis can present with no definite cardiac symptoms.

Oftentimes, sub-acute bacterial endocarditis presents as part of sepsis with fever, chills, and low back pain. Sometimes infected vegetation can be seen on an echocardiogram.

Sometimes, sub-acute bacterial endocarditis presents and manifests itself with general malaise, weakness and intermittent low-grade fever and anemia. If serial blood cultures are drawn, a positive drug culture will eventually be found and the diagnosis of sub-acute bacterial endocarditis can be established.

The treatment of bacterial endocarditis is Vancomycin to cover for Staph coagulase, positive MRSA, ceftriaxone for other gram-positive cocci, and Fortaz to cover for organisms such as pseudomonas. There are other combinations of antibiotics, which can also be quite effective in treating this infection.

The main reason to always give the patient Vancomycin at presentation is that there is significant percentage of Staphylococcus organisms that are resistant to penicillin-like medications, such as Nafcillin, Kefzol, MRSA, and Oxacillin.

Once the culture and sensitivity results are back from the lab, then Nafcillin can be switched for the Vancomycin, assuming that the patient is not allergic to penicillin and that the organism is shown to be sensitive to the Nafcillin. Vancomycin is much more expensive than Nafcillin. In addition to antibiotic treatment, proper fluid management, proper electrolyte management and antipyretic for fever and nasal oxygen must be included as part of the treatment.

Intravenous drug abusers must also be given medication such as methadone to forestall the development of drug withdrawal.

Many drug addicts use alcohol to supplement their drug addiction needs. These patients, when acutely ill, must be watched closely for seizures, which, if they develop, can complicate the patient's overall clinical picture.

Treatment of liver disease in drug addicts is dictated by the clinical condition of the individual patient. If the drug addict presents with acute hepatitis, fever, chills, nausea, vomiting, abdominal pain and elevated liver function tests, the patient ought to be placed in isolation with hepatitis precautions being adhered to. In this setting, the prothrombin time is most important.

This is so because the prothrombin time is a measure as to how well the liver is able to function. The sicker the liver, the higher the prothrombin time will be. If the prothrombin time is elevated, then 10 mg of Vitamin K SC ought to be given in the deltoid with applied pressure both as a test and as a treatment.

The prothrombin time should be repeated 6–12 hours later.

If the prothrombin time is corrected back to normal after the Vitamin K, it means that the patient still has good liver function left though the liver is tender and the liver tests are abnormal. Further, it also means that the patient though may have abnormal platelet count, and does not have DIC.

Treatments with IV fluids, anti-fever medications such as Tylenol, anti-itching medication, anti-vomiting medication ought to be provided to control these particular symptoms. If the patient is not vomiting, is able to eat, and the prothrombin time is normal, it is advisable to treat the patients who have hepatitis at home while monitoring his or her vital signs and liver function tests.

Chronic liver disease, such as chronic active hepatitis and chronic persistent hepatitis, are treated either aggressively or supportively in a conservative way. In the case of chronic active hepatitis, treatment will be provided after liver biopsy and based on the symptoms of the patient and the findings on the liver biopsy.

The most frequently used treatment for patients with chronic active hepatitis and symptoms of chronic active hepatitis with documented liver biopsy are alpha Interferon.

The degree of inflammation seen in the liver biopsy documents the severity of the liver disease. In chronic persistent hepatitis, there is minimal inflammation with no fibrosis in the liver and the liver tests are either slightly or moderately elevated chronically. In chronic lobular hepatitis there is mild to moderate inflammation and mild fibrosis. In chronic active hepatitis there is, as stated above, moderate severe inflammation and moderate to severe fibrosis of the liver.

Patients who abuse intravenous drugs can also develop acute hepatitis A because of intravenous drug use, though less so than hepatitis B and C, but it can occur. There are no chronic sequelae of hepatitis A. It is a good idea for patients who are chronic abusers of drugs to be vaccinated with the hepatitis virus A vaccine, which is available.

In addition, drug addiction is a major psychiatric disease that affects the mind in a very significant way. Once addicted to drugs, these individuals are mentally dependent and emotionally dependent on the drugs and become very preoccupied with when and where they are going to find money for their next fix and their entire preoccupation is related to their drug activities.

The behavior of individuals who are addicted to drugs is totally irrational, particularly when they are under the influence of drugs.

They lose complete control of their humanity; they will do anything under the influence of these drugs. Under the influence of drugs, blacks and men are capable of engaging in a multitude of immoral and illegal activities that have negative impacts on them, their families, and society as a whole.

Individuals who are addicted to drugs are mentally dependent on these drugs. The addiction to drugs preoccupies them totally. Their humanities are no longer their own; their lives are controlled by the drugs that they are addicted to. They are constantly scheming, lying and committing crimes of different types to get money to buy the drugs that their brains crave. Getting the next fix to satisfy their craving is the most important thing in their lives because they have lost complete control of their beings.

When under the influence of these drugs, they are capable of committing a multitude of illogical, irrational and illegal acts.

Drug addiction in blacks is a major problem in U.S. society, and it contributes to the destruction that occurs in the families of these blacks who fall victims to the awful power of drug addiction.

It is important for those in government to proactively undertake actions and create policies that are designed to get to the root causes of drug addiction problems in all their aspects. It is quite clear that present policies of building jails and throwing people in them and treating those people like animals are not working.

You cannot treat a psychological medical problem with jail or "three strikes, you are out" policies. Those policies are designed to get politicians, and district attorneys and judges elected at the expense of the people who are suffering from mental, medical, and physical problems. Those who commit crimes ought to be punished for the crimes they have committed. While in jail, they ought to be given treatments for their addiction and its associated problems.

They should be given a real chance of rehabilitating themselves and they ought to be taught trades of different types that would enable them to be wage earners once they have completed their sentence and back in society.

It is also important to realize that once a drug addict, always a drug addict and, that being the case, long-term psychological treatment ought to be made available to these individuals after they have left jail.

Treatments that are necessary are costly, but they are important, and drug prevention programs, educational programs dealing with the prevention of drugs are very important. Programs to prevent the dissemination of drugs within the communities where those blacks live are very important. The federal and state governments need to spend the billions of dollars that are necessary to fund those programs to help them to become successful.

It is important that drug addiction seminars begin at the earliest grades in schools across the country, so that children can become sensitized to the ravages that drug addiction can cause, as a way to let them know what the facts really are, so that when people approach them trying to get them involved in drugs, they will say "no".

As it is right now, the incidence of drug addiction in schools across the country is high and begins at the earliest age, in elementary school up through middle school and high school.

It is crucial that the educational system join forces with the government agencies to try to encourage drug prevention and drug education programs in elementary schools, middle schools, and high schools. In college, there is also a significant evidence of drug use going on, but these are young adults who choose to do these things to themselves. It is wrong, but they are at an age where they can make their own decisions.

They also should be encouraged to give up drug use or not to start at all, because once a person starts using drugs, it is very difficult to give it up because drug addiction is so overwhelming that these individuals are weakened by the force of the addiction. The colleges also ought to organize drug prevention seminars on their campuses for the benefit of students and faculty, and most definitely confidential drug treatment programs ought to be offered and must be made easily available for college students who are using illicit drugs, to help them give up their habits. It is hypocritical to sweep it under the carpet and pretend that it does not exist.

To help individuals who are addicted to drugs, it requires money, it requires better governmental involvement, and it requires better involvement of the educators, the clergy, and other members of society working as a team to attack a scourge that is destroying significant numbers of people in society.

CHAPTER 76

VIRAL HEPATITIS IN IN AFRICAN AMERCAN MEN

There are five main types of viral hepatitis

Hepatitis A
Hepatitis B
Hepatitis C
Hepatitis D
Hepatitis E

HEPATITIS A

Hepatitis A is transmitted in stools to human when they eat contaminated foods with hepatitis A
Other Foods that are frequently contaminated with hepatitis A include
Raw shellfish
Fecal contaminated fruits
Fecal contaminated green vegetables
Fecal contaminated water etc.

Other ways to get infected with hepatitis A include:

Sexual contact
Blood transfusion (rarely)
Blood products (rarely)
Intravenous Drug addiction
Tattooing etc.
Worldwide 1.5 million people become infected with hepatitis A every year and 80,000 people become infected with hepatitis A every year in the U.S.
Once this virus enters into the body, the incubation period (the time it takes the virus to begin to cause symptoms) is 2-6 weeks.

Symptoms of hepatitis A include:

Weakness
Fatigue
Nausea
Vomiting
Diarrhea
Loss of appetite
General body aches
Fever
Chills
Right sided-abdominal pain

Evaluations of hepatitis A include:

History and Physical examination
Hepatitis A, B, C, D, E profile
CBC
Complete chemistry profile
GGTP
Urinalysis
PT/INR
PTT
Abdominal ultrasound etc;

Signs of hepatitis A include:

Tenderness of the right of the upper abdomen
Enlarged liver
Enlarged spleen
Dark urine
Yellowness of the skin
Yellowness of the eyes
Abnormal liver function tests
Dark urine
Positive hepatitis blood test

Treatments for hepatitis A include:

Bed rest
Zofran or Kytril for nausea and vomiting
NSAID's for fever (if platelets count is normal)
Avoid Tylenol if the liver is failing
IV fluid with D5W1/2 (if the patient is too sick to eat he or she should admitted to the hospital)

If the PT/INR is elevated the patient must be admitted to the hospital because, the liver may be failing.

If the patient is able to eat and the PT/INR is positive, it is best to keep the patient at home to avoid spreading the virus to people in the hospital.

The patient's CBC, complete chemistry, and PT/INR should be monitored closely for several weeks.

Hepatitis A does not cause chronic liver disease. Prevention of hepatitis A include (30million Americans travel every year to countries where hepatitis A is prevalent)

Proper hygiene
Avoid eating raw shellfish
Avoid drinking contaminated water
When traveling to developing countries get vaccinated against hepatitis A.

Vaccines that are in use to prevent hepatitis A are:

Twinrix
Havrix
VAQTA.

CHAPTER 77

HEPATITIS B IN
AFRICAN AMERICAN MEN

—◦◦◦◦◦—

Worldwide hepatitis B infects two billion people and 1.5 million people die every year from hepatitis B. Source: WHO. Hepatitis B is the most common cause of liver disease in the world. In the U.S. 12 million people have hepatitis B and 1.2 million people have chronic hepatitis B and 5000 people die every year from hepatitis B. Hepatitis B is transmitted through infected blood, blood products, IVDA and other body fluids. There are 8 different genotypes of hepatitis B and different genotypes of hepatitis B are found in different parts of the world. All 8 genotypes of hepatitis B are common in the U.S.

Risk factors for hepatitis B include:

Blood and blood products transfusion
Intravenous drug abuse
Semen
Saliva
Unprotected sexual intercourse
Infants of mothers who are infected with hepatitis B (hepatitis B can be transmitted from infected mothers to infants during child birth)
Using tooth brush of people infected with hepatitis B
Babies born to mothers infected with hepatitis B

Once the hepatitis B virus enters into the blood stream of the individual being infected, it takes 40-150 days or an average of 12 weeks for the first symptoms to appear. (Incubation period) Some people infected with hepatitis B never develop acute symptoms, but may go on to be carrier of hepatitis B and some go on to develop chronic persistent hepatitis B.

Signs and symptoms of hepatitis B include:

Fatigue
Poor appetite
Nausea
Vomiting
Abdominal pain
Jaundice (Yellow color of the skin)

Itching
Fever
Chills
Headache
Dark urine
Abnormal CBC
Abnormal liver function tests (elevated SGPT, SGOT, Alkaline Phosphataste, PT, INR, PTT, and bilirubin)
Positive blood test for hepatitis B antibody

Evaluations of hepatitis B include:

History and physical examination
CBC
Complete chemistry profile
GGTP
PT/INR
PTT
Urinalysis
Blood test for hepatitis B antibody
PCR/RNA
Hepatitis B viral load
Abdominal ultrasound
Liver biopsy etc

Treatments of hepatitis B include:

Zofran for nausea and vomiting
                or
Kytril for nausea vomiting
                or
Compazine for nausea and vomiting

Tylenol for fever (low dose only, and no Tylenol if the liver shows signs of failing)

NSAID's for fever (no NSAID's if the platelets count is low)

Benadryl for itching

IV fluid with D5W1/2 normal saline
                or
IV with D5 normal saline

If the patient is not able to eat and vomiting, he or she should be admitted to the hospital If the PT/INR and PTT are elevated, he or she should be admitted to the hospital because this is a sign of liver failure.

If the patient is able to eat, and the PT/INR is normal, the patient should be kept at home to avoid spreading the hepatitis to the hospital staff.

About 5-10% of individuals who develop acute hepatitis B goes on to develop chronic hepatitis B. Chronic hepatitis B causes cirrhosis of the liver and some people go on to have cancer of the liver.

Chronic persistent hepatitis is manifested mainly by persistent mild to moderate elevation of liver function tests, such as bilirubin, SGOT, SGPT, alkaline phosphatase and the GGTP (gamma glutamine transpeptidase) and no major physical findings nor symptoms. On the other hand, chronic active hepatitis is an active inflammatory liver disease with elevation of liver function tests, increased serum ferritin along with malaise, weakness, anemia, and sometimes-palpable liver with right-sided abdominal pain and at times persistent low-grade fever.

Sometimes chronic active hepatitis goes on to develop cirrhosis of the liver with portal hypertension, hyperspleenism, pancytopenia, and esophageal varices. Once the esophageal varices develop, recurrent upper gastrointestinal bleeding can occur.

One of the many chronic complications of hepatitis B in these individuals who develop cirrhosis is hepatocellular carcinoma (cancer of the liver). This cancer in this setting occurs usually 10 to 30 years after the individual becomes sick with hepatitis B.

Fulminant hepatitis with acute liver failure can occur with hepatitis A, B, C, D, E or G. Acute management of hepatitis includes supportive care, careful IV fluid management, careful monitoring of liver function tests, including the prothrombin times, platelets, red blood cells and serum ammonia level.

Dietary management in acute hepatitis is very important, which includes a low-protein diet and low salt. Management of chronic liver disease also includes attention to diet with low protein, low salt, with close attention to liver function tests including the PT, platelet, red cell count and ammonia level. These individuals ought to be given anti-itching medications such as Benadryl, Periactin etc.

The reason for the itching is because the liver is too sick to be able to properly get rid of bile salts, and these bile salts accumulate in the blood, causing severe itching. It is also important that individuals who have chronic liver disease stay away from antiplatelet medications such as aspirin, and NSAIDS.

It is also important not to give them too much Tylenol to patients who have cirrhosis of the liver. Large doses of Tylenol have the propensity to make their liver disease worse.

One has to be very careful to prevent bleeding from the gastrointestinal tract from occurring, because any amount of blood placed in the GI (blood contains protein) tract will be broken down into ammonia by actions of bacteria in the gut.

Because the ammonia cannot be picked up properly by the sick liver, the end result is elevated level of blood ammonia.

High elevated level of ammonia in the blood can cause the patient to become somnolent, confused at times, and if treated promptly and properly can lead to the development of the comatose state.

High ammonia level is treated with low protein diet and Lactulose to induce diarrhea to cleanse the bowel of the stools that contain too much ammonia and other toxic waste matters.

Neomycin 4-12 grams per day can be used to kill as many bacteria as possible to decrease the bacterial load in the gut thereby decreasing the production of ammonia to improve the state hepatic encephalopathy.

Rifaximin 550mg twice per day is the most effective medication available to treat hepatic encephalopathy in combination with lactulose 20 grams twice per day.

Medications in use to treat hepatitis B are

Alpha interferon-2a
PEGylated Interferon-2a (Pegasys)
Adefovir
Lamivudine
Enteccavir
Telbivudine
Tenofovir
Vaccines in use to prevent hepatitis B are
Recombivax B and Engerix-B

CHAPTER 78

HEPATITIS C IN
AFRICAN AMERICAN MEN

Worldwide 170 million people are chronically infected with hepatitis C and 350,000 people die every year from hepatitis C. About 3.2 million people in the U.S. are infected with hepatitis C and 15,000 people die every year in the U.S. from hepatitis C. 75% of adults American who are infected with hepatitis C are baby boomers born between 1945 and 1965.

There are 11 different geno types of hepatitis C, 1-6. Genotype is more common in the U.S. 70-90% of people infected with hepatitis C in the U.S. is infected with genotype 1a and 1b. People who are infected with genotype 1 of hepatitis C respond best to treatments and genotype 1b is highly associated with a high incidence of liver cancer.

"Hepatitis C genotype 1 is the prevalent with 83.4 million infections accounting for 46.2% of all cases worldwide." HCV genotype 3 is the second most common with 54.3 million (30.11%) global infections, HCV genotype 2, 6,5 million cases, genotype 4, 15 million cases and genotype 6, 9.8 million cases worldwide. Sources: WHO

Risks for hepatitis C include:

Contaminated blood
Contaminated blood products
Unprotected sexual intercourse with people infected with hepatitis C
Accidental needle sticks
Intravenous drug addiction
Sharing needles
Tattoos
Piercing
Acupuncture with contaminated instruments
Organ transplants
Long -term hemodialysis
HIV infection
Health care workers
Infants born to mothers infected with hepatitis C.
Once become infected, it takes 2 weeks up to 6 months before symptoms develop.

Signs and symptoms of hepatitis C include:

Fever
Chills
Fatigue
Decrease appetite
Nausea
Vomiting
Headache
Itching of the skin
Abdominal pain
Dark urine
Jaundice
Joints pain
Total body pain
Yellowness of the eyes
Yellowness of the skin

About 80% of individuals who become infected with hepatitis C have no symptoms. About 75-85% of people who just become infected with hepatitis C go on to develop chronic hepatitis C and 70% of these people develop chronic liver disease; and 5-20% of them develop cirrhosis of the liver.

5% of people who develop cirrhosis of the liver because of hepatitis C die of cancer of the liver. Over all, hepatitis C is responsible for 25% of all people who die of cancer of the liver. Source: WHO

Evaluations of hepatitis C include:

History and physical examination
Blood test for hepatitis C antibody
Rapid diagnostic test (RDTs) this test is new
Point of-care tests (POCTs) this test is new
CBC
Complete chemistry profile
PT
INR
PTT
Urinalysis
Abdominal ultrasound
FibroScan
Hepatitis C RNA-PCR
Hepatitis C Viral load
Hepatitis genotype
Liver biopsy

HepaScore
HCV FibroScore

Treatments for hepatitis C include:

Bed rest
Kytril for nausea and vomiting
        or
Zofran for nausea and vomiting
NSAID's for fever if platelets are normal
        or
Tylenol for fever if PT/INR is normal
Benadryl for itching
If the PT/INR is normal and patient can eat, he or she should be treated at home
If he or she is vomiting and cannot eat, he or she should be hospitalized
If the PT/INR, PTT are elevated, this is an indication that the liver may be failing, he or she must be hospitalized

Once in the hospital the patient must be placed in isolation for the protection of other patients a.nd the hospital staff.

At home the patient must used a personal bathroom to avoid spreading the hepatitis to other people in the house or apartment.

Pegylated interferon
Ribavirin
Telaprevir
Boceprevir
Simeprevir costs "about $60,000 over the course of treatment". Ritonavir 100mg with ABT-450 (experimental by Abbott's) Source: Wall Street Journal 10/16/12
Sofosbuvir was just approved by the FDA to treat hepatitis C. This drug appears to cure hepatitis C after a 12 weeks course of treatment. However, it costs $1000 a pill or "$84,000 for a 12-week full course of treatment." The Washington Post 4/28/14
Genotype 1 hepatitis C requires treatment for 1 year
Genotype 2 and 3 can be treated for 6 months
Harvoni (ledipasvir and sofosbuvir) for genotype 1 of hepatitis C approved by the FDA costs $1,125 per pill.
On December 2014, the FDA Approved VIEKIRA for treating hepatitis C (the medication costs about $84, 000 dollars for a six weeks course of treatment.)
Sofosbuvir and Velpatasvir in combination is very effective in treating Genotype 1 or 3 Hepatitis C
Sofosbuvir with Velpatasvir in combination is very effective in treating Genotype 1 to 6 Hepatitis C. "The FDA just approved glecaprevir and pibrentasvir for treatment of hepatitis C genotypes 1 through 6 in previously untreated adults with or without mild cirrhosis." This medication can be used for 8 weeks.

Hepatitis D is contracted in the ways as do hepatitis B and C and causes the similar problems to the liver as do hepatitis B and C. However, hepatitis D requires the presence of hepatitis B for its replication.

Hepatitis E is contracted in the same ways as do hepatitis A. There are 20 million people in the world who are infected with hepatitis E. Similar to hepatitis A, hepatitis E does not cause chronic liver diseases.

Other types of hepatitis include:

Alcoholic hepatitis
Drug induced hepatitis
Autoimmune hepatitis
Primary billiary cirrhosis
Primary sclerosing cholangitis
Primary hemochromatosis
Secondary hemochromatosis etc;

CHAPTER 79

CIRRHOSIS OF THE LIVER IN AFRICAN AMERICAN MEN

—◄◄◄◄∪∩►►►—

Worldwide over 500 million people suffer from liver diseases and in the U.S. 5.5 million people have cirrhosis of the liver and every year 25,000 people in the U.S. die of cirrhosis of the liver.

Cirrhosis of the liver develops because different things happen to the liver that causes inflammation to develop. Once the inflammation becomes chronic, then scaring of liver tissues takes place resulting in the development of cirrhosis.

The different things that cause cirrhosis of the liver include:

Alcohol abuse
Obesity
Hepatitis B
Hepatitis C
Hepatitis D
Fatty liver disease
Primary biliary cirrhosis
Hemochromatosis
Primary sclerosing cholangitis
Biliary atresia
Cystic fibrosis
Wilson disease
Lupus erythematosus
Rheumatoid arthritis
Mixed connective tissue diseases
Glycogen storage disease
Parasitic infestation etc;

Signs and symptoms of cirrhosis of the liver include:

Fatigue
Poor appetite
Weight loss

Easy bleeding
Easy bruising
Nosebleed
Thrombocytopenia (low platelets count)
High prothrombin time
High partial thromboplastin time
Upper gastrointestinal bleeding (from esophageal varices)
Bleeding from the gums
Nausea
Abdominal pain
Jaundice
Yellowness of the eyes
Yellowness of the skin
Enlarged liver
Enlarged spleen
Itching
Spider animate
Redness in the palm of the hands
Break through vaginal bleeding
Enlarged breasts in men
Small and shiny testicles
Edema of lower legs
Fluid in the abdomen (ascots)
Anemia
Leucopenia (low white cells)
Low Folic acid level
Low B12 level
High reticulocytes count
Dark urine
Clay color stools
High aldosterone level in the blood
Erectal dysfunction etc

Evaluations of cirrhosis of the liver include:

History
Physical examination
Vital signs
Body weight
CBC
Reticulocytes count
Complete chemistry profile
Hepatitis A, B, C and D profile in the blood
Viral load for hepatitis B and C
PCR/RNA for hepatitis B and C

Genotype for Hepatitis C (there 11 known genotypes of hepatitis C)
Genotypes of hepatitis B (there 8 known genotypes of hepatitis B)
ANA
Rheumatoid factor
ESR
PT/INR
PTT
Urinalysis
GGTP
Serum folate level
Serum B12 level
Blood alcohol level
Serum Copper level
Stools for ova and parasites
HIV/AIDS 1 & 2 blood tests
VDRL blood test for syphilis
Sweat test for cystic fibrosis
Genetic test for cystic fibrosis
Molucular genetic testing for collagen storage disease
Abdominal ultrasound
Abdominal CAT Scan with contrast
Abdominal MRI with IV contrast
FibroScan
Liver biopsy
HepaScore
HCV FibroScore

Complications of cirrhosis of the liver include:

Portal hypertension
Hypersplenism
Esophageal variceal
Upper gastrointestinal bleeding
Anemia
Ascites
Swollen legs
Itching
Jaundice
Vaginal bleeding
Erectal dysfunction
Hemorrhoids
Rectal bleeding
Higher incidence of infection
Hepatic encephalopathy

Hepatic encephalopathy can develop because the liver fails and is not able to remove toxic materials that are piled up inside it. In addition, hepatic encephalopathy can develop because of GI bleed placing blood in the colon. When blood is put in the colon in the setting of cirrhosis of the liver, bacteria in the colon break down the protein in the blood resulting in the production of large quantity of ammonia, which makes the hepatic encephalopathy worst and hepatic coma can result.

As mentioned above, the most effective medications available to treat hepatic encephalopathy are Rifaxamin 550mg by mouth or via NG tube twice per day and Lactulose 20 grams twice per day by mouth or via NG tube.

Cancer of the liver (cancer of the liver due the complications of hepatitis B kills up to 2 million people per year in the world and is the fourth leading cause of deaths in the world. In the U.S. 25,000 people die every from cirrhosis of the liver due complications of alcohol abuse and hepatitis B and C mainly.

Definitive treatment for cirrhosis of the liver is liver transplant. Every year 6,000 liver transplants are done in the U.S. and 21,000 liver transplants are done worldwide annually.

CHAPTER 80

ASTHMA IN AFRICAN AMERICAN MEN

One in 12 individuals in the U.S. have asthma. That represents 8% of the U.S population or 25 million Americans who suffer from asthma. Each day 11 people in the U.S. die of asthma and 4,000 individuals die annually of asthma.

"Asthma affects 7.5% of adults, resulting in 1.8 million hospitalizations and 10.5 million physician office visits per year. Asthma is more common in black (8.7%) and Puerto Rican Hispanic (13.3%) individualas than in white individuals (7.6%) and is associated with higher mortality in blacks than in whites (25.4 vs 8.8 per million annually.)" Source: JAMA July 18, 2017 Volume 318, Number 3

Worldwide there are 300 million people with asthma and 250,000 people die every year from asthma.

Asthma is more common in Black, Hispanics and other minority men than in white men and in 2015 there were 2.6 million blacks with asthma in the U.S. Asthma is 20 percent more common in black women than in Black men. Hispanic and other minority men have the highest mortality rates from asthma than any other racial groups. The death rate is 2.5 times higher in Black, Hispanic and other minority men compared to white men.

Blacks, Hispanics and other minority men are hospitalized 3 times more often than white men are and black men die of asthma three times more frequently than whites men do. Each year 3 million people visit emergency room because of asthma, 500,000 get hospitalized because of asthma and 10 million out patient visits are made because of asthma. Each year 14 million school days are missed because of asthma attacks in children.

About half of asthma cases develop before age 10 and about one-third of asthma cases develop before age 40. Most cases of allergic asthma begin in early childhood and frequently are associated with family history of asthma, rhinitis, eczema, hay fever, bronchitis, and emphysema.

Many cases of asthma are genetically transmitted. The other common form of asthma is called idiosyncratic asthma, meaning that the individuals who suffer with this type of asthma have no family history of asthma and no history of hay fever, negative skin types were tested, and there is normal IgE level in their blood.

There is still another group of blacks with a mixed form of asthma, with features of both allergic asthma and idiosyncratic asthma.

Risk factors for asthma include:

Genetic
Children
Women
Men
Living in urban areas
Poor urban air quality
Poverty
Poor education
In door allergens
Out door allergens
Smoking
Dwelling with roaches, mice, rats, moles and old and pealing paints
Housedogs
House cats
House birds
High humidity in housing due lack fan and air condition during summer time
Dampness/cold in housing due to lack of heat during wintertime
Stress
Obesity
Upper airway infection
Chronic sinusitis
Gastroesophageal reflux disease (GERD)
Racial discrimination
High unemployment
Inferior medical care etc

Symptoms of asthma include:

Coughing
Wheezing
Shortness of breath
Tightness in the chest
Rapid heart rate
Sneezing
Stuffy nose
Runny nose
Sore throat
Headache
Insomnia
Difficulty in speaking;

What happens in asthma that causes the asthmatic patient to have trouble in breathing is that the bronchioles inside the lungs become obstructed to different degrees, because of being exposed to either one of several irritants. Bronchioles are tube-like structures that are located inside the lungs through which air is channeled in and out the lungs.

The irritants that affect the inside of the bronchioles because swelling and inflammation and secretion of mucoid-like materials to develop. The result is that air gets trapped inside the bronchioles, resulting in shortness of breath, wheezing, marked difficulty in breathing and a feeling of an impending doom.

The wheezing sound that is heard when an asthmatic breathes is due to air fighting to get through the narrow passages that have been created by mucous plug, edema, and swelling inside the bronchioles. The inflammation that occurs at the cellular level is mediated by T lymphocytes that secrete type 2 T-helper cytokines like interleukins 4, 5, and 13. Interleukin 4 and 13 regulate the production of IgE. High-affinity IgE receptor on mast cells mediates the release of histamine, prostaglandins, leukotrienes and inflammatory cytokines, along with interleukins 5 mediation of eosinophils, result in an overall inflammatory process that starts off the asthmatic attack.

Many things can bring on acute asthma attacks; some are allergenic, environmental, infectious, occupational, and pharmacological and some are emotional.

The most frequent form of allergic asthma is seasonal and is associated with hay fever and pollens. Other allergens that can precipitate acute asthma attacks are such things as animal dander, feathers, dust, mites, molds, paints, roaches, mice, rats, and exposure to cats and dogs. Exercise and, in particular, breathing cold air can precipitate an acute asthmatic attack. It is believed that the high incidence of asthma seen in poor communities is the result of the poor living conditions associated with poverty.

Many of these individuals live in poorly ventilated, roach- and rat-infested apartments. The high level of crime seen in these communities' forces those who live there to stay behind closed doors to shield themselves from the daily problems associated with living in these communities and under these conditions.

Roaches carry over their body's irritants and materials that get carried by the air that, when breathed by the asthmatics, precipitate asthmatic attacks. Rats and mice that live in these apartments, no doubt, leave droppings that, when they get airborne, also can be inhaled and participate in bringing about most asthmatic attacks. All these outlined allergens, when inhaled, can precipitate asthmatic attacks.

Environmental factors associated with high incidence of asthma are seen in industrial areas where factories and industrial machines emit sulfur dioxide and nitrogen oxide combining with air, which, when breathed, causes pulmonary diseases of different types, including asthma. Upper airway infection is the most commonly associated precipitating factor triggering asthma attacks. The common infections that frequently precipitate asthmatic attacks are the common cold, which is brought on by rhinoviruses and parainfluenza viruses in adolescents, adults and in young children.

Other infections that can trigger acute asthmatic attacks are respiratory syncytial virus, bacterial infections, such as bacterial bronchitis, bacterial pneumonia, and bacterial sinusitis are all associated with the precipitation of asthmatic attacks. Different types of viral sinusitis, viral bronchitis, and viral pneumonias are also frequently associated with the precipitation of asthmatic attacks.

Occupational exposure plays a major role in both the causation and in the precipitation of asthma. The lists of precipitating materials that blacks can be exposed to that can cause asthmatic attacks are almost endless. Some of the known industrial materials that are associated with the causation and precipitation of asthma attacks are laundry detergents, different types of fumes, coffee beans, nickel, and platinum dust, etc.

A multitude of pharmacology product drugs, when used by asthmatics, can bring on an asthmatic attack. Some of the most common drugs that can set off an asthmatic attack are aspirin, beta-blockers, and some coloring medications, such as red dye number 3, and sulfur medications. There is a syndrome of asthma, nasal polyps, and aspirin allergy. Some of these people can also have a similar reaction when they ingest NSAIDs.

It is, therefore, always prudent to ask these folks the question, "Are you allergic to aspirin or NSAIDs or have ever taken those medications before with no problem?" before prescribing them for any person who suffers with asthma.

Another common precipitant of asthmatic attacks is exercise. Exercise-induced asthmatic attack seems to be associated with the coldness of the air being breathed in. It is, therefore, not a good idea for asthmatics to participate in sports such as skiing, ice-skating and ice hockey. Sports activity where the air is warm is fine. If an asthmatic person wishes to participate in these activities, he or she would be wise to get advice from his or her physician as to what to do to prepare himself or herself to partake in them.

Another frequent trigger of asthmatics is emotional stress. The mechanism for this form of asthmatic attack precipitant is not altogether clear, but the overall mental turmoil associated with stress is capable of triggering an asthma attack.

Before starting the evaluation, quickly listen to the lungs for air movement and the heart to check the rate and the rhythm of the heart, and give her nasal oxygen and an injection of epinephrine subcutaneously. Now proceed with the evaluation.

How to evaluate a person presenting with an asthma attack:

1. First the physician must take a history from the patient to find out several things.
2. It is important to watch how the patient is breathing.
3. Does he have labored breathing?
4. It is important to watch how the patient is speaking.

5. Can he hold a sentence and for how long?
6. How does he look?
7. Does he look tired?
8. Ask the question how many hours ago did the attack start?
9. What medication did he take before presenting?
10. Are the nasal passages stuffed up?
11. Is he coughing up sputum?
12. If yes, what color is the sputum whitish, yellowish, or greenish or bloody?
13. Does he have a fever, chills or body aches?
14. Ask whether he has just been exposed to any of the possible irritants outlined in the preceding paragraphs.
15. Is he wheezing?
16. Does he have shortness of breath?
17. Is he gasping for air?
18. Does his lip look bleu?
19. Do a peak flow test immediately
20. Do arterial blood gas (ABG)
21. Give him oxygen immediately
22. Give him dose of 0.5 cc of 1:1000 solution of epinephrine immediately SC
23. Begin nebulizer treatment immediately
24. Establish IV access immediately
25. Begin IV fluid

Then quickly do a peak flow, using the breathing meter. Try to ascertain the patient's previous known base peak flow. Do an arterial blood gas to determine whether she is retaining carbon dioxide or not. If so, quickly prepare for possible intubation of the patient to secure the airway, to prevent sudden respiratory arrest. Get a good IV line started to provide medications such as fluid and steroid.

Start Alupent nebulizer treatment immediately and continue these treatments every 4–6 hours until the patient is better. Steroid is the backbone and most effective treatment in asthma, but it takes about 6 hours before it starts to work. Get a chest x-ray; look for pneumonia, bronchitis, congestive heart failure, and pneumothorax, which, if present, will complicate the patient's management.

As part of the ER evaluation of the asthmatic patient, a CBC and SMA20 chemistry profile ought to be done. The decision as to whether to admit the patient who presents with an asthmatic attack depends on how the patient looks clinically, how good the peak flow is, and how improved is the examination of the lungs.

If after several hours in the ER with significant and appropriate treatments having been provided without significant improvement in the overall clinical state of the patient, then the patient ought to be admitted for more prolonged treatments. An improved peak flow is good objective evidence that the asthmatic patient has gotten better. One of the controversial issues of the treatment of acute asthma associated with upper airway infection is whether to add antibiotics, either by mouth or intravenously.

Some much-respected experts in infectious diseases say, "Don't use antibiotics because the organisms responsible for the infection are viruses," yet there are some who say, "Yes, antibiotics ought to be used."

The reason given is that the inflammation that the viral infection causes breaks down the protective membranes within the lining of the upper airway.

Once the protective membranes are broken down, local bacteria proliferate, resulting in a superimposed mixed bacterial-viral upper airway infection, precipitating and complicating the asthmatic attack. Even when the upper airway of the asthmatic is irritated with a noxious material, the resulting inflammation can cause the protective membranes to lose their integrity, allowing the bacteria that live in the upper airway to set up an acute asthmatic attack, requiring antibiotic treatment.

The way to diagnose asthma is by:

1. The history
2. Physical examination
3. The chest x-ray and
4. The FEV (forced expiratory volume in 1 second), after administration of 2 puffs of a beta-adrenergic medication and showing that the airway obstruction has been reversed by 15% or greater increase in the FEV. Examination of the chest of the asthmatic patient usually demonstrates different types of wheezes, both inspiratory and expiratory wheezes. Shortness of breath with a fast respiratory rate (normal respiratory 15–20 per minute), the heart rate/pulse rate is fast, 100 or greater per minute. Frequently, the patient uses her abdominal muscles to help to breathe.
5. The peak and ABG are crucial to show whether a person is retaining carbon dioxide or not. An asthmatic who is retaining carbon dioxide is n the process of dying and needs to be intubated immediately. Ordinarily, asthmatics have low carbon dioxide because of rapid breathing, so, when they are retaining carbon dioxide, it means that either bronchospasm and or mucus plugs are preventing exchange of oxygen causing carbon dioxide retention. This condition is called hypoxemia.
6. The chest x-ray usually shows hyper inflated lungs in asthmatic patients.

Treatments of asthma include

Some of the medications used to treat asthma:

Immediate response medications Nebulizer treatments

1. Epinephrine 0.3–0.5 ml. of 1:1000 solution subcutaneously
2. Alupent inhaler
3. Proventil inhaler

4. Albuterol inhaler
5. Bronchodilators in aerosol solution 0.4%–0.6%
6. Xopenex inhaler
7. Maxair inhaler
8. Vantolent inhaler
9. Atrovent inhaler
10. Serevent
11. Prednisone
12. Theophylin
13. Theo-Dur
14. Medrol

Long acting asthma medications include:

1. Salmeterol inhaler
2. Beclovent
3. Vanceril
4. Azmacort
5. Flovent
6. Advair Diskus
7. Aerobid
8. Azmacort
9. Symbicort
10. Qvar
11. Flovent HFA

Leukotriene Modifiers is new family of medications being used to treat asthma.

Among these medications are:

Singulair
Zyflo
Zyflo CR
Zafirlukast
The FDA to Asthma has just approved Mepolizumab IV or SC
Exacerbations.

Asthma is a chronic inflammatory lung disease and, as such, requires different types of medications working via different mechanisms to treat it both acutely and chronically. One of the most common medications used to treat asthma are steroids.

Different types of steroid preparations are used to treat asthma intravenously, by mouth, or via inhalation technique. Steroid is indispensable in the treatment of asthma.

Frequently used intravenous steroids in the treatment of acute asthmatic attacks are Solu-Medrol

Decadron
Solu-Cortef

Prednisone by mouth and by inhalation is also frequently used in the treatment of asthma.

Different irritants, when inhaled, cause an acute inflammatory reaction to occur within the bronchioles (tubes that carry air through the lungs).

Steroid works to decrease that inflammatory reaction, thereby preventing the swelling, mucus production, and spasm within the bronchioles, tissues and other tubes inside the lungs.

The spasm and the mucus plugs that occur within the bronchioles prevent airflow from getting in and getting out of the lungs.

The different medications used to treat asthma decrease the spasm, the inflammation and the production of mucus, allowing air to move easier within the lungs, relieving the acute symptoms will improve the overall incidence of asthma in black men. The annual cost of asthma is 56 billion dollars in the U.S. (2017)

CHAPTER 81

TOBACCO SMOKING AND ITS NEGATIVE EFFECTS ON THE HEALTH OF AFRICAN AMERICAN MEN

Billion people in the world use tobacco. In the U.S. 42.1 million people smoke cigarettes. Worldwide, 6 million people die of cigarettes smoking every year and in the U.S. there are 480,000 deaths from tobacco smoking. Source: CDC

According to the CDC smoking causes more deaths each year than all the conditions listed below combined.

"Smoking causes 14 million related ailments". Research from the Center for Tobacco Products at the US Food and Drug Administration published in JAMA Internal Medicine, has found that around 14 million major medical conditions are the result of smoking." "Smoking harms nearly every organ in the body, often causing multiple serious illnesses such as emphysema, diabetes and colon cancer." "The study also found that smoking is linked to 2.3 million heart attacks, 1.3 million cases of cancer, 1.2 million cases of stroke and 1.8 million cases of diabetes." Sources FDA and CDC

"HIV/AIDS
Illegal drugs use
Alcohol use
Motor vehicle injuries
Firearm-related incidents"

"More than 10 times as many U.S. citizens have died prematurely from cigarettes smoking than have died in all the wars fought by the United States during its history. Smoking causes about 90% (or 9 out of 10) of all lung cancer deaths in black men. About 80% (or 8 out of 10) of all deaths from chronic obstructive pulmonary disease COPD in black men are caused by smoking. Cigarette smoking increases risk for death from all causes in black men and. The risk of dying from cigarette smoking has increases over the last 50 years in men in the United States." Source: CDC According to the CDC,"smoking is estimated to increase the risk of coronary heart disease by 2 to 4 times, stroke by 2 to 4 times, lung cancer in men by 25 times." More than 5.5 trillion cigarettes are made worldwide every year.

"20.5% men and 15.8% women smoke cigarettes
17.3% of adults aged 18-24 years smoke cigarettes
21.6% of adults aged 25-44 years smoke cigarettes
19.5% of adults aged 45-64 years smoke cigarettes
6.9% of adults aged 65 years and older smoke cigarettes."
"21.8% of American Indians/Alaska Natives smokes cigarettes

10.7% of Asians (non-Hispanic; excludes Native Hawaiians and Pacific Islanders) smoke cigarettes
18.1% of Blacks (non-Hispanic) smoke cigarettes
12.5% of Hispanics smoke cigarettes
19.7% of Whites (non-Hispanics) smoke cigarettes
26.1% of multiple race individuals smoke cigarettes."
"24.7% adults with 12 or less years education (no diploma) smoke cigarettes
41% of adults with a GED diploma smoke cigarettes
23.1% of adults with a high school diploma smoke cigarettes
9.1% of adults with an undergraduate college degree smoke cigarettes
5.9% of adults with a postgraduate college degree smoke cigarettes."

"27.9% of adults who live below the poverty level smoke cigarettes
17.0% of adults who live at or above the poverty level smoke cigarettes."
Source: CDC

"Tobacco use was more common among black men (26.2%) than women (15.4%). Rates were highest among 25 to 44 year olds (25.2%) and lowest among adults aged 65 years or older. By education level, tobacco use was highest adults with a general education Development certificate (43.8%) and lowest among those with a graduate degree (6.3%) By geographic region, prevalence was highest in the Midwest (23.9%) sand lowest in the west (19%). "Source: MMWR Morb Mortal Rep. 2014, 63(25): 542-547.

Tobacco smoking is a very dangerous habit. Cigarettes and other tobacco products contain chemical that cause diseases in people who use them and in those who are near them when they are smoking.

"Tobacco smoke contains over 4,000 different chemical, at least 250 are known to cause cancer in human because of the carcinogens they contain, and many are poisonous." Source: Health Education Authority (UK) Lifesaver

A partial list of harmful chemicals found in cigarettes includes:

"Benzene
Formaldehyde
Ammonia
Acetone
Tar
Nicotine

Carbon Monoxide
Arsenic
Hydrogen Cyanide act; "
Source: Health Education Authority (UK) Lifesaver.

Nicotine addiction is one of the major problems associated with tobacco smoking.

Signs and symptoms of nicotine withdrawal include:

Anxiety
Tobacco craving
Irritability
Rapid heart rate
Elevated blood pressure
Palpitation
Sweating
Headache
Fatigue
Nausea
Insomnia
Difficulty concentrating
Depression
Increased hunger
Weight gain
Erectile dysfunction
Infertility

"Every 6 seconds a person dies from a tobacco related disease and every six seconds 10 people die from a tobacco related disease. 20% of deaths in the U.S. are from tobacco. More than 600,000 nonsmokers die each year from secondhand smoke worldwide, and 1/3 of them are children. 50,000 people die every year in the U.S. from second hand smoking. Tobacco industry revenue was $664 billion in 2010, greater than the GPD all, but 18 nations."

"More than 293 billion cigarettes were purchased in the United States in 2011, with Three companies selling nearly 85% of them." Source CDC

"Smoking attributable economic costs in the U.S. are estimated to be between $289 to 332.5 billion
$132.5 to 175.9 billion for direct medical care of adults
$151 billion for lost productivity due to premature deaths
$5.6 billion for lost productivity due to exposure to secondhand smoke" Source: ACS 2/13/14.

In 2017, the total annual economic cost of smoking is estimated to be 467 billion dollars in the U.S. and worldwide the annual estimated cost of smoking is 1 trillion dollars.

Evaluations of cigarettes /other smokers include:

History and physical examination

Chest x-ray
CT of the chest
CBC
Complete blood chemistry profile
Urinalysis
EKG
ABG
Forced Spirometry
Peak flow evaluation
Pulmonary function test

Complications of tobacco smoking include:

COPD/Emphysema
Chronic bronchitis
Lung cancer
Head and neck cancer
Cancer of mouth
Cancer of the pharynx
Cancer of the tongue
Cancer of the throat
Cancer of the pancreas
Cancer of the urinary bladder
Cancer of the kidney
Cancer of the esophagus
Breast cancer
Cancer of the stomach
Leukemia
Liver cancer
Colorectal cancer
Cancer of the small bowel
Cancer of adrenal gland
Cancer of uterine cervix
Hypertension
Pulmonary hypertension
Atherosclerosis
Heart attacks
Heart failure
Strokes
Liver disease
Peptic ulcer

Peripheral vascular disease
Amputation of toes
Amputation of fingers
Amputation of feet
Amputation of legs
Addiction to nicotine
Erectal dysfunction
Miscarriages
Atopic pregnancy
Premature births
Sudden infant death syndrome
Stillbirth
Orofacial clefts in infants
Peridontal disease
Cavities
Gum disease
Eye disease
Increase incidence of pulmonary infection
Infertility in women because tobacco smoking poisonous effects on the ovaries
Possible association with dementia
Depression
Poor appetite
Secondary polycythemia
Pulmonary failure
Death

Chewing and smokeless tobacco are extremely harmful to human health's as well and same is true with e-cigarette.

Medications to prevent smoking include:

Xyban
Chantrix
Wellbutrin
Nortriptyline
Nicorette gum
Nicoderm patch etc;

Non-medication methods to stop smoking include:

Going cold turkey
Psychotherapy etc;

The most important thing as far as smoking is concerned is not to begin smoking, because tobacco products contain nicotine which is an extremely addicting drug and most people find it near impossible to give it up.

CHAPTER 82

EMPHYSEMA/COPD IN AFRICAN AMERICAN MEN

Chronic Obstructive Pulmonary disease COPD/Emphysema is divided in 2 parts COPD and Emphysema. COPD occurs because of recurrent exposure of lung tissues and bronchioles to irritants from tobacco smoking such as cigarettes and cigars. In pure Emphysema, it is the alveolar that are damaged preventing air exchange to occur. Every year tobacco smoking is responsible for 6 million deaths in the world.

In 2017 there are 12.7 to 14.7 million people with COPD/Emphysema in the U.S. and probably there are another 12 million people who have COPD/Emphysema do not yet diagnosed. Source: NHLBI March 31, 2011. Each year 120,000 people die of COPD/Emphysema in the U.S. and the yearly cost of COPD/Emphysema is 49.9 billion dollars Source: National Institute of Health.

Worldwide 600 million people have COPD/Emphysema and every year 2.74 million people die of COPD/Emphysema and COPD/Emphysema is the 5th leading cause of deaths in the world.

" Approximately 1 in 12 people worldwide are affected by asthma or chronic obstructive pulmonary disease (COPD); once regarded as two distinct disease entities, these two conditions are now recognized as heterogeneous and often overlapping conditions.

The term "asthma-COPD overlap syndrome" (ACOS) has been applied to the condition in which a person has clinical features of both asthma an COPD." Source: N Engl. J MED 373; 13 NEJM.org September 24, 2015

Risk factors for COPD/Emphysema are:

Cigarette smoking
Cigar smoking
Air pollution
Industrial exposure to pollution
Black lung/coal miners' lung
Gold mining
Alpha-1-antiprypsin deficiency (responsible for 2% of COPD)

Cystic fibrosis
Cotton textile workers
Exposure to cadmium
Exposure from welding fumes
Exposure to isocyanides
Exposure to silica dust
Exposure to asbestos
Sugar cane cutters
Sugar cane mills workers
Recurrent pneumonia etc;

In COPD, the inflammation that results due to the irritating effect of cigarette/tobacco smoking or other pollutants from the air causes secretion of thick mucous that blocks the free flow of air in and out of the lungs, making very difficult for people with COPD to breath.

Emphysema and Chronic Obstructive Pulmonary Disease in Blacks in the US:

Adult blacks in the U.S. who smoke by age and level of education are as follows:

Age 18 to	24 24.5 percent
25 to 44	25.6 percent
45 to 64	22.5 percent
65 and older	11.2 percent
Whites who smoke	23.6 percent
Blacks who smoke	21.6 percent
Hispanic blacks who smoke	13.3 percent
American Indian/Alaskan/Native blacks who smoke	38.1 percent
Asian/Pacific/Islander blacks who smoke	9.9 percent

10.7% of blacks with 8 years education or less smoke cigarettes.
34.3% of blacks with 9 to 11 years of education smoke cigarettes.
24.1% of blacks with 12 years of education smoke cigarettes.
22.8% of blacks with 13 to 15 years of education smoke cigarettes.
11.2% of blacks with 16 and more years of education smoke cigarettes.

Source: National Health Interview Survey, 1998, National Center for Chronic Disease Prevention and Health Promotion, Center for Disease Control Prevention.

Presently there are about 55 millions smokers in the U.S.

Tobacco smoking is a very dangerous habit. Cigarettes and other tobacco products contain chemical that cause diseases in people who use them and in those who are near them when they are smoking.

"Tobacco smoke contains over 4,000 different chemical, at least 50 are known to be carcinogens (cause cancer in humans), and many are poisonous." Source: Health Education Authority (UK) Lifesaver

The list of harmful chemicals found in cigarettes includes:

"Benzene
Formaldehyde
Ammonia
Acetone
Tar
Nicotine
Carbon Monoxide
Arsenic
Hydrogen Cyanide act; "
Source: Health Education Authority (UK) Lifesaver

Symptoms and complications of COPD/Emphysema include:

Chronic cough
Sputum production (in chronic bronchitis)
Dyspnia
Wheezing
Tiredness
Weight gain in bleubloater
Weight loss in pink puffers
Pulmonary hypertension
Pulmonary embolism
Right heart failure corpulmonale

Left heat failure (when the right heart fails the left will eventually fail)

Cushing disease due to chronic steroid use
Osteoporosis due to chronic steroid use
Aseptic necrosis with arthritis due steroid use
Depression due in part due to steroid use
Psychosis due to steroid use
Elevated blood sugar due steroid use in pre-diabetics/diabetics
Peptic ulcer due to chronic steroid use
Acute exacerbation due to bacterial, and viral infections (usually 25% of the infections are bacterial, 25% are viral and 25% are a combination of bacterial and viral.

Cigarette smoking is the number-one cause of lung diseases. There are two general forms of COPD/Emphysema: one form is the pink puffer and the other form is the blue bloater. The pink puffer type is the so-called dried emphysema. It is called dried emphysema because people with pink puffer cough a lot, but no sputum comes up. These individuals are called pink puffers because they breathe with a pursed lip to force the air into their lungs and their lips look puffed.

In addition, they have barreled chests and they are usually thin in stature. Another distinct feature that differentiates pink puffers from blue bloaters is that pink puffers usually do not retain carbon dioxide because they are continuously puffing it out.

On the other hand, blue bloater COPD/Emphysema patients are usually obese; they cough up copious amount of sputum, their lips are blue and retain carbon dioxide. The toxic effects of the tobacco, which the smokers inhale, damage the substance of the lungs, resulting in a multitude of anatomical abnormalities causing trapping of air.

It is the trapping of air and the stiffness of the lung that cause the patients with emphysema so much difficulty in breathing. Frequently, people with emphysema develop right-sided heart disease, complicating their overall cardiopulmonary state.

The incidence of tobacco use increased significantly in people in the last 40 years, and the result is that lung diseases of different types and severity have increased accordingly. Prominent among these lung diseases are chronic bronchitis, asthma, lung cancer and frequent pneumonia. Because the effects of tobacco damage the inner lining of the lungs, bacterial growth is favored and frequent lung infections develop which can lead to different degrees of respiratory decompositions.

Very often, when people with COPD/Emphysema develop pneumonia, the respiratory system becomes decompensated, resulting in the need for the individuals to be placed on the respirator. The incidence of adult respiratory distress syndrome (ARDS) increases in pe0ple who smoke.

In the year 2017, 222,500 will be diagnosed with lung cancer and 155,870 are expected to die of lung cancer in the U.S. Source: Cancer Facts &figures ACS 2017 In 2017, 13,720 black men will be diagnosed with lung cancer and 9,710 black men are expected to die of lung cancer in the U.S. Source: Cancer Facts and Figures ACS 2017 Lung diseases in people are associated with tobacco smoking, air pollution, exposure to industrial pollutants, exposure to asbestos and anti-trypsin deficiency etc.

Exposure to asbestos can lead to the development of a type of cancer called mesothelioma. Characteristic of asbestosis of the lungs is calcification of the lining of the lungs. Emphysema frequently results in end-stage lung disease. End-stage lung disease causes pulmonary hypertension, right ventricular heart failure, distended neck veins, swollen abdomen, swollen lower legs, large liver and cardiac arrhythmias of different types, which contributes, often times, to the death of affected people.

Exposure to several other noxious materials is also known to cause damage to the lungs that can lead to COPD/Emphysema in people. One well-known example is coal miner lung disease. Other examples include exposure to inhalation of cotton fibers by people who work in cotton mills; a similar lung disease can develop in people who work in sugar cane fields/ factories as described above.

How to evaluate people with COPD/emphysema

The first thing to do is to take a good history from the man to ascertain his symptoms and what kind of noxious materials or environment he may have been exposed to. It is important to find if she smokes tobacco, if it is via cigarettes, cigars, or pipe. What type of work he or does? If he does not smoke, it is important to find out whether his wife or her husband, boyfriend, girlfriend or significant other, with whom he or she is frequently in close contact, smokes tobacco.

It is also important to find out if he is exposed to tobacco smoke from his co-workers on the job.

The next thing to do is to carry out a complete physical examination, paying close attention to the following:

1. Is he very thin?
2. Is he fat?
3. Is he short of breath?
4. Is he constantly coughing?
5. Is the cough dry or productive of sputum?
6. Are his lips blue or pink?
7. Does he purses his lips when he breathes or not?
8. How hard is his breathing?
9. Can he or carry a sentence through without stopping to catch his or breath?
10. Is he or using accessory abdominal muscles to help him to breathe?
11. Does he have clubbed fingers?
12. On listening to his lungs, how well is he moving air?
13. Are there rales or wheezes heard in his lungs?
14. On listening to the heart, are the heart sounds distant?
15. Are the heart sounds heard best below the breastbone?
16. Is the heart rhythm regular or irregular?

In people who have the dried type emphysema (pink puffer), the heart sounds are distant and very difficult to hear and the air movement is difficult to hear, as well.

The best way to hear the heart beats in these individuals is below the breastbone area. This is so because in this type of emphysema, the position of the heart is shifted to that area.

The heart frequently beats irregularly in emphysema patients because of an abnormal rhythm called atrial fibrillation. Other abnormal heart rhythms such as premature atrial and ventricular contractions are also quite common in patients with emphysema /COPD.

These cardiac abnormalities occur because of a combination of lung and heart malfunctions that emphysema causes. Rales are heard by listening to lungs because of heart failure, which causes fluid to accumulate within the lungs.

The most common chamber of the heart that fails in people who have emphysema/ COPD is the right ventricle. When the right ventricle fails, the bulk of the work is left to the left ventricle, which ultimately fails as well, resulting in biventricular failure.

After the history and physical examinations are completed, several tests have to be done to document the fact the patient does have emphysema.

The first tests to do are a chest x-ray, followed by spirometry, and arterial blood gas, and pulmonary function test.

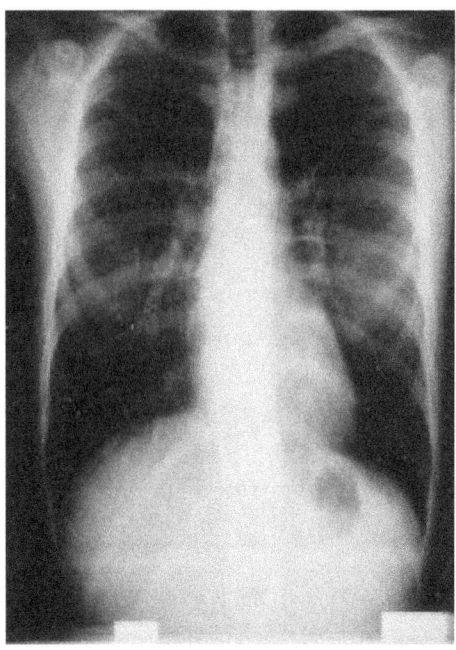

Figure 82:1–Normal chest X-ray in non-smoker

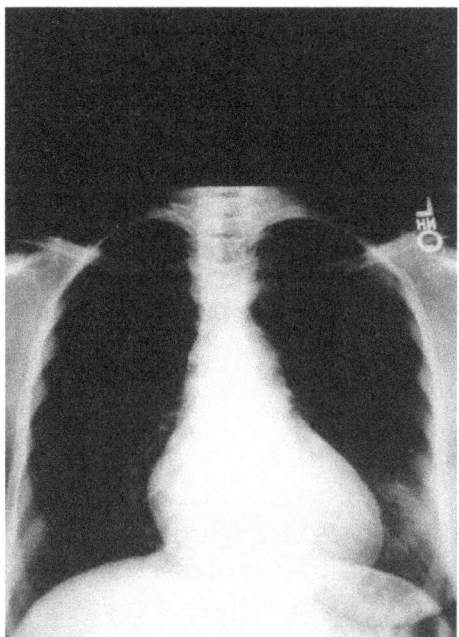

Figure 82:2– Abnormal chest X-ray in smoker with emphysema

Chronic Obstructive Pulmonary Disease –COPD/Emphysema is the number forth cause of death in the U.S. There are 12 million individuals with COPD in the U.S. and there are about 12 million more individuals with COPD who are yet to be diagnosed.

Frequently both arterial blood gas and the pulmonary function tests are abnormal in COPD/Emphysema patients.

When COPD/Emphysema is discovered in a non-smoker with no exposure to secondary tobacco smoke and no exposure to industrial air pollution, etc., it is likely to be due to a hereditary condition known as alpha-1-antitrypsin deficiency. There is a commercial blood test available to test for alpha-1- antitrypsin level in the blood.

People with chronic bronchitis/emphysema/COPD develop infection in the lungs very frequently, as well as infection of the upper airway. The very nature of this disease predisposes these people to those infections.

The most frequent bacterial and viral organisms causing upper air way/lungs infections in these people are as follows:

Haemophilus influenzae
Haemophilus parainfluenzae
Streptococcus pneumonia
Moraxella catarrhalis
Klebsiella pneumoniae
Serratia marcescens and
Pseudomonas

Rhinoviruses
Corona virus
Influenza viruses

Frequently, these infections are mixed infections, associated with more than one bacterial organism causing the infection. Frequently, these upper airway infections start out with viral URI and become complicated with a secondary bacterial infection. Any infection affecting the airway of people with chronic bronchitis/emphysema/COPD usually causes their pulmonary status to become decompensated resulting in difficulty of breathing and anoxia. If the infection in the upper airway is not treated early and aggressively with antibiotic, the result oftentimes is the development of pneumonia.

Pneumonia and its complications are frequently the cause of death of individuals who suffer from chronic bronchitis/emphysema/COPD. The effects of tobacco smoking and other inhaled toxins damage the tissues of the lungs and the chronic nature of these diseases places these individuals in an immuno-suppressed state, which predisposes them to the development of pulmonary infections of different types and severity.

The microorganisms that most frequently cause pneumonia in people with emphysema/COPD are the following:

Haemophilus influenzae
Haemophilus parainfluenzae
Streptococcus pneumonia
Moraxella catarrhalis
Klebsiella pneumoniae
Serratia marcescens
Pseudomonas
Staphylococcus aureus
Methecillin resistant staph aureus (MRSA)

Rhinovirusis and corona viruses are responsible for the majority of upper airway infections. Influenza viruses also cause a significant percentage of URI. URI causes exacerbation of COPD/Emphysoma. All these microorganisms can cause pneumonia further worsening the clinical status of COPD/Emphysema.

How to evaluate a patient with emphysema for pneumonia

The first thing to do is to take a good history from the patient. Ask him, are you coughing and for how many days? Is the cough productive? What is the color of the sputum? Is the sputum yellow, green, and dark green, bloody, or whitish? Do you have a fever? Are you having chills? Does your chest hurt when you cough? Are you having headaches? Is your nose stuffed? Do you have a runny nose? Do you have generalized body aches and pain? Who else is sick in your household? Do you have birds in the house? Have you traveled recently out of the country or to other states in the USA? Do you have night sweats? Have you lost weight? Do you have poor appetite? The next thing to do is a physical examination.

When a physician suspects pneumonia in a patient, the most important parts of the physical examination are as follows:

1. The respiratory rate: Is it greater than 20?
2. The pulse rate: Is it 100 or greater?
3. Is the blood pressure normal or is it abnormally low?
4. Is the patient using abdominal muscle to help in breathing?
5. Does the patient look pale? Is the skin warm and moist?
6. How sick does the patient look?
7. Is the temperature below 98.6°F or 100 .4°F or greater?
8. How fast is the heart rate?
9. How do the lungs sound?
10. Is the patient moving air well?
11. Are there pneumonia sounds (rales) in the lungs? If so, where are they located in the lungs?
12. Is the patient wheezing?

Once the physical examination is completed, the next step is look at the chest x-ray. Are there infiltrates in the lung fields?

What do those infiltrates look like? What does the arterial blood gas look like? Is the patient hypoxic (low oxygen)? In the case of the patient with emphysema, is he or she retaining carbon dioxide? If so, how much? Is the patient producing sputum? What is the color of the sputum? Is it yellow? Is it green? Is it bloody? Alternatively, is it whitish? On the other hand, is it a mixture of all these colors?

Once the physical examination has been completed, the next thing to do is to order some tests.

The most appropriate tests to order are the following:

1. Chest x-ray
2. ABG
3. Spirometry
4. EKG
5. CBC
6. Chemistry profile (SMA 20)
7. 2 sets of blood cultures
8. Sputum gram stain
9. Sputum culture and sensitivity
10. Peak flow evaluation
11. Pulmonary function test (once patient is stable)

Once these tests have been ordered, treatment for pneumonia/COPD can be started.

1. The type of IV and amount of fluid that is given to these patients depends on the level of dehydration that the patient presents with. Usually Dextrose with normal saline or half normal saline, either alone or with dextrose at a reasonable rate of 125 cc per hour can be started. If the patient is a diabetic, half normal saline or normal saline can be given at the same rate.
2. Oxygen can be given via nasal canals of 2–3 liters per minute in patients who have pneumonia and no emphysema. If the patient has emphysema/COPD and pneumonia, it is best to give oxygen via venti-mask, to prevent too much oxygen from being administered, since, in a patient who is suffering from emphysema, such as a blue bloater who retains carbon dioxide, too much oxygen can cause more carbon dioxide to be retained. The higher the level of carbon dioxide in the body, the sicker he or she will become.

If this high concentration of carbon dioxide is allowed to persist, several major complications, including inability of the heart and brain to function properly, can develop.

Frequently, patients with emphysema who have pneumonia develop respiratory failure, necessitating placement on the respirator for breathing assistance.

Acute medications for COPD/Emphysema include:

Nebulizer treatments
Short- acting medications
Ventolin HFA
Albuterol
Xopenex
Atrovent
Long-acting medications
Serevent
Spiriva
Foradil

Inhaled steroid medications include:

Pulmicort
Flovent

Combination inhaler medications include:

Symbicort
Advair
Oral medications include:
Prednisone
Singulair

Theophylline
Steroid IV
Nebulizer treatments

The next step is to administrate antibiotics intravenously. If the patient comes from home, then a protocol that provides antibiotic coverage for community-acquired pneumonia is put into place. Examples of the intravenous antibiotics that can be used are the following:

a. Ceftriaxone, 1 or 2 grams every 24 hours, or
b. Levaquin, 500 mg. IV every 24 hours, or
c. Penicillin G, 10 to 20 million units daily in divided doses of IV, or
d. Ampicillin, 2–4 grams every 6 hours IV or,
e. In penicillin-allergic patients, Cipro, 400 mgs. IV daily, or
f. Erythromycin, 500 mg. IV every 6 hours or
g. Tequin, 400 mg IV daily for 7-10days
h. Ceftazadine 1-gram IV q8h plus
i. Vancomycin 1 gram IV q12h plus
j. Zosyn 3.375 grams IV q6h
k. Doribax 500mg IV q8h
l. Cefepime 2 grams IV daily
m. Zyvox 600mg IV q12h (MRSA)
n. Bactrim IV in Pneumocystis carinii 15-20 mg/kg/day q6-8h for 14 days
o. Zithromax 500 mg per day has recently been found to be very effective in COPD patients to prevent pulmonary decompensation

Even though the patient is coming from the community, the health profile of the patient determines whether the patient gets started on one or more antibiotics. The types of work the patient does for a living, as well, where the patient may have been prior to getting sick, also determines whether she gets started on one or more antibiotics and what type of antibiotics are used to start treatment.

Erythromycin is an excellent antibiotic to use, especially in the setting where atypical pneumonia and organisms such as legionella is suspected. Once the result of sputum gram stain/culture is back, antibiotic treatment is adjusted according to the results of these two tests.

People who are coming from a nursing home or who are in the hospital, and who develop pneumonia, are treated with different antibiotics, because bacterial organisms such as pseudomonas and staphylococcus for which specific antibiotics are required for treatment, frequently colonize these people.

The best antibiotic to use to treat pseudomonas is Ceftazidime and the best antibiotic to use to treat staphylococcus/methicillin resistant staphylococcus-MRSA is Vancomycin. Examples of IV antibiotics that can be used to treat hospitalized patients with pneumonia and their usual doses are as follows:

1. Ceftriaxone, 1–2 grams IV every 12 to 24 hours
2. Cefotaxime, 1–2 grams IV every 8–12 hours
3. Cefuroxime, 750 mg IV every 8 hours
4. Cipro, 400 mg IV every 24 hours
5. Erythromycin, 500 mg IV or by mouth every 6 hours
6. Imipenem, 500 ml IV every 6 hours
7. Nafcillin, 2 grams IV every 4–6 hours
8. Penicillin G, 2 million units every 6 hours IV
9. Vancomycin, 1 gram IV every 12 hours
10. Flagyl, 500 ml IV every 6 hours
11. Clindamycin, 600 ml IV every 8 hours
12. Levaquin, 500 ml IV once per day
13. Ceftazidime, 1gram IV every 8 hours
14. Tequin, 400mg IV every 24 hours
15. Bactrim DS, one tablet 2 times per day or IV Bactrim when the situation calls for it.
16. Doribax 500mg IV q8h
17. Cefepime 2 grams IV daily

In the office setting, Levaquin, Tequin, Zithromax, Cipro, Avelox, Biaxin, and Bactrim DS can be used as a single antibiotic, to treat appropriate individuals for pulmonary infection. Other medications that are used to treat patients with pneumonia and emphysema include: steroid IV or by mouth; Ventolin inhaler; Albuterol inhaler Alupent treatment; Maxair inhaler; Serevent; Flovent; and Singulair by mouth, etc. together with oxygen, IV fluid, cough syrup and pulmonary toilet.

Viral pneumonia is treated with IV steroid, Alupent treatment, IV fluid, oxygen; cough syrup, and pulmonary toilet. In patients with chronic lung disease and viral pneumonia, broad-spectrum antibiotics must be added to their treatments to cover for the possibility of secondary bacterial infection which inevitably always becomes part of the pulmonary infection. If it is determined that the clinical picture is that of pure viral pneumonia, then the antibiotics can be stopped.

This determination can sometime be made through viral titers. As for fungal infection of the lung, this diagnosis is more appropriately established with specimen taken during bronchoscopic examination with biopsy/brushing, and then treatment can be started with Amphotericin B or Fluconazole.

Pneumocystis carinii pneumonia (PCP) is more commonly seen in patients with AIDS. The diagnosis is usually made by the history, the clinical picture with breathing difficulty, hypoxemia, fever, chills, night sweat, weight loss, the chest x-ray characteristics, the propensity for oxygen desaturation on exercising, O_2 concentration under 70, alveolar-arterial oxygen gradient over 35, elevated LDL and the recovering of the PCP organism on pulmonary washing or on lung biopsy.

Acute PCP is treated with IV Bactrim and IV steroid or steroid by mouth for 21 days. Pentamidine IV can also be used in patients who are allergic to Bactrim. Pentamidine has serious cardiac, kidney, and pancreatic complications, including severe hypoglycemia (low blood sugar).

CHAPTER 83

PNEUMONIA IN AFRICAN AMERICAN MEN

Pneumonia is an infection of the lung that can be caused by bacteria, virus, fungus, protozoa and sometime by aspiration of chemical materials.

The most common bacterium that causes pneumonia is Streptococcus pneumonia.

Streptococci include
Alpha hemolytic streptococcus
Beta hemolytic streptococcus
Pneumococcus

These organisms come from people's throats where they live or people get pneumonia When people cough near them and they inhale the organism causing the pneumonia into they lungs.

Staphylococcus is another bacterium that frequently causes pneumonia.
Staphylococcus include
Staphylococcus Aureus
Staphylococcus epidermidis
Methicillin-resistant staphylococcus Aureus (MRSA)
Vancomycin Resistant Staphylococcus aureus (VRA)
MRSA is resistant penicillin and penicillin like antibiotics
VRA is resistant to Vancomycin
Both Streptococcus and Staphylococcus are gram-negative organisms.

Other bacteria that frequently cause pneumonia are gram-negative bacteria.

These Gram- negative organisms that frequently cause pneumonia include:

Haemophilus influenza
Pseudomonas aeruginosa
Klebsiella pneumoniae
Escherichia coli
Moraxella catarrhalis

Serratia
Legionella etc;

Atypical bacteria that can cause pneumonia include:

Chlamydophilia pneumoniae
Coxiella burnetii mycoplasma pneumoniae

Once the bacteria enter into the lung tissues through inhalation, they multiply causing an acute inflammatory reaction inside the lungs. The inflammation inside the lungs interferes with the exchange of oxygen, resulting in a state of hypoxemia.

The elderly, infants, and people with diseases such as cancer, diabetes COPD, Asthma, cystic fibrocystic and AIDS or otherwise immunosuppressed are prone to getting pneumonia. In addition people who are in the hospitals or live in nursing homes are at high risk of getting pneumonia.

Signs and symptoms of pneumonia include:

Cough (productive of greenish or yellowish sputum)
Fever
Chills
Headache
Chest pain
Rapid breathing
Rapid heart rate
Sweating
Weakness

Evaluations of pneumonia include:

History and physical examination (rales/pneunmonic sounds are heard in the lung affected by pneumonia during examination of the lung with the stethoscope)

Chest x-ray
CBC
Sputum Gram stain
Sputum culture
Blood culture
Nasal swab for MRSA
Complete chemistry profile
ABG
EKG
Chest x-ray of a patient with bacterial pneumonia

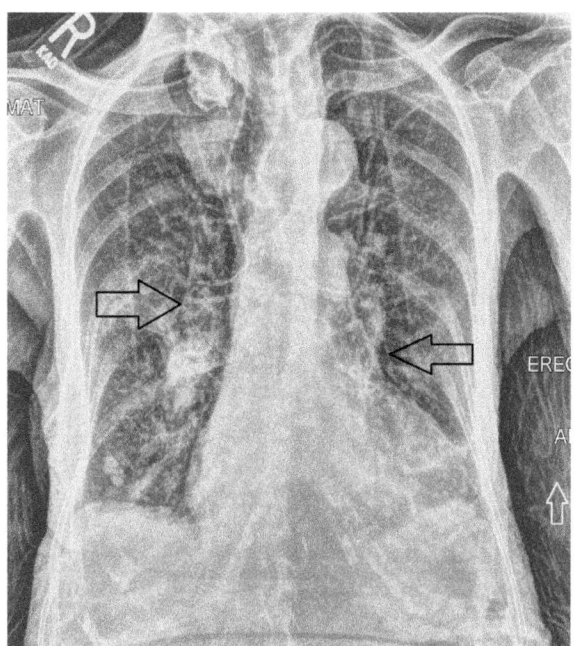

Figure 83:1 *Example of pneumonia in both lungs.*

Treatments of bacterial pneumonia include:

Nasal Oxygen
Intravenous fluid with DW5/normal saline or DW5 with ½ normal saline, or normal saline or ½ normal saline

Antibiotics treatments are dictated by the underline medical condition or conditions of the patient, or whether the patient is coming from the community, nursing home, in the hospital, the age of the patient or whether the patient is immunosuppressed or not.

In clinical practice, when a patient presents with pneumonia broad spectrum antibiotics are given empirically until result of the sputum culture is back from the bacteriology laboratory. Result of the sputum Gram stain gives important information by letting the physician know whether the bacterium causing the infection is Gram negative or Gram positive, but this information is not enough to be used to make a definitive antibiotics treatment.

The best antibiotics to treat these patients are:

Ceftazidime 1 gram IV qh 8 hours and Vancomycin 1 gram IV Q12 hour
or
Ceftriaxone 1 gram IV q12 hour and Vancomycin 1 gram IV q 12 hour
or
Levaquin 500mg IV q 24 hours and Vacomycin 1 gram IV q 12 hour
or
Cipro 400mg IV q 12 hours and Vancomycin 1 gram IV q 12 hour

or

Zoszyn 3.375 grams IV q 6 hour and Vancomycin 1 gram IV q 12 hour

or

Nafcillin 1 gram IV q 6 hour and Vancomycin 1 gram IV q 12 hour

or

Penicillin G 600,000 to 1 million units per day and Gentamycin 1.5 mg/kg q 12 hour

Other antibiotics that available to treat pneumonia in combination or singly include:

Cubicin
Erythormycin (very good to treat Ligionair pneumonia)
Pipercillin
Zithromax
Biaxin
Avelox
Keflex
Ceftin
Imipenem
Meropenem
Primaxin
Augmentin
Ampicillin
Amoxicillin
Bactrim DS (good to treat MRSA as well)
Clindamycin
Flagyl
Doxycycline etc.
Zyvox for VRA or MRSA (this medication is very expensive and Vacomycin is used more frequently for MRSA).

Patients in the hospital who develop pneumonia must be treated for Pseudomonas till proven otherwise. The same is true for patients residing in nursing home and other health care facilities. Nursing home patients must also be treated for MRSA till proven otherwise. Nasal swab can easily rules out MRSA.

People living at home who present to emergency rooms with pneumonia must also get tested for MRSA with nasal swab because there have been several cases of MRSA pneumonia reported in the medical literature.

Prevention of pneumonia is a very important clinical maneuver to do to prevent certain types of pneumonia. The elderly and people who are immunosuppressed ought to be vaccinated to prevent Pneumococcal pneumonia.

The people who need to be vaccinated include:

The elderly (people over age 60)
People with no spleens such as people with sickle cells disease
People whose spleens were surgically removed
People with HIV/AIDS
People with other immunosuppressive disease

The Vaccines that are in use are:

Pneumovax
Prevnar 13
Flu vaccination

In addition, patients being treated for pneumonia should have blood test to rule out TB in particular, if these patients come from areas where TB is prevalent or if they are immunosuppressed.

All patients with HIV/AIDS, who have pneumonia, should be evaluated for Pneumocystis caranii pneumonia (PCP).

Viral pneumonia is a very common type of pneumonia in all age groups.

The viruses that can cause pneumonia include:

Influenza A
Influenza B
Parainfluenza virus
H1N1 virus
Respiratory syncitial virus RSV
Herpes simplex virus
Varicella-zoster virus
Adenovirus
Measles virus
Rubella virus
Cytomegalovirus (CMV)
Corinavirus (Severe acute respiratory syndrome virus (SARS)

Signs and symptoms of viral pneumonia include:

Cough
Fever
Chills
Body aches
Chest pain
Weakness

Shortness of breath
Flu like symptoms
Headache
Rapid heart rate
Rapid respiratory rate (breathing fast)
Runny nose
Sore throat
Poor appetite
General malaise
Rales/Pneumonic sounds on examination of the lungs (may or may not present)
Infiltrate seen on chest x-ray

Evaluations of viral pneumonia include:

History and physical examination
Chest X-ray
CBC (the white cells count may be slightly high, normal, or low and the number of lymphocytes and monocytes may be high, and atypical lymphocytes may be present)
Nasal swab for influenza A or B
Viral titers in the blood for influenza A, B, herpes, Adenovirus, Varicella virus and for H1N1 virus depending on the clinical setting
Complete chemistry profile
ABG
EKG

Treatments of viral pneumonia include:

IV fluid with D5W/normal saline or D5W1/2 normal saline or plain normal saline
Nasal Oxygen
Tylenol for fever
Non-steroidal anti -inflammatory drugs (NSAID's) don't give Aspirin to children with pneumonia
Cough syrup
Amentadine
Tamiflu
Rimantadine
Ribavirin
Acyclovir (for herpes simplex virus)
Gancyclovir (CMV)

The best way to prevent viral pneumonia is to be vaccinated against adenovirus, herpes simplex, herpes zoster, measles, adenovirus, rubella, influenza A an B, SARS, H1N1, and the flu virus.

People who are sixty or older, young children and those who are immunosuppressed should get the flu shot every year.

CHAPTER 84

SARCOIDOSIS IN AFRICAN AMERICAN MEN

Sarcoidosis is a very common inflammatory disease of unknown etiology that frequently affects the lungs and many other organs in the body. The lungs are the most frequently affected organs with sarcoidosis and most definitely the most important organ to be affected by this disease. Sarcoidosis is much more common in Blacks, Hispanics, and Northern Europeans than Whites and Asians.

Worldwide the incidence of sarcoidosis is up to 50 per 100,000 and in the U.S. the incidence of sarcoidosis is up 40 per 100,000.

Sarcoidosis affects Blacks 3-4 times more often than other ethnic groups and it occurs in ages 20-40 and there appears to be a family connection.

The most frequent signs and symptoms of pulmonary sarcoidosis are the following:

1. Shortness of breath
2. Coughing
3. Wheezing
4. Fever
5. Night sweats
6. Weight loss
7. Chest pain
8. Fatigue
9. Enlarged lymph nodes
10. Rash
11. Nodules
12. Blurry vision
13. Pain in the eyes
14. Sensitivity to light
15. Conjunctivitis
16. Frequent urination
17. Hypercalcemia
18. Kidney stone
19. Seizure

20. Bell's palsy
21. Palpitations
22. Irregular pulse
23. Swollen joints
24. Hoarseness
25. Hypercalcemia
26. Kidney stone
27. Hematuria

Infiltrates and nodules of different sizes can be seen on chest x-ray. The pulmonary function test is abnormal in pulmonary sarcoidosis. In time, there will be the development of pulmonary fibrosis.

The diagnosis of sarcoidosis is usually established by taking a biopsy of a pulmonary nodule during a bronchoscopic examination or by biopsying a palpable lymph node. The characteristic histopathological finding on tissues taken from a person with sarcoidosis is non-caseating granuloma. The angiotensin-1-converting enzyme blood test is usually elevated in blacks suffering from sarcoidosis. Sarcoidosis is a multi-system disease that affects many organs in the human body.

Clinical manifestations of sarcoidosis pulmonary sarcoidosis

Sarcoidosis has the potential to affect all organs in the body and its manifestations may be felt throughout the body.

The organs most frequently affected are the following:

1. The lungs
2. The lymph nodes
3. The eyes
4. The skin
5. The upper respiratory tract
6. The liver
7. The spleen
8. The bone marrow
9. The kidney
10. The heart
11. The nervous system
12. The endocrine system
13. The gastrointestinal tract
14. The exocrine glands and
15. The musculoskeletal system etc.

Evaluations of pulmonary sarcoidosis include:

History and physical examination
CBC
Complete chemistry profile
Urinalysis
Angiotensin-1- converting enzyme
ESR
Chest x-ray
Chest CT
Spirometry
ABG
Pulmonary function test
Skin biopsy
Lymph biopsy
Bone marrow biopsy
Eye examination by Ophthalmologists
Bronchoscopy
Lung biopsy

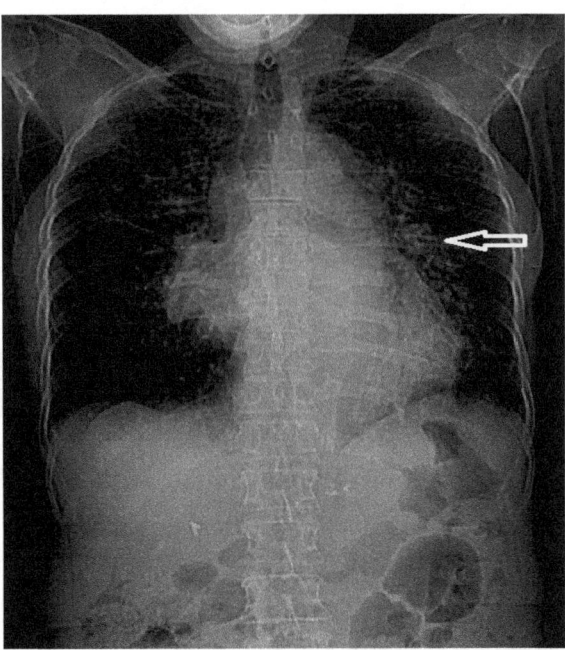

Figure 84:1-Chest x-ray in a patient with pulmonary sarcoidosis with a mass and nodules in the lung.

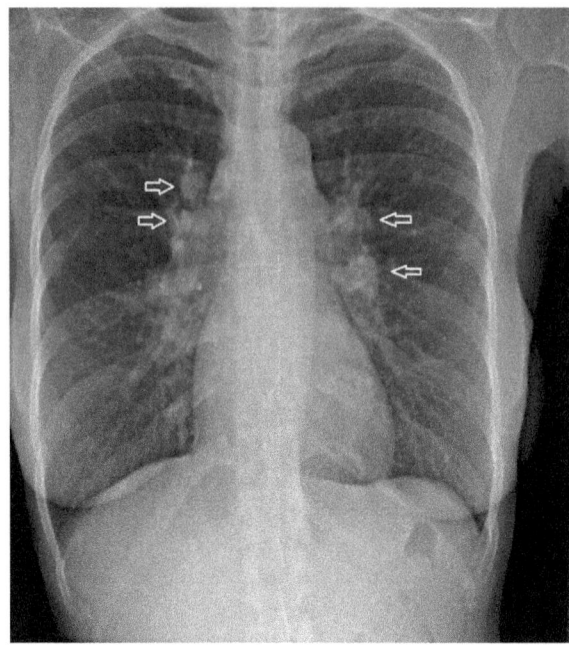

Figure 84:2 Chest x-ray showing multiple enlarged hilar nodes in a person with sarcoidosis.

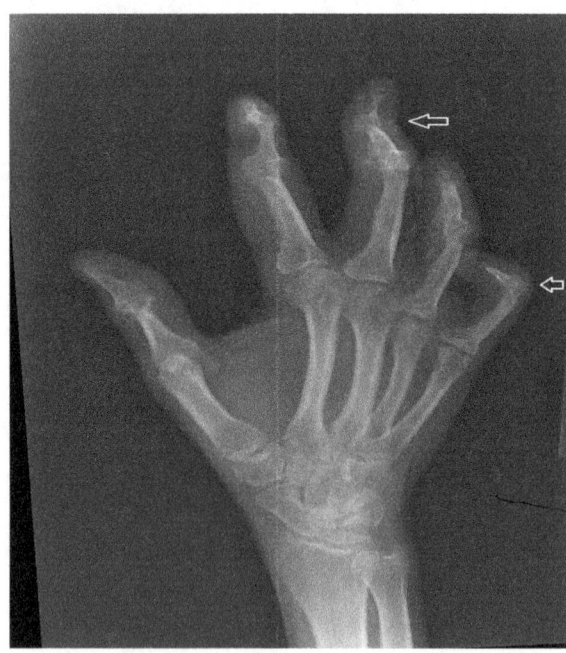

*Figure 84:3 x-*ray of right hand of a person with sarcoid arthropathy showing severe deformities and bones destructions.

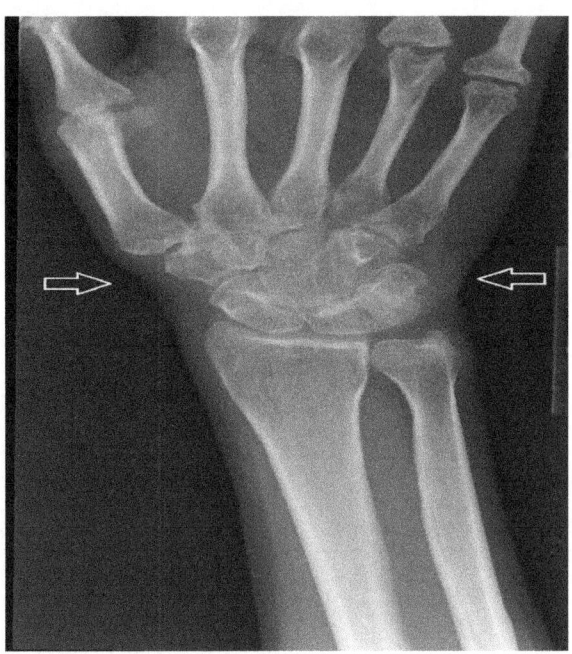

Figure 84: 4 x-ray of the right hand of a person with sarcoid artrhopathy showing deformities bones destruction.

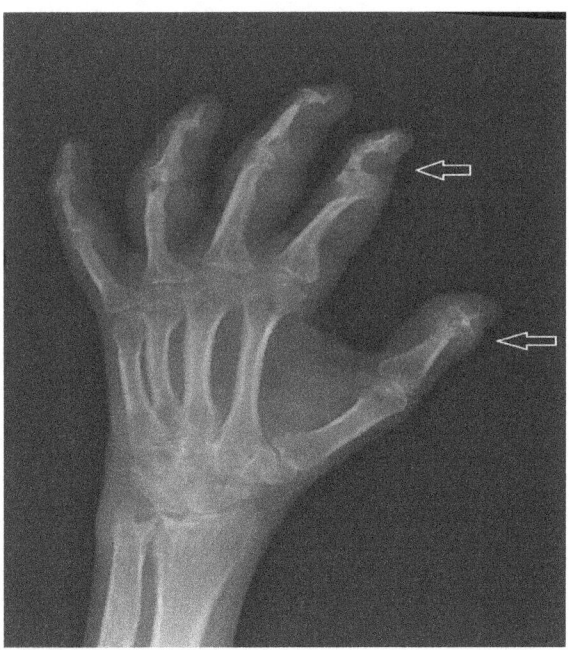

Figure 84: 5 x-ray of the left hand of a person with sarcoid arthropathy showing bones deformities

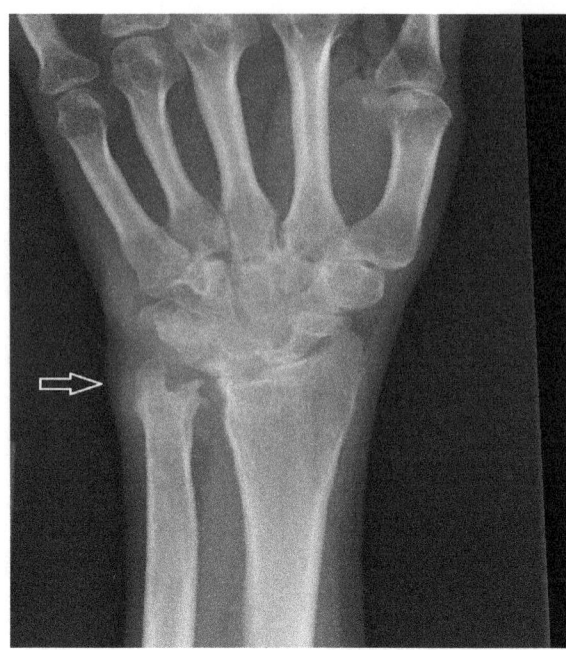

Figure 84: 6 *x-ray of the left wrist of a person with sarcoid arthropathy showing bones deformities*

Sarcoid arthropathy is a very complication of sarcoidosis and is usually treated with steroid and NSAIDs.

About 90% of people with sarcoidosis have their lungs involved with the disease process. Approximately, 50% of these individuals develop permanent lung abnormalities and about 15% develop pulmonary fibrosis, and a significant percentage of these people go on to die of respiratory failure.

Fever of unknown origin is frequently due to sarcoidosis. Weight loss, night sweats, general weakness, and poor appetite can be seen in sarcoidosis.

Blurry vision and bleeding into the eyes can also occur in sarcoidosis 25% of the time.

The usual types of the eye problems that are frequently seen in sarcoidosis are uveitis, detached retina, etc. When the eyes are affected, sore eyes and dryness of the eye can develop and if left untreated, blindness is the usual result.

Kidney stones with acute back pain and kidney stones in the urine can occur in sarcoidosis because of high serum calcium. Sarcoidosis is frequently associated with hypercalcemia (high serum calcium), and when the calcium is high in the blood, it can precipitate in the kidneys, resulting in calcium kidney stones.

Multiple and different joints and muscles can get involved in sarcoidosis, resulting in severe pain, arthralgias, arthritis, and different bone abnormalities. Carpal tunnel syndrome can also be seen in sarcoidosis. Muscle weakness, such as polymyositis, has also been described in sarcoidosis.

Sarcoidosis can involve the heart 5% of the time. The parts of the heart most frequently affected by sarcoidosis are the left ventricle, the conductive system causing complete heart block etc. Both congestive heart failure and different types of cardiac arrhythmias can also occur in sarcoidosis.

The neurological system is commonly affected by sarcoidosis and in about 5% of the time a neurological finding is documented. Damage to the nerve resulting in Bell's palsy (paralysis of one side of the face) can be seen in sarcoidosis. Damage to the liver and spleen can also occur in sarcoidosis resulting in enlargement of both the liver and spleen, causing significant abnormalities in liver functions and white blood cells, red blood cells, as well as platelets.

The bone marrow is involved in about 40% of cases of sarcoidosis.

The manifestation of the bone marrow involvement with sarcoidosis is reflected by anemia, leukopenia, and thrombocytopenia.

The skin is commonly involved in sarcoidosis in up to 20%–25% of the cases.

Among the most commonly seen skin lesions in cases of sarcoidosis are erythema nodosum and alopecia. Enlargement of the lymph nodes is quite frequently seen in sarcoidosis. Mediastinal nodes are enlarged in about 90% of patients with sarcoidosis. Other nodes that are frequently enlarged in sarcoidosis are axillary notes, cervical nodes, inguinal nodes, etc.

Several laboratory tests can be abnormal in sarcoidosis; examples are low white blood cells, low red blood cells, low platelets, high serum calcium, and high sedimentation rate.

Treatments of sarcoidosis include:

Steroid
Cytoxan
Imuran
Nasal oxygen
Kidney stone medications
Medications for hypercalcemia
NSAIDs for joints pain
Steroid eye drops etc;

Complications of Sarcoidosis include:

Hypercalcemia
Kidney stones
Kidney failure
Bell's palsy
Heart block
Peptic ulcer (high serum calcium causes over secretion of Gastrin, which is associated with the development of peptic ulcer)
Frequent urination
Lung cancer
Thymoma
COPD
Seizure
Pulmonary failure
Death

CHAPTER 85

THROMBOPHILIA IN AFRICAN AMERICAN MEN

Thrombophilia is a condition that when it exists in a person blood causing the blood to become thick. The thickness of the blood (hypercoagulable state) can result from many conditions.

The conditions that can cause hypercoagulable state include:

Cancer –resulting in Trousseau syndrome
Elevated homocysteine level
Anti-thrombin III deficiency
Protein C deficiency
Protein S deficiency
Elevated lipoprotein-a
Prothrombin mutation G 20210A
Factor V Leiden mutation
Lupus anticoagulant
Anti-cardiolipin antibody
Elevated Fibrinogen
Elevated Factor VIII
PA1-1 mutation
MTHFR DNA Analysis
B12 deficiency
Folic acid deficiency
Vitamin C deficiency (although low Vitamin C is not a thrombophilia per se, it is
Known to cause recurrent miscarriages)
Taking birth control pills to prevent pregnancy
Taking birth control pills prevent pregnancy
Using IM estrogen to prevent pregnancy
Using birth control pills to regulate menstrual period
Taking estrogen as treatment for post menopausal symptoms
Using hormones to treat prostate cancer
Using testosterone in any forms

Other conditions that predispose people to the development of DVT are:

Traveling long distances by planes or by cars
Lying in bed in the hospital after surgery
Anyone of the things listed above when abnormal can cause the affected person to have a thrombophilia and thus becomes hypercoagulable. Thrombophilia predisposes a person to the development of DVT and pulmonary embolism.

All types' cancers can cause Trousseau syndrome (clot formation), but the most common cancers that are more frequently associated with the development of DVT/Pulmonary embolism are:

Cancer of the pancreas
Cancer of the stomach
Cancer of the colon
Cancer of the prostate
Cancer of the lung
Melanoma
All hematological malignancies etc;

The way cancer causes DVT/Pulmonary embolism is that the cancer cells secrete a series of procoagulant proteins, and once these procoagulant proteins enter into the blood stream, they create a state of hypercoagubilty resulting in the formation of clots.

Sometimes the first presentation of cancer is DVT/Pulmonary embolism. So, if a person presents with DVT/Pulmonary embolism and no obvious cause or causes can be found, then an evaluation ought to be carried out looking for the presence of cancer in the body.

Complications of thrombophilia include:

DVT
Pulmonary embolism
Stroke
Myocardial infarction
Renal vein thrombosis
Ischemic colitis
Blindness
Miscarriages
Microvascular disease of the brain
TIA
Seizure etc;

Evaluations of thrombophilia includes:

History and physical examination
CBC
Complete blood chemistry profile
Urinalysis
PT, PTT and INR
Complete hyperpecoagulable profile (see the list of thrombophilias above)

CHAPTER 86

DEEP VEIN THROMBOPHLEBITIS IN AFRICAN AMERICAN MEN

Every year 2.5 million people develop DVT in the U.S. Most of the time pulmonary embolism occurs because a person develops deep vein thrombophlebitis (DVT) in an extremity or extremities and a piece of the clot brakes off and migrates to the lung causing pulmonary embolism to occur.

DVT occurs because of a thrombus (clot) that develops in the venous system (low flow system). The thrombus that develops in the venous system is a red thrombus (red clot). This red thrombus is composed of red blood cells and debris.

Thrombi that develop in the high flow system (arterial system) are white thrombi. White thrombi are composed of white blood cells and platelets.

Risks and causes of DVT include:

Cancer
Thrombophilia
Hypercoagulation
Low protein C
Low protein S
Low anti-thrombin III
Positive Lupus anticoagulant
Anti-cardiolipin antibody
Elavated Lipoprotein a
Elavated homocysteine
Positive Factor V Leiden antibody
Positive Prothrombin G20210A
Positive MTHFR
Positive PA1-1mutation
Taking birth control pills
Taking post menopausal hormones
Taking testosterone hormone to treat ED
Taking hormones to treat prostate cancer
Major trauma

Cancer of all types
Polycythemia Vera
Secondary polychythemia
Essential thrombocythemia
Myelofibrosis
Pregnancy (According to the literature DVT occurs 85% in the left leg during
Pregnancy as compared to 55% in the left leg in non-pregnant women
DVT develops roughly in 2 pregnancies in every 1000 pregnancies.
Roughly 80% of postpartum DVDs occur up to 3 weeks after delivery
Post major surgical procedures
Lying for long period of time in the hospital bed
Flying long distances by plane
Driving long distances by car etc.

Signs and symptoms include:

Swelling in the leg
Swelling in the arm
Unexplained pain in the leg
Unexplained pain in arm
Redness and tenderness over legs or arms etc;

How to evaluate a person for DVT

History
Physical examination
Ultrasound of the affected extremity
D-dimer
CBC
Complete metabolic profile
PT, INR
PTT
Chest x-ray
EKG

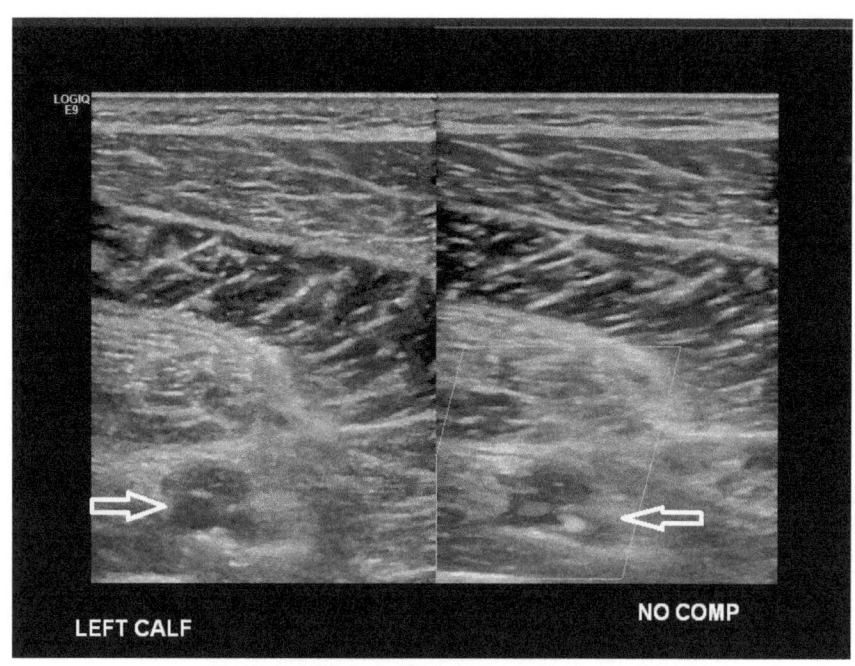

Figure 86:1 DVT left calf

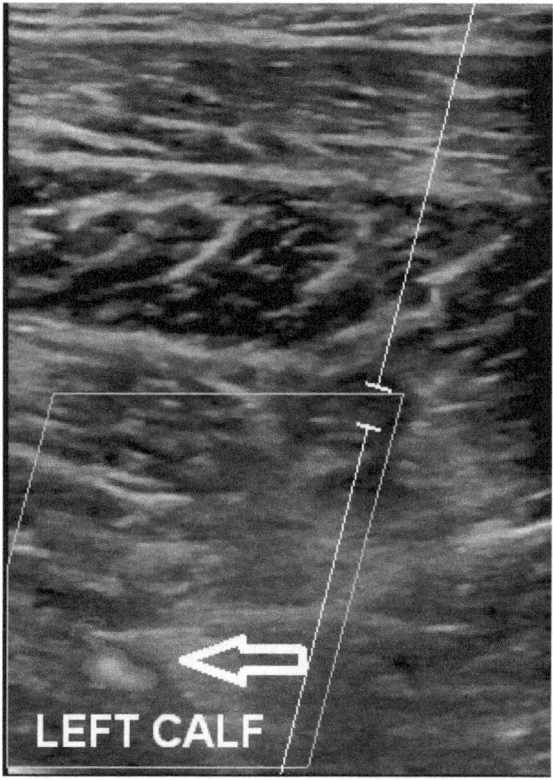

Figure 86:2 **DVT left calf**

Treatments of DVT

The mechanism that causes clot formation leading to DVT and pulmonary embolism and other clotting problems are:

Clots form in both the arterial system (high flow system) Venous system (low flow system)

The clots that form in the arterial system are called white clots because they are composed of white cells and platelets mainly. The clots that form in the venous system are called red clots because they are composed of red cells debris mainly.

Knowing that they are red clots and white clots and what they compositions are and where they develop in the body is of utmost importance because these different clots are treated with different medications.

Clots in the high flow/arterial system are composed mainly of white cells and platelets and are treated with Aspirin, heparin, or coumadin mainly. Clots in the low flow/venous system are composed mainly of red cells and debris and are treated with heparin, Lovenox, and coumadin.

Aspirin and Plavix are not very effective in preventing clots in the venous system (low flow system) because these types of clots are deficient in platelets. Aspirin and Plavix prevent clot formation by preventing the aggregation of platelets.

Other medications in use to treat and to prevent DVTs include: (factor Xa inhibitors such as the medications listed below)

Xarelto
Pradaxa
Apixaban
Argatroban
Fondaparinux
Idraparinux etc.

These medications are good to prevent clot formation in both the arterial and venous systems. Inferior venacava filter is used to prevent pulmonary embolism in certain clinical settings.

Once it is established by ultrasound that the person has DVT, then anti-coagulation

must be started first with heparin IV. The reason why it is preferable to begin anti-coagulation with heparin is because heparin has anti-inflammatory property that helps to decrease the inflammation that DVT causes.

While on heparin, it is important to monitor daily PTT and CBC and stool hemoccult. The reasons for daily PTT and CBC are to monitor the levels of red blood cells and platelets. If the red blood cells dropped from baseline, it means that the person is bleeding from the heparin. If the PTT is elevated near 70 second, 80, or 90 second, it does not matter much. Because, once the PTT is elevated at the level 45-50, it means that all the factors in the intrinsic pathway are already affected maximally.

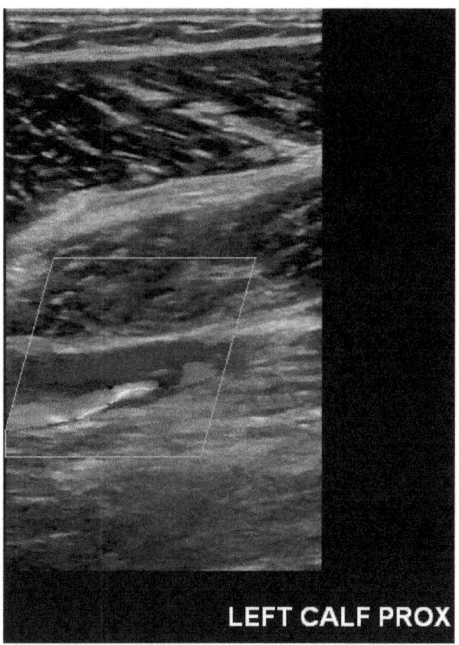

Figure 86:3 Left calf DVT

What is most important is when the PPT remains in the normal range even though the patient is on full dose of. In this case, it means that the person is so actively clotting that he or she is secreting massive amount of platelet factor IV. Platelets factor IV is anti-heparin. In this case, the dose of heparin needs to be increased.

If the platelets dropped by 50% from baseline, it means that the person has developed Heparin induced thrombocytopenia and the heparin must be stopped immediately.

In this case, the person must be started on Argatrobin as per protocol and at the appropriate time, the person can be started on Coumadin to complete the course of treatment.

Individuals who developed heparin -induced thrombocytopenia must never again be treated with heparin and Lovenox.

DVT is treated for a total 12 weeks. However, if it is determined that a person develops DVT because of a Thrombophilia, then that person must remain on prophylaxis anticoagulation for life.

When DVT or Pulmonary embolism develops in the setting of Trousseau syndrome, namely because the person is suffering from cancer, Coumadin should never be given to treat the DVT/Pulmonary embolism because it will not work.

Coumadin does not work in Trousseau syndrome because the cancer cells overwhelm the blood system by damping massive amount of procoagulant proteins into the blood that are constantly causing clotting to occur.

The way to treat DVT/Pulmonary embolism in the setting of Trousseau syndrome is to use heparin or lovenox as anticoagulant.

Better still, is to treat the cancer. Once the cancer is treated, the hypercoagulable state / Trousseau syndrome should resolve. It is important to keep in mind that DVT/Pulmonary embolism may be the presenting sign of cancer.

Therefore, when cause cannot be found to explain why someone has DVT/Pulmonary embolism, a full and complete work up ought to be carried out looking for cancer in that person.

CHAPTER 87

PULMONARY EMBOLISM IN AFRICAN AMERICAN MEN

Every year 600,000 individuals in the U.S. develop pulmonary embolism, resulting in 300,000 deaths. About 60,000 individuals die yearly in the U.S. because of undiagnosed pulmonary embolism whose diagnosis are determined at autopsy.

Most of the time pulmonary embolism occurs because a person develops deep vein thrombophlebitis (DVT) in an extremity or extremities and a piece of the clot brakes off and migrates to the lung causing pulmonary embolism to occur.

Every year in the US 2.5 millions individuals develop DVT.

Conditions that predispose people to DVT or pulmonary embolism include:

1. Obesity
2. Birthcontrol
3. Hormone replacement therapy
4. Post-surgery immobilization
5. Multiple trauma
6. Immobilization after a stroke
7. Hypercoagulable state due to cancer of different types
8. Deep vein thrombophlebitis (DVT)
9. Polycythemia vera
10. Post-partum state
11. Elevated homocysteine level
12. Anti-thrombin III deficiency
13. Protein C deficiency
14. Protein S deficiency
15. Elevated lipoprotein-a etc
16. Pulmonary embolism can occur without DVT in extremities

The most frequent symptoms of pulmonary embolism consist of:

1. Shortness of breathes
2. Tachycardia (rapid pulse rate)
3. Pleuretic chest pain

4. Sweating
5. Paleness
6. Restlessness
7. Coughing
8. Coughing up blood
9. Pain in calf muscles
10. Syncopal episode
11. Fever
12. In massive pulmonary embolism/saddle embolism, sudden death can occur

Following the history and physical examination, the most important tests to do to confirm the presence of pulmonary embolism consist of:

1. Arterial blood gas (ABG)
2. D-dimer
3. Chest x-ray
4. Ultrasound of the lower extremities
5. Ultrasound of upper extremities
6. Lung Scan
7. CT angiogram
8. EKG

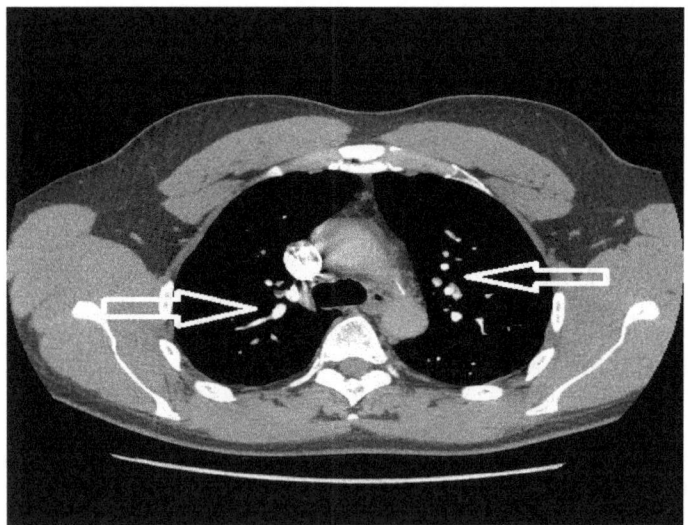

Figure 87:1 Bilateral pulmonary emboli

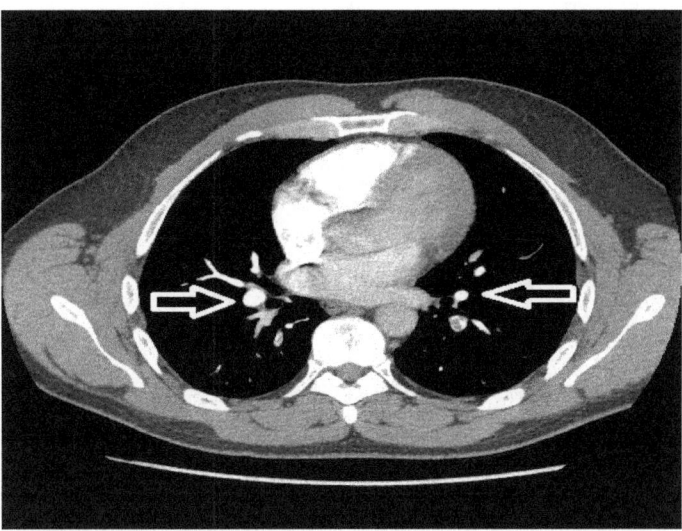

Figure 87:2 bilateral pulmonary emboli

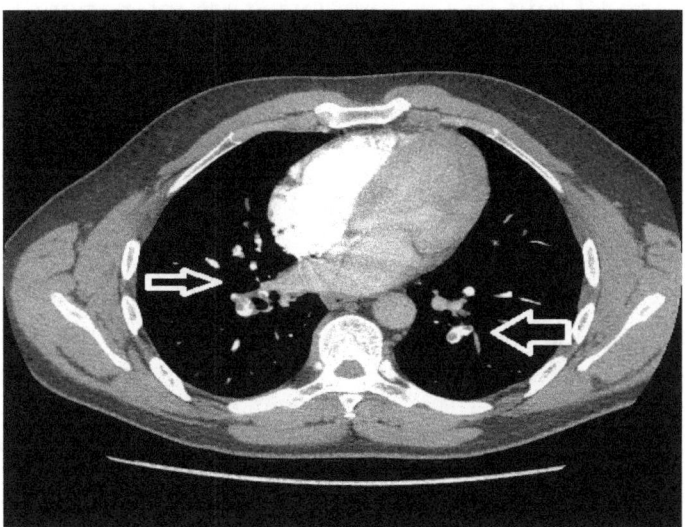

Figure 87:3 bilateral pulmonary emboli

The most definitive test to do to establish the diagnosis of pulmonary embolism is the pulmonary angiogram, but this test is hardly ever necessary nowadays because D-dimer; ultrasound of the lower extremities and the high probability lung scan are sufficient to arrive at the diagnosis of pulmonary embolism. The D-dimer blood test is extremely important because when pulmonary embolism is present, this test is positive.

Whenever a clot is formed anywhere in the body, the clots release plasmin in the blood stream which in turn causes d -Dimer to become elevated. D-dimer is not specific for DVT or pulmonary embolism because, it is also elevated in pregnancy, sepsis, and DIC.

However, if the lung scan is read as high probability for pulmonary embolism, the D-dimer is elevated, and if the ultrasound of the extremity shows a DVT, the possibility that the patient has pulmonary embolism is greater than 90%.

Computed Tomographic Pulmonary Angiography is also a very good test that can show the presence of pulmonary embolism.

Treatment for pulmonary embolism:

The treatment choice for pulmonary embolism is intravenous heparin. However, before starting heparin, several blood tests must be done:

1. Prothrombin time (PT)
2. Partial thromboplastin time (PTT)
3. Hematocrit
4. Platelet count
5. Stool for hemoccult

The importance of the PT and PTT is to ensure that the patient's coagulation system is working normally, so as not to precipitate bleeding. The importance of the platelet count is 1) to make sure the platelet count is not too low prior to starting heparin; 2) to have a baseline normal platelet count. The rationale for establishing that the baseline platelet count is normal is that in the event that if the platelet count drops to 50% of the baseline platelet count that means that the patient is developing platelet-induced thrombocytopenia.

Therefore, the heparin administration must be stopped immediately.

Lovenox and other high molecular weight heparin can also cause heparin-induced thrombocytopenia sometimes therefore, are not good alternative to regular heparin.

Heparin induced thrombocytopenia occurs because an antigen/antibody reaction.

The best way to evaluate HIT is to test for anti-platelets antibodies. However this test takes several days to come from the lab and is not always positive even tough HIT exists. Drop in the platelets count by 50% from base is much more important in making the diagnosis of HIT because daily platelets count can be done.

HIT can cause thrombosis to occur in about 2-5% of people causing stroke or acute myocardial infarction (heart attack).

Once HIT is suspected, heparin must be stopped immediately. The anticoagulant Argatrobin must be started IV to anticoagulate the person.

In the setting of HIT, Coumadin must never be used. Doing so can lead to major clinical catastrophe such as acute cold limb syndrome, cercrosis of the breast and possibly death.

The reason this happens is because the HIT causes an acute hypercoalugable state and giving Coumadin to patient makes the hypercoagulable worse resulting in diffuse clotting.

Everyone who gets Coumadin becomes hypercoagulable immediately because the ½ life of factor VII is 4-6. Factor X ½ life is 48 hours, and Factor II ½ life is 72 hours. These factors are vitamin K dependent factors, Coumadin decreases them sequentially, and while this process is going on, the person on Coumadin remains hypercoagulable until all of these factors are depleted. Once all of them are depleted coagulation occurs. That is why adding Coumadin to acute HIT is contraindicated.

The only medication approved in the U.S. to treat HIT is Argatroban.

This medication is given IV. Once the platelets count becomes normal, then and only then can Coumadin be given to complete the course of anticoagulation treatment.

The reason why it is necessary to check the hematocrit every day in a patient receiving heparin is that the heparin can cause bleeding to occur and a drop in hematocrit would document that.

Checking the stool for blood every day is important, because if the stool is positive for blood, it means that the patient is bleeding and the heparin must be stopped.

Once these tests are done, then heparin can be infused as a 5000 units bolus IV, followed by 1000 units per hour intravenously. While on heparin, the patient must be monitored with daily PTT and CBC.

It is a good idea to keep the patient with pulmonary embolism on heparin for 7 to 10 days. Then Coumadin ought to be started while the patient is still on heparin. After 5 days of the Coumadin by mouth, the heparin can be stopped if the prothrombin time and the INR (international normalized ratio) are therapeutic. This protocol of treating with heparin for 7-10 days and begin Coumadin as just described applies to male patients as well.

The Coumadin is continued for 6 months to 1 year. Anticoagulation may need to be continued for life, if the pulmonary embolism is associated with a hereditary hypercoagulable state (thrombophilia).

Factor Xa inhibitors like Xarelto given 15mg twice per day for 6 months or 20mg Daily for 12 weeks to treat pulmonary embolism;

Prevention of DVT/Pulmonary embolism:

It is very important that people make sure they are screened for the presence of thrombophilia as part of their routine medical evaluation. Knowing whether or not an individual has does not a thrombophilia dictate what medication he or she can or cannot take? As mentioned before, there are several common medications such as birth control pills and other estrogenic medications that anyone with any type of thrombophilia should avoid, because these medications can precipitate clots formation in a thrombophilic person.

In addition, if a thrombophilic person must travel long distances either by air plane or by car, he or she should be anticoagulated daily with Lovenox while traveling to prevent DVT/Pulmonary embolism.

One of the most frequent complications of anticoagulation treatments is bleeding.

To avoid bleeding people should be tested before any anticoagulation treatment is started with.

PT/INR
PTT
CBC/Platelet count

Once bleeding is detected, the anticoagulation medications or antiplatelets medications must be stopped immediately. And if necessary, Fresh frozen plasma (FFP) should be given if heparin/lovenox is responsible for the bleeding. Vitamin K IV should be given if Coumadin is responsible for the bleeding. In certain cases where the bleeding is profuse and excessive, FFP should be given. FFP works in 2-3 hours to stop bleeding, while vitamin K takes 12-24 hours to stop bleeding.

If Aspirin/Plavix or NSAIDs is responsible for the bleeding, Desmopressin (DDAVP) should be given to stop the bleeding. DDAVP 20mcg in 50cc of normal saline over ½ hour stops the bleeding in 1 ½ hour. DDAVP works to stop the bleeding by increasing the factor VIII Von Willebrand by 15-20% and this enough to transiently correct the qualitative platelet abnormality caused by the anti-platelets medication.

The effects of Aspirin/Plavix on the platelets last 7-10 days in the body, the effects of NSAIDs on the platelets last only 6 hours in the body.

CHAPTER 88

BLEEDING DISORDERS IN AFRICAN AMERICAN MEN

The most common bleeding diseases in the world include:

"Von Willlerdrand disease 1, 2 and 3 (70 million people in the world have Von Willebrand disease and 1.5 million people in the U.S. have Von Willebrand disease.) "
Hemophilia A -factor VIII deficiency
Hemophilia B -factor IX deficiency
Immune thrombocytopenic purpura ITP
Fibrinogen deficiency- factor I deficiency
Afibrinogenemia
Hypofibrinogenemia
Factor II deficiency-Prothombin
Factor V deficiency
Factor VII deficiency
Factor X deficiency
Factor XI deficiency
Factor XIII deficiency
Platelet disorders
Glanzman thrombasthenia
Bernard-Soulier syndrome
Gray platelet syndrome
Wiskott-Aldrich syndrome
Platelet storage pool disease
Combined factor deficiencies
a-2antiplasmin deficiency
a-1 antitrypsin deficiency
Ehlers-Danlos syndrome
Osler-Weber-Rendu syndrome
Vitamin C deficiency
Scurvy."
Coumadin treatment with secondary bleeding
Factor X inhibitors medications with secondary bleeding

Vitamin K deficiency occurs very frequently in people who are sick in the ICU/CCU in the hospital and being treated with IV antibiotics and are not able to eat, or in people who are not eating, but are on chronic antibiotics at home on in the Nursing Home.

Ninety percent of vitamin K in the body is taken in foods that people eat and ten percent is produced by actions of bacteria in the large bowel. So, when people are very sick and are receiving antibiotics and are not able to eat, it takes, but a few days (about 7 days) for them to become vitamin K deficient. Once they become vitamin K deficient, they are at risk for bleeding. One of the most common causes of bleeding in the ICU/CCU is vitamin K deficiency. Patients who are IV antibiotics in ICU/CCU ought to be given 10mg of IV vitamin k once per week to prevent bleeding.

All of the above listed abnormalities can cause people to bleed profusely including:

Cirrhosis of the liver

Disseminated intravascular coagulopathy

Von Willebrand disease as stated above is the most common bleeding disorder in the world and there are three different types of Von Willerbrand disease type 1, type 2 and type 3.

Type 1 Von Willebrand is the most common type, and 3 out 4 people with Von Willerbrand have type 1. Type 1Von Willwerbrand is the mildest type. In type 1 Von Willerbrand both Von Willerdand factor and factor VIII l levels are low.

Type 2 Von Willebrand has 2A, 2B, 2M and 2N subtypes.
In type 2 Von Willerbrand the Von Willerbrand factor does not well.

In type 3 Von Willerbrand there is no there no Von Willerbrand factor and factor VIII is low. Type 3 Von Willerbrand is the severest type and most serious type.

Evaluations of Von Willerbrand disease include:

History and physical examination
CBC
Complete blood chemistry profile
Bleeding time (must be off aspirin for 7 to 10 days and off NSAIDs for 2 days before the test is done)
Complete Von Willerbrand profile
PT
PTT
Urinalysis
ABO blood typing

Treatments of Von Willerbrand include:

Desmopressing (DDAVP) 20 mcg in 50cc of normal saline IV over ½ hour
or
DDAVP via nasal inhalation
or
DDAVP SC
Blood transfusion as needed
Platelets transfusion as needed
Vitamin K SC or IV for too high PT due Coumadin
Fresh Frozen Plasma to treat high PT due to Coumadin
Andexanet Alfa is very effective to reverse bleeding due factor X inhibitors.

Idiopatic Thrombocytopic Purpura or Primary Immune Thrombocytopia is an autoimmune platelets abnormality that cause people to bruise easily and bleed. ITP affects both children and adults.

ITP develops when the body develops antibodies against platelets resulting in an antigen antibody reaction.

The antigen antibody complexes that are formed on the surfaces of the platelets in the body cause the destruction of the platelets by the spleen, the liver and wherever there are reticuloendothelial and parenchyma cells in the body.

Worldwide, there are 10 million people who have ITP and about 30.000 people in the U.S. have ITP.

The causees of ITP are unknown, but can occur after viral infection like measles, mumps and upper respiratory viral infection. In addition, ITP occurs in about 52 percent of people who have H. Pylori gastritis. ITP occurs 2 times more frequently in women compared to men.

Signs and symptoms of ITP include:

Bruising
Petechia on arms and legs
Heavy bleeding when cut
Nosebleed
Bleeding from the gums
Rectal bleeding
Hematuria
Heavy menstrual bleeding
Iron deficiency anemia
Weakness
Tiredness
Low platelets
Positive H. Pylori antibody in the blood etc;

Evaluations of ITP include:

History and physical examination
CBC
Blood smear to look the quantity of platelets on the smear
Complete blood chemistry profile
Anti-platelets antibodies
PT/INR
PTT
Bone marrow smear
Bone marrow biopsy
H. pylori antibody test

Treatments of ITP include:

Steroid
Intravenous immunoglobulin
Rituxan
Splenectomy
Nplate

Bleeding is the most serious complication of ITP including bleeding in the brain. Spontaneous bleeding does not occur when the platelets count is above 20.000 People with ITP should not take Aspirin or NSAIDs.

CHAPTER 89

TUBERCULOSIS IN AFRICAN AMERICAN MEN

Tuberculosis is one of the world's most common infections that affect the lungs.

"In 2010, a total of 11,181 tuberculosis (TB) cases were reported in the United States." MMWR 2010 More than two billion people, equal to one third of the world's population, are infected with TB bacilli. "Each year, over nine million people around the world get infected with TB and almost two million TB related deaths are recorded worldwide. TB is a leading killer among people living with HIV." Source: WHO Source: WHO

"TB remains a major threat to health around the world.
In 2013, there were an estimated 11 million prevalent cases, and an estimated 9.0 million incident cases occurred globally. An estimated 1.1 million incident cases occurred among people living with HIV. 550,000 occurred among children, and 3.3 million occurred among women.
TB caused approximately 1.5 million deaths and in 2014, 1.1 million people died of TB in the world.
Worldwide, of which 210,000 were due to MDR TB and 360,000 were among people living with HIV".

In 2015, there were 9 million in the world infected with TB.

The incidence of TB infection is highest in Asia because 4 billion of the population lives in Asia, as result there are altogether 5 million cases or 75% of TB cases occur in 22 countries of Asia. The incidence of TB is high in Africa mainly due to the AIDS epidemic there. 1 billion of people live with TB in Africa.

Blacks and other minorities are 8 times more frequently affected with tuberculosis than whites are. "In 2007, TB was reported in 4,470 blacks in the U.S." the World Health Organization reported that 9 million cases of tuberculosis occurred worldwide each year and that 1.6 million people died in the world from tuberculosis during that same period.

A significant percentage of the people who died of TB were also infected with HIV/AIDS. About 98% of these cases of tuberculosis occurred in the developing countries of the world.

About 10% of new tuberculosis cases that occur in the U.S. occur in individuals who were skin test positive for TB, (latent TB) therefore this group of individuals serves as a reservoir for new TB cases.

The organism that causes tuberculosis is mycobacterium tuberculosis. Infected individuals can transmit the TB organism to uninfected people through droplets that come from the lungs when they cough.

Once the TB organism enters into the lungs of the person being infected, it locates itself in the upper/posterior part of the lung, where the oxygenation of that area of the lung favors its growth.

Symptoms of pulmonary tuberculosis include:

1. Fever
2. Chills
3. Weight loss
4. Loss of appetite
5. Night sweats
6. Cough
7. Hemoptysis (coughing blood)
8. Shortness of breath

Findings on physical examinations may be positive for enlarged lymph nodes, large spleen, large liver, fever, and evidence of weight loss.

Evidence of fluid in the lungs may show evidence of fluid around the heart (cardiac tamponade pericardial effusion). x-ray findings frequently seen in tuberculosis include:

1. Infiltrate seen on chest x-ray
2. Cavity seen on chest x-ray

Non-specific laboratory tests that may be abnormal in pulmonary tuberculosis:

1. Low white blood cells
2. High white blood cells
3. Low red blood cells (anemia)
4. Low platelet count
5. High platelet count
6. High serum calcium
7. High alkaline phosphatase
8. High serum protein
9. Low serum albumin
10. High LDH (lactic dehydrogenase)
11. Low serum sodium due syndrome of inappropriate antidiuretic hormone (SIADH)

Specific laboratory tests that are positive in pulmonary tuberculosis are as follows:

1. Acid fast bacteria (AFB) seen on stain of sputum coughed up by the patient.
2. Acid fast bacteria (AFB) seen on stain of washing/tissues taken during bronchial examination of the lungs/pleural biopsy of pleural fluid.
3. M. tuberculosis organism grown on AFB culture six weeks after it is plated on appropriate culture medium.
4. AFB organism seen on lymph node biopsy from patients suspected of suffering with tuberculosis
5. AFB DNA probe (PCR) this test can confirm M Tuberculosis quickly.

The pathological finding seen on tissue specimens taken from an individual suspected of suffering from tuberculosis is caseating granuloma.

Positive sputum for AFB does not necessarily mean that the person has M. tuberculosis because mycobacterium avium intracellulare (MAI) also stains positive for AFB. However, using DNA probe test, MAI can be differentiated from M. tuberculosis quickly.

How to test the skin for TB

When an individual has been exposed to a person infected with tuberculosis, the first thing to do is to plant a PPD 5TU on the person's arm. If the PPD is positive and the person being tested has not been vaccinated with BCG this then raises the possibility that the individual may in fact have been exposed to TB. This finding has an even stronger meaning if the person being tested is known to have had a negative PPD in the past.

The PPD test must be read within 48 hours to 72 hours from the time it was planted and does not always provide definitive answer.

The following blood tests are much more accurate in diagnosing TB.

The Interferon-Y release Assays (IGRA),
T-SPOT.TB
QuantiFEROn-TB Gold

The FDA has approved a new test for TB called Xpert MTB/RIF. This test is an assay and is able to identify M tuberculosis with 98.1% accuracy and is simultaneously able to diagnose Rifampin resistant TB 97.6% of the time. In addition, this test provides results in 2 hours, while the old Tb test takes up 3 months to give a result. Source: FDA, 7/26/2013

Four percent or 360,000 of the 9 million new cases of TB around the world are resistant Rifampin. Source: WHO

When any of these tests are positive, the next thing to do is a chest x-ray. If the chest is positive for TB, then the person is treated for TB. If on the other hand, the chest x-ray is negative, the person then is to be given prophylaxis with Isoniazid (INH) 300mg daily for

6 months together with Vitamin B6 one tablet per day, or Rifampin 300mg twice per day for 4 months.

TB can affect all organs in the human body and Symptoms can mimic many diseases. Therefore, it is always prudent for physicians to include TB in their differential diagnoses when evaluating individuals with complicated symptoms.

Another stage of TB is Latent TB infection (LTBI); in this stage TB individuals have positive mantoux skin test. These individuals usually think their positive mantoux or PPD skin test is due BGC vaccination received in childhood. However, when the QuantiFERON TB Gold test is done using their bloods, it is usually positive in many of them, and if their chest x-rays are negative, that means that they in fact have LTBI. LTBI is treated with Rifampin 300mg twice per day for 4 months.

Treatments for M tuberculosis

The medications that are used to treat M. tuberculosis include:

Rifampin
Isoniazid
Pyrazinamide
Ethambutol
Streptomycin

The usual period of time that individuals are treated for TB is 9–12 months. The usual adult doses of these medications are: 1) Isoniazid 150 mg by mouth twice a day; 2) Rifampin 300 mg by mouth twice per day; and 3) Pyrazinamide 25mg/kg per day by mouth and Ethambutol 15 mg/kg body weight per day by mouth and Streptomycin 10–15 mg/kg body weight per day. Usually after the first month of treatment the sputum becomes negative for AFB.

During treatment for TB, complete blood count and liver function tests must be done every 6–8 weeks to monitor for possible low platelets, low white blood cells, low red cells count, and medication-induced hepatitis with elevated liver function tests.

Multiple drugs resistant TB remain a major problem in the treatment of tuberculosis Globally. "In 2012, and estimated 450,000 people developed MDR-TB in the world. It is estimated that about 9.65 of these cases were XDR-TB." Source WHO

Once MDR-TB is suspected because of failure to respond to Isoniazide and Rifampin, the sputum or other specimens should be sent to the microbiology laboratory for culture and sensitivity.

The sensitivity test will identify which anti-TB medications the TB organism is sensitive to.

In the U.S. the FDA for treatment of MDR-TB approves bedaquiline
"At a dose of Weeks 1-2: 400mg daily by mouth

Weeks 3-24: 200mg three times per week, for a total of 600mg per week." Source CDC

CHAPTER 90

MALARIA IN AFRICAN AMERICAN MEN

It is estimated that 300-500 million people worldwide become infected with malaria each year and 1 million people in the world die of malaria of malaria yearly: Source CDC 1500 cases of malaria are reported annually in the United States. These cases occur in people who traveled to countries where malaria is endemic.

Malaria is a parasite that is carried by mosquitoes and humans get infected with Malaria when mosquitoes carrying the malarial parasites bite them. Malaria can also be transmitted by blood transfusion in rare occasions.

It is the female malaria organism that feeds on mammals including humans. The female malaria releases the infectious material as she bites to suck the blood. The infectious material is released through her saliva into the blood stream and enters into red blood cells. From there the infected red blood cells go to the liver-hepatocytes, where it is reproduced asexually again and again and the morozoites for of the malarial organism gets transmitted back into the blood stream again.

Malaria is develops mainly in tropical and subtropical countries.

The countries where malaria is most often found are:

Africa
Asia
The Americas
South East Asia

Malaria is common in these countries because these countries have high humidity and rain, conditions, which are perfect for malaria to grow.

Malarial disease is highly associated with poverty. The people who are mostly affected by malaria live in poor conditions that predispose them to being infected by malaria.

Most of them live in poorly constructed houses that offer no protection from malaria. To be protected from malaria requires living inside nets that shield them from being bitten by malaria. In addition, certain repellents that can kill malaria need to be used to spray areas that harbor malaria. In addition, using nets to shield people from being bitten from malaria is necessary. Travelers to malaria-infested countries are at high risk of becoming intercepted with malaria.

The five commonly known malarial organisms are:

Plasmodium falciparum
Plasmodium vivax
Plasmodium ovale
Plasmodium malariae
Plasmodium knowlesi (more prevalent in South East Asia)

P. Falciparum is the most virulent malarial parasite and the severe form of malarial disease.

Once a person becomes infected the malarial parasites/sporozoites, the sporozoites travel from the through the blood to the liver. In the liver the sporozoites mature into mezoites. From the liver the parasites re-enter the blood stream and infect red blood cells. They remain inside the red blood cells for 48-72 hours. After 72 hours, the red blood cells burst open (hemolyze) releasing more infecting more red blood cells with malarial parasites. This process goes on and on for as long as the infected person remains infected with malaria.

Ninety per cent op people who die of malaria are African children. Seventy per cent of malarial infections are the result Plasmidium Falciform, twenty per cent are due to Plasmidium Vivax and five per cent are due to Plasmidium malariae and Plasmidium Ovale.

After infection symptoms of malaria infection usually develops within 10 days to 4 weeks. However, symptoms can develop up to 1 year after infection. Symptoms occur in a cycle of 48 to 72 hours.

Symptoms of malaria include:

Fever
Chills
Sweating
Headache
Nausea
Vomiting
Muscle cramps/pain
Anemia
Bloody stools
Hemolysis
Jaundice
Seizure
Coma etc;

Evaluations of malaria include:

History
Physical examination
CBC with differential count
Malarial blood smear
Complete chemistry profile
Reticulocytes count
Serum LDH
PT/INR, PTT
Urinalysis
Chest x-ray
EKG
Abdominal ultrasound (to look at the liver and spleen)

Treatments of malarial infection depend on the type of malarial parasites responsible for the infection and the severity of the infection.

Acute P. falciparum infection is a medical emergency and needs hospitalization for treatments to be given.

Treatments for acute malaria infection include:

Bed rest
Vital signs
Nasal Oxygen
IV fluid with D5 Normal saline at 150cc per hour
Blood transfusion if necessary
IV Quinidine or Quinine plus IV Doxycycline or Doxycycline by mouth
                              or
Clindamycin IV
                              or
Artesunate IV in developing countries is being used to treat Falciform malaria
Artesunate is not approved for use in the U.S.
A new drug "(Spiroindolone KAE609 30mg daily for 3 days seems very effective against Falciparum and Vivax malaria)" Source: New England Journal of Medicine, July 31, 2014
Monitor Fibrinogen, PTT to rule out DIC
Monitor renal profile
Monitor peripheral blood smears to look schistocytes.
Polymerase chain reaction (PCR) can also be used to identify specific types of malarial organisms. Prevention of malaria is extremely important.

Many people who live in countries and areas of the world where malaria is common have antibodies to malaria, but travelers to these countries and areas do not have antibodies to malaria. Therefore, people who are going these countries and areas where malaria is endemic, need to take anti-malaria medications 1-2 weeks before traveling and 4 weeks upon returning.

Different anti-malaria medications are used for different countries.

People traveling to Africa, South America, Latin America, Central America, the Caribbean, Asia, Indian sub-continent, and the South Pacific should take either Mefloquine, Chloroquine, Doxycycline, Malarone, or Hydroxychloroquine, Primaquine. Anti-malaria prophylaxis medications should be taken 1-2 weeks before traveling. Once per week while in that country and for once per week for 4 weeks upon returning. Before taking anti-malaria medications, people should be tested for G6-PD deficiency.

Complications of Malaria infection include:

Cerebral malaria
Seizure
Coma
Pulmonary edema
Hemolysis
Severe anemia
DIC
Kidney failure
Rupture of the spleen
Enlargement of the liver
Hypoglycemia
Deaths.

CHAPTER 91

PARASITIC INFESTATION IN AFRICAN AMERICAN MEN

Parasitic infestation is the 6th most common disease in the world and parasitic diseases outrank cancer as the number one killer in the world. Source: WHO About ½ to 1/3 of the world 7.4 billion people are infested with one type of parasites or another.

Some of the most common parasites that infest humans are:

Toxoplasma Gondii 3-3/12 billion people in the world are infested
Ascaris 807 million people
Hookworm 740 million people in the world are infested
Round worm (Trichuris trichiuria) 1 billion
Tapeworm 75 million
Tenia solium pork tapeworm
Tenia saginata beef tapeworm
Diphyllobothrium fish tapeworm
T. Solium larvae can sometimes go to the brain headache and seizures (Neurocysticercosis)
Hymenolepis NANA Dwarf tapeworm is the most common human tapeworm, it is estimated that 75 million people are carriers and 25% of children in some parts of the world are said to be infected by it. Most recently it has been documented in the literature that H. NANA has caused cancer in a person with HIV infection.

Pinworm 200 million
Whipworm 1.5 billion
Schistosomiasis 230 million people are treated yearly for this worm Source: WHO
Entamoeba histolytica 500 million people in the world
Giardia lamblia 200 million
Cryptosporidium causes about 748,000 infections yearly and worldwide is one of the common diarrheal diseases in the world. This infection is most common in people with AIDS worldwide.
Other intestinal infections seen in AIDS causing diarrhea include
Cytomegalovirus, Tospora Belli
Other enteric parasitic infections include Cyclospora, Microsporidia, and Toxoplasma etc;

Intestinal parasitism is quite common in people who originate or travel to the tropics or who live in the rural parts of the southern United States. Intestinal parasitism is also commonly seen in people who migrated to the United States from Southeast Asia and other third world countries where poor sanitation and poverty are prevalent.

Parts of the world where parasitic infestation is most ofen found include:

Africa
Southeast Asia
North Africa
India
China
Indonesia
The Americas
The Middle East etc;

It is estimated that hookworms infest about 740 million in the world and the daily blood loss is estimated at 7 million liters. Two million people in the United States are infected with hookworm. Ascaris infestation is a very common parasitic infestation.

The Signs and symptoms of intestinal parasitic infection are many and can manifest as

Nausea
Vomiting,
Constipation
Diarrhea
Weakness
Dizziness
Headache
Chronic
Cough,
Skin rash
Generalized itchiness
Bloody stools
Iron deficiency anemia
Bloating
Hematemesis (Chinese Flukes)
Flu like symptoms
Fever
Cramping and Gas
Weight loss
Itching around the anus (mostly at night)
Foul smelling stools
Passing worms in the stools
Irritable bowel syndrome
Joints pain

Muscles ache
Elevated IgG
Eosinophelia on peripheral blood smear
Allergy dermatitis
Nervousness
Anxiety
Insomnia
Headaches
Seizures (due to Cysticercosis of the brain due to Taenia Solium-Pork Tape worm)
Transverse Myelitis of the spinal cord (due Schistosomiasis mansoni's eggs in the spinal cord)
B12 deficiency
Depression
Poor memory (due to B12 deficiency)
Dementia (due to B12 deficiency)
Intestinal obstruction (due large worms)

In recent years, there has been a greater increase in intestinal parasitism brought about by the AIDS epidemic. People who are immunosuppressed are more prone to be infested by parasites of all types including Giardia lamblia, amoeba, etc.

Strongyloides stercoralis a round worm whose larvae can get into the venous system of the blood stream and migrate to the lungs. They recycle in lungs and can spread to multiple organs including the brain, the heart etc causing fever, chills, abdominal pain and shock and often time death. People infected with strongyloides when placed on steroid for one reason or another, can develop acute systemic strongyloides. Therefore, before placing a person at high risk for strongyloides on steroid, stools for ova and parasites or serum antibody for strongyloidis should be done.

Evaluations of intestinal parasitic infestation include:

Physical examination
CBC
Complete chemistry profile
Stools for ova and parasite
Toxoplasma titer
Strongyloides titer
HIV test
Urinalysis
Serum B12
Chest x-ray
Brain CT
Brain MRI
EEG
EKG etc;
Medications available to treat intestinal parasitic infestation include:

Mebendazole
Albendazole
Diethylcarbamazine
Ivermectin
Praziquantel
Pyrantel pamoate
Piperazine citrate
Flagyl
Levamisole
Metrifonate
Oxamniquine

These different medications are recommended by the WHO to use to treat different individual intestinal parasites.

It is up to the treating physicians to choose which medications to use to treat which worm. Some of these people, due to poverty, walk barefooted, exposing their feet to fecal materials, permitting parasites to enter into their bloodstream and, with no water available to wash hands after bowel movements, hands soiled with parasite-contaminated stool that provides an entry point for intestinal parasitism and all its serious medical complications. Proper hygiene with hand washing with water and soap and walking with shoes or sandals and eating properly coked foods will help to decrease the incidence of intestinal parasitism.

However since there is so much poverty in the world forcing people to live in deplorable conditions, it is doubtful that intestinal parasitic infestation will ever be eliminated.

Another common parasitic infestation that causes a lot of people to suffer throughout the world is tapeworm (Taenia solium) disease of the brain known as neurocysticercosis. According to the WHO, there are about 2 million people in the world who are suffering from this condition. The countries where neurocysticercosis is prevalent include Africa, Asia, Latin America and other developing countries. The black men who have neurocysticercosis (Tapeworm brain disease) have recurrent seizures. The available medications to treat Tapeworm of brain disease include Albendazole to kill the worms and Dexamethasone to reduce the inflammation and anti seizure medications. Source: JAMA, May 15, 2013 –Vol 309, No 19.

CHAPTER 92

TICK BORNE DISEASES/LYME DISEASE IN AFRICAN AMERICAN MEN

The most common thick born diseases in U.S. are

Lyme disease
Babesiosis
Ehrlichiosis
Rocky Mountain spotted fever
Anaplasmosis
Rickettsia parkeri rickttsiosis
Southern tick-associated rash illness (STARI)
Tickborne relapsing fever (TBRF)
Tularemia
364D rickettsiosis Source: CDC

The most recently discovered tick borne disease in Northeastern United States is Borrelia miyamotoi Disease, it is carried by deers. The most common symptoms of BMD is fever, myalgia, flu-like illness, rash and headache etc.; Doxycycline is the drug of choice to treat BMD.

Tick-borne diseases are found abroad as well.

Crimean-Congo hemorrhagic fever
Imported tick-borne spotted fevers
Tick-borne encephalitis (TBE) Source: CDC

The different ticks that cause tick-borne diseases are

Rocky Mountain spotted fever (American dog tick, Rocky Mountain Wood tick, Lone star tick, Brown dog tick.

Brown dog tick (Rickettsia parkkeri rickettsiosis)
Blacklegged tick (Ixodes scapularis) deer tick (anaplasmosis, babesiosis, and Lyme disease)
The lone star tick (ehrlichiosis, tularemia)

Signs and symptoms and complications of Lyme disease and other tick borne diseases include:

Skin rash (macular, popular, erythema migrans, Bull's eye rash, (300,000 people are affected by Lyme disease every year in the U.S.)
Muscle aches
Headache
Fatigue
Fever
Chills
Fatigue
Joints pain
Heart block (Lyme disease)
Cardiac arrhythmia
Pericarditis
Myocarditis
Meningitis (Lyme disease)
Hepatitis
Anemia
Seizure
Arthritis
Bell's palsy (Lyme disease)
Memory loss (Lyme disease)
Paralysis (Lyme disease)
Chronic fatigue (Lyme disease)
Depression (Lyme disease)
Insomnia (Lyme disease)
Paralysis
Dementia

Evaluations for tick-borne including Lyme diseases include:

History and physical examination
CBC
Complete chemistry profile
Blood titers/ Western blot for the suspected tick-borne disease
Blood culture
Malarial smear
Blood titers for babesiosis
VDRL
Urinalysis
ESR
Chest X-ray
Brain CT
EKG

24 Hour Holter monitor
EEG
Dermatology consultation etc;

Antibiotics in use to treat tick-borne disease include:

Doxycycline
Mepron
Amoxicillin
Erythromycin
Tetracycline
Azithromycin
Ceftriaxone IV
Cefuroxime IV
Other treatments are provided for individual complications.

Prevention of tick-borne diseases includes:

Dress with light color cloths so that the tick can be seen
Wear socks up to knees
Wear high booths
Remove shoes and socks before entering the house
Make dogs and cats do not bring ticks in the house
Use repellents with DEET to kill ticks
Individuals with fair skin must examine their skins looking for tick when they come from Tick infested areas. In particular, look for the baby tick called Nymph (it is white and as such can be missed easily). It is very infectious.

If a tick is found on the skin, use a tweezers to remove it without breaking it. You should check with your physician immediately to seek treatment, and anyone Who thinks he or she has tick-borne disease should seek medical treatment for his or her physician immediately.

CHAPTER 93

HEADACHE AND MIGRAINE IN AFRICAN AMERICAN MEN

Head ache is one of the most common maladies that has affected mankind since the beginning of time. Headache is much more common in blacks and other minorities than whites. In the U.S. 28 million individuals suffer from headache.

World wide there are several hundred millions people who suffer from headache. Nine out of 10 people in the world suffer from headache sometime in their lives.

Some of the most common headaches are:

1. Tension
2. Migraine headache
3. Cluster headache
4. Sinus headache
5. Cervical spine arthritic disease headache

Some of the medical conditions that can cause headache are:

1. High blood pressure
2. Brain aneurism
3. Severe anemia
4. Polycythemia
5. Lyme disease
6. Lupus (SLE)
7. Rheumatoid arthritis
8. Mixed collagen vascular disease
9. Viral meningitis
10. Fungal meningitis
11. Neuro syphilis
12. Sepsis
13. Temporal arteritis
14. Cryptococcal infection of the brain
15. Toxoplasma infection of the brain
16. Histoplasma infection of the brain

17. Herpes simplex infection of the brain
18. Cytomegalovirus infection of the brain
19. Parasitic infection of the brain
20. Malarial infection of the brain
21. Encephalitis
22. Brain abscess
23. Vasculitis of the brain
24. Stroke
25. Cancer of the brain
26. AIDS brain disease
27. Osler, Weber, Rendu disease of the brain (AVM) causing bleeding
28. Sub-dural hematoma
29. Multiple Sclerosis
30. Viral syndrome
31. Migraine
32. Tension headache
33. Cluster headache;

Tension headache is the most common form of headache.

Tension headache is more common in blacks and other minorities than whites. It affects 90 percent of blacks and other minorities and 70 percent of whites. It affects people between the ages of 20-50 more.

Symptoms of tension headache are:

Tension headache can cause a dull pain around the forehead and some time the pain can radiate to the back of the neck and shoulder.

The evaluation of patients with tension headache includes:

1. A complete history and physical examination
2. CBC
3. Erythrocyte sedimentation rate (ESR)
4. SMA 20 chemistry profile
5. Urinalysis
6. ANA
7. VDRL blood test for syphilis
8. HIV/AIDS blood test
9. Lyme disease blood test
10. Chest X-ray
11. CT scan of the brain with or without IV contrast
12. MRI of the brain with or without contrast
13. MRI of the cervical spine

The most common medications used to treat tension headache are:

Aspirin Non-steroidal anti-inflammatory drugs NSAID (such as ibuprofen, Naproxen, Advil etc.) Some patients respond to muscle relaxant or tricyclic antidepressant.

The next most common headache is Migraine headache.

Risks of migraine headache include:

Female sex Genetic transference, if both parents suffer from migraine, there is a 75 percent chance that an offspring will also suffer from migraine.

If one parent suffers from migraine, there is a 50 percent chance an offspring will also suffer from migraine.

Migraine usually begins in childhood, adolescent and in early adulthood.
It is believe that migraine is caused by a combination of vascular dilatation and constriction of blood vessels in the brain.

Some of the things that known to be able to bring on symptoms of migraine are:

1. Fatigue
2. Hunger
3. Changes in the whether
4. Emotional stress
5. Foods such as
6. Nuts
7. Cheese
8. Chocolate
9. Avocados
10. Alcohol consumption etc;

Symptoms of migraine include:

1. Throbbing pain in the head
2. Nausea
3. Vomiting
4. Sensitivity to light
5. Numbness in the face
6. Tingling of the face and lip
7. Weakness of arm or leg etc.
8. An attack of migraine headache can last for several hours and up to several days.
9. Close to 60% of people who suffer with migraine can have one or more attacks per month, 28 million individuals suffer from migraine in the U.S.
10. 11 million of them are made disabled by the severity of these migraine attacks.

11. Roughly, 175 million workdays are lost yearly as a result migraine attacks in the U.S. impacting the economy greatly.

The evaluation for migraine headache includes:

1. A history and physical examination
2. CBC
3. Erythrocyte sedimentation rate (ESR)
4. SMA-20 chemistry profile
5. Urinalysis
6. VDRL for syphilis
7. HIV/AIDS blood test
8. Lyme disease blood test
9. Chest X-ray
10. CT scan of the brain with or without IV contrast
11. MRI of the brain with or without IV contrast

Medications in use to treat migraine headache include:

1. Aspirin
2. NSAID
3. Cafergot
4. Midrin
5. Imitirx
6. Replax
7. Zomig
8. Fiorenol
9. Fiorocet
10. Beta Blocker such as Inderal
11. Calcium channel blocker such as Procardia
12. Compozine or Zofran for nausea and vomiting etc.

Another form of headache is cluster headache.

The pain associated with cluster headache usually comes on suddenly and frequently subsides just as quickly.

The evaluation for cluster headache includes:

A complete history and physical examination

1. CBC
2. ESR
3. SMA-20 chemistry profile
4. Urinalysis
5. ANA

6. VDRL blood test for syphilis
7. HIV/AIDS blood test
8. Lyme disease blood test
9. Chest x-ray
10. CT scan of the brain with or without IV contrast
11. MRI of the brain with or without IV contrast

Medications in use to treat cluster headache include:

1. IM Imitrex
2. Zomig
3. Dihydroergotamine either IM, IV or intranasal
4. Fiorocet

Some people respond to surgery to cut the trigeminal nerve to relieve symptoms of chronic cluster headache.

Cervical spine arthritic headache results from severe arthritis of the cervical spine or, herniated cervical disc.

Evaluation of cervical arthritis headache includes:

1. History and physical examination
2. CBC
3. SMA-20 chemistry profile
4. ESR
5. ANA
6. Serum uric acid level
7. MRI of the cervical spine
8. Referral to a neurologist/neurosurgeon/orthopedist

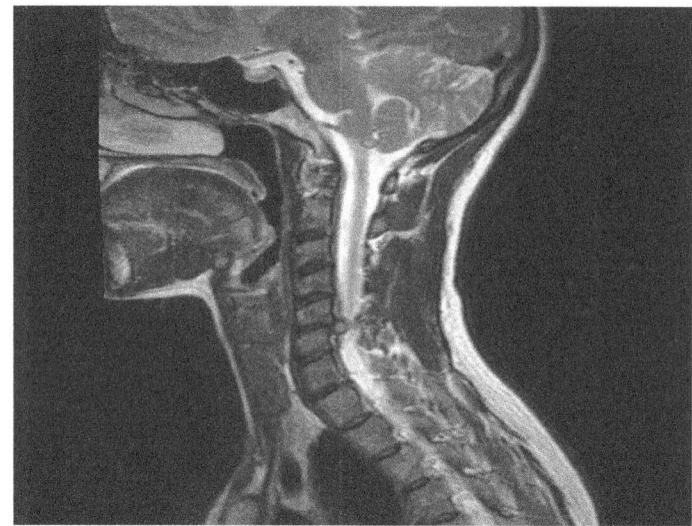

Figure 93:1 **MRI** *of cervical spine demonstrating an extruded disc herniation at C5-C6 (see arrow):*

Treatments of cervical arthritis headache include:

1. NSAID
2. Heat pad
3. Neck collar
4. Analgesia as necessary to control pain

How to detect, evaluate, and treat the medical conditions that can cause headache

To detect hypertension as a cause headache:

1. Take the person's blood pressure using the blood pressure cuff.
2. Do a CBC, SMA20, Urinalysis, Chest x-ray, and EKG

How to treat the hypertension associate headache:

1. Use a thiazide diuretic if the person's kidney function is normal.
2. Add either an ARB such as Cozaar or a calcium channel blocker such Cardizem if the diuretic is not sufficient to control the blood pressure.
3. Decrease salt intake to a between 3-4 grams sodium per day.
4. Exercise and weight management is important in controlling blood pressure.

How to detect brain aneurism associated headache:

How to detect brain aneurism associated headache:
Take a complete history from the patient.

Do a complete physical examination
Do Brain MRI with IV contrast
If an aneurism is detected, the patient must be referred to a neurosurgeon for surgical
Intervention to treat the brain aneurism and relieve the headache

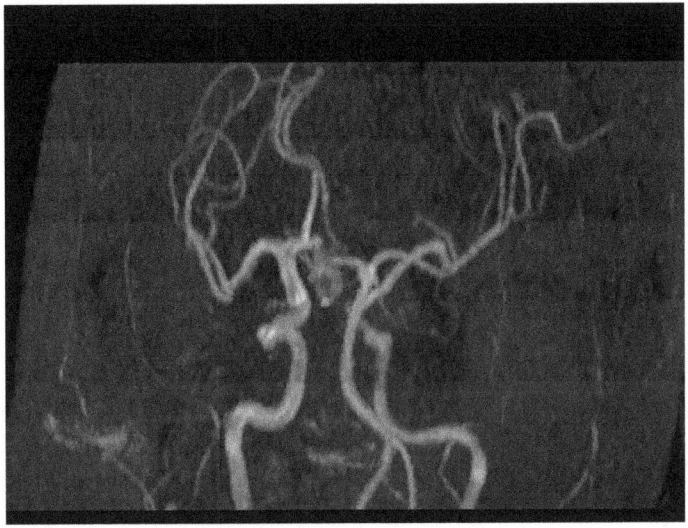

Figure 93:2 **MR** *Angiogram demonstrating an aneurysm of the anterior
communicating artery (See arrow):*

How to detect anemia-associated headache:

1. Take care a history from the patient
2. Do a complete physical examination
3. Do CBC

(See chapters on anemia for evaluation and treatments of different anemias)

If severe anemia is found, such as a hematocrit of between 15-20 per cent, the patient,
cannot deliver oxygen properly to the brain which, can cause headache to occur.

How to detect Polycythemia associated headache:

1. Take a history from the patient.
2. Do a complete physical examination
3. Do a CBC
4. Do a SMA20 chemistry profile
5. If the hematocrit is found to be 60% or above, the polycythemia evaluation ought
   to be carried out to determine whether the polycythemia is primary or secondary.
6. Polycythemia causes the red blood cells level to be too viscous preventing blood
7. Oxygen from moving with ease through blood vessels to deliver oxygen to the brain
   and other organs in the human body.

8. The viscosity of the can cause both headache and stroke to occur.
9. Treatments of polycythemia are complex and are determined based on the type of polycythemia and the cause.

How to detect and treat Lyme disease associated headache:

1. Take a complete history from the patient
2. Do a complete physical examination
3. Do a Lyme disease Elisa and Western blot blood test and these are positive
4. Do a CT scan of the brain
5. Do a lumbar puncture and send the spinal fluid for Lyme disease antibody test and culture
6. Treatments of Lyme disease meningitis include IV Ceftriaxone and Doxycycline by mouth and pain medication.

How to detect and treat Lupus (SLE) associated headache:

1. Take a complete history from the patient
2. Do a complete physical examination
3. Do a CBC
4. Do an SMA20 chemistry profile
5. Do a ESR
6. Do an ANA
7. Do a double stranded DNA
8. Do a brain CT scan
9. Do a lumbar puncture
10. Send the spinal fluid to the lab for ANA, double stranded DNA, glucose. Protein
11. Cell count, Gram stain, and culture.
12. Treatments for lupus associated head (meningitis) include usual medications used to
13. Treat lupus plus steroid and pain medication.

How to detect and treat Rheumatoid arthritis associated headache:

1. Take a complete history from the patient
2. Do a complete physical examination
3. Do CBC
4. Do SMA20 chemistry profile
5. Do a ESR
6. Do an ANA
7. Do a Rheumatoid factor
8. Do double stranded DNA
9. Do MRI of the cervical spine
10. Do CT Scan of the brain
11. Do a lumbar puncture

Send the spinal fluid for ANA, Rheumatoid factor, glucose, protein, cell counts, Gram stain and culture.

Treatments of Rheumatoid arthritis associated headache include the usual medications used to treat RA plus steroid.

If the headache is due to herniated cervical spine, then, the patient needs to be evaluated by a neurosurgeon. In addition, the patient needs treatment with NSAID plus pain medication.

How to evaluate and treat Mixed Connective Tissue Diseases associated headache:

1. Take a complete history from the patient.
2. Do a complete physical examination
3. Do a CBC
4. Do SMA20 chemistry profile
5. Do ERS
6. Do ANA
7. Do ENA
8. Do RNP
9. Do rheumatoid factor
10. Do double stranded DNA
11. Do CT scan of the brain
12. Do MRI of the cervical spine
13. Do lumbar puncture
14. Send spinal fluid for ANA, rheumatoid factor, double stranded DNA, glucose, protein, cell counts, Gram stain and culture.

How to evaluate and treat temporal arteritis associated headache:

1. Take a complete history
2. Do a complete physical examination
3. Get the Eye doctor to do complete eye examination
4. Do an ESR
5. Start patient on Steroid immediately to prevent blindness.
6. Doing surgery to section the temporal artery to diagnose temporal arteritis is very inaccurate.

How to evaluate and treat viral meningitis associated headache:

1. Take a complete history
2. Do a complete physical examination
3. Do CBC
4. Do an SMA20 chemistry profile
5. Do an ESR
6. Do blood tests for viral profile
7. Do HIV1/HIV2 blood tests

8. Do Blood culture
9. Do Chest x-ray
10. Do brain CT
11. Do a lumbar puncture
12. Send spinal fluid for cell counts, Gram Stain, both bacteria, viral and fungal cultures,
13. Glucose and protein
14. Start treating patient with Ceftriaxone IV and Vacomycin IV if he or she is not allergic to penicillin.
15. If the patient is allergic to penicillin, Levaquin IV can be added to IV Vancomycin till the results of microbiological tests are back from the laboratory.

How to evaluate and treat bacterial meningitis associated headache:

1. Take a complete physical examination
2. Do a complete physical examination
3. Do CBC
4. Do an SMA20 chemistry profile
5. Do Urinalysis
6. Do an ESR
7. Do Blood culture
8. Do Urine culture
9. Do HIV1/HIV blood tests
10. Do chest x-ray
11. Do EKG
12. Do brain CT
13. Do a lumbar puncture
14. Send spinal fluid for cell counts, Gram stain, bacterial culture, viral culture, fungal culture, TB culture, AFB stain, glucose, and protein.
15. Start treatment with Ceftriaxone IV and Vacomycin or Penicillin G IV, Fortaz and Vacomycin. Rifampin plus Ampicillin IV can also be used depending on the patient's profile and age till the results of the microbiological laboratory are back.

How to evaluate and treat fungal meningitis associated headache:

1. Take a complete history
2. Do a complete physical examination
3. Do a CBC
4. Do an SMA20 chemistry profile
5. Do urinalysis
6. Do ESR
7. Do blood culture
8. Do urine culture
9. Do HIV1/HIV2 blood tests
10. Do VDRL
11. Do blood test for CMV
12. Do blood tests for herpes simplex type 1 and type 2

13. Do blood test and blood smear for malaria
14. Do PPD skin test for TB
15. Do chest x-ray
16. Do EKG
17. Do brain CT
18. Do MRI with IV contrast
19. Do a lumbar puncture
20. Send spinal fluid to the lab for cell counts, Gram stain, fungal culture, bacterial culture,
21. Viral culture, TB culture, AFB stain, HIV1/HIV2 tests, Cryptococcal antibody, Toxoplasma antibody, Histoplasma antibody, Candida, Aspergillus, India ink test, do tests for protozoa, Herpes simplex, Cytomegalovirus and VDRL, Parasitic organisms, glucose and protein
22. Start treatment with IV Amphotericin B or Fluconazole and provide treatments based on the results of laboratory and X-ray results.

These types of infections are most frequently seen in individuals who are inmmunosuprssed, such as people who have AIDS or people who have been treated with chemotherapy.

How to evaluate and treat brain cancer associated headache:

Take a complete history
Do a complete physical examination
Do MRI of the brain with IV contrast

The different brain tumors that can be found include:

1. Glioma
2. Astrocytoma
3. Meningioma
4. Acoustic neuroma
5. Oligodendroglioma
6. Glioblastoma multiforme
7. Medulloblastoma
8. Metastatic cancer frequently occurs in the brain as well etc;

Some of the most common cancers that can metastasis to brain include:

1. Lung cancer
2. Breast cancer
3. Colon cancer
4. Prostate cancer
5. Melanoma
6. Lymphomas
7. Leukemias etc;

If a tumor is found in the brain, the patient needs to be referred to a neurosurgeon for a brain biopsy and removal of the cancer.

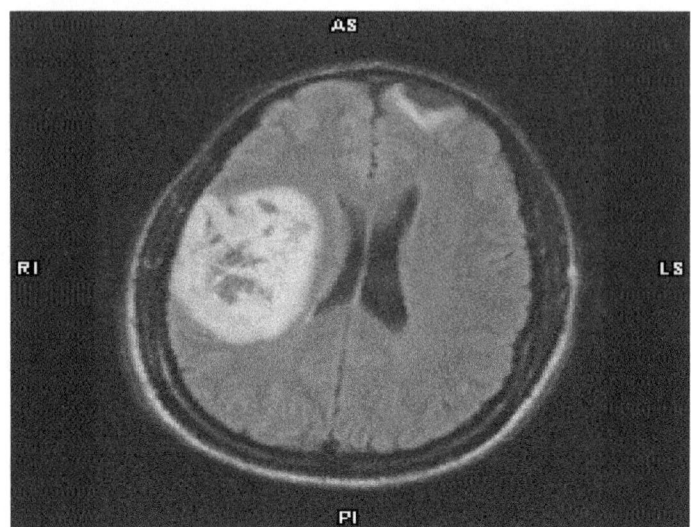

Figure 93:3 Axial MRI image demonstrates a glioblastoma multiforme of the right cerebral hemisphere. There is also evidence of old traumatic injury at the left frontal pole:

At times it may be necessary to obtain a consult from a neurologist to examine the patient and do a lumbar puncture, using a thin needle to avoid herniation of the brain.

The spinal fluid obtained from the patient must be sent to the laboratory for

1. Cytology
2. Glucose
3. Protein
4. LDH
5. Cell counts
6. Gram stain and culture.

Treatments of brain cancer associated headache include:

1. Surgical resection
2. Radiation therapy
3. Chemotherapy
4. Steroid IV or by mouth
5. Pain medication etc;

CHAPTER 94

THYROID DISEASES IN AFRICAN AMERICAN MEN

The thyroid gland is located at the base of the neck. The normal functions of the thyroid gland are under the control of the pituitary gland, which produces the thyroid-stimulating hormone, and the hypothalamus, which produces thyroid -releasing hormone. These two hormones working in concert stimulate the thyroid gland to secrete thyroxin, which is necessary for the functions of all organs and parts of the human body.

Hypothyroidism appears to be more common in Whites and Hispanics compared other ethnic groups and it is more common in women than men.

The most common diseases of the thyroid gland include:

Thyroid goiter
Hypothyroidism
Sub–clinical hypothyroidism
Hashimoto thyroiditis
Hypothyroidism with Mixed edema
Hyperthyroidism
Graves' disease
Thyroid nodules
Thyroid cancer

THYROID GOITER

The thyroid goiter produces thyroxin. Worldwide, there about 1 billion people who are deficient in iodine.

Worldwide, about 200 million people develop goiter and most of these people live in the developing countries of the world. Many of them live high elevation and mountainous areas where they have no access to sea water and loss of iodine from the soil that washed away by rain etc. Sea water contains small amount of iodine, and they do not have access to foods that are iodine supplemented? Iodine deficiency and thyroid goiter do develop in a small percentage people who live in the developed countries as well

There are three different types of goiters: simple goiter, nontoxic goiter and, toxic goiter. Simple goiter is quite common and is due to lack of iodine in the water and diet of those who are affected. Simple goiter causes enlargement of the thyroid gland. Toxic goiter occurs when the thyroid gland is enlarged because of either an acute inflammation of the thyroid gland or thyroid cancer. Hashimoto's thyroiditis can also cause thyroid goiter also.

Symptoms of thyroid goiter include:

Swelling in the neck
Swelling of the of the neck on one side or both side of the neck
Difficulty swallowing
Hoarsness
Pressure on the esaphagus
Deviation of the trachea
Sub-external goiter as seen on chest-xray

Evaluations of thyroid goiter include:

Palpation of the thyroid gland
Ultrasound of the thyroid gland (sometime thyroid goiter is sub-sternal and cannot be palpated)
Radioactive iodine uptake of the thyroid gland
Serum T4 and TSH
Anti thyroid antibodies

Treatments of thyroid goiter include:

Surgical removal of the thyroid goiter
Iodine replacement (daily requirement of iodine is 60mcg daily)
Syntroid 50mcg by mouth daily

CHAPTER 95

HYPOTHYROIDISM AND SUB-CLINICAL HYPOTHYROIDISM IN AFRICAN AMERICAN MEN

The most common causes of the hypothyroidism include:

Iodine deficiency
Thyroid Goiter
Hashimoto thyroiditis
Radioiodine treatment for hyperthyroidism
Radioiodine treatment for thyroid cancer
Surgical removal of the thyroid gland
Medical treatments of hyperthyroidism
Congenital hypothyroidism
Radiotherapy to the neck area to treat cancer
Congenital thyroid disease
Subclinical hypothyroidism
Pituitary disorder
Exposure to atomic bombs such as what happened in Japan, and nuclear accident such as Chernobyl.

Sub-clinical hypothyroidism is the most common type of hypothyroidism, it affects 8.0% in women and 3% in men, and the causes and symptoms are the same as outlined above and the evaluations are the same.

However, in sub-clinical hypothyroidism the serum T4 is normal, but the TSH is elevated. This is why sub-clinical hypothyroidism is referred to as normal T4 hypothyroidism.

Worldwide, there are about 1 billion people who have iodine deficiency. This occurs because most of these people live in the developing world in high elevation areas with no access to seawater or foods that contain iodine. Iodine deficiency can cause thyroid goiter.

Symptoms of hypothyroidism include:

Fatigue
Constipation
Weight gain
Cold sensitivity
Dry skin
Weakness
Thining of hair
Hair loss
Bradycardia
Depression
Poor memory
Hoarsness
Deep voice
Swollen face etc;

Evaluations of hypothyroidism include:

History and physical examination
Serum T4 and TSH
CBC
Complete blood chemistry profile
Thyroid ultrasound
EKG etc;

Treatments of hypothyroidism include:

Synthroid
Levothyroxine

Complications of hypothyroidism include:

Braycardia
Fatigue
Anemia
Goiter
Depression
Peripheral neuropathy
Myxedema
Congenital hypothyroidism
Cretinism etc;

CHAPTER 96

HASHIMOTO THYROIDITIS IN AFRICAN AMERICAN MEN

Hashimoto thyroiditis is an autoimmune disease. It is about 7 times more common in women than men. Hashimoto thyroiditis causes hypothyroidism.

Symptoms of Hashimoto thyroiditis include:

Fatigue
Constipation
Weight gain
Hair loss
Brittle nails
Depression
Swelling of joints
Painful joints
Slow heart rate (Bradycardia)
Infertility
Puffiness of face
Anemia

In addition, Hasimoto thyroiditis can be associated with other autoimmune Diseases such as:

Pernicious anemia
Systemic Lupus erythematosis
Rheumatoid arthritis
Vitiligo
Sjogren syndrome
Malabsoprtion of the bowel resulting in B12 deficiencies;
Therefore, when ever hypothyroidism is diagnosed without obvious explanation,
it is required that serum anti-thyroid antibodies are tested for to be sure the person
being evaluated does not have Hasimoto thyroiditis causing the hypothyroidism.
Hypothyroidism occurs because of failure of the thyroid gland to produce
enough thyroid hormone.

Evaluations of Hashimoto Thyroiditis include:

History and physical examination
CBC
Complete metabolic chemistry profile
T4 and THS
ANA
Anti-thyroid antibody
Anti-mitochondrial antibodies
Serum B12
ESR
Direct Coomb's test
Thyroid sonogram
Fine needle thyroid biopsy
Rheumatoid factor etc;

Treatments of Hashimoto's Thyroiditis include:

Synthroid etc;
Hypothyroidism is sometimes seen in association with lupus, vitiligo, rheumatoid arthritis and pernicious anemia. Sometimes the neck becomes painful and a person may think he or she has an ordinary sore throat, and sometimes it occurs with no symptoms at all. Both acute and sub-acute thyroiditis can lead to either transient or permanent hypothyroidism.

CHAPTER 97

HYPOTHYROIDISM ASSOCIATED WITH MIXED EDEMA

Mixed edema due hypothyroidism develops because of very or complete absence of thyroxin in the body of the affected individual. It occurs in about 0.1% of people who have hypothyroidism. The mortality rate in mixed edema is as high as 40%.

Causes of mixed edema include:

Pituitary gland failure
Hypothalamus failure
Inability of the thyroid gland to produce thyroxin

Drugs and other medical conditions that cause the development of mixed edema in a hypothyroid person include:

Lithium
Narcotics
Sedatives
Anesthesia
Stroke
Infections
Trauma
GI bleeding
Heart failure
Failure of patients to take syntrhoid
Hypothermia etc;

Symptoms of Mixed edema coma include:

Hypothermia
Seizures
Hallucinations
Disorientation
Marked swelling all over the body
Enlargement of the tongue

Loss of hair
Loss of part of eyebrows
Shortness of breath
Bradycardia
Heart failure
Pleural effusion
Fluid around the heart
Constipation
Anemia
Electrolytes abnormalities
Deep voice
Coma etc;

Evaluations of Hypothyroid-Mixedema-coma include:

History and physical examination
T4 and TSH
CBC
Complete blood chemistry profile
Serum B12
Anti-thyroid antibodies
ANA
Rheumatoid factor
ESR
Urinalysis
Chest x-ray
EKG
Echocardiogram
Brain CT
Brain MRI
EEG
Abdominal ultrasound
Ultrasound of the extremities etc;

Prevention and treatments of hypothyroid-mixed edema-coma includes:

Frequent physical examination by a physician
Frequent testing of T4 and TSH
Treatment with synthroid
Treat all medical symptoms associated with hypothyroid- mixed edema
Treat all medical problems caused by hypothyroid- mixed edema etc;

CHAPTER 98

HYPERTHYROIDISM IN
AFRICAN AMERICAN MEN

Hyperthyroidism is divided in two major parts:

1. Hyperthyroidism due to excessive production of thyroid hormones, resulting in the clinical hyperthyroid state
2. Grave's disease has three parts:

    a. A large goiter
    b. Large protruding eyes (exophthalmos)
    c. Skin abnormalities (dermatopathy)

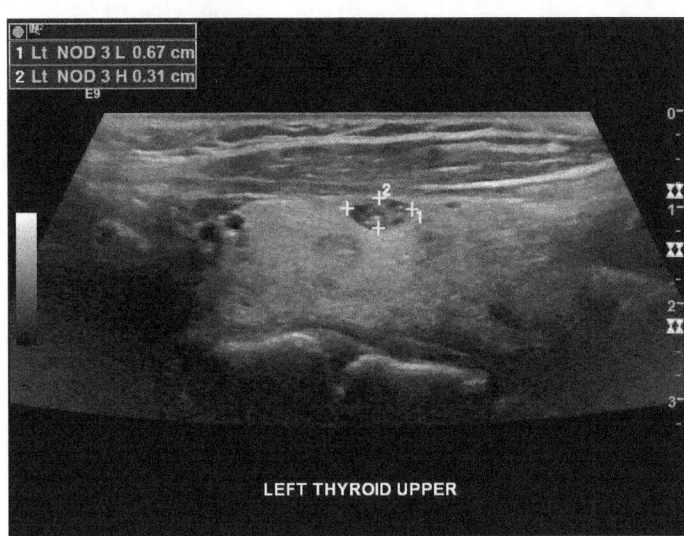

Figure 98:1 Examples of thyroid nodules on sonogram

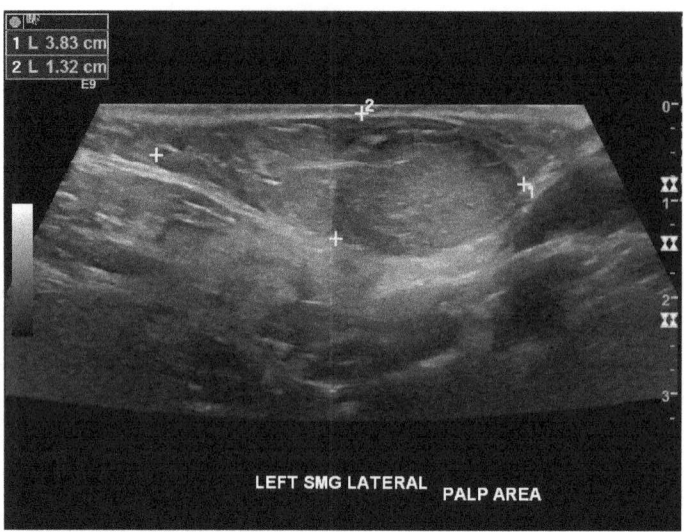

Figure 98:2 Example of thyroid nodules on sonogram

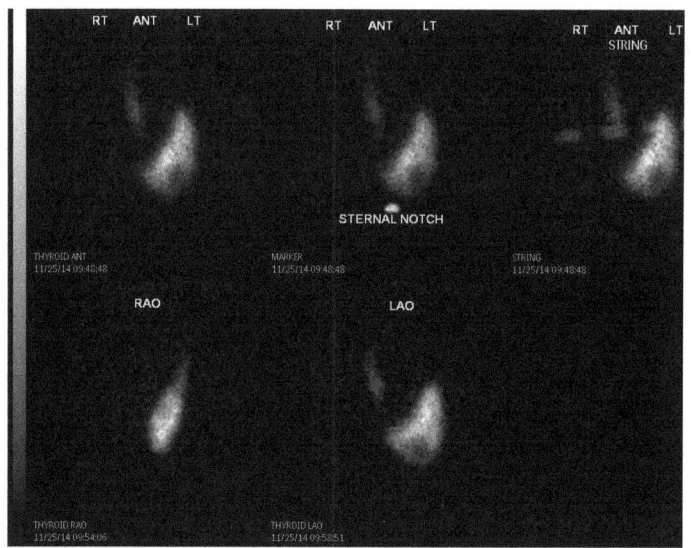

Figure 98:3 example of thyroid nodules on Iodine uptake Scan Symptoms, evaluations, and treatment by hyperthyroidism

The symptoms of hyperthyroidism (overactive thyroid gland) are as follows:

Weight loss
Diarrhea
Agitation
Insomnia
Palpitations
Cardiac arrhythmia
Chest pain

Shortness of breath
Poor appetite
Weakness
Depression
Nervousness
Sweatiness
Warm feeling
Psychosis
Mental confusion
Poor memory
Dementia
Thyroid storm etc;

The usual findings on physical examination of people who are suffering from hyperthyroidism/Graves' disease includes:

1. Large thyroid gland, tender or non-tender
2. Protruding eyes
3. Fine, smooth skin
4. Sweaty palms
5. Fast pulse rate
6. Irregular heartbeat
7. Fluid in the lungs
8. Heart murmur.

Laboratory evaluations in hyperthyroidism consist of:

1. Serum T4, TSH, free T4 and T3
2. ANA
3. B12
4. CBC
5. Reticulocytes count
6. Liver Function Tests
7. Anti-thyroid antibody and anti-microsomal antibodies
8. Thyroid Scan
9. Thyroid ultrasound

In hyperthyroidism, serum T4, T3 and free T4 are high and serum TSH (thyroid-stimulating hormone is low).

There is a subgroup of hyperthyroidism called apathetic hyperthyroidism (or T3 thyrotoxicosis) with high serum T3 and low serum TSH, seen often in elderly people.

These people usually become bed-bound and show no obvious signs of overactive thyroid, except for a fast heart rate, weakness, poor appetite, and poor memory.

The fast heart rate and the apathetic look in the patient's face are the red flags that overactive thyroid is responsible for the patient's total body weakness which, if left untreated, can lead to the death of the affected person.

CHAPTER 99

GRAVE'S DISEASE IN AFRICAN AMERICAN MEN

Graves' disease is a form of hyperthyroidism (overactive thyroid) state, during which the thyroid gland is enlarged and tender. The eyes are markedly enlarged (exophthalmos); the skin areas that are affected are thickened and edematous. The swelling around the eyes is due to infiltration by lymphocytes and mononuclear cells. Graves' disease occurs commonly. Graves' disease may be an autoimmune disease.

"Graves disease is the most common cause of persistent hyperthyroidism in adults. Approximately 3% of women and 0.5% of men will develop Graves disease during their lifetime." JAMA December 15, 2015 Volume 314, Number 23

There exists a link between Graves' disease, Hashimoto's disease, hypothyroidism, pernicious anemia and vitiligo etc.

The evaluations of Graves' disease (hyperthyroidism) are as described earlier. The treatments of Graves' disease are the same as that of other forms hyperthyroidism.

The different types of treatments used to treat hyperthyroidism are as follows: high

1. Surgical removal of part of the thyroid
2. Medication to suppress the thyroid glands' ability to produce thyroid hormone
3. Steroid IV or PO
4. Radioactive iodine to destroy the thyroid glands

Treatments that are preferable to treat hyperthyroidism in women who are pregnant are surgical removal of the thyroid gland or administering Propylthiouracil by mouth. In women who are not in childbearing age or who are elderly, radioactive iodine is preferable.

For people who present with hyperthyroidism and a fast heart rate, Inderal by mouth is given to slow the rate of the heart down to prevent cardiac compensation and possible cardiac arrhythmia that can develop if the heart rate is allowed to remain fast.

Whether or not the treatment is given inside the hospital or in the office setup depends on the judgment of the treating physician and or how sick the patient looks.

The next thing to do is to give medication to shut down the production of thyroid hormones. The most frequently used anti-thyroid medications are Propylthiouracil and Tapazole. The usual dose of Propylthiouracil is 100 to 150 mg every 6 or 8 hours, by mouth. Propylthiouracil works to decrease the symptoms of hyperthyroidism by preventing the conversion of T4 to T3 in the bloodstream. Tapazole works to decrease the symptoms of hyperthyroidism by inhibiting the production of thyroid hormone by the thyroid gland.

The usual dose of Tapazole is 30–40mg in divided doses 2–3 times per day by mouth.

In the acute hyperthyroidism state to prevent the so-called thyroid storm, large doses of Dexamethasone 2 grams every 6 hours IV can be given in addition, to reduce the level of T4 in the body, thereby improving the overall condition of the affected person.

Either Propylthiouracil or Tapazole can be used for up to 2 years, while a decision is being made regarding a long-term modality of treatment. During the administration of these medications, a complete blood count must be done every month or so, because leukopenia and low platelet count can develop.

When it is decided based on clinical facts and the appropriate patients that radioactive iodine is the treatment modality, an endocrinologist will administer the proper dose of radioactive iodine to the patient to destroy the thyroid gland.

Following the administration of the radioactive iodine, the patient will be monitored for many years, waiting for the development of the hypothyroidism state, which is guaranteed to develop in time. When the T4 and TSH evaluation indicates that the patient has developed hypothyroidism, then Synthroid by mouth for life will be given to her.

CHAPTER 100

PRIMARY HYPERPARATHYROID DISAESES IN AFRICAN AMERICAN MEN

There are 4 parathyroid glands in the human body and they are located in the neck. The role of the of the parathyroid glands are to secrete parathyroid hormone (PTH) to keep a proper level of calcium and phosphorus in the body.

Parathyroid hormone (PTH) plays a key role in both Vitamin D and magnesium levels in the human body.

When one or more of these glands developed an adenoma (a benign) tumor, or when hyperplasia develops in these glands, the serum calcium becomes elevated. On rare occasions, cancer can develop in the parathyroid gland causing elevated serum calcium as well.

Primary hyperparathyroidism

"Primary hyperparathyroidism is caused by a solitary adenoma in 80% to 85% of cases and genetic endocrine disorder in 10 % to 15% of cases, less than 1% of primary hyperparathyroidism is due to parathyroid cancer." Source: American Journal of Medicine October 2011, volume 124 Number 10

Primary hyperparathyroidism develops in 1 in 1000 people in the U.S. secondary Hyperparathyroidism develops usually in people with chronic kidney failure causing low level of vitamin D is in the body.

Risks for primary hyperparathyroidism include:

Idiopathic hyperparathyroidism
Familial hyperparathyroidism
Obesity
Menopause
Depression
Multiple endocrine neoplasia type 1
Treatment with lithium
Radiation treatment to the neck etc;

Hyperparathyrodism is more common in women than men.

Many patients with primary hyperparathyroidism are asymptomatic. Those with symptoms usually have serum calcium in the range of 12 mg/dL or 14 mg/dL. Serum calcium higher than 15 mg/dL can cause serious symptoms.

Symptoms of primary hyperparathyroidism include:

Fatigue
Weakness
Seizure
Cardiac arrhythmias
Osteoporosis
Abdominal pain
Frequent urination
Kidney stones
Bones and joints pain
Depression
Loss of appetite
Nausea
Vomiting
Muscle soreness
Muscle weakness
Constipation
Dementia
Increase thirst
Dyspepsia
Peptic ulcer
Anemia
Osteitis fibrosa cystica
Urinary frequency
Memory loss
Anxiety etc.

Parathyroid hormone increases serum calcium level in the blood by bleaching calcium from bones, which in turn leads to osteoporosis, kidney stones etc. In addition, there is increased calcium absorption from the diet, as well as increased kidney reabsorption of calcium caused by a high level of 1,25-hydroxy vitamin D.

The evaluation of a person suspected of having hyperparathyroidism include:

History and physical examination
CBC
Complete metabolic (chemistry) profile including serum calcium
Urinalysis
24 hours urine calcium

Serum IGG, IGM, IGA, IGD
Serum immuno electrophoresis
Urine immuno electrophoresis
Serum PTH
Serum Phosphorus level
Serum magnesium level
EKG
Chest x-ray
Chest CT
Bone density
Ultrasound of the neck
Sestamibi Scan
Endoscopic examination of the stomach
Surgical Consult

If the parathyroid hormone is elevated or normal, and serum calcium is high along with low serum phosphorus, the diagnosis of primary hyperparathyroidism is confirmed. The next most important non-surgical test to do to fully establish the diagnosis is to show parathyroid adenoma on the Sestamibi nuclear test.

Treatments of Primaryhyperparatroidism:

Once these things are done, the next step is surgical intervention to remove the adenoma from the parathyroid gland or glands.

If the parathyroid glands are found to have hyperplasic tissues in them, the surgeon will remove some of glands as a treatment. Surgeons always leave on parathyroid gland so that the patient can have parathyroid endocrine function. If the patient refuses surgery and is not able to have surgery, Sensipar (cinacalcet) can be used to treat patients with high calcium due to primary hyperparathyroidism. The usual dose of Sensipar is 30 mcg per day by mouth.

People with primary hyperparathyroidism seem to suffer more serious complications because there are always delays in making their diagnoses due to lateness in presentation for medical evaluations and treatment.

CHAPTER 101

SECONDARY HYPERPARATHYROIDISM IN AFRICAN AMERICAN MEN

Secondary hyperparathyroidism is more common in blacks and other minorities than in their white counterparts because blacks and other minorities suffer more from hypertension and diabetes mellitus than do whites.

Hypertension and diabetes frequently cause chronic kidney failure, and kidney failure causes secondary hyperparathyroidism.

Secondary hyperparathyroidism is due to low serum calcium, low vitamin D and low magnesium in the body.

Conditions that cause low calcium and secondary hyperparathyroidism include:

Kidney failure
Dietary calcium deficiency
Vitamin D deficiency
Malabsorption
Low magnesium

Lactose intolerance is very common in all ethnic groups. People with lactose intolerance are able to tolerate dairy products in their diets. Dairy products contain vitamin D and calcium.

Vitamin D is made in the body under the skin by the action of the rays of the sun and the darker the skin the more difficult it is for the rays of the sun to penetrate the skin to stimulate the production of vitamin D. Nine percent of Blacks and other people with dark skin have low vitamin D. Seventy percent of Whites and Asians have low vitamin low.

Parathyroid hormone (PTH) is needed for calcium metabolism and the concentration of calcium in the blood stream controls the secretion of parathyroid hormone. When the circulating calcium is low and the level of phosphate is high the parathyroid is left unchecked and over secretes parathyroid hormone.

The over secretion of PTH leads to removal of calcium from bones causing osteomalacia, low phosphorus, low magnesium. This complex of abnormalities can cause renal tubular acidosis (kidney disease) because of excretion of excess magnesium and phosphorus in the urine.

Magnesium is needed in normal amount in the blood stream in order for the parathyroid gland to function normally.

Low serum magnesium, low phosphorus, low calcium and low vitamin D cause over activation of the Parathyroid glands leading to secondary hyperparathyroidism, osteomalacia and if severe Rickets.

Rickets/Osteomalacia is treated with vitamin D, magnesium, and neutrophos by mouth.

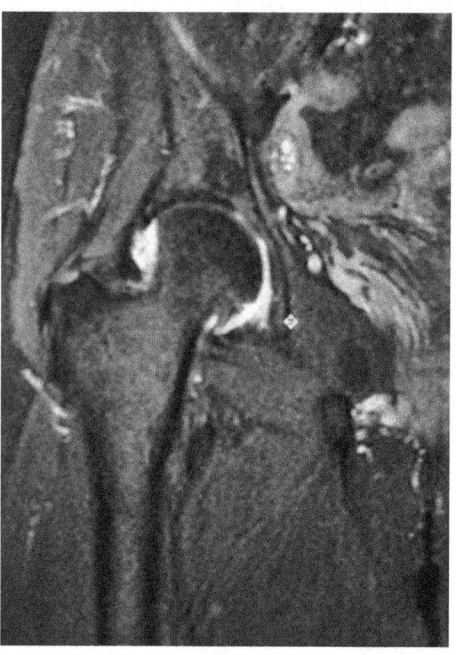

Figure 101:1 *MRI of the bone of an adult person with Rickets' Osteomalacia due to secondary hyperparathyroidism.*

The treatments of secondary hyperparathyroidism include:

Calcimimetic is approved by the FDA to treat hypocalcaemia due to cancer of the parathyroid gland and secondary hyperparathyroidism.

Sensipar 60mcg per day is used to treat people with primary and secondary hyperparathyroidism and kidney failure.

Tertiary hyperparathyroidism

Tertiary hyperparathyroidism develops when the parathyroid secretes parathyroid hormone for a very long time due secondary hyperparathyroidism insipte of medical treatments. The treatment of choice of tertiary hyperparathyroidism is surgical removal of the parathyroid adenoma.

CHAPTER 102

VITAMIN D DEFICIENCY IN AFRICAN AMERICAN MEN

Ninety percent of African Americans, Hispanics and other people with dark skins and seventy five percent of white people have either vitamin D deficiency or vitamin D insufficiency. Seventy percent of white Americans are vitamin D deficient and seventy-five of the world population suffers from vitamin deficiency. Poor diet is responsible for a significant percentage of low vitamin D.

The reasons for low vitamin D include:

Lack of sun exposure
Darkness of skin
Lactose intolerance
Diet deficient of vitamin D containing foods
Chronic pancreatitis
Malabsorption
Primary hyperparathyroidism
Secondary hyperparathyroidism
Rickets
Kidney failure
Liver failure
Low serum magnesium

The darkness of the skin of Negroes and all people whose skins are dark makes it very difficult for the sun's rays to penetrate their skins to stimulate the production of vitamin D whose precursor is located under the skin on one hand. On the other hand, seventy five percent of Negroes suffer from lactose intolerance to one degree or another preventing them from eating or drinking dairy products that contain lactose. There are 2 main forms of vitamin D in the human body, vitamin D2 and vitamin D3.

Negroes and other dark skin people who live in tropical countries and specially those work in the farms and other outdoor occupations have good level of vitamin D because of the fact their skins are more exposed to the rays of the sun than those who live the developed countries and have less sun exposure.

Seventy percent adults in the world population suffer from lactose intolerance. Fifty million Americans suffer from lactose intolerance. "Seventy percent African Americans, Jewish, Native Americans, Mexican Americans and ninety percent of Asian Americans suffer from lactose intolerance."

When the precursor of vitamin D is 7-Dehydrocholesterol under the skin is exposed to UVA rays of the sun, it becomes stimulated and produced cholecalciferol Vitamin D, which provides 90% percent of the vitamin D that human beings need.

Once in the body, vitamin D3 is taken to the liver through the blood stream where it is converted to vitamin D2 25-hydroxyvitamin D2 or calcidiol, then the calcidiol goes to kidneys to be converted to calcitriol, the active form of vitamin D, 125-Dihydroxyvitamin D.

Vitamin D has many functions in the human body including absorption of calcium and phosphorous from the gastrointestinal tract for bone health.

Other sources of Vitamin D include:

Cheese
Milk
Eggs
Salmon
Sardines
Herring
Mackle
Cod liver oil
Tuna
Cereal
Beef liver
Some mushrooms etc.

Some of the diseases that low vitamin D can cause include:

Lactose intolerance
Secondary hyperparathyroidism
Osteoporosis
Kidney disease (low vitamin D can cause kidney disease and chronic kidney causes low vitamin D)
Hypertension (low vitamin D causes over activation of the rennin angiotensin aldosterone system which causes high blood pressure)
Low serum phosphorous
Low serum magnesium
Low serum calcium
High parathyroid hormone
Osteomalacia
Renal tubular acidosis

Rickets
Obesity
Seasonal Affective Disorder (this condition occurs during winter months when there is lack of sun light, it is treated with light therapy)
Immunodeficiency etc;

Lactose in.tolerance occurs in all racial groups, but is more common in Blacks and other dark skin people.

This condition develops when the enzyme lactase, which is located in the wall of the bowel, is deficient making it hard if not impossible for the sugar lactose, which is found in all dairy products to be broken down, leading to abdominal cramps, excessive gas and diarrhea.

The end result is that people who are lactose intolerant avoid dairy products in their diets causing them to become vitamin D deficiency/insufficiency.

Other medical conditions that are associated with low vitamin D include:

Diabetes mellitus
Cancer
Heart disease
Congestive heart failure
Multiple sclerosis
Dementia
High serum potassium
Bone fractures
Kidney stones
Tetany
Infertility
Recurrent miscarriages
Erectal dysfunction
Depression etc.

Evaluations of vitamin D deficiency/insufficiency include:

History and physical examination
Serum 25-hydroxyvitamin D
Complete blood chemistry profile
Serum parathyroid hormone
Serum magnesium
Serum phosphorous
CBC
Complete blood chemistry profile
Urinalysis
Chest x-ray

EKG
Bone density
Skeletal survey
Kidney stone abdominal CT protocol
The normal of 25-hydroxyvitamin D 3 is 30 ng/mL to 100 ng/mL
Vitamin D deficiency exists when the blood level is 1ng/mL to 10 ng/mL
Vitamin D insufficiency exists when the blood level is 11ng/mL to 29 ng/mL

Treatments of vitamin D include:

Treatments of vitamin D deficiency level 10 or less are vitamin D 50,000 units twice per week for 8 weeks and eating vitamin D rich foods.

Treatments of vitamin D insufficiency level 10 – 15 ng include vitamin D 50,000 units twice per week for 8 weeks and treatments for vitamin D level from 15 ng/mL to 25ng/mL include vitamin D 4000 units daily and for vitamin D level 26 ng/mL to 29 ng/mL and vitamin D level of 29 ng/mL to 30 ng/mL can be treated with vitamin D2000 units daily and eating vitamin D rich foods.

After 8 weeks of treatments the blood level of vitamin D should repeated and treatments with vitamin D adjusted according to the level.

It is a good idea for Blacks and all dark skin people to have their level of vitamin D tested regularly because ninety percent of them 90% of them and 75% of other people have low vitamin D. More than one in two black adults and one out of three other American adults have elevated blood pressure, and as outlined above, the lower their vitamin D levels the harder it is to control their blood pressures.

Low vitamin D over activates the renin angiotensin-aldosterone system leading to secondary hyperaldosteronism, which causes salt and fluid retention resulting in hypertension.

High blood pressure is the number one disease in black people and 1 in three American adults suffers from hypertension and 1 in two Black American adults suffers from hypertension and most of them have either untreated or poorly treated blood pressure to begin with, and when you add low vitamin D to that equation, Blacks and these other hypertensive individuals in America and around the world have zero chance of living healthy lives.

The 50,000 units dose of vitamin D have to be prescribed, but other doses can be bought over the counter and lactose free milk and other dairy products and be bought by those who have lactose intolerant and Lactaid can also be taken by lactose intolerant people.

Prevention of low vitamin D:

African Americans, other black people around the world and people who have dark skin and all people have to make an effort to get more sun exposure and must play closer attention to their diets by eating more vitamin D rich containing foods.

For those who cannot tolerate dairy products can use Lacaid to prevent the symptoms of lactose intolerance.

CHAPTER 103

HEMOPHILIAS IN AFRICAN AMERICAN MEN

Hemophilia A is a disease caused by a deficiency of factor VIII. This deficiency prevents the blood from clotting. Hemophilia is inherited as an X-linked recessive trait. The gene is defective on the x chromosome. Hemophilia A is seen mostly in males because males have only one X chromosome and that X chromosome is always the carrier of the disease.

Women have two X-chromosome so, if one X chromosome were to be defective for factor VIII, the other X chromosome would work well to prevent hemophilia A in women.

Worldwide, there are 6.9 milllion people with hemophilia and 80% of them have hemophilia A. and 20% have hemophilia B.

In the U.S. 20,000 people have hemophilia and 20% of them have hemophilia B and 80% have hemophilia A. "75% of people with hemophilia do not know they have it".

Signs and symptoms of hemophilia A include:

Easy bruising
Nosebleed
Bleeding from the gums
Bleeding into joints
Hematuria (blood in the urine)
Blood in the stools
Vomiting blood
Heavy and prolonged bleeding when cut
Heavy and prolonged bleeding after surgery
Heavy and prolonged bleeding after tooth extraction
Spontaneous bleeding etc

Evaluations of hemophilia A include:

History and physical examination
Prothombin time (PT is normal in hemophilia A)
Partial Thromboplastin time (PTT is high in hemophilia A)

Factor VIII level (In hemophilia A factor VIII level is low)
Bleeding time (is normal in hemophilia A)
Fibrinogen level (is normal in hemophilia A)
HIV 1 and 2 blood tests
CBC
Complete blood chemistry profile
Serum ferritin
Urinalysis
Stool hemoccult
ABO blood typing
Type and screen
Hepatitis A, B, C, E. screen
VDRL

Treatments of hemophilia A include:

Hepatitis A and B vaccinations
Factor VIII concentrate
Fresh frozen plasma
Blood transfusion
Desmopressing (DDAVP) for minor surgical procedures

Hemophilia B or factor IX deficiency is an X-linked recessive disease with the abnormality located on the X chromosome. Worldwide there are 400,000 people with hemophilia and 20% or 80,000 of them have hemophilia B.

In the U.S. there are 18,000 people with hemophilia and 20% or 3,600 of them have hemophilia B. Hemophilia affects mainly men. Women who carry the abnormality on one of their two X chromosomes for hemophilia B are carriers and usually do not manifest the bleeding abnormality because women have two X chromosomes and as such, the good x chromosome protect them from the clinical manifestation of the disease.

Hemophilia B or factor IX deficiency affects men only because men have one X-chromosome and that X chromosome carries the hereditary abnormality in men who are at risk for the disease.

Signs and symptoms of hemophilia B include:

Bruising
Nosebleed
Bleeding gums
Blood in the urine
Blood in the stool
Excessive bleeding after circumcision
Gastrointestinal bleeding
Heavy and prolonged bleeding after cut

Heavy and prolonged bleeding after tooth extraction
Heavy and prolonged bleeding after surgical procedures
Spontaneous bleeding;

Evaluations of hemophilia B include:

History and physical examination
Prothrombin time (PT is normal in hemophilia B)
Partial Thrombostatin time (PTT is high in hemophilia B)
Factor IX level (In hemophilia B factor IX level is low)
Fibrinogen level (is normal in hemophilia B)
Bleeding time (is normal in hemophilia B)
HIV 1&2 blood test
VDRL
CBC
Complete blood chemistry profile
Urinalysis
Serum ferritin
Stool hemoccult
Hepatitis A, B, C, E screen
ABO blood typing
Type and screen

Treatments of hemophilia B include:

Factor IX concentrates
Fresh frozen plasma
Blood transfusion
Hepatitis A and B vaccination;

CHAPTER 104

PRIMARY POLYCYTHEMIA VERA IN AFRICAN AMERICAN MEN

Plocythemia Vera is an incurable chronic blood disease that results in the production of too many reb blood cells, platelets and white blood cells by the bone marrow. (Pancytosis)

The most significant manifestation of P. Vera is the over production of red blood cells rendering the blood too thick. P. Vera usually affects people 60 or over but, there are exceptions. About 100,000 people are living with P. Vera in the U.S. and million more People around the world.

Because the blood is so viscous (thick) it cause
Stroke
Heart attack
Thrombosis
Pulmonary embolism etc;

Signs and symptoms of P. Vera include:

Headaches
Dizziness
Weakness
Double vision
Enlarged spleen
Severe burning pain in hands and feet
Itching all over the body
Itching after warm or hot showers or baths
Fullness below left rib cage-due enlarged spleen
Reddish of palms of hands
Redness of face
Bluishness of skin
Gouty arthritic pain in joints
Peptic ulcer

Evaluations of P. Vera include:

History and physical examination
CBC
Complete blood chemistry profile
Serum uric acid
ESR
Serum ferritin in P. Vera the serum ferritin is low to zero because all the iron is used to make red blood cells.
Serum uric acid
Bone marrow aspiration
Bone marrow biopsy
Serum erythropoietin level
Serum JAK 2 kinase (JAK2 mutation is a member Janus kinase family) 100 percent of people with P. Vera has JAK2 mutation.
Abdominal ultrasound
Abdominal CT
Chest x-ray
EKG
D-dimer
ABG
Ultrasound of lower extremities
Lung Scan

Complications of P. Vera include:

TIA
Stroke
Heart attacks
Cardiomyopathy
Congestive heart failure
Budd-Chiari
Hepatic vein thrombosis
Renal vein thrombosis
Retinal arterial/ vein thrombosis
General arterial thrombosis
Myelofibrosis
Dementia
Acute myelocytic leukemia
Gout
P. Vera is more common in Jews of European extraction as compared to other ethnic groups.

Treatments of P. Vera include:

Phlebotomy
Hydroxyurea
The FDA has just approved Ruxolitinib to treat Polycythemia Vera.

CHAPTER 105

SECONDARY POLYCYTHEMIA IN AFRICAN AMERICAN MEN

Secondary polycythemia is a condition during which the level of red blood cells in the circulation is too high.

The conditions that cause secondary polycythemia include:

Living at high altitude
Hypoxia due to COPD/emphysema
Sleep Apnea
Hypernephroma
Hepatoma
Dehydration
Atrial septal defect
Patent ductus arteriosus
Ventricular septal defect
Aortic stenosis
Pulmonary stenosis
Atrioventricular canal defect
Tetralogy of Fallot
Transposition of the great arteries
Totanomalous pulmonary venous return
Tricuspid atresia
Persistent truncus arteriosus
Hypoplastic left heart
Pulmonary atresia
Ebstein's anomaly
Hemoglobin Chesapeake
Hemoglobin Kempsey
Pheochromocytoma
Cushing's syndrome
Anabolic steroid
Exccessive use of Procrit/Epogen
Dehydration etc;

Every year there are about 1.5 million new cases of congenital heart disease in the world. The cyanosis associated with congenital heart disease causes secondary polycythemia. In hypernephroma and hepatoma too much erythropeitin is produced leading to too much red blood cells in the circulation resulting in polycythemia and hyperviscosity.

Evalutions of secondary polychytemia include:

History and physical examination
CBC
Complete blood chemistry profile
Urinalysis
Hemoglobin electrophoresis
Plasma Erythropoeitin level
Plasma Catecholamine level
Serum uric acid
Arterial blood Gas (ABG)
Pulmonary function test (PFT)
Chest x-ray
EKG
Echocardiogram
Abdominal ultrasound
Abdominal CT etc.

Treatments of secondary polycythemia include:

Medical treatments of the underline problem or problems causing the secondary polycythemia
Surgical treatments of the underline problem or problems causing the secondary polycythemia
Cessation of the use anabolic steroid
Cessation of the use of Procrit/Epogen, unless prescribed by a physician.
Phlebotomy as needed (removal of blood)

Complications of secondary of secondary polycythemia include:

Stroke
Myocardial infarction (heart attack)
Congestive heart failure (CHF)
Renal vein thrombosis
Retinal vein thrombosis
Arterial thrombosis
Gout etc;

CHAPTER 106

ESSENTIAL THROMBOCYTHEMIA IN AFRICAN AMERICAN MEN

Essential thrombocythemia is a rare blood disease characterized by over production of platelets by megakariocytes in the bone marrow. Every year about 7,000 people are diagnosed with essential thrombocythemia in the U.S. and several hundred thousand people across the world have essential trhombocytemia.

Signs and symptoms of essential thrombocythemia include:

High platelets count
High white cells count
Normal red cells count (hematocrit)
Normal serum ferritin (This is the absolute key point in differentiating between P. Vera and ET) In P. Vera the serum ferritin/serum iron is low to zero and ET the serum ferritin/iron is Normal. In P. Vera all the iron is used to make red blood cells.
Nosebleed
Gum bleed
Gastrointestinal bleed
Throbbing of hands
Throbbing of feet
Burning of feet
Burning of hands
Petechiaes over lower legs (little red dots over lower legs)
Burning of legs (due to the occlusion small arterioles –erythromelalgia)
Enlarged spleen
Positive JAK2 in 50% of people with ET
Normal serum ferritin
No evidence of myelofibrosis

Evaluations of essential thrombocythemia include:

History and physical examination
CBC
Complete metabolic chemistry profile
LDH

753

ESR
Serum ferritin
JAK2
Bone marrow aspiration
Bone marrow biopsy

Treatments of essential thrombocythemia include:

Hydroxyurea
Anagrelide
Aspirin (for erythromelalgia)
" Telomerase Inhibitor Imetelstat in Patients with Essential Thrombocythemia ."

Complications of essential thrombocythemia include:

Myelofibrosis
Acute myelocytic leukemia
Stroke etc;

CHAPTER 107

MYELOFIBROSIS IN AFRICAN AMERICAN MEN

Myelofibrosis is a myeloproliferative disease that develops when abnormal hematopoietic produce cytokines such as fibroblast growth factor from the megakyocytes causes replacement of normal hematopoietic cells in the bone marrow by collagen fibrosis. This process prevents production of normal new blood cells in the bone marrow resulting in chronic pancytopenia.

The body's response to this process is to make the cells that the bone marrow is not able to make and make them in the spleen resulting in marked enlargement of the spleen.

About 200,000 of people in the U.S. are living with myelofibrosis and several hundred thousands more around the world.

Signs and symptoms of myelofibrosis include:

Low white blood cells
Low red blood cells
Low platelets
Low reticulocytes count
High MCV
Fatigue
Easy bruising
Easy bleeding
Bone pain
Enlarged spleen
Enlarged liver
Abdominal fullness
Left sided abdominal pain due to enlarged spleen
Pallor
Shortness of breath due anemia
Congestive heart failure due to the anemia
Susceptibility to infection due to low white cells
High serum uric acid due to rapid cell turns over
Gout etc;

Evaluations of myelofibrosis include:

History and physical examination
CBC
Complete metabolic chemistry profile
Reticulocytes count
JAK2 screening
Bone marrow aspiration
Bone marrow biopsy
Abdominal sonogram
Abdominal CT
Abdominal MRI

Treatments of myelofibrosis include:

Blood transfusion
Procrit
Epogen
Prednisone 40mg per day
Danazol 600mg per day
Thalidomide 50mg per day
Ruxolitinib is recently approved by the FDA as an inhibitor of JAK1 and JAK2 to treat the splenomegaly and its symptoms in myelofibrosis
"Telomerase Inhibitor Imetelstat in Patients with Myelofibrosis."

Complications of myelofibrosis include:

Acute myelocytic leukemia
Pneumonia
Sepsis
Congestive heart failure
Bone marrow failure
Death.

CHAPTER 108

PARKINSON DISEASE IN AFRICAN AMERICAN MEN

Parkinson disease is a form of degenerative disease of the central nervous system. The constellation of symptoms seen in Parkinson disease is the of the death of dopamine Generating cells in the subtantia nigra part of the midbrain, why these cells die, no one knows. In addition, Parkinson disease is characterized with accumulation of alpha-synuclein protein and Lewy bodies in the neurons in the midbrain. Parkinson disease develops in people who are 50 years and older.

A recent report published in Current Biology, "brain cells in Parkinson's disease exhaust themselves and prematurely". BBC News 8/28/15 Causes of Parkinson disease include genetic and abnormal mutations seen in LRRK2 and recurrent trauma to the brain such as that seen in Boxers and some other sports.

Parkinson disease is classified as:

Primary
Idiopathic
Secondary or acquired
Hereditary
Age
Sex (PD is more common in men than women)
Exposure to herbicides
Exposure to pesticides and other toxins

Worldwide, there are 10 million living people with Parkinson disease and in the U.S. there are 1 million people living with Parkinson's disease.

Early symptoms of Parkinson disease include:

Shaking (tremors)
Rigidity of muscles
Impaired posture and balance
Loss of autonomic movements
Slow movements (bradykinesia)

Difficulty walking
Speech changes
Writing changes

Late symptoms of Parkinson disease include:

Thinking problems
Behavior problems
Depression
Hallucinations
Delusions
Apathy
Anxiety
Psychosis
Indifference
Sensory problems
Sleep disorder
Difficulty swallowing
Constipation
Urinary incontinence
Abnormality in smelling
Pain
Speech disorder
Mood disorder
Cognition disorder
Decreased facial expression
Binge eating
Drop in blood pressure
Dizziness
Fatigue
Overuse of medications
Hyper sexuality
Pathological gambling
Dementia etc;

Evaluations of Parkinson disease include:

History and physical examination
Neurological examination by a neurologist
Examination by a Psychiatrist
Brain CT
Brain MRI with and without IV contrast
Diffusion MRI of the brain
Measurement of dopaminergic function using PET Scan or SPECT radiotracers
CBC

Complete metabolic chemistry profile
Urinalysis
T4 and TSH
Serum B12
RPR
PPD skin test
HIV 1 and 2 blood tests
PSA in men
Chest x-ray
Abdominal CT etc;

Prevention of Parkinson disease includes:

Vitamin C
Vitamin D
Caffeine consumption
Tobacco smoking (nicotine seems to stimulate dopamine production (however tobacco is bad for people's health and ought to be avoided).

Treatments of Parkinson disease include:

Amantadine 100mg bid
Levadopa 25/100 mg
Carbidopa 10/100 mg bid
Sinemet 50/200
Rivastigmine 1.5 mg bid
Entacapone 200mg
Tocapone 100mg
Rasagline 0.5mg
Selegiline 1.25mg
Cogentin 0.5mg
Trihexphenidyl 2mg
Ropinirole 0.25 mg
Mirapex 3mg
APOKYN injection .02ml
Mirapex 0.25mg
Beomocriptine 2.5mg
The FDA to treat Parkinson disease has just approved Rytary
Fixed Body Sensors can be used to properly "quantify the quality and duration of different daily activities".
DBS surgery to treat Parkinson disease.

CHAPTER 109

SPORTS ASSOCIATED /POST TRAUMATIC BRAIN INJURY IN AFRICAN AMERICAN MEN

Sport associated acute and chronic brain injury is very common and can lead to Parkinson's disease, dementia and many other serious neurological complications

The sports associated with brain injuries include:

Boxing
NLF football
Soccer
Ice Hockey
Wrestling
Martial arts
Rugby
Basketball
Softball

"Of 23,566 reported injuries in the 10 sports during the 3-year study period, 1219 (5.5%) were MTBIs. Of the MTBIs, football accounted for 773 (63.4%) of cases; wrestling, 128 (10.5%); girls' soccer, 76 (6.2%); boys' soccer, 69 (5.7%); girls' basketball, 63 (5.2%); boys' basketball, 51 (4.2%); softball, 25 (2.1%); baseball, 15 (1.2%); field hockey, 13 (1.1%); and volleyball, 6 (0.5%). The injury rates per 100 player-seasons were 3.66 for football, 1.58 for wrestling, 1.14 for girls' soccer, 1.04 for girls' basketball, 0.92 for boys' soccer, 0.75 for boys' basketball, 0.46 for softball, 0.46 for field hockey, 0.23 for baseball, and 0.14 for volleyball. The median time lost from participation for all MTBIs was 3 days. There were 6 cases of subdural hematoma and intracranial injury reported in football. Based on these data, an estimated 62,816 cases of MTBI occur annually among high school varsity athletes participating in these sports, with football accounting for about 63% of cases."

"JAMA July 25, 2017

Clinicopathological Evaluation of Chronic Traumatic Encephalopathy in Players of American Football

"**Findings** In a convenience sample of 202 deceased players of American football from a brain donation program, CTE was neuropathologically diagnosed in 177 players across all levels of play (87%), including 110 of 111 former National Football League players (99%)."

"**Results** Among 202 deceased former football players (median age at death, 66 years [interquartile range, 47-76 years]), CTE was neuropathologically diagnosed in 177 players (87%; median age at death, 67 years [interquartile range, 52-77 years]; mean years of football participation, 15.1 [SD, 5.2]), including 0 of 2 pre–high school, 3 of 14 high school (21%), 48 of 53 college (91%), 9 of 14 semiprofessional (64%), 7 of 8 Canadian Football League (88%), and 110 of 111 National Football League (99%) players. Neuropathological severity of CTE was distributed across the highest level of play, with all 3 former high school players having mild pathology and the majority of former college (27 [56%]), semiprofessional (5 [56%]), and professional (101 [86%]) players having severe pathology. Among 27 participants with mild CTE pathology, 26 (96%) had behavioral or mood symptoms or both, 23 (85%) had cognitive symptoms, and 9 (33%) had signs of dementia. Among 84 participants with severe CTE pathology, 75 (89%) had behavioral or mood symptoms or both, 80 (95%) had cognitive symptoms, and 71 (85%) had signs of dementia. Source: JAMA. 2017;318 (4):360-370."

The most common TBIs in sports are cerebral contusion, second impact concussions, dementia pugilistica, and hematomas, Parkinson's disease, seizures etc.

Symptoms of concussion include:

Physical abnormalities
Cognitive abnormalities
Emotional abnormalities
Sleep disturbances
Headache
Irritability
Fatigue
Dizziness
Nausea
Vomiting
Memory loss
Posttraumatic amnesia
Loss of consciousness 10 percent of the time
Players suspected of suffering from concussion most be removed from the game and must undergo
a concussion protocol.

Signs of immediate cerebral contusion include:

Headache
Slurred speech
Nausea
Vomiting
Dilated pupils
Restlessness
Memory loss
Seizures etc;

Post game symptoms concussion include:

Loss of consciousness
Severe headaches
Loss of consciousness
Coma
Evaluations of concussion include:
History
Physical examination Neurological examination by a neurologist
Brain CT
Brain MRI
EEG

Complications of sport associated traumatic brain injury (TBI) include:

Chronic Traumatic Brain (CTB) occurs in about 20 percent of professional boxers
Dementia Pugilistica (Punch-Drunk Syndrome)
Hematoma
Chronic Traumatic Encephalopathy (CTE)
Parkinson 's disease
Depression
Insomnia
Anger
Irritability
Psychosis
Loss of appetite
Headache
Vision difficulty
Tremor
Poor hygiene
Confusion

"87 out 98-deceased NFL's player's brains revealed evidence of chronic traumatic encephalopathy

In another published study conducted at Boston at the Boston University School of Medicine 33 out of 34 NFL's players who died revealed CTE."

"4500 former NLF players have joined a class action lawsuit against the NFL alleging that it had covered up a growing body of evidence about the preponderance of head-trauma related CTE in ex-NFL players."
Suicide

Treatments of Chronic traumatic brain injury include:

Pain medications
Sleeping medications
Anti-depression medications
Anti-Psychotic medications
Anti-Parkinson medications
Aricept
Namenda
Namzaric
Anti-headache medications etc;

To decrease /eliminate the incidence of sport associated traumatic brain injury, newer head gears/helmets should be used, and newer rules should be instituted to decrease the incidence of blows to the head. In addition, sticker concussion protocols must be created and enforced to prevent players who suffer with concussion from returning on the field play too soon.

CHAPTER 110

DEMENTIA IN AFRICAN AMERICAN MEN

Dementia is a disease that affects people all over the world.

Worldwide 6.2% or 44.4 million people have dementia, 8.8% of women and 3.1% men have dementia. In the U.S. 7.7 million people have 85 or older have dementia. Alzheimer's disease affects 5.2 million people in the U.S.

"According to a just published report, the worldwide incidence of AD has increased to 47 millions AP 8/26/15."

Forty to fifty percent of people who have dementia have micro-vascular or multi-infarct dementia. 3 % of people ages 65-74 have dementia, 47% of people over age 85 have dementia.

"Nearly one-third of dementia cases preventable based on lifestyle factors, report finds

The Washington Post 7/20, 2017 reports a study presented on Thursday at the Alzheimer's Association International Conference in London found that nearly one-third of the world's dementia cases are preventable through managing "factors such as education, hypertension, diet, hearing loss and depression over the course of a person's lifetime." Researchers found that controlling the factors could reduce one's risk of developing dementia by 35 percent."

"HealthDay 7/18, 2017 reports that the CDC "report [pdf] found that nearly one in four adults with diabetes didn't even know they had the disease, and less than 12 percent with prediabetes knew they had that condition." CDC Director Brenda Fitzgerald, MD, stated, "More than a third of US adults have prediabetes, and the majority don't know it." In a news release, Fitzgerald added, "Now, more than ever, we must step up our efforts to reduce the burden of this serious disease." "

The different types and causes of dementia include:

Alzheimer's disease
Multi-infarct dementia
Parkinson's disease associated dementia
Down's syndrome
Autism
AIDS dementia

Metabolic disorders
Hypoglycemia (recurrent)
Hypothyroidism
B12 deficiency
Low vitamin D
Lewy body dementia (1.5 million Americans have Lewy body dementia)
Pick's disease of brain dementia
Frontotemporal dementia
Normal pressure hydrocephalus dementia
Progressive supranuclear palsy dementia
Corticobasal degeneration dementia
Creutzfeldt-Jakob disease dementia
Neuro-syphillis

Many elderly people who suffer with dementia do so because of Vitamin B12 deficiency that was not diagnosed and treated in time. Chronic hypothyroidism can also cause dementia. After 5 years without treatment with B12 in those who are B12 deficient, its symptoms are not reversible.

There are 77 million adults with hypertension in the U.S. and 30-40% of these individuals do not know that they have hypertension. 1 in 3 adults in the U.S. have hypertension and 1 in 2 adults Negroes/Blacks have hypertension in the U.S.

Forty percent of all deaths in Negroes/Blacks in the U.S. are due to hypertension. Of all the people with Hypertension in the U.S. only about 20-30 of them being treated for hypertension.

As far as Blacks with hypertension is concerned, only about 19-20% of them are getting treated for Hypertension. And, of that number only a very small percentage are receiving the proper medications to treat their hypertension. Hence, once of the reasons for such high incidence of hypertension associated deaths, multi-infarct disease and dementia in African Americans.

In other words, many physicians in the U.S. do not know how to treat hypertension in Negroes/Blacks, Asians, Hispanics, Native Americans and other people of color. They simply were never taught how to do it the proper way. The plain and honest truth is that those who taught them dont know how to do it themselves. They never bother to take the necessary time and effort to learn the difference that exists in the basic physiology of Caucasians and Blacks and other non -Caucasians that dictates the need for the treatments of high blood pressure to be different between different racial groups.

In medical schools and during residency, they use only the Caucasian model to treat hypertension, as they do for many other diseases. This is not only wrong, it is gravely wrong and need to be changed, if proper medical care is to be given to people of all ethnicities.

Of the 7.4 billion people who inhabit the world in 2017, 4 billion live in Asia, 1.1 billion live in Africa and close 1 billion live in North America and other places where Caucasians do not live.

Therefore, since the majority of the world population is non -Caucasians, how can one justify using only the Caucasian model to teach medical students, interns and residents how to practice medicine? It just simply does not make sense.

In fact, millions of white Americans are not being treated with the right medications to treat their blood pressures either because many of them are not getting thiazide water pills as part of their blood pressure regimen.

Essential hypertension develops in humans because the body retains too much salt. (See chapter 1 on hypertension to learn the best way to treat hypertension.)

The vast majority of Negroes/Blacks with dememtia do not have Alzheimer's disease. Most of them have dementia due untreated or poorly treated high blood pressure resulting in micro-vascvular disease of the brain also known as multiple small vessels/small infarct of the brain resulting in dementia and all its associated symptoms and complications.

Signs and symptoms of dementia include:

"Memory loss
Difficulty with complex tasks
Difficulty communicating or finding words
Difficulty with planning and organizing
Difficulty with coordination and motor functions
Problems with disorientation, such as getting lost
Personality changes
Inability to reason
Inappropriate behavior
Paranoia
Agitation
Hallucinations"

Evaluations of dementia include:

History and physical examination
CBC
Complete chemistry profile
T4 and TSH
Serum B12
HIV 1&2 blood tests
VDRL
PPD
Vitamin D 25 level

Urinalysis
Chest-x-ray
EKG
ANA
ESR
Brain CT
Brain MRI/MRA
SPECT MRI of brain
PET Scan of the brain
Consultation with a neurologist;

Treatments of dementia include:

Aricept
Namenda

Injection of B12 when level B12 is low, B12 deficiency causes degeneration of myelin sheaths that cover the nerves within the white matter of the brain resulting in dementia and many other problems in the human body.

In addition, low B12 can occur in elderly people because of dryness of salivary glands in the elderly as a normal aging process and because of atrophic gastritis that occurs in the elderly. About 5 million elderly people in the U.S. have B12 deficiency

Another common cause of dementia is hypothyroidism. Hypothyroidism is a common cause of dementia in the elderly.

Complications of dementia include:

Memory loss
Delusions
Hallucinations
Depression
Anxiety
Insomnia
Poor judgment
Inability to interact socially
Poor hygiene
Wandering
Inability to communicate
Poor appetite
Inability to feed oneself
Death

CHAPTER 111

ALZHEIMER'S DISEASE IN AFRICAN AMERICAN MEN

Alzheimer's disease is neuro-degerative-psychiatric disease. Worldwide there are 40 million people with Alzheimer's disease and 5.2 million people in the U.S. has AD. Alzheimer's disease usually affects people starting at age 65, but there are people age 40-50 who develop Alzheimer's disease. Alzheimer's disease is the leading cause of dementia. Alzheimer's disease is both more common and more severe in women than men. According to the CDC, Alzheimer's disease is the 6th leading course of death in the U.S.

"Alzheimer's Deaths On The Rise, CDC Says"
USA Today 5/25, 2017 reports data from the CDC published in the Morbidity and Mortality Weekly Report indicate "more people are dying from Alzheimer's disease."

"Reuters 5/25, 2017 reports that the data indicated "93,541 people died from Alzheimer's in the United States in 2014, a 54.5 percent increase compared with 1999." Over "that period, the percentage of people who died from Alzheimer's in a medical facility fell by more than half to 6.6 percent in 2014, from 14.7 percent in 1999." (The researchers also found that "the number of people with Alzheimer's who died at home increased to 24.9 percent in 2014, from 13.9 percent in 1999.")"
Source: CDC May 2017

Alzheimer's develops in stages such as:

Pre-dementia
Early dementia
Moderate dementia
Advanced dementia

Signs and symptoms of AD include:

"Memory loss
Repeat statements and questions over and over, not realizing that they have asked the question before
Forget conversations, appointments or events, and not remember later
Routine misplace possessions, often putting them in illogical locations
Eventually forgot the names of family members and everyday objects.

Depression
Anxiety
Social withdrawal
Mood swings
Distrust in others
Irritability and aggressiveness
Changes in sleeping habits
Wandering
Loss of inhibitions
Delusions, such as believing something has been stolen".

About 5 percent of all cases of Alzheimer's disease have a genetic basis.
Several genes have been discovered that are said to be associated with AD.
Among these genes are:
The genes that encode for amyloid APP and presenillins 1 and 2

The APP and presenillins increase the production of a protein called A β42, this is responsible for senile plaques.
E4 allele of apolipoprotein E (APOE), about 40-80% of individuals with Alzheimer's disease has at least one APOE 4 allele

The APOE 4 allele increases the risk of a person getting Alzheimer's disease by 3 times in people who are heterozygote and by 15 times in people who are homozygote.
The TREM2 mutation increases the risk of AD by 3 to 5 times.

The different hypotheses to explain different causes of AD include:

Amyloid hypothesis
Cholinergic hypothesis
Tau hypothesis
Herpes simplex 1
Dietary copper
Low vitamin D

The cholinergic hypothesis states that AD develops because of synthesis of the Neurotransmitter acetylcholine. The amyloid hypothesis states that extra cellular beta-amyloid deposits in the brain cause AD, APOE4 causes excessive build up of beta amyloid in the brain. The Tau hypothesis states that hyperphosphorylated tau proteins are paired with other thread proteins to form neurofibrillary tangles inside nerve cell bodies in the brain, which ultimately leads to the death of brain cells.

Alzheimer's disease causes loss of neurons and synapses in the cerebral cortex and sub cortical regions of the brain. The loss of neurons results in atrophy of these affected regions of the brain, which include degeneration of the temporal and parietal lobes and part of the frontal cortex, cingulated gyrus, and brainstem. These different abnormalities are responsible the cognitive abnormalities seen in Alzheimer's disease.

Evaluations of Alzheimer's disease include:

History and physical examination
Observations of the person behaviors and mannerism
History from family members and caregivers
Neurological examination by a neurologist
Psychiatric consultation
Brain CT
Brain MRI with IV contrast
SPECT imaging of the brain
PET Scan of the brain
Chest x-ray
EKG
CBC
Complete chemistry metabolic profile
T4 and TSH
Serum B12
VDRL
Vitamin D 25 level
ESR
ANA
PPD

Treatments of Alzheimer's disease include:

Namenda 10 mg PO daily
Aricept 10mg PO daily
Namzaric 10mg per day
Razadyne 4mg or 8mg PO daily
Exelon 1.5mg, 3 mg PO
Psychotropic medications
Anti-anxiety medications
Anti-insomnia medications
Good nutrition

The stress on caregivers of people with Alzheimer's disease is enormous. People with advanced Alzheimer's disease require 24 hours help with all daily living activities such as toileting, dressing, eating, sleeping etc;

There are no effective preventive measures available that can prevent Alzheimer's disease, but change in life style, clean living like regular exercises, good diet, dancing, music, no alcohol abuse, no tobacco use, no obesity and constant intellectual activities like reading books etc, keep the brain actively occupied and can prevent the onset of dementia/ Alzheimer's disease. The total annual health cost of Alzheimer's disease in the U.S. in 2014 was 220 billion dollars and worldwide, Alzheimer's disease cost was 604 billion in 2014.

CHAPTER 112

EPILEPSY (SEIZURE) IN AFRICAN AMERICAN MEN

Epilepsy or seizures are a group of neurological disorders manifested by epileptic seizures. Worldwide there are 65 million people suffer from epileptic seizures and in the U.S. there are 6.2 million people who suffer with epileptic seizures.

"Despite the availability of more than 20 different anti- seizure drugs and the provision of appropriate medical therapy, 30% of people with epilepsy continue to have seizures."

Epileptic seizures are more common in men than women. Hispanics, Blacks suffer more from seizures than do Whites. 60 percent of seizures cause convulsion and 40 percent of seizures causes no convulsion.

The most common types of focal seizures are:

Dyscognitive focal seizures
Simple focal seizures"

The most common types of generalized seizures are:

Absence seizures (petit mal seizures)
Tonic seizures
Tonic seizures
Clonic seizures
Myoclonic seizures
Atonic seizures
Tonic-clonic seizures (grand mal seizures

Risks of seizures include:

Family history
Age (most seizures develop in childhood and in people 60 year or over)
Injury to the head
Stroke
Microvascular disease in the brain

Dementia
Meningitis
Diffuse strongyloides of the brain
Cysticercoids of the brain
Amebiasis of the brain
Brain abscess
Encephalitis
Toxoplasmosis of the brain
Toxocariais
AVM of the brain
Brain cancer
Malaria of the brain
AIDS of the brain
Neuro-syphilis
TB of the brain
SLE
Hypoglycemia (low blood sugar)
Hepatic failure
Hyperosmolarity
B12 deficiency
Alcohol withdrawal
Hypophosphotemia
Hyponatremia
Diabetic kitoacidosis
Uremia etc;

Symptoms of seizures include:

Generalized jerking movements of legs, arms and body
Confusion
Loss of consciousness
Loss of awareness
Loss of control bowel
Loss of control urination
Biting of the tongue
Chocking by the tongue
Psychotic behavior
Post epileptic state etc;

Evaluations of epileptic seizures include:

History and physical examination
Neurology consults
Neurological examination
CBC

Complete chemistry metabolic profile
Urinalysis
Serum prolactin
T4 and TSH
HIV 1 and 2 blood tests
Lyme disease western blot
VDRL
FTA-ABS
TPP
Brain CT
Brain MR
MRI
PET Scan of the brain
SPECT scan of the brain
EEG
Lumbar puncture
Spinal fluid LDH, Sugar, Protein
Spinal fluid Cultures for bacteria, AFB, and fungus
Spinal fluid Gram stain for bacteria, AFB and fungus

Treatments of seizures include:

Dilantin
Keppra
Dekapote
Phenobarbitol
Valium
Tegratol
Mysoline
Valproic acid
Several States in the U.S have authorized the use of Marijuana to treat seizures.
" Cannabis has been used medically for millennia and was used in the treatment of epilepsy of epilepsy as early as 1800 B.C. in sumeria."

Non-medications treatments of seizures include:

Hemispherectomy
Anteromedial temporal resection
Multiple subpial transaction
Corpus callosotomy etc;

Complications of seizures include:

Depression
Car accidents
Falling
Fractures of bones
Sub-dural hematoma from trauma to head during falls
Epidural hematoma from trauma to head during falls
Drowning
Sudden death
Status epilepticus
Aspiration pneumonia
Chocking
Tongue biting etc;

CHAPTER 113

NEURO-SYPHILIS IN AFRICAN AMERICAN MEN

Worldwide there are 12 million people who are infected with syphilis and there are about 600,000 people who have neuro-syphilis.

Neuro-syphilis develops when people who are infected with syphilis go without antibiotic treatments. Neuro-syphilis affects the brain and spinal cord. It's caused by the spirochaete Treponema pallidum organism. Neuro-syphilis usually develops 10 to 20 years after infection occurred and develops in 25% - 40% of untreated individuals.

The four types of neuro-syphilis are:

Tabes dorsalis
Meningovascular
General paresis
Asymptomatic

Signs and symptoms of neuro-syphilis include:

Confusion
Disorientation
Dementia
Abnormal gait
Blindness
Depression
Psychosis
Headache
Memory loss
Irritability
Mood disturbances
Incontinence
Numbness of toes
Numbness of feet
Numbness of legs
Catatonia

Seizure
Tremors
Poor concentration
Muscle weakness
Muscle atrophy
Muscle contraction
Abnormal reflexes
Argyll Robertson pupils
Coma
Death

The different stages of syphilis are:

Chancre
Primary syphilis
Secondary syphilis
Tertiary syphilis
Congenital syphilis
Neuro-syphilis

Evaluations of syphilis include:

History and physical examination
CBC
Complete chemistry profile
Urinalysis
VDRL (Veneral disease research laboratory)
RPR (Rapid plasma regain test)
FTA-ABS (Fluorescent treponemal antibody absorption test)
TPPA (Treponema padllidum particle agglutination assay)
MHA-TP (Microhemagglutination assay)
Dark field microscopy
Lumbar puncture
Spinal fluid VDRL, FTA-ABS and TPPA
Spinal fluid protein
Spinal fluid protein
Spinal fluid LDH
Spinal fluid culture
Spinal fluid gram stain
PPD
HIV 1 and 2 blood tests
Head CT
MRI of brain, spinal cord and brain stem

Treatments of neuro-syphilis include:

Procaine penicillin 2.4 million units IM daily
Plus Probenecid 500mg by mouth four times per day for 10-14 days
or
Aqueous crystal penicillin G 24 million units daily divided into 4 million units IV every 4 hours for 10-14 days.
Individuals who are HIV infected must be treated for longer period of time.
Repeat VDRL, FTA-ABS ought to be repeated every 3, 6, 12, 24 and 36 months.
Lumbar puncture to get CSF fluid to examine with VDRL and FTA-ABS ought to be done every 6 months.

Complications of Neuro-syphilis include:

Individuals with AIDS and syphilis must always be treated for neuro-syphilis
Headache
Sizures
Paralysis
Psychosis
Depression
Coma
Death

ABOUT THE AUTHOR

Valiere Alcena M.D., M.A.C.P. is a practicing physician, medical scholar, medical educator, and author.

He is a Professor of Medicine at the Albert Einstein College of Medicine, Bronx NY and Adjunct Professor of Medicine, New York Medical College, Valhalla N.Y.

He is an attending physician at Montefiore Hospital Center in the Bronx, NY.

He is also an attending physician at White Plains Hospital Center in White Plains, NY.

On May 15, 2008, Dr. Alcena was inducted into the American College of Physicians as MASTER-MACP in a ceremony held in Washington, D.C. (Mastership in Medicine is the highest level in the profession of Medicine that any physician in the world can achieve).

On October 19, 2010, Dr. Alcena was elected Fellow of the Royal Society of Medicine in London, England (Royal Society of Medicine was founded in 1773).

Dr. Alcena is a TV Producer and TV Journalist. He is the producer and host of the award winning weekly TV program Discussing Problems and Issues of Health with Dr. Alcena (The longest running TV health show in the New Tri-State region - on the air since 1992)

He is also the producer and host of the weekly TV program: White Plains Community Health Fair Speaks Dr. Alcena is the Chairman Emeritus of the White Plains Cable Access Commission.

Dr. Alcena founded the Minority medical Students Affair Committee (MAC) at Albert Einstein College of Medicine in 1969 and is still the Chairman of that Committee. This was the first such committee of his kind in the U.S.

Dr. Alcena created the first Community Health Fairs in the State of New York and in the U.S. He has published numerous articles in the scientific literature.

Dr Alcena published the article that first recommended the creation of community health centers in the U.S.

Dr. Alcena is credited as the physician who originated the idea that male circumcision would decrease the incidence of HIV/AIDS. Dr. Alcena wrote the article about AIDS and circumcision in August of 1986 in the NY State Journal of Medicine. This idea has prevented several million people from becoming infected with HIV/AIDS (6.3 million" between"

2006-2007). Close to 1 million deaths have also been prevented during that time because of male circumcision. Time Magazine named the idea of "Male circumcision #1 among the Top 10 medical breakthroughs for the years 2007".

In 2007, Dr. Alcena was named ICM teacher of the year at Albert Einstein College of Medicine. In 2000, Dr. Alcena received "The Community-Based Excellence in Teaching Award" by the American College of Physicians.

In 1996 he was the winner of the "Ten Year Community-Based Outstanding Teacher Award" from the American College of Physicians.

Dr. Alcena first published the idea of the need for the creation of community health centers in the United States to serve the Ghetto Poor while a medical student at Albert Einstein College of Medicine in the Bronx N.Y.

Dr. Alcena has made many major discoveries, and published many other ideas and concepts that have made major contributions to the field of Medicine in the 20th and 21st centuries and have saved countless lives throughout the world.

Dr. Alcena is recognized as the pioneer who first exposed the health care disparity that existed and still exists in minorities in the United State of America. He wrote about it in 1994 in his first book. Dr. Alcena is the recipient of the PIONEER HEATH CARE DISPARITY AWARD - THE VOICE FOR THE ELIMINATION OF HEALTH CARE DISPARITY PRESENTED BY WESTCHESTER, PUBLIC, PRIVATE PARTNERSHIP FOR AGING SERVICES at a ceremony held at Pace University Law School in White Plains, NY on June 11, 2005.

In May 2014, VALIERE ALCENA, M.D.,M.A.C.P. was cited as leader in Internal Medicine, Hematolgy, Medical Oncology and community service, was chosen by the Albert Einstein College of Medicine Chapter of the Students National Medical Association (SNMA) as one of four most Notable and Outstanding minority Physicians in the history of Medicine in the United States of America and have done the most and made the most contributions to advance health care for Black People in the U.S. Two of the other three Physicians cited lived in the 18th century and one lived in the 19th century.

The SNMA did this during the celebration of its 50th anniversary.

On May 2ND 2017, Valiere Alcena, M.D., M.A.C.P. was inducted into the Leo M. Davidoff Society of excellence in Teaching at the Albert Einstein College of Medicine.

The Leo M. Davidoff excellence in Teaching Society is the most prestigious that exists at AECOM and only medical students can recommend medical educators for induction into this society.

In addition, Dr. Alcena has received several dozen other awards over the years from many academic, governmental and, community organizations. Dr. Alcena has his medical office in White Plains, New York where he practices General Internal Medicine, Hematology, and Medical Oncology.

The followings are the many Books that Dr. Alcena has written

1. The Status of Health of Blacks in the States of America- A Prescription for Improvement (1992)
2. The Third World Tropical Diet, Health Maintenance, and Medical Management Program (1994)
3. African American Health Book (1994)
4. AIDS the Expending Epidemic, What the Public Needs to know: A Multi Cultural Overview (1994)
5. African American Women's Health Book (2001)
6. Women's Health and Wellness for the Millennium (2002)
7. Women Health and Wellness for the New Millennium Second Edition Hard Cover 2002
8. Men's Health and Wellness for the New Millennium (2007)
9. The Best of Women's Health (2008)
10. Health Care Disparity in the United States: An Urgent Call for Universal Health Insurance & A Public Health Insurance Plan (2009)
11. Triumph and Tragedies of Haiti and Its People (2010)
12. Health Care Disparity in the United States of America. (2011)
13. THIRD WORLD HEALTH CARE IN A FIRST WORLD COUNTRY (2011)
14. The Tragic History of Haiti (2011)
15. Black people and medical diseases 2012
16. The most common medical diseases seen in black people and how best to diagnosed and treat
17. Black people and medical diseases the root causes of health care disparity
18. African Americans and medical diseases An American Health Care Crisis That is Crying For Help and Actions 2013
19. Anthology of Medical Diseases 2013
20. Health Status of African Americans 2014
21. Health Status of African Americans Second Edition 2014
22. The Best of Clinical Medicine for the Twenty First Century 2015
23. The ART and Practice of Modern Clinical Medicine 2016
24. Living in the Shadow of Blackness as A Physician and Health Care Disparity in The United of America 2017
25. African American men's Health 2017

CPSIA information can be obtained
at www.ICGtesting.com
Printed in the USA
BVHW04*0025150318
509901BV00001B/1/P

9 781495 820946